Unraveling Cancer

Cancer Prevention Even After Diagnosis

Charles A. Lewis, MD MPH

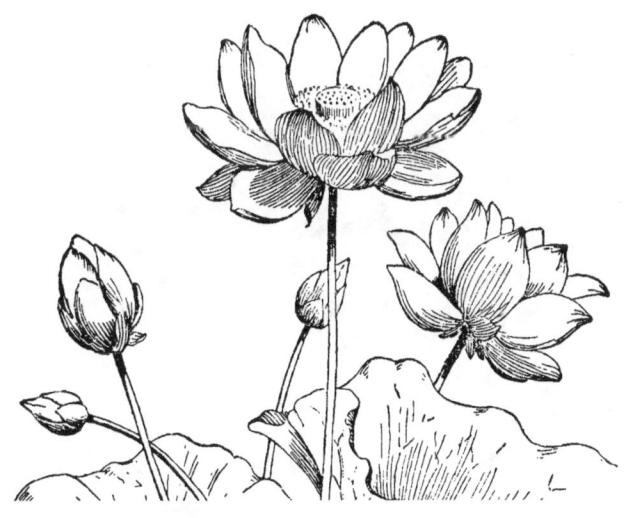

A HOPE Book
Health Outreach, Prevention, and Education

Psy Press
Est. 1978

Copyright © 2016, 2018 by Charles A. Lewis

ALL RIGHTS RESERVED. This book contains material protected under International and Federal Copyright Laws and Treaties. Any unauthorized reprint or use of this material is prohibited. No part of this book may be reproduced or transmitted in any form or by any means, electronic or mechanical, including photocopying, recording, or by any information storage and retrieval system without prior written permission of the publisher except for the case of brief quotations embodied in reviews and certain other noncommercial uses permitted by copyright law.

LIMIT OF LIABILITY AND DISCLAIMER OF WARRANTY: The information and opinions provided in this book are believed to be accurate and sound at the time of publication. The contents of this book should be considered as information to be weighed alongside other medical data, and should not be construed to be medical advice. Each individual is different. Medical decisions should be tailored to the patient and their situation; this cannot be done from a text. Individuals are advised to discuss disease prevention and treatment plans with their physician before taking actions that may affect their health. The author and publisher are not liable for harm resulting from misuse of this book or its contents. The information herein is provided "as is." Psy Press makes no representation or warranties with respect to the accuracy, timeliness or completeness of the contents of this book and specifically disclaims any implied warranties.

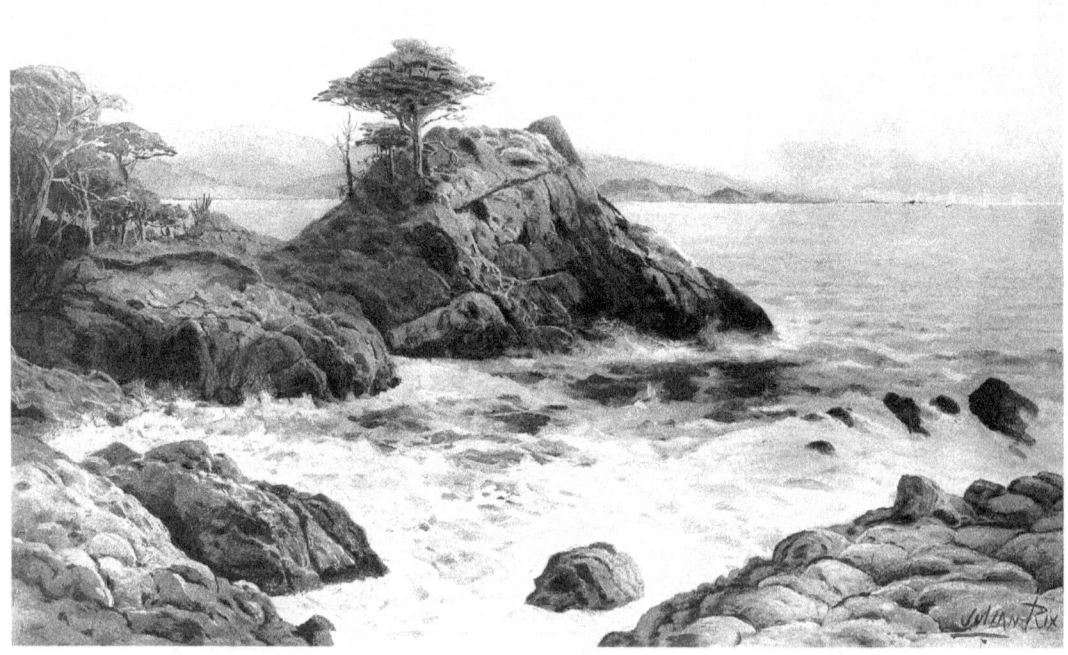

Dedicated to those who work to improves the lives of children they most likely will never meet.

Psy Press™
Carrabelle, Florida
PsyPress📖email.com
EDITION 1.02A
On Demand Publishing
ISBN: 978-1535593724

Table of Contents

1: Spoiler Alert 1

2: Cancer Vocabulary 7

3: Biochemistry 101 18

4: What Causes Cancer? 25

5: The Great Cell Cycle 41

6: Carcinogens 49

7: Cancer Causation 60

8: Hereditary Cancers 65

9: Infectious Causes of Cancer 73

10: Tobacco 91

11: Alcohol 96

12: Obesity 119

13: Exercise 133

14: Diet and Cancer 149

15: Meat and Heat 153

16: Percivall Pott and the Flue of Death 155

17: Heterocyclic Amines 159

18: N-Nitrosyl Compounds 173

19: Maillard and other Heat Reaction Products 180

20: Red Meats and Iron 189

21: Fungal Toxins 192

22: Ionizing Radiation 198

23: Stress Response Elements 206

24: Garlic, Broccoli, and Mustards 221

25: Fats 234

26: Fruits and Vegetables 243

27: Fiber 256

28: Liver Cancer 275

29: Other Environmental Causes 284

30: Sleep 291

31: Breast And Colorectal Cancer Screening 312

32: Breast and Ovarian Cancer Risks 323

33: Bladder Cancer 336

34: MTOR 339

35: Hacking mTOR and AMPK 359

36: Chemotherapy 367

37: Modified Fasting 388

38: Hyperthermia 403

39: Non-Genotoxic Medications 414

40: After the Diagnosis 416

Appendix A: Foods Allowed in the *Sanafast*™ Diet 420

Appendix B: Ceramide and S1P 423

Appendix C: Stress Management 429

References 435

1: Spoiler Alert

This book draws upon recent understanding of not only how we can prevent cancer, but also how to slow its growth, and prevent cancer reoccurrence. Rather than slowly doling out the essential and most salient information on how to avoid cancer (a far more practical approach than heroic battles against advanced cancer), here are many of the central lessons of the book right up front, in headline, bumper-sticker form. Understanding and use of this information can help avoid misery, ruin, and death from cancer. These are not teasers, but rather summary statements of the main concepts from this book on how to prevent cancer, slow its growth and prevent its recurrence after treatment. Okay, so they are teasers.

❈ A Mediterranean diet with extra virgin olive oil may cut the risk of breast cancer in by more than half. Eating an ounce of mixed tree nuts a day also appears to strongly decrease breast cancer development.[1] (Details in Chapter 32)

❈ Most vitamin supplements increase cancer risk and recurrence. Most vitamin supplements decrease survival in cancer patients.

❈ All cancers are caused by genetic mutations; however, only about 6 percent of the population inherits a "cancer gene." Even among these people, additional mutations are required to cause cancer. For an adult-onset cancer, it generally takes 5 to 10 cancer-causing mutations to turn a cell into a cancer cell.

❈ Mostly, inherited cancer genes raise the risk of cancer development, but that risk is significantly impacted by lifestyle and diet.

❈ Cells are most susceptible to cancer-causing mutations during growth; *childhood and adolescence* are a time of very high susceptibility to carcinogens. The lifetime risk of cancer can be lowered by avoiding exposure to cancer-causing agents during childhood and adolescence.

❈ Garlic and cruciferous vegetables, such as cauliflower and broccoli, decrease cancer risk and slow cancer growth in some cancers, however, if these vegetables are overcooked (boiled) they provide little, if any, benefit at all. (Details in Chapter 24)

❈ Children and adults need different diets to optimize health.

❈ Having a waist circumference greater than 31.5 inches (80 cm) for a woman or more than 37 inches (94) for a man increases the risk of cancer considerably from that of having a slimmer waist. This risk can be lowered by certain types of exercise. (Chapters 12 and 13)

❋ Exercise decreases the risk of cancer and cancer recurrence but only if the exercise is vigorous enough to cause shortness of breath. Chapter 13 explains the type and amount of exercise required to get the most benefits from the least amount of work and time.

❋ Adults who exercise alone are less than half as likely to maintain an exercise routine. Find a buddy to exercise to keep you going.

❋ Chapters 13 also explains how the infirm, indulgent, and indolent, and the languid, listless, lackadaisical, and lethargic can achieve many of the health the health benefits of exercise just by luxuriating in hot (100° F to 106° F –37.8° C to 41.0° C) baths.

❋ Lack of quality sleep is a risk factor for cancer and speeds cancer growth. (Chapter 30)

❋ Shift-work and fluorescent lighting after dark can raise the risk of colon and other cancers. (Chapter 30)

❋ Using oral contraceptives (OCs) for five years lowers the risk of ovarian cancer, but many OCs raise the risk of breast cancer. Table 32-5 lists OCs that do not increase breast cancer risk.

❋ Excess fructose, especially from sweet beverages such as soda pop, and high-fat diets increase the propensity for obesity and increase the risk of cancer. (Chapter 12)

❋ Two cups of coffee a day lowers the risk of liver cirrhosis and its progression to hepatic cancer. (Chapter 28)

❋ Mutagens that cause cancer also cause faster aging. In the U.S.A., the most common dietary mutagen is not meat, but rather meat that has been cooked at excessive temperatures. Hamburger is the riskiest meat in terms of potential for high quantities of carcinogenic compounds. (Chapter 17)

❋ A sensation of more than a mild relaxation from the effects of alcohol is likely associated with an increased risk of cancer. Intoxication with alcohol definitely is. Enough alcohol to cause a hangover is even worse. (Chapter 11 gives the 411)

❋ There are extremely effective vaccines available that prevent cancer. More than a quarter of a million young women die each year from cervical cancer, a disease for which there is an effective vaccine, but the vaccine is only effective when parents vaccinate their children while they are young. Universal vaccination for Hepatitis B could prevent over 750,000 liver cancer deaths a year. (Chapter 9)

❋ Most stomach cancer is caused by a common bacterial infection that can be treated with antibiotics. (Chapter 9)

☀ Initial cancer-causing mutations may occur over 30 years before a cancer manifests, or as little as two years. Cancer prevention takes a long-term lifestyle, not a diet to get into a swimsuit for a holiday.

☀ More than a quarter of all cancer cases in the U.S. are caused by tobacco. Children exposed to tobacco smoke are at increased risk of leukemia when young and at increased risk of other cancers as adults. Women exposed to second-hand smoke are at increased risk of breast cancer. (Chapter 10).

☀ Screening for intestinal adenomas (polyps) can reduce the risk of colorectal cancer by more than half – but only if you select a doctor with a high *Adenoma Detection Rate*. Ask for the doctor's Adenoma Detection Rate before scheduling your sigmoidoscopy or colonoscopy. Details are given in Chapter 31.

☀ Individuals that form colon polyps and those diagnosed with colon cancer may cut the risk of metastasis and cancer death in half by taking an 81 mg baby aspirin a day. (Chapter 25)

☀ Patients can decrease both the long-term and transient toxic side-effects of chemotherapy by preconditioning with exercise and diet. Broccoli, cauliflower, and garlic are some of the foods that can help protect the patient. (Chapter 36)

☀ Occasional fasting can promote renovation of the organelles in the cells of the body, making them healthier, decreasing free radicals, and thus reducing the risk of cancer. More in Chapter 37.

☀ Fasting before chemotherapy and radiation therapy can lessen the side effects from treatment. (Chapters 36 and 37)

☀ Exposure to carcinogens is extremely dangerous for cancer patients as they are much more susceptible to developing mutations; these additional mutations often make the cancer more aggressive and more resistant to treatment.

☀ Nearly 20% of all new cancers diagnosed in the U.S. occur in previous cancer patients.[2] Cancer survivors can lower this risk.

☀ Even when someone already has incurable lung cancer, quitting tobacco can more than double the time he or she has left. Even if a smoker has had the good fortune to have been cured of smoking-induced cancer, continuing to smoke increases their risk of new and more aggressive cancers.[3] Chapter 10 gives advice on quitting.

☀ Most cancer risk factors promote the growth and progression of tumors, just as or even more potently after a cell turns into cancer. Cancer progression is accelerated by these risk factors.

✹ Cancer cells have poor genetic stability. Carcinogens cause mutations more easily in cancer cells, and additional mutations often make the cancer more aggressive and less responsive to treatment. If a person continues to be exposed to the risk factors that caused thier cancer, the cancer will be less likely to respond to chemotherapy and more likely to come back and grow faster.

✹ Following a cancer prevention lifestyle after cancer has been diagnosed can save the life of the person with cancer. It's not too late to make a difference.

If you want a clear and simple prescription for lowering cancer risk, adopt a vegan diet, get vigorous exercise, sufficient sleep, and avoid obvious risks such as smoking. Add some olive oil and nuts to the daily diet. Simple. But for those who enjoy a carnivorous lifestyle, it becomes more complicated. Meat does not have to be carcinogenic – the risk is mostly created when meat is prepared wrong. This book explains the why and how to do it right. It provides details that give a better understanding of cancer causation, how to prevent it, and after it occurs, how to slow its growth.

I can be lazy, and recognize that most people have areas in their life where they are less than perfect in sticking to an ideal, healthy lifestyle. I would not be a very good physician if the only patients I could help get better were those with the self-control of a saint and the discipline of a Zen warrior. So why not make this as easy as possible?

One of the major influences on whether or not people follow healthy lifestyles is how easy it is for them. How many young men graduate high school in California and then decide to move to West Virginia to be coal miners? Coal miners make it their career choice because it is the most reasonable option available to them, and because they see those around them making similar choices. The same occurs with diet and exercise. On average, people living in Honolulu live longer than people in most other places, not because they are genetically or morally superior, but because sunshine, outdoor activity, seafood, and fresh produce is more easily available to them, and they have less exposure to toxins as compared to those living in Cucumber, West Virginia. A healthy lifestyle is easier in Capri, off the coast of Italy, than it is Moscow, an impact that creates a nearly 20-year difference in average longevity.

My goal is to help people adopt a lifestyle that avoids disease. To be successful in this, the changes in lifestyle need to be as easy and effective as possible. Very few people are going to follow a diet that is difficult, inconvenient, expensive, unpalatable, or that leaves them feeling weak or hungry. Diets that do these things are recipes for failure. A diet should make people feel better, and accomplish this within days. Otherwise, people will likely abandon it. The exercise target needs to be within reach or people will find excuses to skip it. The changes in behavior promoted, need to provide short-term as well as long-term rewards.

A vegan diet cuts cancer risk but is not an efficient way to do it, and vegans don't live as long as do vegetarians that eat fish.[4] This book explains how to improve upon the benefits provided by a vegan diet to make it work even better, and how to garner the fruits of a vegan diet for those who eat meat.

As adults, we need our eight hours in bed and seven and a half hours of quality sleep. Some people feel fine with fewer hours of sleep; mostly, these individuals are less sensitive to feeling the effects of the chemicals in our blood that make us feel tired. When these people get less than sufficient sleep, even though they may feel fine, they have the same negative impacts on performance, reaction time and health as those who feel fatigued with the same limited amounts of sleep. Short-changing sleep increases appetite and promotes obesity – a risk factor for many types of cancer. Short-changing sleep increases inflammation and increases the growth of most cancers. (Chapter 30)

Numerous studies have shown *decreased cancer survival* in those taking nutritional supplements. There is some evidence that certain vitamins can help *prevent* cancer before it has formed. However, many vitamin and mineral supplements increase cancer growth, even at a time when the cancer is too small to be detected. As a rule, cancer patients and those over 50 should avoid vitamin supplements, and instead, get their vitamins from a nutritious diet. For these people, vitamin supplements should be used as medicine to treat deficiencies documented by medical testing. Vitamin D generally lowers cancer risk, and deficiency is endemic in adults; thus, it can be safely used by most adults. (Chapter 23)

Another goal of this book is to demystify cancer. Cancer and its treatment have its own vocabulary. Chapter 2 is a glossary and reference for help in understanding what this book and the patient's doctor are talking about. The book explains how environmental, infectious, and dietary exposures increase or prevent cancer risk. With this knowledge, we can build a reasoned approach to prevent, impede, and perhaps vanquish cancer. For an even deeper understanding, there is some toe-dipping into molecular biology. I know you do not want to miss the gooey, sweet center of this book that explains why the evil pink robots destroy their makers, and how to stop them.

Once certain cancer-promoting mutations have developed in a cell line, the mechanisms that protect healthy cells from mutations often don't work well. Thus, cancer cells mutate much more readily than do normal cells. This is why chemotherapy may work at first, but later fail, and why cancer can go from slowly growing to very aggressive after chemotherapy. Chapter 36 explains how a cancer patient can prepare for chemotherapy so that they have less short-term and long-term side-effects from treatment. It explains what a cancer patient can do to prepare for cancer treatment to make it as effective as possible the first time around, by slowing the cancer's growth and making it more susceptible to cancer treatment. Most chapters have a summary that the reader can skip ahead to for those times you feel my verbosity has gotten out of hand.

Unfortunately, nothing in this book is a cure for cancer, and little in this book will help with late stage, aggressive cancers. However, avoiding mutagens and slowing tumor growth, as can help prevent or delay the transition of a cancer into more aggressive stages. Nothing in this book should be interpreted as a suggestion that a cancer patient delay or forgo cancer treatment or seek alternative medicine (AM) remedies after the diagnosis of cancer.

❈ In a study of patients using unconventional, unproven cancer treatments from nonmedical personnel, the five year death rates were twice as high as for those getting conventional cancer treatment. The difference in death rate was explained by delays or refusal of conventional therapies.[5]

❈ *In a study of cancer patients, those who chose AM therapies as the sole treatemnt for cancer had a death rate 2.5 times higher than those accepting conventional therapies. For those with colorectal cancer the death rate was 4.5 times higher and for breast cancer it was 5.7 times higher for AM.* The risk associated with AM was higher among more educated patients.[6]

Let this serve as a warning to patients that the information provided herein is meant to complement conventional cancer treatment, including surgery, chemotherapy and radiation. Cancer treatment should not be delayed to give alternative or complementary therapies a chance to "cure" the cancer. Cancer is complex and even with great effort and resources, difficult to cure or even slow.

This book is not intended to, nor can it, replace a physician. A patient's doctor understands the specifics of their condition and situation; this book does not. Those diagnosed with cancer should seek a physician they trust and follow their doctor's advice. Each cancer is different, and treatment needs to be tailored to the patient.

2: Cancer Vocabulary

The diagnosis of cancer is harrowing and accompanied by a vocabulary of frightening medical terms that the patient and family will likely be unfamiliar with. I doubt that this section will make things any less scary, but at least, understanding what is being discussed is helpful. It allows for the making of more informed decisions and helps provide the patient and family a better sense of control of the situation. Also included in this glossary are some biology definitions to help understand the content of this book. I admit the chapter is pretty boring; I promise it gets better.

Cancer Terms

Tumor: A tumor is a mass. It can refer to any mass in the body that does not belong there. Nearly 20 years ago, I published a recommendation that this term be reserved to indicate unregulated tissue growth, such as cancer or growth of a benign neoplasm.[7] It is an unfortunate term that originally referred to nodules formed by tuberculosis. It is confusing to patients; by the standard definition, any mass or cyst can be called a tumor, including a large zit.

Cyst: A fluid-filled mass.

Benign Tumors: An aberrant mass of cells grow in a confined area forming a localized mass, but without the metastatic potential to invade or spread to other areas. A benign growth can cause problems as it puts pressure on other tissues. A benign tumor in the brain can take up limited space and impede normal blood flow or compress or distort brain tissue, impairing its function. Benign tumors can cause pain by stretching the lining around the bone (the periosteum) or around other tissues. Although a cancer can begin within a benign tumor, the risk of cancer developing in a benign tumor is not much higher than it is for cancer to develop in normal tissues.

Cancer: Cancer is an abnormal growth of cells that are unregulated, and able to invade and grow in other tissue.

Neoplasm: This term comes from Greek for "new formation" and refers to an abnormal tissue growth. Neoplasia is the abnormal proliferation of cells. It can be benign, in situ, malignant, or of undetermined significance.

Malignant: In non-medical terms, malignant means malicious, vengeful, cruel, and spiteful. In medical terms, it refers to the cruelty of dangerous, virulent, invasive growth. In regards to a neoplasm, malignant refers to tumor cells that can invade and destroy nearby tissues, or spread (metastasize) to distant organs. A malignant neoplasm is a cancer.

Metastasis is the spread of a primary cancer to sites beyond the organ in which it originated. Breast and prostate cancers can metastasize, often to the long bones, such as the femur or the ribs, sooner than to other organs. Sometimes the diagnosis of cancer is only made after a fracture of a weakened bone occurs. Colon cancer often spreads to the liver.

Invasive Cancer: A cancer that has spread beyond the organ of its origin.

Dysplasia: An abnormal change in the appearance or function of cells for their site. For example in cervical dysplasia, also known as cervical intraepithelial neoplasia (CIN), there is an unusual number of immature cells present on the mucosal surface, as seen on a pap smear. With this, there is an increased risk of transformation into squamous cell carcinoma.

Proliferation: The growth in the number of cells.

Metaplasia: Conversion of the cell type from the normal one for that tissue to a different cell type. In Barrett's esophagus, the squamous (flat) cells lining the esophagus undergo metaplasia, converting into tall columnar cells. Metaplasia is a risk factor for cancer.

Mutations: A change in the DNA of a cell that can pass on to subsequent generations of that cell.

Somatic Mutation: A mutation in the genes of one or more cells, usually stem cells or progenitor cells of the body, that were not inherited from a parent.

Germline Mutation: A mutation that is passed in the genetic materials from parent to child, and thus, can be inherited and passed generation to generation. Since a germline mutation can be a new mutation in a single germ cell, the parent may not have this mutation in their own genome.

DNA Adducts: Certain chemical compounds have a proclivity to bind to DNA, forming DNA adducts. These adducts can damage the DNA and cause breaks in the DNA during DNA replication. They can impair DNA repair mechanisms, and bind to the DNA in a way that prevents gene transcription. Many DNA adducts are mutagens and carcinogens.

Mutagens: Mutagens are compounds or forces that cause changes in the DNA. Examples are chemical compounds that damage the DNA or forces such as ultraviolet or X-ray radiation, which can break the DNA strand. Mutations may occur as a result of the binding of a chemical to the DNA or from errors occurring during repair of a disrupted DNA strand. Mutations may also occur from oxidizing agents or wavelengths of electromagnetic energy that damage the DNA or impair the function of DNA repair or transcription proteins. A mutagen can affect the activity of a protein or enzyme without causing cancer.

Carcinogens: Some mutagens are carcinogens. Mostly, mutagens act in carcinogenesis when they inhibit transcription or function of regulatory genes that control cell growth. A compound that causes mutations in regulatory genes is a carcinogen. Often, cancer is caused by damage that impairs the function of proteins that regulate cell reproduction.

Risk Factor: Any agent or exposure that raises the probability of an unwanted event, such as the occurrence of a disease.

Risk Ratio: Studies usually express the amplitude or effect size of a risk factor as a ratio. For example, people who are exposed to a particular chemical risk factor may be twice as likely to develop a disease. This would be expressed as a 2:1 risk ratio, or a relative risk of 2.0. A relative risk (RR) of 1.2 indicates a 20 percent increase in risk. A risk ratio of 0.6 indicates a 40 percent reduction in risk as compared to the unexposed group. Thus, when the RR is less than one, the exposure has a negative or preventive effect. A risk ratio of 1.0 means that the exposure does not affect disease occurrence.

Variance: Studies provide statistical estimates based on a sample of patients and examine only some of the possible exposures that may influence disease. The variance can be understood as the effect of unexplained risk and preventive factors as well as "noise" and imprecision error in the study.

Confidence Interval: The variance in risk-response in a study is quantified by the "confidence interval" (CI) which gives the predicted range of risk imparted by a risk factor. The CI is usually expressed as the 95% probability range of relative risk. For example, the CI may be 1.4 to 2.1 in a study. This would mean that the risk for those exposed to a factor was raised between 40 to 210 percent. If the CI includes 1.0, (for example 0.8 to 1.9), it means that the risk factor did not meet statistical significance that it changed the outcome.

Meta-analysis or meta-study: These are studies that analyze the results of multiple studies. In medicine, they are often used in order to give a comprehensive assessment of risk, by looking at the results of studies that have been performed in different populations and have used different research techniques and measurements. For example, one study may look at the risk of diet on prostate cancer diagnosed by PSA testing while another may look at the same dietary factors on the risk of death from prostate cancer. If the risk factor has a similar effect in both cases, it is more likely to indicate that the risk factor causes the disease. Other meta-analyses may only look at studies with very similar risks and outcomes to get a more precise assessment of risk amplitude.

Incidence: The number of *new cases* of a disease diagnosed usually expresses as a population ratio, such as 210 cases per 10,000 persons, during a single year.

Prevalence: Number of current cases of a disease, usually expressed as a population ratio, present in the population. Prevalence rates convey the number of people alive with the disease. They are usually used for chronic diseases such as diabetes where people live many years with the condition. If the average person survived 5 years with a disease, the prevalence would be five times the incidence rate.

Interactions: Sometimes adding two risk factors for cancer only raises the risk slightly, because the factors overlap – leading to the same process. Other times, the risks add to each other. In other situations, the risks create an *interaction* or synergy that multiplies the risk.

Gene: A segment of the DNA that codes for a specific protein. The human genome codes for about 19,000 to 23,000 genes. Unrelated humans share a 99.9 percent similarity to each other. We also share a 96% similarity with chimpanzees and a 50% genetic similarity with the chimp's favorite fruit, the banana.

DNA Transcription: The copying of a gene as mRNA so that a protein can be transcribed. This is explained in Chapter 3.

Transcription Factor: A protein that binds to two specific areas of a DNA strand, forming a loop, and that then promotes or inhibits the transcription of the genes contained within that loop of DNA. For example, sexual differentiation between males and females results from the activity of a transcription factor, TDF, on the Y chromosome. It, in turn, controls the production of other transcription factors that upregulate or downregulate the production of numerous proteins that control sexual development and sex hormone response. Several transcription factors are important in cancer development.

Cytoplasm: The main compartment of a cell, as opposed to the nucleus. The cytoplasm is the principal area of cellular metabolism. It is composed of the cytosol and the organelles.

Cytosol: The gel-like matrix composed of numerous proteins and enzymes that fill the cell.

Allele: A normal variation in a given gene within the population is called an allele. Some alleles cause traits that are easy to see such as blue or brown eyes or curly or straight hair. Others are not easily visible. Some gene alleles affect how avidly we metabolize toxins and medications. These alleles are not considered defects, and do not cause disease, but may affect how we interact with foods, medications or toxins we are exposed to. Several alleles can impact our personal risk of cancer; one of the reasons I recommend we get to know our personal genome.

Cytochrome P450: "CYP 450's" or "p450's" are enzymes found in plants, animals, fungi, and bacteria that help process molecular compounds. We humans have 57 p450 genes. The CYP's are important in the metabolism of xenobiotics (chemical compounds from outside of the body such as medications and toxins), often by oxidation of the compound. CYP's are also essential in the synthesis and breakdown of cholesterol and steroid hormones, including vitamin D3, as well as for the metabolism of eicosanoids.

Eicosanoids: Fatty acid derived signaling molecules that participate in inflammation and blood flow control, including prostaglandins thromboxanes and leukotrienes.

Apoptosis: An adaptive cellular function for programmed cell death for the destruction of damaged or unneeded cells.

Ubiquitination: A cellular process in which proteins are tagged for recycling.

Diagnosis: The Latin root "gnosis" means knowing. A diagnosis is a determination that a specific disease is present. Since medical insurance may not pay for testing needed to confirm a diagnosis, the term diagnosis has come to mean that a disease is highly suspected from clinical data, such as physical exam and symptoms, even though confirmatory testing has not yet been done.

Pathology: Pathology is the study of disease, but the term is used for several things, most commonly, the behavior of the disease or the microscopic examination of the affected tissue. In cancer, the pathologic diagnosis using microscopic examination is important for determining the cancer type and subtype, as well as the spread of the disease. Thus, pathology reports guide treatment decisions. Pathology also includes blood tests and can include genetic testing of the cancer.

Onco-: Mass or tumor. Oncology is the study of cancer. An oncologist is a doctor that specializes in cancer treatment.

Prognosis: A prognosis is a prediction of what the outcome will be, based on past experience with similar patients with the condition.

Symptoms: The effect of disease felt by the patient.

Signs: The effects of disease that can be observed by the doctor. Signs are any disease related clues that can be seen, heard, felt or smelled as a result of the illness, and may include changes in behavior, heart sounds, feeling a lump or changes in body odor.

Chemotherapy: Chemotherapy or "Chemo" is the use of chemicals, often toxic chemicals, to treat cancer. Historically, these have been agents that are especially toxic to rapidly growing cells and less toxic to other cells. Since cancer cells are constantly reproducing, these toxins have much greater impact on cancer cells, but it also damages other cells that grow quickly, such as the cells of the hair follicles. This is why the hair may fall out after chemotherapy. It also damages the rapidly growing cells lining the intestine, thus causing nausea and diarrhea.

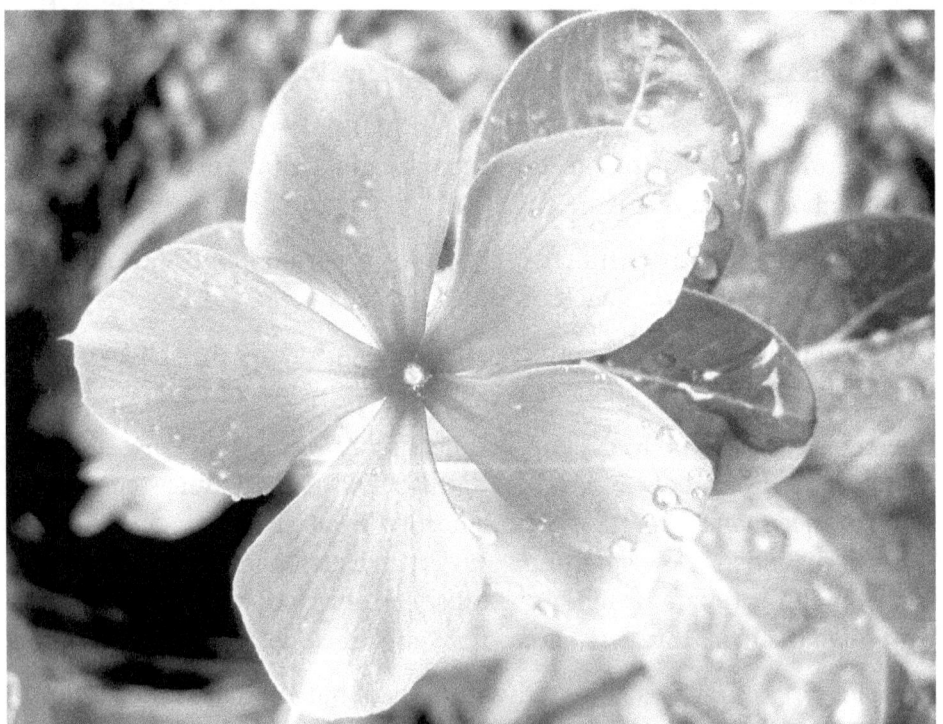

Figure 2-1: Fun Fact: Vincristine and vinblastine are chemotherapy agents used in the treatment of Hodgkin's lymphoma and leukemia. These compounds are derived from the Madagascar rosy periwinkle, *Catharanthus roseus,* a common but toxic garden flower, such as this one, from my front yard. It was formerly classified in the genus *Vinca*, thus explaining the names of the medications

Some chemotherapy acts by blocking the effect of growth-stimulating hormones. Medications that decrease sex hormone production are used to slow cancer growth. Leuprorelin (Lupron) is in the treatment of prostate and certain breast cancers, and tamoxifen, which acts as an anti-estrogen is used in premenopausal, hormone-sensitive breast cancers. Other medications are bonded to a second molecule that is more readily absorbed into tumor cells than normal cells; this allows the drug to concentrate in the cancer and cause less toxicity to normal cells. Paclitaxel is sometimes bonded to the fatty acid DHA to have this effect. These medications may provide safer chemotherapy with less severe side effects.

Induction chemotherapy: The use of drugs for the treatment of cancer in a patient that has not been previously treated, with the intent of curing the cancer.

Adjuvant therapy: Refers to additional treatment. An example is chemotherapy after surgical removal of a breast tumor, where there is no direct evidence of invasive disease, however, and chemo is given when there is a substantial risk that some cells may have escaped the tumor.

Neoadjuvant therapy: Rather than given as a follow-up, chemo is given before the main treatment. An example of this would be the use of chemo to shrink a thyroid tumor prior to surgery.

Consolidation chemotherapy: A follow-up booster dose of chemo for a patient in remission, used with the intent of keeping the patient in remission. The same drugs used in induction are used for consolidation therapy.

Complete remission: A response to cancer treatment that has successfully eliminated all signs of the cancer; however, cancer cells may still be present in the body and the cancer may return. Cancer is usually not considered to be cured unless there has been no evidence of disease for 5 years.

Partial Remission: The cancer has responded and gotten smaller. The patient may be able to take a break from treatment until there is evidence of new growth of the cancer.

Palliative treatment: Palliative treatment is medical care that is provided in order to give relief from the symptoms of a disease, but not intended to cure or even to slow the progression of the disease. In cancer, palliative treatment may be provided to help with pain, or to shrink a tumor. Shrinking a lung cancer tumor may allow the patient to breathe better and help prevent the collection of secretions in which bacteria can thrive, and thereby cause infection. Thus, palliative treatment of lung cancer can help breathing and help prevent pneumonia but is not intended to slow or cure the cancer.

Radiation therapy: Radiation therapy, aka radiotherapy, like some chemotherapy, is especially injurious to rapidly dividing cells. During cell reproduction, a new copy of the DNA must be made so that each cell has its own copy. During the copying process, radiation can cause such severe damage to the DNA that it prevents the cell from completing the process of dividing. The radiation also damages existing proteins in these cells. Unfortunately, the radiation also cooks some of the surrounding tissue.

Radiation: X rays and gamma rays are forms of electromagnetic radiation, as is light. And like a beam of light, radiation can be focused into a beam and used to kill cancer cells in a limited area. This is usually done in Stage II or Stage III cancers where it is focused on the tumor and the lymph nodes downstream from the affected organ. Radiation therapy is also used in Stage IV cancers, but here, it is mostly used as palliative treatment to shrink, rather than cure cancer.

Cancer recurrence: Refers to cancer that was in remission (inactive or apparently "cured") coming back.

Cancer reoccurrence: Refers to a brand spanking new cancer in a patient with a previous cancer. An example would be a breast cancer patient later developing a new cancer in a different breast or a different type of cancer.

Cytokine: Cytokines are small proteins that are important molecular signals from one cell to another. They help regulate inflammation and immune function. For example, some cytokines control the class of inflammatory cells that respond to an infection, while others quell inflammation.

Cancer Screening: Cancer screening tests are used for the *secondary prevention* of cancer: early disease detection at a time that the disease can be cured (oftentimes by simple surgical excision of the lesion) or its impacts limited. With colonoscopy, a doctor can see and remove precancerous polyps from the colon. Cologaurd™ stool tests detect hemoglobin from red blood cells and DNA alterations from colon cells in the feces and is useful for screening low-risk individuals for polyps and early cancers. Pap tests screen for cervical dysplasia, a stage of disease development that allows a surgical cure. Although cancer screening can greatly decrease the incidence of invasive cancers, these tests are imperfect and may produce both false positive and false negative tests. The rational use of screening mammograms is discussed in Chapter 31.

Cancer Staging

Two main cancer staging systems describe how advanced the cancer is. The general scheme for staging for solid tumors is:

Stage 0: Early, also known as cancer in situ. Carcinoma in situ (CIS) refers to neoplastic cells that remain in the area of their origin. These are often early stages of cancer or precancerous lesions. In Stage 0, there is a growth of abnormal, dysplastic cells present, usually on a surface, but they have not invaded into other layers of normal tissue. When cancer in situ is discovered on the surface, as it might be for the cervix of the uterus with a pap smear, it can be easily treated, sometimes just with freezing the cells and watching to make sure it does not return. Most carcinoma in situ can be thought of as precancerous lesions. Depending on the site and tissue type, some are low risk, but others are at high risk of progression and transformation to cancer if left untreated.

Stage I: The tumor is localized within the organ of origin, and has not spread to other tissues. This represents an early diagnosis, usually made through screening, such as breast cancer found early through mammography. Many stage I cancers can be cured just by surgical excision of the lesion.

Stage II: In Stage II cancers, the cancer has grown and has spread within the organ of origin. This is where cancer gets its name, the same name as the astrological sign of the crab. As cancer grows, it often has many small pointy legs, like a crab, growing into the surrounding tissue. In stage II cancer, the growth has infiltrated into the organ, spreading out arms from the original lesion. Stage II cancer treatment may include surgical removal of the affected area when possible, plus radiation and chemotherapy.

Stage III: Stage III cancer is in a late stage of localized growth. There may be evidence that cancer cells have begun growing and seeding other tissues. The cancer cells are no longer just growing locally; they are migrating out of the organ of origin and are invasive.

Lymph nodes are part of the immune system. Specialized white blood cells (WBCs) live in the various tissues in the body looking for evidence of infection. When they find an antigen, a protein they recognize as not being of the body's genetic make-up, they carry it down a lymphatic channel to a lymph node, where it can be processed, and the body can develop an immune response to the antigen.

Cancer cells commonly get caught in the lymph nodes downstream from a cancerous growth and begin to grow. From here, cancer can release cells into the bloodstream. In stage III, cancer cells are found in the lymph nodes downstream from the tissue with cancer. For the breast, these include lymph nodes in the axilla (armpit), but may also include those along the sternum (breastbone) and behind the collarbone, depending upon where the tumor is in the breast. When a diagnosis of cancer is made, part of the staging process involves removing some nearby lymph nodes and microscopic examination of them, to look for cancer cells. If they are found here, it is very likely that cells have spread to other parts of the body. Stage III cancers thus require systemic treatment, such as chemotherapy, to control the growth of or kill cancer cells that may have spread to other parts of the body.

Stage IV: In Stage IV cancer metastatic lesions are found. Cancer cells from the original (primary) cancer have developed new tumors in distant organs. This is strong evidence of aggressive cancer and that the immune system has failed to recognize the cancer. At this stage, it becomes likely that the cancer will continue to seed itself from secondary lesions to even more areas. Thus, the treatment of stage IV cancer may be very aggressive, or merely palliative.

TNM Staging

The TNM system (Tumor, Node, Metastasis) is another staging system. It is a bit more detailed and complex; it is used by doctors to communicate the progression of the cancer and data on how the information was determined. The staging is classified by prefixes that tell how the diagnosis was made: "c" is for clinical diagnosis and "p" is for pathology, when the diagnosis was made by microscopic examination of tissue taken from the patient. "P" is thus a confirmed diagnosis. Other prefix modifiers are included below.

TNM Prefixes:

- c: Clinical diagnosis
- p: Pathology confirmed diagnosis
- y: Assessment after chemotherapy
- r: Recurrent
- u: Determined by ultrasound.

Tx: Tumor not evaluated

T0: no sign of tumor

Tis: Carcinoma in situ (CIS)

T1: Early local invasion of the tumor into the primary organ

T2: Tumor locally invasive deeply in the primary organ

T3: Tumor spread to the outer edge of the primary organ

T4: Spread locally through and beyond the primary organ

Nx: Lymph nodes have not been evaluated

N0: Tumor cells are absent from regional lymph nodes

N1: Neoplastic cells have spread to some regional lymph nodes

N2 and N3: Neoplastic cells spread to more numerous regional or widespread lymph nodes.

M0: No metastatic lesions

M1: Cancer has metastasized to distant organs.[8]

A pT2N0M0 stage would mean that the cancer is a pathology-confirmed, early invasive cancer that has not spread to the lymph nodes, nor metastasized.

The TNM system is used for most cancers other than brain tumors and those cancers arising from blood cells, such as lymphomas and leukemias.

3: Biochemistry 101

DNA and Protein

In case that you have forgotten, or slept through your biology classes, here is a brief, bare-bones primer on DNA and proteins. Cancer is caused by alterations in how certain proteins function and this section should help in understanding the how and why.

Genes are segments of the genome that contain the code for building proteins. Humans have about 20,000 protein coding genes which code for about 60,000 proteins and peptides (tiny proteins). The genome is the entire database encoded into the DNA sequence of our 23 pairs of chromosomes.

DNA (deoxyribonucleic acid) is a double-stranded helix with the rails composed of alternating phosphate (PO4) and pentagon-shaped 5-carbon sugar residues. The name of these sugars is 2-deoxyribose. Each sugar has one of four nucleobases, adenine, cytosine, guanine or thymine, attached by a strong covalent bond. Each of these nucleobases pairs, by way of hydrogen bonding, exclusively with only one other nucleobase: *adenine* pairs only with *thymine* and *guanine* only pairs with *cytosine*. The hydrogen bonds (shown as dotted lines in Figure 3-1) are weak, and allow the double strand to be unzipped into two strands so that the DNA can be read and duplicated, and then zipped back into place.

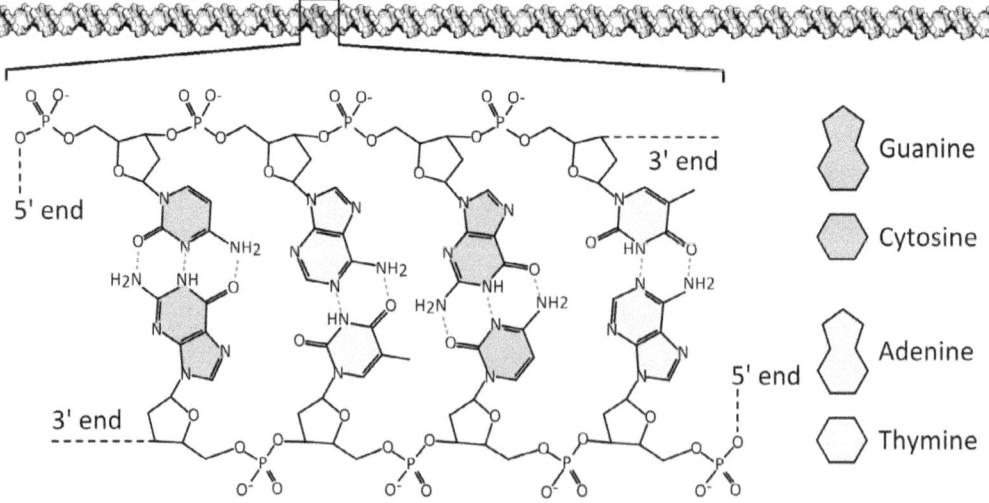

Figure 3-1: DNA Structure[9]

The pairing of bases allows the complementary side of the DNA to act as a template for repairing the DNA if there is a single strand break during DNA transcription; all that is needed to repair the break is to replace the complementary nucleobase. This exclusive pairing also allows for duplication of the DNA during cell division.

Each sequence set of three nucleobases in a gene, when transcribed to messenger RNA (mRNA), codes for a particular amino acid to be placed in a protein. There are also stop sequence triads that tell the ribosome that the protein translation has been completed.

Proteins are made up of chains of amino acids. There are around 500 amino acids (AA), but our bodies use only a small number of these. Only 22 amino acids, those listed in Table 3-1, are incorporated into the proteins of plants, animals, and fungi. These 22 AA's form all proteins; similar to how only 26 letters plus 10 numeric characters convey the myriad ideas expressed by the English language. The AA's are strung together in various orders and lengths during the formation of the proteins

Animals cannot synthesize AA's; however, we have the capacity to modify several amino acids from our diets into other AAs. Nine amino acids are considered essential; we need them pre-formed in our food because we cannot make them. Additionally, we have insufficient capacity to convert essential amino acids into the AA's arginine, cysteine, and tyrosine, to sustain rapid growth. Thus, these amino acids are considered essential for children.

Table 3-1: Protein Forming Amino Acids

Essential	Nonessential	
Histidine	Alanine	Glutamine
Isoleucine	Arginine*	Glycine
Leucine	Asparagine	Proline
Lysine	Aspartic acid	Serine
Methionine	Cysteine*	Tyrosine*
Phenylalanine	Glutamate	
Threonine	*Essential for children	
Tryptophan	Post-Translational	
Valine	Citrulline, Hypusine Selenocysteine	

In addition to forming proteins, AA's have many other functions. Glutamate is an excitatory and d-serine an inhibitory neurotransmitter. Serotonin and melatonin are formed from tryptophan, and histamine is formed from histidine. The catecholamines, such as epinephrine, are formed from tyrosine. Methionine forms the methyl donor S-adenosylmethionine (SAMe) which becomes homocysteine.

Building Proteins

To build new proteins, an RNA copy of a gene for the induced protein is transcribed in the nucleus. Induction of new proteins occurs as a result of signaling from the cell. These signals allow the formation of the proteins the cell needs so that not all the possible proteins in the genome are continually made. The result of transcription is a long mRNA molecule that is a copy of a section of the DNA for a gene. The mRNA exits the nucleus and moves into the cytosol, the main area of the cell, to be translated into a protein. In the translation process, the mRNA feeds through ribosomes.

The genetic code, transcribed from the DNA to the mRNA strand has nucleic acids sequenced to code for specific amino acids. The four nucleic acids in RNA are adenine (A), cytosine (C), guanine (G), and uracil (U). Triplets of nucleic acids, called codons, code for the various amino acids to incorporate the correct sequence of amino acids in the protein. A triad of the four possible nucleic acids in a sequence allows for 64 (4^3) possible codons. Some AA's are coded by only one codon while other AA's are coded by two or three codons. There are one start codon and three stop codons that signal the beginning and the end of the protein chain.

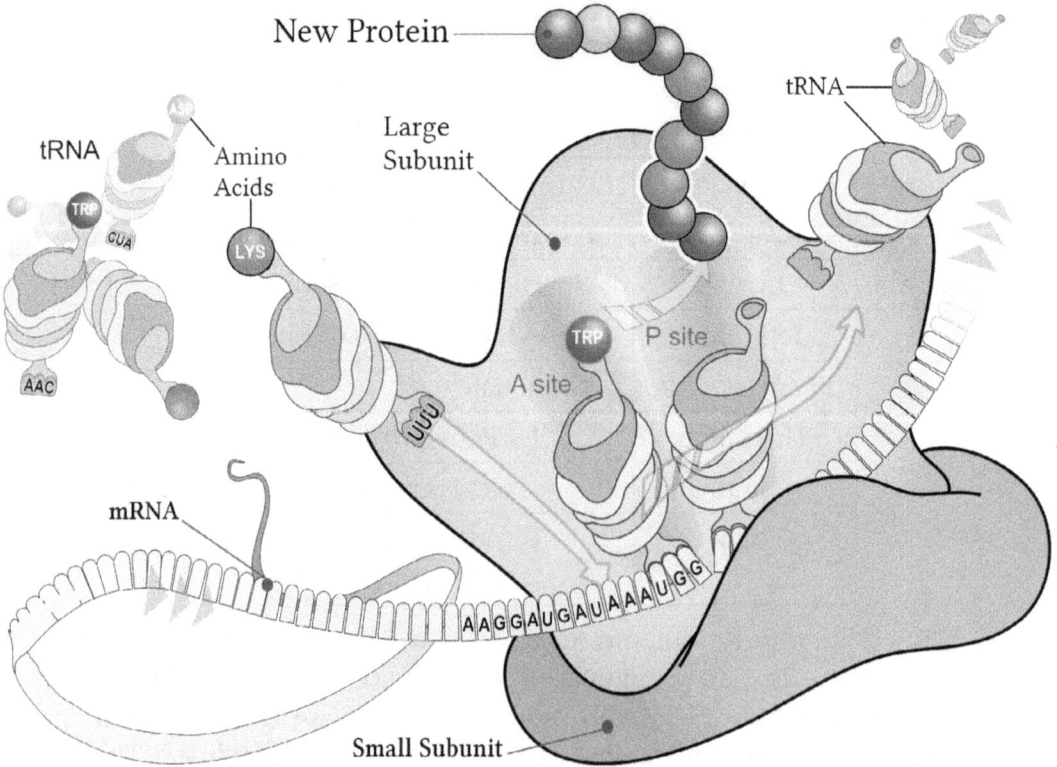

Figure 3-2: Ribosome and Protein Formation[10]

Before mRNA can be fed through the ribosome and translated into protein, a small hairpin-shaped loop at the front end of the mRNA has to be trimmed off. The mRNA moves through the ribosome, and like an assembly line, one AA is added at a time to the protein chain, as shown in Figure 3-2. For each codon in the mRNA, there is a transfer RNA (tRNA) which delivers its AA to the ribosome. The tRNA that matches the next codon to be read by the ribosome delivers its amino acid, and the AA forms a covalent bond to the end of the forming protein chain. Most protein assembly takes place with the ribosome attached to the endoplasmic reticulum (ER), and the protein strand is fed directly into the ER so that further processing of the protein can take place.

Proteins start as a chain but are carefully folded into 3-dimensional shapes in the ER. The primary structure of a protein is the order of the amino acids in the protein chain as held together by covalent bonds. The secondary protein structure results from much weaker hydrogen bonds. A covalent bond in a protein chain is like a weld, while a hydrogen bond is like the adhesive on a Post-it® note, or blue painters tape. Hydrogen bonds are fairly easy to break apart and reattach.

These weak bonds cause "sticky" areas along the protein chain that help the proteins to fold-up and stay in a three-dimensional shape. One of the reasons the sequence of various AA's in the protein is so critical is that specific AA's determine the form and function of the protein. The sequence of the various amino acids and the hydrogen bonds cause the proteins to form α-helices, β-sheets, and loops, in very specific conformations that give a protein its "secondary structure," as illustrated in Figure 3-3. If the wrong AA is placed in a protein, one of the many things that can go wrong is that it may change how the protein gets and stays folded. This may alter the protein's function and how long it lasts before being recycled.

In addition to hydrogen bonds, pairs of sulfur-containing amino acids (cysteine and methionine) can form disulfide bonds that also help to shape and determine the function of proteins. These S:S bonds have about 40 percent of the binding energy of a covalent bond, and thus are easier to break and reform than covalent bonds, but are many times stronger than hydrogen bonds.

Since one protein strand may include several secondary conformational areas, including both α-helices and β-sheets and curves, the overall structure of a protein is referred to as its "tertiary structure".

Figure 3-3: Protein Structure

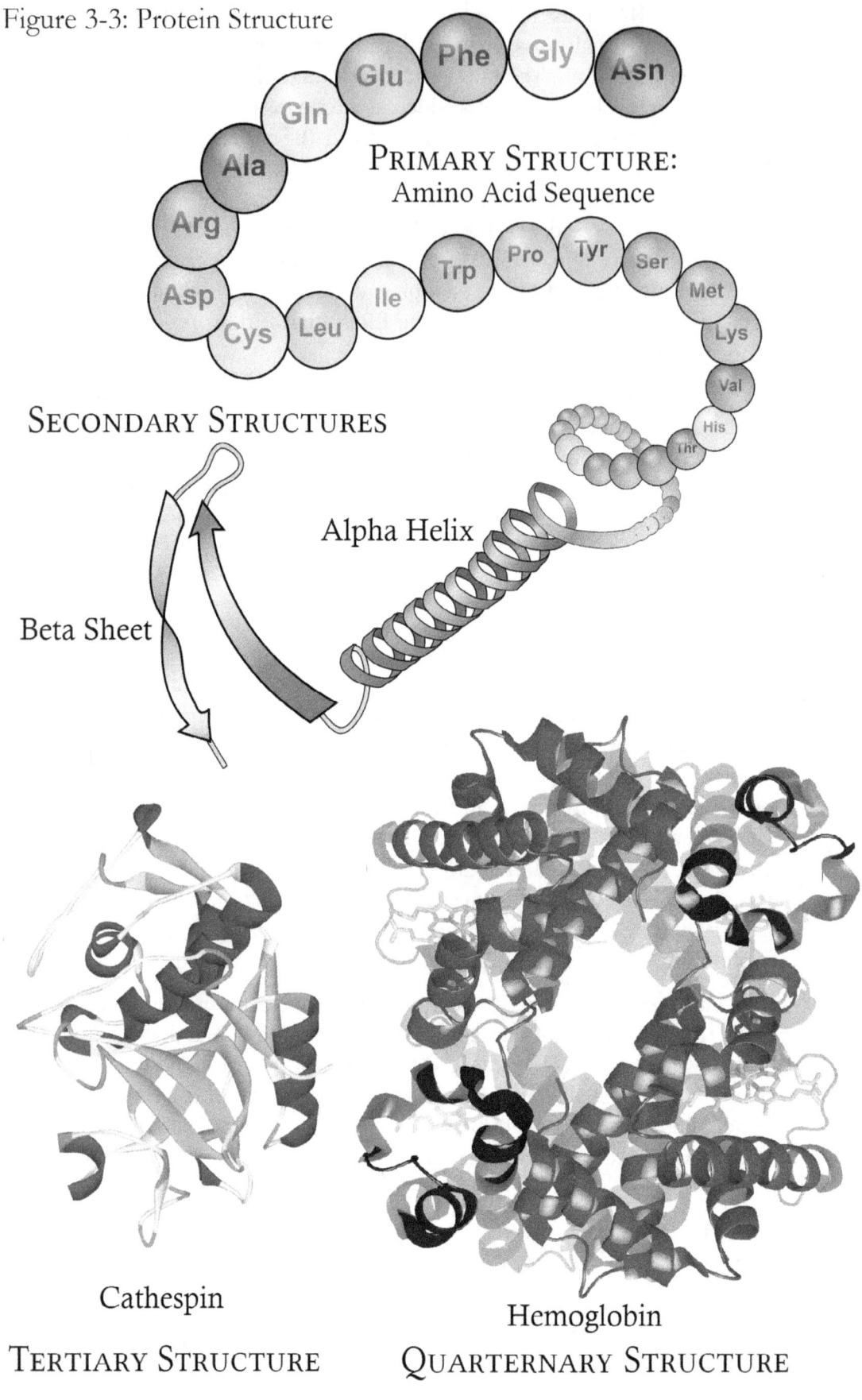

Many large proteins are composed of more than one protein chain; the combined protein structure is the quaternary structure. Many cellular processes are controlled by proteins joining or letting go of their quaternary partnership with other proteins. Hemoglobin, the molecule that carries oxygen in the blood, is illustrated above. It is a quaternary protein composed of four tertiary proteins.

Proteins have many functions. For example, collagen is a structural protein. Enzymes are proteins that catalyze reactions, such as cutting or joining molecules at very specific points. The hormone insulin is a signaling protein. Proteins can serve these functions by acting as simple nanomachines. For example, a protein may grab a molecule, and hold it in a particular position. The protein may then change its conformation, effecting a change in the molecule, releasing the molecule, and then the protein may change back to its original conformation so that it can repeat the action. Proteins function as transmembrane portals, such as calcium channels and glucose transporters; as ligands, such as immunoglobulins; as movers such as myosin and actin in muscle; as builders such as ribosomes which build the proteins; as editors, such as DNA repair proteins; and as receptors such as the Fas ligand.

Many proteins that have enzymatic activity function by breaking and reforming disulfide (S:S) bonds, and thereby, changing the conformation of the protein. S:S bonds are essential in many proteins, as the bond can be broken and reformed, allowing it to have a toggle-like action. Muscles work by having one protein grab a second protein, change conformation, release, and grab again further along the second protein chain. In this repetitive action, the first protein ratchets along a second protein, like a farm jack or ladder.

By linking several simple nanomachines together, complex nanomachines can be assembled. An example of such a nano-machine is the flagellum of a bacterium. Protein nanomachines form a tail that spins like a high-speed propeller, allowing the bacteria to swim through the fluid. Microtubules as nano-machines help sort and separate the chromosomes into opposite poles of the cell before cellular division.

Most single-gene hereditary diseases are caused by dysfunction of proteins, usually from the substitution of one amino acid for another. These changes can result in the misfolding of a protein that affects its activity. A substitution can also change how quickly a protein is degraded. Even if a protein functions normally, if it is degraded more quickly, it will cause an impairment of its function.

Disease can also be caused by proteins that degrade too slowly and have an increased functional activity.

Cancer is caused by genetic mutations that affect protein functions. Most of the mutations that cause cancer affect proteins that control cellular reproduction, DNA repair mechanisms, responses to stress, and apoptosis.

4: What Causes Cancer?

Not a day goes by in which I don't make billions of mistakes. Fortunately, most go unnoticed.

The adult human body is composed of about 37 trillion cells. Most of these, the 26 trillion red blood cells and 1.5 trillion platelets, almost don't count when it comes to cancer.[11] More relevant, are the fifty billion white blood cells and the four trillion solid tissue cells that form our organs.

Among the cells that form solid tissues, some are very stable; these cells form while we are young, and are irreplaceable. Several of these cell types are pretty much done growing by the time we are three years old. These cells are sometimes called "immortal cells," not because they live forever, but because they are adapted to last a lifetime. Those we grow as children and adolescents comprise most of those we will ever get.

The "immortal" cells include the neurons in our brains; our large muscles, including the heart; and most of the cells of the retina. When these are damaged, recovery is poor. We can grow a modest number of new nerve, heart and muscle cells from stem cells; however, this process is quite limited. Since the reproduction of these cells is extremely constrained, they are not candidates for cancer beyond childhood.

Most of our cells are not static. The majority of the cells in our body are short-timers; some only live a few days, and thus have to be replaced – every few days. Some of our cells have considerably longer replacement cycles, and last for weeks, months, or even years, as outlined in Table 4-1.

While almost all of the neurons you still have left in your brain have been there since you were three, the cells lining your intestine aren't even the ones you had a week ago; those cells get replaced about every five days. Other, structural cells of the intestine, forming of connective tissue, last much longer, on average, about 16 years.[12] The cells lining the prostate gland are changed out about every 500 days.[13] Liver cells are replaced about once a year; which allows the liver to recover from abuse and damage, but also makes it susceptible to metaplasia. As adults, bone and muscle cells are replaced less than once a decade. The muscle cells of the heart are replaced very infrequently.

The lifespan of most white blood cells is measured in days. Neutrophils, a type of white blood cells that fights infection, live about three days unless they have enjoyed a fine meal of bacteria, in which case they self-destruct within 12 hours. Another type of white blood cell, basophils, last about a week, and eosinophils, which fight parasitic infections, live about three weeks. Most of the B-cells, those that produce antibodies to help fight infections, live from a few days to several weeks.

Table 4-1 Typical Cell Replacement Cycles[12]

G_1 Phase Cells:	Constantly Growing
White blood cells (WBC's): basophils, eosinophils, neutrophils	10 to 72 hours
Stomach mucosa cells	2 days
Male sperm cells	3 days
Colon mucosa cells	4 days
Small intestinal mucosa cells	5 to 7 days
Platelets	7 to 10 days
Skin epidermal cells	2 to 4 days
Red blood cells (RBC's)	120 days
G_0/G_1 Phase Cells:	Cells that Take Growth Rest Breaks
White blood cells: Lymphocytes	60 days to more than a year
Macrophages	Months to Years
Liver cells	8 to 16 months
Pancreas cells	One year or more
Prostate gland cells	500 days
Connective tissue	12 - 20 years
Smooth and skeletal muscle cells	25 years
Bone cells	25 to 30 years
Cardiac myocytes	300 years?
Cortical neurons	Not normally replaced

While it is very nice to be able to replace worn-out cells with young, active, healthy cells, it does present some difficulties. Since the immortal cells cannot divide, they rarely cause cancer in adults. It is the cells that get replaced most frequently that can become cancer.

The red blood cells (RBC) have an average lifespan 120 days. Platelets function for and require replacement, every seven days. Even though red blood cells and platelets are the most numerous cells of the body, they are weirdos. They are formed by precursor cells but mature into cells that don't have a nucleus, and they are incapable of reproducing themselves. These cells are drones with an ingenious safety feature; they cannot be hijacked to become viral cells as they lack the mechanisms required for viral replication. And even though exposed to continuous oxidative stresses, they cannot mutate into cancers.

As outlined in Table 4-2, the type of cancer depends on the cell type the cancer originated from. The most common human cancers form from epithelial cells. These are the cells that make up the skin, the mucous membranes and the lining of the intestines and glands. These cells are replaced very frequently. Epithelial cell cancers are known as carcinomas; they comprise 85 percent of all human cancers.

Squamous cells are flat epithelial cells. They make up our outer skin cells and line the airways and the esophagus, and can give rise to cancers in these areas: skin, esophagus, and lungs. Another class of epithelial cells lines the inside of glands and produce secretions. When these give rise to cancer, they form adenomas, such as the cancers of the breast, prostate, and intestine, kidney, and lungs. The third type of epithelial cells, known as transitional cells, line the urinary bladder. Thus, epithelial cells can form squamous cell carcinomas, adenocarcinomas, or transitional cell carcinomas. The second most frequent set of cancers arise from white blood cells which are also replaced quickly. Cancers of the white blood cells (leukemias) or lymphatic cell (lymphomas) comprise about seven percent of adult cancers.

Table 4-2: Cell of Origin for Various Cancers

Epithelial Cells	
Squamous Cells	Squamous cell carcinoma
Glands	Adenocarcinomas
Transitional cells (Urinary Bladder)	Transitional cell carcinoma
Liver cell (hepatocytes)	Hepatocarcinoma
White Blood Cells	
Leukocytes	Leukemia
Lymphocytes	Lymphomas
Connective Tissue	
Bones, Muscles, Cartilage	Sarcomas

Much less common are cancers arising from the connective tissue: bones, muscles, and cartilage. These are called sarcomas, and they make up about one percent of cancers. They occur more commonly when these tissues are growing, and thus, these cancers represent a higher proportion of cancer cases diagnosed in children and teenagers.

In our heart and minds (and eyes) are some cells (cardiac muscle cells, neurons, and retinal cells) that rarely reproduce after their growth period. You can accurately determine the average age of the neurons in the cerebral cortex of your brain by looking at your driver's license,[14] as about half of those neurons formed before your birth and the other half formed and stopped reproducing by your fourth birthday.

The heart needs to grow to fit the body, but even in young adults, less than one percent of heart muscle cells are replaced each year, and this slows to less than half a percent a year with aging. Fewer than half of the cells in the heart muscle are replaced during an adult's lifespan.[15] However, there is some increase in heart muscle cell replacement after injury.[16]

Cells that don't normally reproduce after maturing are referred to as post-mitotic cells. We need to take good care of them. If we lose them, there is minimal recovery of these cells. That is why many diseases of aging are caused by the accumulation of damage to neurons (dementia), cardiac myocytes (heart failure), and retina (glaucoma). These tissues have very limited ability to grow new cells. On the bright side, since post-mitotic cells do not reproduce, they do not become malignant.

It is to our advantage that we don't replace neurons. If we did, with each replacement we would lose the connections that neurons make with each other, and along with those links, we would lose our knowledge, memories, and personality. We would cease to be us, cease to recognize our childhood friends, and we would need to relearn constantly. If retinal cells were replaced, along with their connections to the ganglion cells which transmit information to the brain, our vision would be a blur until we learned to reorganize the visual input into an image. If cardiac muscle cells were to reproduce quickly, we would lose the connections that allow rhythmic contractions of the heart and be at increased risk of fatal dysrhythmias.

But what about brain cancer? These are not rare. Most of the cancers found in bones or brain, however, are cancers that have spread to these areas, by metastasis, rather than originating in them. The cancers that do originate in the brain are rarely from neurons, but rather from support cells that have white blood cell or epithelial cell origins, such as gliomas, astrocytomas, and meningiomas. Rarely, neurons do transform into cancer, (medulloblastomas). These arise from neural stem cells and mostly occur in young children during the time when neurons are actively increasing in number.

Thus, the cells that are most likely to turn into cancer are those that divide most frequently. The epithelial cells and white blood cells have short replacement cycles. This means that they are more frequently exposed to the risk of reproduction errors, and it is these cells that are most susceptible to cancerous alterations.

Mutations

And this is how I make my billions of mistakes a day.

Even as adults, we are forming over 7 billion white blood cells and about 10 billion epithelial cells every day. When the body makes new cells, there is a tiny risk of making errors. When cells reproduce, each new cell needs a copy of the genome, the database encoded into our DNA. Even though the process is 99.999999% accurate, there is an error rate of about one base pair error per one hundred million base pairs copied.[17] Every time the DNA is copied for new cells, it has to copy the entire three billion base-pair code in the human chromosomes.

Recall that the DNA contains four different base pairs of nucleic acids that act like an alphabet, made up of adenine (A), cytosine (C), guanine (G) and thymine (T); there are only four letters in this alphabet. But sometimes during copying, typographical errors are made. Each new cell needs a full copy of the genome, and on average, while making a copy, about thirty mistakes are made in the copy and paste process.

Luckily, we have a DNA repair mechanism that catches and correctly restores 99 percent of those errors. That limits the error rate to only three errors for every ten new cells. Not so bad, except that we make 30 billion new nucleated cells each day. We are back to nine billion errors a day, and that many typos can spell trouble.

Fortunately, most errors are not significant. The vast majority of our genome is like space between the stars. Genes only occupy about 1.5 percent of the genome. We have about 20,000 genes that we use. These code for proteins that our body is made up of and that control our metabolism. Additionally, we carry around approximately 13,000 ancestral genes that we never use. Are these genes for making feathers, gills, tails and dorsal fins? Perhaps, but less tantalizing, many of these have to do with the sense of smell. For example, sixty percent of our olfactory receptor genes never get used. As a result, humans have a much poorer sense of smell than other mammals that use more of these proteins. We hire dogs for this job instead. Also, some of these ancestral remnants may represent metabolic processes such as making vitamin C or processing uric acid in the way most other animals do, but primates do not. In any case, errors made in these genes do not present a problem; they are like spelling mistakes in old books that no-one ever reads.

> Aside: Most primates stopped making the enzyme uricase long ago. Silencing this gene allows us to store fat more easily and helped primates survive an ice age 14 million years ago caused by a pair of large meteor impacts in what is now Europe. We also gave up making vitamin C from glucose, but rather learned how to recycle it. This is another energy saving process that helps us survive ice ages when fruits are rare, and food is in short supply.

A considerable portion of the DNA helps gene regulation and protein synthesis and processing. These areas contain some important information, but large areas of the DNA are highly variable repeat sections where spelling mistakes usually have no impact. Thus, most of the genome is resilient to DNA substitution errors, where one nucleotide is substituted by one of the other three choices.

> Some non-protein coding areas of the DNA code for microRNA (miRNA). These small segments of RNA are usually from the same area of the gene for the mRNA being transcribed. The miRNA can bind to the mRNA and prevent it from moving through the ribosome to form protein and marking it for destruction. This helps regulate protein transcription, by limiting how long the mRNA sticks around and how many times it gets read by the ribosomes. A mutation in the DNA that alters the miRNA could bind to the wrong mRNA, blocking it, or cause the miRNA to fail in eliminating mRNA; either could cause disease. MicroRNA is not specific to an individual protein, but rather affects clusters of proteins that are transcribed together. Some cancers may be associated with miRNA mutations, but more commonly, the impact of miRNA in cancer is due to mutations in proteins that transport or process the miRNA, inhibiting the inhibition they do.
>
> MicroRNA can be detected in the blood and have some utility in understanding aberrant protein production by tumor cells, and thus, may be useful for selecting medications to target the cancer.[18]

Even when an error is introduced into a gene, it may occur in areas where it does not affect protein function. Many errors that might affect proteins in an adult cell may be for proteins that particular cell will never make. For example, although a cell in the intestinal mucosa contains the genes needed for making specialized proteins used in teeth, hair and the lens of the eye, it will never need to make these proteins. Thus, an error arising in these genes only makes a difference if they occur in germ cells that are carried into the next generation.

It is mostly mutations in genes that regulate growth, DNA replication, and DNA repair that cause cancer. Rarely, but obviously not rarely enough, mutations occur in very specific areas of a tiny percentage of our 20,000 genes in a way that dysregulates the cell's reproduction mechanisms, causing a cancer-driving mutation. Less than 500 human genes, less than 2.5% of genes, are involved in the development of cancer. These genes are known as oncogenes (cancer genes). Oncogenes do not cause cancer; they prevent it. It is mutations in these genes and the dysfunction of their proteins that causes cancer. Since a mutation in a gene has to occur in a specific area of the gene to induce a cancer-causing dysfunction, even in these genes, most mutations don't cause cancer.

Thus, we are likely only making about a few million new mutations that could cause cancer a day. Pretty slim odds right? Not all cells are good at reproducing. It is mostly stem cells and precursor cells that split into cells capable of serial division. It is these that are most likely to become cancerous. Now the number of significant errors starts to seem manageable, likely only in the range of 1,000 errors or so a day.

Unlike us, bacteria engage a strategy of using frequent mutations to enhance their survival advantage. They can spare a few billion runts to get one bacterium that can adapt to a new or changing environment. It is like doing a billion experiments in one night to get one right answer. But bacteria can do it quickly, and replace their number with the new, improved bacteria in a couple of days. What are a few billion bacteria? That many fit into a half gram probiotic capsule. This mutation strategy, however, is not effective for complex, slowly reproducing organisms.

Where have all the old cells gone?

If we are growing billions of new cells every day, where do they go? We get 216 billion new red blood cells and 200 billion platelets a day, and thus, retire about the same number. These are removed by other cells, mostly in the liver, spleen and lymphatic tissues. The cells are broken down, and the materials are mostly recycled. Some materials, such as bilirubin, are waste products that are eliminated from the body.

Most cells retire themselves. When cells get old and worn out, are injured, are not working correctly, or have completed their job, they voluntarily self-destruct in a programmed process called *apoptosis*. Different stimuli can trigger apoptosis. Typically, however, cells undergo this process when they have collected sufficient markers of cell aging. This prevents sick, inefficient cells from reproducing or even just hanging out. When solid cells undergo apoptosis, the neighboring cells take note and fill in the gap left behind.

Several forms of cell removal and death have been described, and the various forms rely on overlapping mechanisms. The easiest to understand is necrosis.

Necrosis is cell death caused by factors external to the cell. The cell may be stabbed, poisoned, asphyxiated (deprived of oxygen), or have its head cut off. The cell gets murdered, and the body is left as evidence. Surgery may be required to remove any large areas of necrotic, non-viable tissue. In necrosis of small areas of tissue, white blood cells can carry away the tissue remains. Scarring often occurs in the healing of the surrounding tissues.

Several other forms of cell death might be considered physiologic or programmed cell death (PCD). In these, the cell retires and participates in its own removal.

Apoptosis is programmed cell death that involves the activation of specific proteins made by the cell that causes a controlled cascade of events leading to cell auto-destruction. Special proteins are made or released that cause the DNA to condense, and the nuclear membrane to dissolve. The cell forms fragments that are easily consumed by tissue macrophages. Apoptosis is the normal process for replacement of cells when they reach retirement age or are otherwise no longer needed. It does not elicit an immune response.

Pyroptosis or Paraptosis: Similar to apoptosis, pyroptosis occurs as a response to intracellular infection and paraptosis as a response to protein errors which often occur in cancer cells. Here, the programmed shutdown of the cell begins in the cytosol and often does not include nuclear fragmentation or DNA condensation. The cell usually swells and detaches from its neighbors. Paraptosis and pyroptosis induce an immune response.

Autophagic Cell Death: Autophagy is a process in which the cell recycles its internal organelles. This normal replacement helps keep cells young and vital. It is like changing the spark plugs or timing belt on a car when these parts get worn out. Autophagy is impelled by nutrient deprivation and certain stressors. Autophagic cell death can occur if excessive autophagic signaling occurs as a pathologic process. This may occur, for example, in cells where toxins inhibit protein production.

An overview of differences in PCD is given in Table 4-3. PCD actually occurs as a continuum of intrinsic, nuclear-mediated and extrinsic, cytosolic-mediated apoptosis. Numerous internal and external factors influence whether a cell undergoes apoptosis, and when the vote to undergo apoptosis is ratified, the auto-destruct process begins.

In the pure *intrinsic, nuclear pathway*, proteins in the nucleus vote on whether the cell lives or retires. If p53 or other promoters of apoptosis find mistakes in the DNA, they can stop DNA synthesis and send a signal into the cytosol of the cell initiating the breakdown of the cell. Thus, this pathway protects us from cancer as it helps keep many cells with DNA problems from reproducing. Growth factors and hormones vote against intrinsic apoptosis.

In the *extrinsic, cytosolic pathway*, the cell responds to stressors and signals in the cytosol as well as to influences external to the cell. This pathway evolved to participate in immune defense and helps prevent the spread of intracellular infections. Extrinsic, cytotoxic T-cells and killer T-cells can also promote PCD, by injecting an enzyme into the target cell that causes breakdown of the DNA and nuclear membrane, as well as through other mechanisms.

The intrinsic apoptotic pathway begins in the nucleus and includes the auto-digestion of nuclear materials. In the *extrinsic, cytosolic apoptotic* pathway there is the secondary destruction of the nuclear components, incomplete digestion of cytosolic materials, and participation of phagocytic immune cells. *The nuclear option prevents immunoreactivity against cellular debris created during PCD, while cytosolic apoptosis enhances it.*

All PCD pathways share many protein mediators and the downstream destruction of the mitochondria. This allows factors from both the nuclear and cytosolic areas to weigh in on PCD, voting yes or no to it, and allows a spectrum of influences to affect the cell's survival or destruction.

Table 4-3: Programmed Cell Death

Extrinsic – Cytosolic Paraptosis and Pyroptosis	Intrinsic – Nuclear Apoptosis
Augmented by external factors	Inhibited by inflammation
Occurs as a cytosolic process	Initiated in the nucleus
Activates immune response	Avoids immune reaction
Doesn't require mitotic crisis or DNA damage	Leaves little Trace
	Often initiated by p53 accumulation

Even when potential cancer-driving mutations occur in a cell, the order in which the mutations develop may determine the cell's fate. A β-catenin mutation can cause proliferation in colon cancer, but if p53 is functional, there is a good chance that the cell will undergo apoptosis and the mutation be eliminated. If p53 gets incapacitated first, followed by a β-catenin mutation, cancer risk is much higher.

Damage and errors to progenitor cells are dangerous. In human females, the number of eggs that mature during a woman's life is quite small; about 500 to 1000. Pretty much all the eggs in the ovaries are formed before a baby girl is born. Thus, the number of mutations in these progenitor cells is small. The DNA of a typical human egg has only about 10 base pair changes from that of the woman. Men produce about 3 million sperm each day for decades. Sperm "bud" from progenitor cells and the number of base pair changes in the sperm increases with age. Sperm may have several hundred DNA sequence errors as man's age increases. But since reproduction is dependent on sperm health, runted sperm usually lose out to healthier sperm. Additionally, many fertilized eggs fail to grow because of DNA errors, and thus the most severely affected germ cells are eliminated. Still, it is estimated that the average child has 350 new mutations in their DNA that were not present in their parents. Each generation, on average, has a 350 base-pair drift further away from our predecessors.

When an error is transcribed into a gene that causes the gene to function aberrantly, it is called a mutation. Mutations can occur in a place that alters the function of a protein or gene regulator that causes the cell to behave differently. Mostly, such differences are not advantageous. Very rarely, a mutation may mean more efficient or better adapted, but almost all mutations are unhelpful. Mostly, they just impair the ability of the cell to do its job.

Animals have a lower mutation rate than might be expected, as we mostly do not do sequential divisions as do bacteria, which repeatedly divide, adding the errors. Most of our new cells "bud" off from progenitor cells; even though the new cell may have an error, most cells do not reproduce.

It is not the intestinal cells that we shed every day that cause cancer, but rather the progenitor cells that they bud from. If the short-lived cells have problems, they are mostly just runts that don't function well, and get eliminated in a short time. It is the progenitor cells that matter.

The likelihood that a tissue begets a cancer is largely influenced by the number of cell divisions of its stem cells. Stem cells are the cells that the progenitor cells develop from. Progenitor cells have a practical limit to the number of times they can bud off new cells, and then they need to be replaced by stem cells. The lifetime risk for cancer-causing mutation is directly related to the number of stem cell divisions for that tissue[19].

Some tissue types with a high number of stem cells division include the cells lining the colon and rectum, pancreatic duct, lungs, and small intestine.

Johns Hopkins cancer researcher Bert Vogelstein points out that the risk of cancer is highly linked with the rate of stem cell division. Similar to the risk of being in a car accident; the more total miles driven, the higher the risk is. He has calculated that 65 percent of the variation in cancer risk between different tissues can be explained by the number of stem cell divisions in those tissues. This suggests that most cancer risk can be explained by random mutations occurring during stem cell division.[19]

If a safe driver drives through town, stopping at red lights and stop signs, and does not cause any accidents, this does not mean that she will not be rear-ended while stopped at a red light by a text-messaging idiot. The chances of such an accident occurring driving through town one time are pretty low. But if the driver makes the same trip several times a day, several days a week over several years, the risk of being rear-ended while stopped at an intersection goes up with the number of stops she makes. More trips, more stops, more exposure; the more risk of being rear-ended.

If 65 percent of cancer site variance is explained by random DNA errors during stem cell divisions, ten percent of cancers being hereditary, and twenty percent caused by viruses and other infections it would seem that we have little way to prevent cancer.

It is very easy to misinterpret this data. What Vogelstein found was that cell turnover is associated with cancer risk. Organs that have many short-lived cells that need constant replacement are at higher risk than organs that have fewer cell replacements. Some tissues are at greater risk for mutation because they have more cells undergoing division. A larger organ, such as the colon or skin is thus at higher risk, as are organs in which the cells are rapidly dividing. If cancer could be simply explained by random errors, it would mean that everybody would have a similar risk of every cancer; we all need to replace our cells. But this is not how it works.

Basal cells, the progenitor cells for squamous cells in the skin, are exposed to a similar amount of UV radiation as are melanocytes, the cells that make skin pigment. The basal stem cells divide more times than perhaps any other cell type; they divide about 50 times more frequently over a lifetime than do melanocytes. This helps explain why the annual incidence of basal cell carcinoma is 146 cases per 100,000 people and while it is around 2.5 per 100,000 for melanoma. If a person is exposed to whole-body X-rays, the cells that are dividing at the time are at highest risk. This explains why one cell type is more susceptible but does not discount UV radiation from the sun as causing skin cancers.

But cancer risk is not just caused by random transcription errors. We know that the risk of cancer increases with age, but stem cell division slows with age. Pretty much everyone alive has a colon, but only about five percent of people develop colon cancer, even if they live to be 100. Not that 5% is a small number; but if we were all at similar risk, why don't we all get it? Individuals who form colon polyps, a precursor to most colon cancer, usually develop many polyps. People that develop a squamous cell carcinoma of the skin usually need annual visits with the dermatologist to burn off multiple lesions. Everyone has a liver, but in Mongolia, that rate of liver cancer in men is extremely high; about one in a thousand men are diagnosed with liver cancer each year. In Iceland, the rate is one in 50,000. It is not just random errors.

Women who develop breast cancer are at much higher risk of developing a second primary breast cancer than are other women. In a follow-up study of 11,000 women diagnosed with breast cancer, nearly 11 percent of them developed a second, new cancer. Excluding any cancers present within a year of the breast cancer diagnosis, these cancers occurred, on average, after seven years. This study did not include recurrence of the original breast cancers; these were new cancers. More than half of the cancers were new breast cancers, but the other nearly half included colorectal, endometrial, and ovarian cancers.[20] These cancers share causality. If a person is at risk of one, they are at risk for the others. Getting one of these cancers proves the person is at high risk of developing other cancers in this group.

In 1880, only New Jersey and Massachusetts had death registries; by 1900, about 40 percent of the country's population was covered. Two-thirds of the United States population lived in cities that had death registries by 1914. The data is most certainly flawed; however, examining the proportion of cancers by site should give an indication of the relative prevalence of various cancers. Between 1900 and 1914 the proportion of cancer deaths from stomach cancer appears to have been on the rise until around 1910, after which it leveled off. By 1914, stomach cancer comprised 24.4 percent of all cancers deaths. In the same year, cancers of the uterus comprised 14.3 percent of cancers, and cancer of the breast 10.3 percent of cancer mortality. Cancer of the lungs comprised only 0.7 percent of cancer deaths[21].

In 1930, when more reliable statistics became available, the death rate for stomach cancer in the United States was about 45 per 100,000, and the mortality rate from lung cancer was about two per

100,000, two deaths per hundred thousand person-years. By 1990, the mortality rate for lung cancer was 59 per 100,000, and the death rate for stomach cancer had fallen to six per 100,000.

In 1914, the death rate from stomach cancer was 35 times higher than the rate of lung cancer mortality. Secular trends for various cancer types among American men since 1930 are shown in Figure 4-1. By 1990, lung cancer mortality was ten times that of stomach cancer. A 350-fold change in risk distribution between these two cancers occurred over the 76 years from 1914 to 1990.

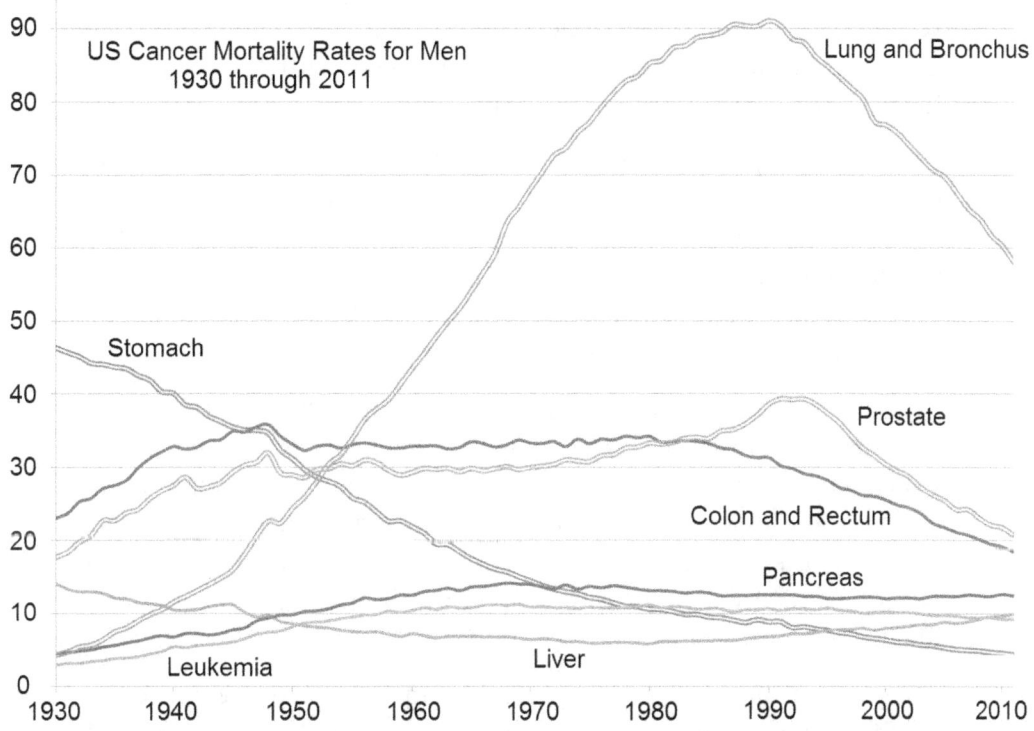

Figure 4-1: Age-adjusted U.S. cancer mortality per 100,000 men.[22]

This reversal in trends is not explained by a large difference in case mortality; treatment even in 1990 was not great for either of these diseases. The reversal of mortality was caused by a change in the incidence (occurrence) of these cancers. Obviously, background errors in stem cell base pair transcription errors do not explain this shift in cancer incidence. The rise in lung cancer was mostly due to the rise in cigarette smoking which occurred during the twentieth century, bolstered by the patriot contributions of cigarettes to U.S. soldiers during the Second World War by tobacco companies as their part of the war effort. The incidence of lung cancer peaked in 1992; by 2011, as fewer people were smoking, the incidence of lung cancer fell by 20 percent. The incidence of prostate cancer, another tobacco-related cancer, peaked in 1992.

The incidence of gastric cancer has fallen greatly in the U.S. In the 1930's, gastric cancer was the most common cause of cancer death in the United States. The incidence of stomach cancer has been slowly falling since then. In 2011, there were 7 cases per 100,000 person-years and the mortality rate was 3.2/100,000.

The incidence of gastric cancer in the U.S. had been rising since at least 1900. Prior to 1923, meat was cured using saltpeter, (potassium nitrate). When saltpeter is used in the curing process, bacteria present in the meat convert nitrate (NO_3) to nitrite (NO_2). At the time, there was no regulation limiting the amount used, and levels were often quite high. Some hotdogs tested at the time had nitrate levels as high as 1400 mg per kilogram. When nitrites are heated during cooking, carcinogenic nitrosamines are formed.

In 1923, the US Department of Agriculture performed experiments and found that it was nitrites that were responsible for meat preservation, rather than nitrates. In 1925, they set rules limiting the concentration of nitrites to 200 mg per kilogram and discouraged the use of nitrates for preserving meats. By 1936, the average nitrite content in cured meat had been lowered by more than three times.[23]

More importantly, about 90% of gastric cancers are caused by infections (Chapter 9). The bacteria, *Helicobacter pylori*, are involved in about 80 percent of stomach cancers. One hundred years ago, nearly every person on the planet had the bacteria *H. pylori* living in their stomach. With improved hygiene and use of antibiotics (to treat other infections) the infection rate has steadily fallen.

Figure 4-2 illustrates that the decline in incidence and mortality rates for gastric cancer have very little divergence. This suggests that the death rate for invasive stomach cancer has not improved as a result of better treatment, but rather, mostly from a lower incidence of the disease.

A decline in deaths from colorectal cancer (CRC) can also be seen in Figure 4-1. Although this reduction is multifactorial, screening and early and more effective treatments explain less than a third of this change;[24] most of the fall in CRC is due to changes in dietary and other environmental risk factor exposure. Red and processed meats are significant risk factors for CRC.[25] Since 1975, average beef consumption in the U.S. has declined from 90 to 53.6 pounds per year and the decline in CRC has followed along with it.[26] The areas of the U.S. with the highest CRC death rates are areas with high poverty rates, diets high in soda pop, red meat and salty snacks; areas where obesity is common and where leisure-time physical activity is uncommon.[27]

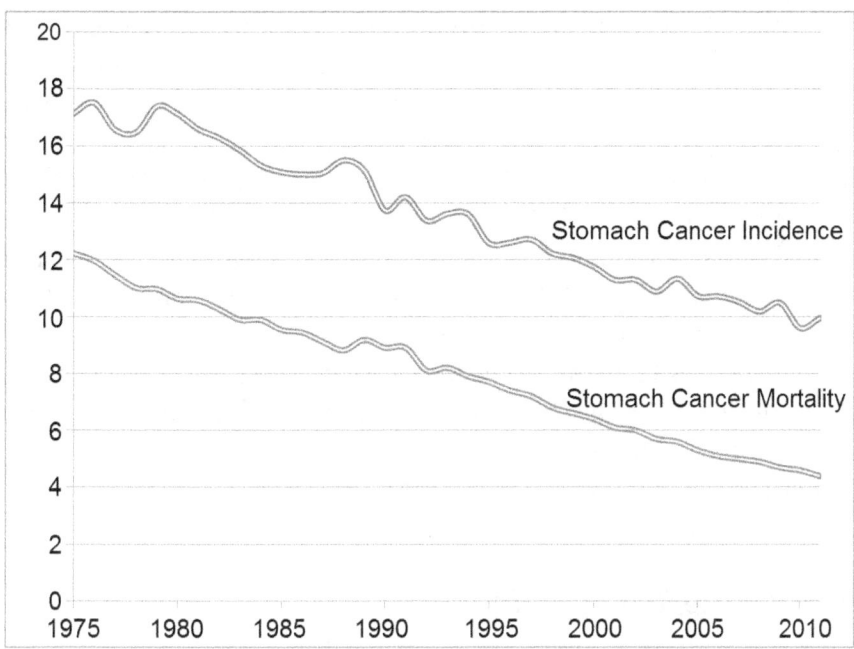

Figure 4-2: Secular trends in stomach cancer incidence and Mortality among U.S. men, 1975 - 2011. SEER data.[28]

We all need to replace billions of WBC's and epithelial cells every day, and we all make billions of "spelling mistakes" that are transcribed into the DNA of the new cells due to random transcription errors. We don't all succumb to cancer, and cancers are not randomly distributed in the population based on the population of cells being replaced.

One reason risk is not the same for everyone is that some people replace their cells more quickly than do others. An important risk factor for cancer is the accelerated turnover of cells due to chronic inflammation or tissue injury. Hepatitis B and hepatitis C infection increase the risk of liver cancer mainly by damaging hepatic cells, causing them to need more frequent replacement. If a person needs to replace 10 million liver cells a day rather than 1 million, they have increased their risk of liver cancer 10-fold.

Another reason that there is diversity in cancer risk is because, in health, our cells are adept at recognizing and eliminating DNA errors that are likely to cause problems. Many of the things we recognize as risk factors for cancer are things that impair the body's ability to repair DNA or to eliminate defective cells. Mostly, we are quite good at eliminating cells that have significant DNA damage or dangerous mutations.

The BRCA1 gene is an oncogene associated with early onset breast cancer. The normal BRCA1 gene does not cause cancer, but quite to the contrary, prevents mutant breast cells from reproducing. It is abnormal, dysfunctional variants of this gene that allow breast and other mutated cells to reproduce. The BRCA1 gene codes for a protein that repairs both single and double-stranded DNA breaks, and is also involved in marking intracellular structures for recycling (ubiquitination). Individuals who inherit impaired forms of the BRCA1 gene are less able to repair breaks in their DNA correctly and less likely to eliminate cells with aberrant DNA, and thus, more likely to accumulate DNA mutations that cause cancer. The BRCA1 protein is highly expressed in the breast, ovary, fallopian tubes and the pancreas. BRCA1 mutations that disrupt DNA repair increase not only breast cancer risk but also increase the risk of cancer in these other organs. BRCA2 is a structurally unrelated protein, but similarly, participates in single-strand DNA repair, and is associated with increased risk of breast, ovarian and prostate cancers.

Summary: Mitogens and Mutagens

Two major factors that increase the risk for cancer are mutagens and mitogens. Mitogens are agents that increase the reproduction of cells, and that promote entry of quiescent cells into the cell cycle. Some of the infectious agents that increase cancer risk do so by promoting a chronic, accelerated turnover of cells. Infected cells that undergo Programmed Cell Death (pyroptosis) are replaced by neighboring cells. Just increasing cell turnover increases cancer risk because it increases the likelihood that an error will be made in a critical section of a gene that codes for a protein that regulates growth or that stops aberrant cells from multiplying. Mutagens are chemical exposures or other forces that create spelling errors in the DNA. Many mutations occur as a result of a background random error rate during transcription.

Secular changes in lung, prostate, stomach, colorectal, and other cancer incidences show that cancer causation is not limited to the effects of random errors in DNA transcription. Most of our efforts for cancer prevention should be directed towards primary prevention by risk reduction.

DNA errors also occur when there are breaks in the DNA strand, and the repair mechanism puts them back together. Usually, DNA repair proteins autocorrect these errors. Occasionally, however, autocorrect creates problems, just as autocorrect for text messaging can change a text from "I walked her home and kissed her tonight" to "I walked her home and killed her tonight."

5: The Great Cell Cycle

I have many good memories of my high school biology class, but almost no memories of anything the teacher taught. There was this sweet blond girl, named Linda Ramirez, who was so much more captivating than that study of mitosis. I am going to assume you can use a refresher.

Figure 5-1 may remind you of something you may have seen in your high school biology class. Pay attention: there will be a test!

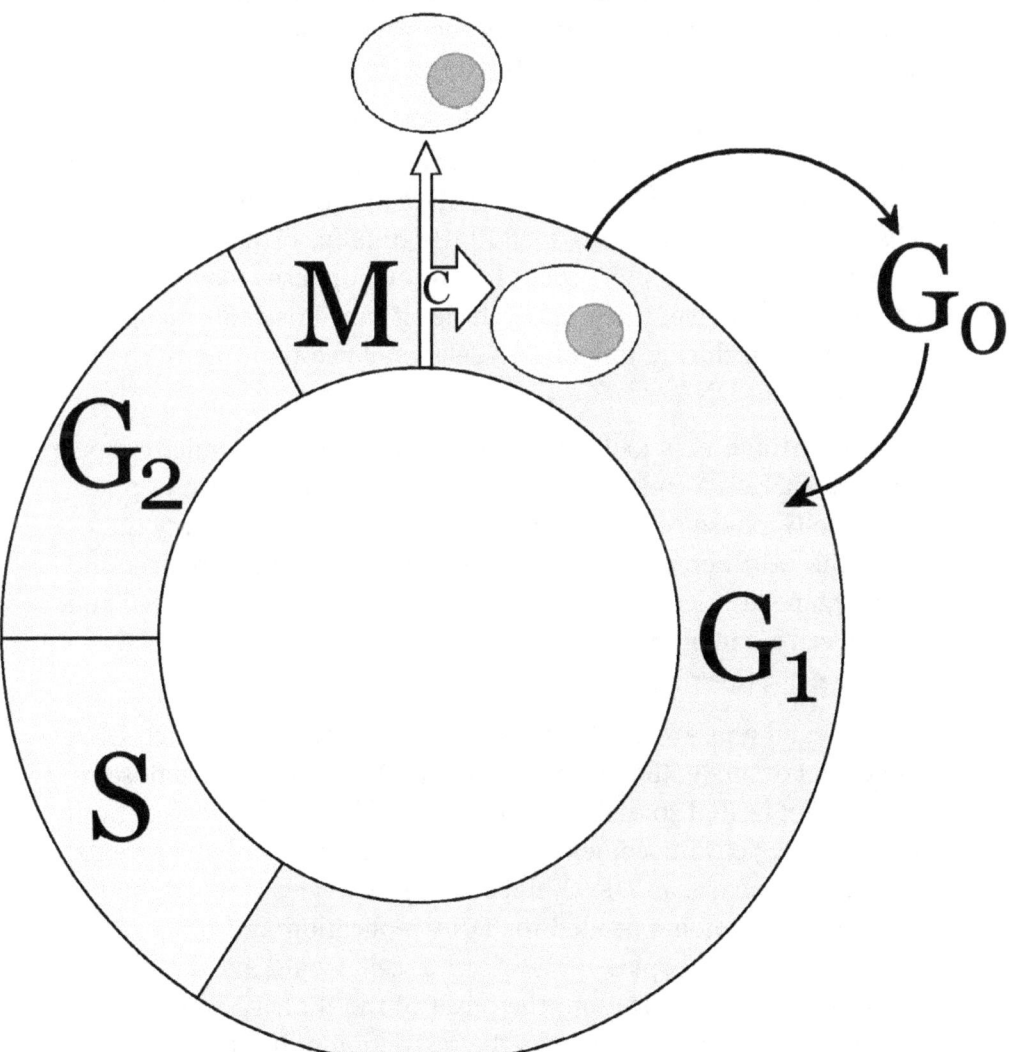

Figure 5-1: The cell cycle.

The cell cycle is the series of events that occur during the duplication and division of one cell into two daughter cells. There are four distinct steps in the cell cycle: *Gap 1, Synthesis, Gap 2, and Mitosis* which lead to cytokinesis, the splitting of the cell into two.

The first phase is known as the Gap phase, as under a microscope, it looks like nothing is happening in the reproductive realm. And in some cells, there is no apparent cell growth.

For long-lived cells, such as the cardiac muscle cells and those of the bone, the Gap phase is the usual state of activity. This is called the **Gap zero phase** (G_0). These cells are referred to as being in a quiescent state, although the cardiomyocytes, neurons, and liver cells (hepatocytes) can hardly be thought of as being on metabolic vacations; these are highly active cells. They are just not growing or preparing to divide. The hepatocytes have a great capacity for self-replacement and do so when needed after injury or loss. Cells entering senescence also go into the G_0 phase.

Many cells temporarily go into the G_0 phase and come out of retirement when new cells are needed. While in health, liver and most kidney cells spend most of their lives in the G_0 phase, but other cells, such as epithelial cells spend little time in, or never enter the G_0 phase. Even though cells in the G_0 phase may be very metabolically active, they have little if any risk of malignant transformation during this phase. Cells may use the time in the G_0 phase to repair DNA errors.

The **G_1 phase** may look similar to G_0 phase under a microscope; however, there is a considerable difference between G_0 and G_1 phase cells. The G_1 phase could be called the Growth phase. During the G_1 phase the cell increases in size. The number of mitochondria and other organelles increases as does the pool of proteins in the cell and in the cell's membrane in preparation for splitting. In actively growing cells, this phase may take as little as 6 to 12 hours.

The second phase is the Synthesis or **S phase**, during which DNA replication occurs within the nucleus. The DNA of each chromosome has to be replicated so that each new cell will have a full copy of both pairs of the 23 chromosomes we humans inherited from our parents. During the S phase, a CDK/Cyclin complex activates transcription of enzymes and proteins needed for DNA replication and other tasks. Since having two copies of DNA in a cell would be dangerous, initiation of DNA replication, the onset of the S phase commits the cell to division. This is known as the restriction point, as there is no turning back. Once the cell has committed to moving from the G_1 to the S phase, the DNA replication occurs quickly. The S phase is a risky time, as this is when mutagens can easily damage the exposed and thus susceptible DNA.

This is the most critical stage of the cell cycle for DNA breaks and the most difficult time for DNA repair. During most of a cell's life, the DNA is wound around histone proteins, and only the sections of

DNA that need to be coded into new proteins are uncoiled and thus exposed. Even if these exposed areas are damaged, the damage is usually to one side of the double strand, so the complementary side of the strand can be used to correct the break with the correct nucleotide. During the DNA synthesis phase, the DNA is much more highly exposed. If both strands of the DNA are broken, it can be guesswork how to repair the DNA. If sections are broken off, they may be repaired, sometimes leaving out or adding bits. During the S phase, the centrosome, an organelle that helps the chromosomes move to the opposite end of the cell, is also duplicated. The S phase typically takes about 6 to 8 hours to complete.

There is a second Gap phase, the **G_2 phase**, following the S phase. During this time, the cell grows more and is actively producing proteins that will be required for the new cells. This phase can be completed in as little as 3 to 4 hours. During the G2 phase, mechanisms in the cell make sure everything is in place for the next steps in cell division.

The G_1, S, and G_2 phases combined are called the *Interphase*. During this time, under the microscope, the cell looks about the same, it is just getting larger.

The next phase in cell division is mitosis, also known as the **M phase**. This phase is a hotbed of activity during which the chromosomes line up in pairs in the middle of the cell, and then one of each pair of identical chromosomes is pushed into opposite ends of the cell. After this is cytokinesis; the cell splits into two, each new cell having a full complement of chromosomes, mitochondria, and other organelles, and all the other proteins that a cell needs.

At the onset of mitosis, the network of microtubules that compose the cell's cytoskeleton during other periods of the cell's life undergo a complete rearrangement and form the mitotic spindles. These specialized microtubules are responsible for guiding the *chromatids,* the condensed DNA strands, into each end of the cell and ensuring that each new cell has the original cell's complete genetic content. A metaphase chromosome consists of a matching pair of chromatids, held together at a central location by a centromere.

Mitosis has several steps (Table 5-1 and Figure 5-2), beginning with prophase. In prophase, the identical pairs of chromatids, replicated during the S-phase, condense within the nucleus to form X-shaped chromosomes that are bound together by a centromere. Next, in prometaphase, the kinetochore-microtubule spindle forms between the centrosomes, attaches to each chromosome at its centromere, and the nuclear envelope disintegrates. In metaphase, microtubules begin moving the chromosomes into the two opposite ends of the cell. In anaphase the microtubules push against each other, elongating the cell. This continues in telophase. Additionally, in telophase, new microtubules push against each other, elongating the cell and pushing a set of chromosomes into each end. The nucleus forms around the chromatids after which the chromatids decondense. Once started, the M phase transpires rapidly, taking about one hour.

Table 5-1 and Figure 5-2: Phases of Cell Division

Steps in Mitosis	Events
Prophase	The DNA condenses within the nucleus into chromosomes. Centrosomes migrate to opposite poles of the cell.
Prometaphase	The nuclear envelope disintegrates, and the kinetochore-microtubule proteins bind to the centromeres of the chromosome (Not illustrated)
Metaphase	Microtubule proteins begin moving the chromosomes into the two opposite ends of the cell.
Anaphase	Microtubules lengthen, causing the cell to elongate, as also shown in Figure 5-3.
Telophase	Microtubules push chromosomes into each end of the cell. New nuclear membranes reform around the chromosomes and the chromosomes decondense.

Interphase   Prophase   Metaphase   Anaphase   Telophase

Finally, the process of *cytokinesis* occurs. Here, the cell begins to contract at the middle of the cell, in the area where the metaphase plate had been, and like a tightening belt, the cell narrows until it becomes divided into two separate cells, each with a nucleus and a full set of parts.

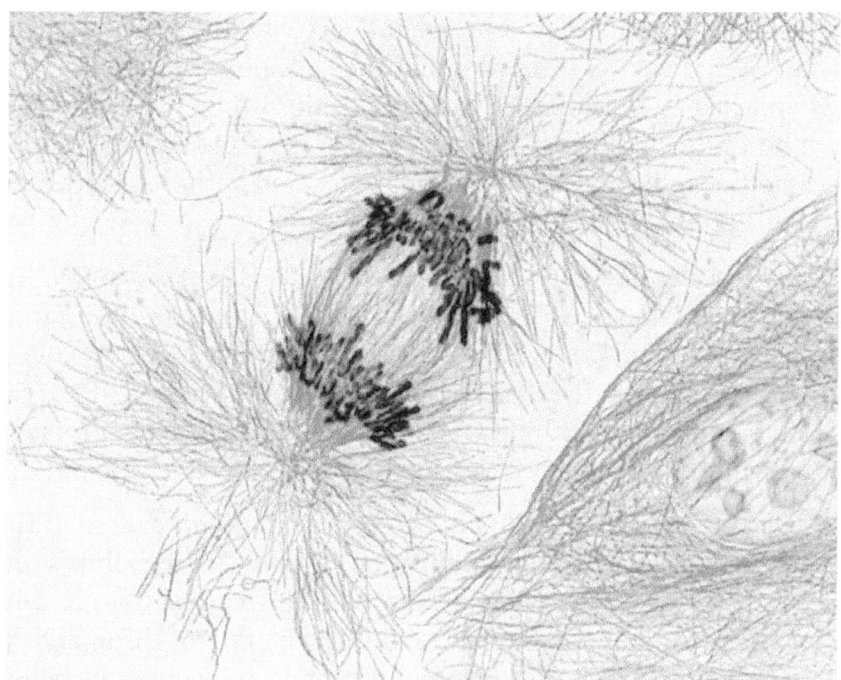
Figure 5-3: Mitotic tubules and chromosomes during anaphase.[29]

Checkpoints

What you were likely not taught in high school, is that the cell cycle has checkpoints with armed guards along the roadway that can arrest the cell cycle process. There are three points along the process that can prevent the process of cell replication from going forward and that can destroy the cell if it does not pass the inspection. The first checkpoint is just a restriction. The cell can remain in G1 for an extended period. The G1 restriction prevents the cell from entering into the S phase until it has built up the resources it needs to make it through the cell division process. This checkpoint makes sure that the DNA is in good condition and that there are sufficient resources to build all the proteins and organelles the cell will need. A protein known as Rb acts as the auditor, preventing entry into the S phase. Rb is named after Retinoblastoma as the Rb gene is often mutated in this form of cancer. Once the cell passes the G1 restriction, there is no turning back – the cell is now committed to cell division; it will either divide into two cells or succumb during the process.

The second checkpoint is in the G2 phase, which acts similarly to the G1 restriction, but with more teeth. The clock is ticking, and the protein, p53, is accumulating. If the checkpoint criteria are not accomplished quickly enough, sufficient p53 will accumulate and trigger apoptosis and death of the cell. P53 is constantly being formed and destroyed in the cell, but its destruction slows during cell division. If cell division proceeds too slowly after entering the S phase, p53 accumulation will promote apoptotic cell death.

The third, and final, checkpoint occurs during mitosis at metaphase. It checks to ensure that the chromosomes are lined up and attached to the spindles correctly so that when the cell divides each new cell will have one of each of the 46 chromosomes. Mitosis does not move into anaphase without this, and within a short time, p53 will accumulate and promote apoptosis.

These checkpoints prevent unhealthy cells, those with DNA or chromosomal damage, or with chromatid missegregation, from surviving and reproducing. These checkpoints play a central role in preventing dysfunctional cells and preventing cancer. P53 can promote apoptosis and destruction of the cell if the problems blocking the checkpoint progression cannot be effectively repaired.

P53 is the most commonly mutated gene in human cancer. If this protein is damaged and cannot function correctly, checkpoint failure may not promote elimination of the cell. This can allow cells with damaged DNA, mutations, or incorrect distribution of chromatids to survive, sneak past the checkpoint, and reproduce defective, potentially malignant cells. The p53 gene is susceptible to mutation as it is transcribed and thus continuously exposed during cell growth and reproduction.

Cancer cells may not go into G_0 but continue into G1 preparation for growth and division, and often ignore the G1/S restriction. This may occur, for example, if there are mutations in the CDK/Cyclin complex that allow the cell to reproduce DNA even when obvious DNA errors are present. CDK/Cyclin thus can act as an oncogene.

> We all start out as a single, fertilized ovum; the cell cycle allows for a single cell to reproduce, doubling 47 times in cell number, into a forty trillion cell organism with sparkling blue-grey eyes, a roguish grin, and a fine wit. ($2^{46} \approx 70$ trillion). Since it only takes about a day for cells to double their number, this could be done in only seven weeks, but for the fine detail of feeding those cells. The final day, like every day before, it would double the animal's size. Thus, it would need enough nutrition to maintain the fetus, plus enough to build a new one of the same size in a day, and need an absorption and delivery system for all that nutrition. Small animals can efficiently turn 10 pounds of food protein into one pound of body protein. Thus, to add five pounds of lean body mass in a day would take consumption of and a digestive system capable of handling and processing 50 pounds of protein. Nine months is a better time frame.

Table 5-2 contains details for geeks and nerds – it lists several of the proteins that are involved in the control of the cell cycle and its checkpoints.

Table 5-2: Cell Cycle Phases and Checkpoints[30]

Gap 1	Cell Growth in preparation for division
G1 Restriction (G1→S)	Is there enough energy? Are there enough building materials? Are there enough parts (organelles) for two cells? Is the DNA in good condition?
	If these criteria are not met, the cell will block the transition from G1 to S. Rb, p107 and p130 are restriction point repressors. They bind to E2F proteins forming complexes (Rb:E2F1, Rb:E2F2, RbE2F3, p107:E2F4 and p130:E2F5) that repress E2F mediated G1→S progression.
	Cyclin D forms a complex with CDK4 and CDK6, which in turn phosphorylate the proteins Rb, p107, and p130, thus promoting the transition to the S phase. When there is damage to the DNA, Chk1 or Chk2 activate p53. P53 activates several proteins, including p21 and p16 that block G1→S progression. P16 disrupts the cyclin D-CDK4 complexes. P21 activates Rb.
	When the cellular mechanisms work correctly, the inhibitors prevent G1→S progression until the DNA damage has been repaired. If the cell cannot repair the damage, p53 induces apoptosis of the cell.
	Once committed to the S phase, there is no turning back.
Synthesis	Reproduction of the DNA strands within the nucleus of the cell.
Gap 2	Further growth of the cell.
G2 Checkpoint (G2→M)	Did DNA replication work?
	Cyclin B-cdc2 (CDK1 homolog) complex is needed for the G2→M transition. DNA damage triggers activation of p53 which activates p21 and 14-3-3 and in turn, inhibits cyclin B-cdc2 complex formation.
Prophase and Prometaphase	Formation and pairing of chromosomes
Metaphase Checkpoint (Spindle Checkpoint)	Are the chromosomes correctly paired?
	Before the cell splits into two daughter cells, each end of the cell will need its own set of chromosomes. In humans, that means 23 different chromosomes, and each new cell will need one of each flavor. The chromosomes pair up and are attached to "spindles." A protein named securin prevents the protein separase from initiating the movement of a chromatid (half of the chromosome pair) into each end of the cell.
	The "anaphase-promoting complex" (APC/C) is an ubiquitin ligase that breaks down securin, and thus allows the transition from metaphase to anaphase, the separation of chromatids into the two ends of the cell. APC/C activity is regulated by several other proteins.
	When the metaphase checkpoint fails or occurs prematurely due to damage of participating regulatory proteins, the chromosomes can missegregate, causing aneuploidy, extra or missing chromosomes in the daughter cells. When aneuploidy is not lethal, it can cause tumorigenesis. Aneuploidy is common in BRCA-1 breast cancer cells and in lung cancer.
Metaphase, Anaphase, and Telophase	Chromosomes are moved into the two ends of the cell, cell elongates, nuclear membranes reform.
Cytokinesis	Cell splits into two

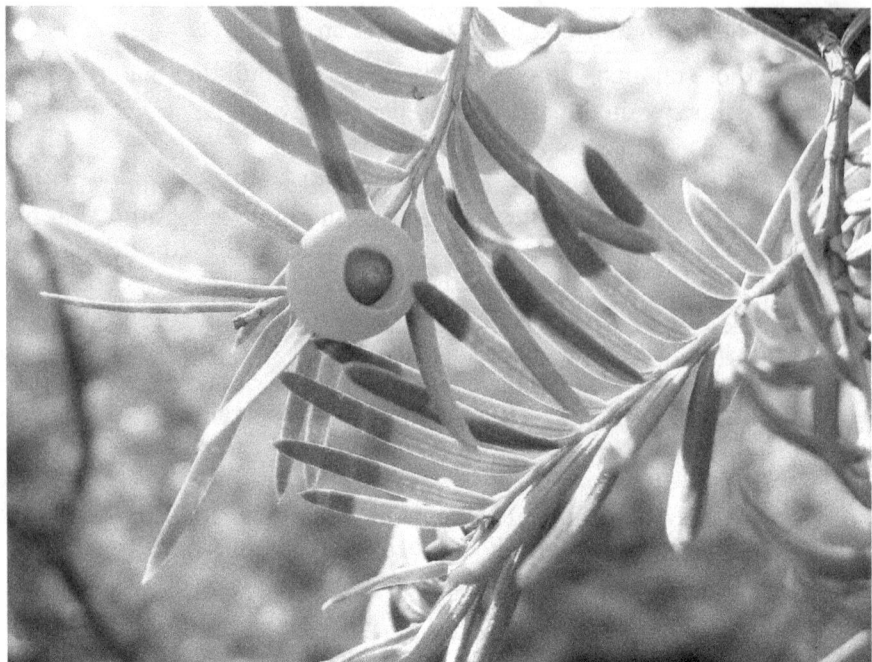

Figure 5-4: A branch of the Pacific yew tree, showing ripe arils

A class of chemotherapeutic agents that includes paclitaxel (Taxol) and docetaxel (Taxotere) prevents mitosis by impeding normal spindle formation through polymerization of the microtubules into non-functioning clusters[31] as well as preventing the dissociation of microtubules from the centrosome.

The Pacific yew tree is the natural source of paclitaxel (Taxol), an effective treatment for ovarian cancer. The bark of the tree was discovered to contain an anti-carcinogenic compound in the 1960's, but it took the bark of four full grown trees to make enough medicine for one patient. The tree quickly became an endangered species. Now, however, the medication is synthetically derived. Yew trees are sometimes called the tree of death because the leaves and seed are quite toxic. The red arils are sweet and edible, but the seeds at the center of the arils and leaves were used for suicide in ancient times.

Another class of agents that includes vincristine and vinblastine, disrupts spindle function and mitosis, destabilizing the microtubules and fragmenting them, as well as detaching the spindle poles. Both these classes of chemotherapeutics act during mitosis and help trigger cell death at the metaphase checkpoint. (These agents are also from a toxic plant, *Catharanthus roseus*, shown in Figure 2-1).

The protein, survivin, collects around the microtubules of the mitotic spindles near the centrosomes and helps stabilize and protect the microtubules. In doing so, it impedes apoptosis. Survivin is commonly over-expressed in cancer cells and induces resistance to chemotherapeutic agents that polymerize or destabilize the microtubules.[32]

6: CARCINOGENS

There are several mechanisms underlying the development of cancer, and most cancers have more than one defective mechanism at play. The National Institutes of Environmental Health Sciences at the NIH have identified ten different mechanisms by which carcinogens cause cancer.[33]

- Act as an electrophile
- Be genotoxic
- Alter DNA repair or cause genomic instability
- Induce epigenetic alterations
- Induce oxidative stress
- Induce chronic inflammation
- Suppress immune function
- Modulate receptor-mediated effects
- Cause immortalization
- Alter cell proliferation, cell death, or nutrient supply.

Electrophiles, such as epoxides, are chemical compounds that can form strong (covalent) bonds with protein, lipids, and DNA, forming protein adducts and DNA adducts. Many, perhaps most, electrophilic human carcinogens are absorbed as pre-carcinogens that are activated by the metabolism, such as cytochrome p450 or other enzymes, into electrophiles.

Genotoxic compounds damage the DNA; they may break the DNA strand or cause cross-linking of the DNA. Nucleotide substitutions or other mutations may occur during the DNA repair process. Certain mutations in specific genes can cause cancer, usually by either inhibiting the elimination of abnormal cells or inducing unregulated growth of cells containing the mutation. DNA adducts can cause substitutions and breaks in the DNA strand. Ionizing radiation (UV, X-ray, and gamma rays), can also cause DNA breaks and errors.

There are a variety of DNA mutations that can occur; point mutations may cause a substitution of a single nucleotide, frameshifts, translocations, deletions, insertions or inversions of the DNA sequence. These mutations can alter or disable the function of the protein transcribed from the altered gene.

Compounds that *impair the DNA repair process,* or that cause genomic instability, similarly cause cancer because they induce mutations by preventing the correct repair of DNA breaks. Some DNA adducts impair the DNA repair process. Cadmium, arsenic, formaldehyde and radiation reduce the fidelity of DNA repair.

Epigenetic alterations can change how easily various genes are expressed. Epigenetic settings can be inherited by daughter cells.

When the cell determines the need for certain sets of proteins, specific signaling molecules in the cell enter the nucleus and induce specific areas of the DNA to unwind from the protein (histones) that helps store and protect the DNA. This exposes the DNA section so that it can be read and transcribed into messenger RNA that is used to make requisite proteins. Typically, the promoter unwinds a section of the DNA that codes for several genes, and thus allows several different proteins to be made that work in unison.

The proclivity for various sections of the DNA to unwind under the influence of promoters is moderated by methylation of the DNA to the histone. The more methylations, the more resistant the DNA is to unwinding. The enzyme histone deacetylase helps free the DNA. The degree of DNA methylation and acetylation of different sections of the DNA varies among individuals and helps us to adapt to our environment. This adaptation or mis-adaptation as the case may be, is known as epigenetic adaptation.

Certain epigenetic adaptations or alterations can influence cancer risk. For example, the protein p53 helps prevent cells with mutations from reproducing. If p53 is highly methylated, it will not be as available for preventing aberrant cells from reproducing. On the other hand, when p53 is freed from its histone, it is much more susceptible to damage and mutation. P53 mutations are the most prevalent mutation found in cancers. Thus, very low or high histone binding can be a risk factor for cancer.

Oxidative stress, from ROS (reactive oxygen species) and RNS (reactive nitrogen species), causes protein, lipid and DNA damage. Damage to proteins and lipids puts increased stress on the cells and favors cell death. Oxidized lipids can act as toxins that age cells. DNA oxidation can cause point mutations and cross-linking that increase the risk of carcinogenesis.

Free Radicals and Oxidative Stress

Free radicals are troublemakers. They incite damage by avidly stealing an electron from another molecule. This causes an imbalance in the victim molecule, which compels it to replace the electron by grabbing it from anywhere it can. Most of the free radicals in our bodies are unbalanced oxygen molecules, such a superoxide, and hydrogen peroxide. There are several different ROS and RNS that act as free radicals in the body.

When ROS damage occurs, it is not a single susceptible molecule which is injured, but rather a chain reaction of stealing electrons from another molecule, and damaging the target molecule and possibly changing its conformation. The target, now missing an electron itself, becomes radicalized and tries to grab an electron from another molecule. During the recovery of the electron, the protein may not return to its original form; so even though it has replaced the missing electron, it may be crippled or dysfunctional.

It is as if you had a kindergarten class where everyone had an ice cream cone, but Tommy gobbles his down, gets an ice cream headache and then wants another. Being a bully, Tommy grabs another kid's ice cream cone and starts eating it. That other child gets upset and steals the ice cream from a third kid while the second child, although having an ice cream cone, is still crying and upset because he had wanted his mango ice cream, but now has strawberry ice cream. The next child does the same thing to yet another kid and is also bent out of shape by the incident. Soon the entire classroom is unhappy. With free radicals, it is not 20 kids in a room; *a single ROS can cause a chain reaction that damages billions of molecules per second.*

Antioxidants are like the nice lady that quickly intervenes, supplying an extra ice cream cone right away, breaking the chain of ice cream cone-snatching, so that things don't get out of hand in the classroom.

Antioxidants are molecules that prevent the oxidation of other molecules. They do this mostly by donating electrons and quenching the free radical. In this process, they themselves become oxidized; however, they are made for this and do not pass the damage along. Most antioxidants can do this because they can exist in more than one redox state; copper can be Cu^{1+} or Cu^{2+} and iron Fe^{2+}, Fe^{3+}, or Fe^{4+}. Sulfur has six potential redox states. The redox state tells how many electrons these metallic ions can hold. The atoms act as antioxidants, not free ions in the cell, but only as a part of an antioxidant molecule. Thus, an antioxidant containing a copper Cu^{2+} can donate an electron and become Cu^{1+}, without damaging the molecule.

Our body makes ROS and RNS on purpose. The white blood cells use ROS to kill bacteria and parasites, as part of the immune mechanisms used for destroying infected cells. However, ROS are also produced by worn-out, poorly functioning mitochondria in the cells. In health, these feeble mitochondria are eliminated. If not, the cell will become senescent and die. We can replace most of the cells in our body, so this is not a problem, except when the cell happens to be one of those troublesome irreplaceable neurons in our brain, muscle cell in our heart, or retinal cell in our eye or cochlea of the ear. It can also be a problem when there is an excessive replacement of cells that increases the risk of mutagenesis and cancer.

One of the jobs of vitamin C, an antioxidant, is to donate an electron to copper-containing antioxidants, restoring their ability to act an antioxidant again. Humans and other primates are quite unusual mammals in terms of vitamin C. For almost all other non-primates, ascorbic acid (vitamin C) is not a vitamin. Most animals can make ascorbic acid themselves. For us, ascorbic acid is a vitamin by definition, as we need it in our diet. Even more remarkable is that an animal of similar mass to a human makes hundreds of times as much vitamin C as we consume in our diet. A goat weighing about the same as an adult human makes about 200 mg of ascorbic acid from glucose per kilogram on a good day, and even more when under stress. That would be equivalent to an adult man taking 14 grams of vitamin C per day when the recommended daily intake is only about 0.1 grams. Fourteen grams of vitamin C in a day would cause bloating and diarrhea in most people as our body does not absorb nearly that amount, and most of it would ferment in the gut.

Why do we need so much less ascorbic acid as an antioxidant than other mammals? Actually, we need just as much.

When vitamin C is oxidized, it is exported out of the cells and into the serum, the liquid part of the bloodstream, in the form of dehydroascorbate – oxidized ascorbic acid. In most mammals, dehydroascorbate is then eliminated by the kidneys. In primates, however, dehydroascorbate is taken up by the red blood cells where it is recycled into vitamin C by the antioxidant glutathione and later released back into the bloodstream.[34, 35] Not only does this trick help to redistribute vitamin C to where it is needed most, but it also saves energy. It is more efficient to recycle vitamin C than build it from glucose. This process saves about the equivalent of 10 days worth of calories per year; a very handy adaptation during an ice age when food is scarce.

Many people take antioxidant supplements as a way to prevent oxidative "stress," the damage caused by ROS. This is a great idea, other than it does not work. Not only does it not help, but some antioxidant vitamins also increase the risk of cancer, heart disease, and mortality.[36] This likely occurs for several reasons. First, it is very hard to get the concentration of an antioxidant above the physiologic level in a cell, the site of ROS damage. Secondly, the antioxidant beta-carotene is converted to vitamin A, which can act as a growth factor that supports the growth of tumor cells. Moreover, antioxidants act slowly in comparison to the speed at which the damage occurs. Perhaps most importantly, antioxidants may decrease the cells reactivity to stress and may prevent sick cells from eliminating themselves through apoptosis. Masking oxidative stress can also inhibit the induction of the cellular stress response, which includes the formation of antioxidant enzymes.

Chronic inflammation increases the production and turnover of white blood cells and raises the production of pro-inflammatory cytokines that can favor apoptosis. This increases cell turnover in the inflamed tissues, thus increasing the risk of mutation. Chronic stress may also promote epigenetic alterations that favor cellular turnover. Inflammation can induce production of enzymes, such as prostaglandin synthase that can transform compounds into electrophiles.

Immunosuppressive agents can cause immune dysfunction and impair immunosurveillance. This can prevent the immune system from recognizing cancer cells and eliminating them.

Protein receptor-mediated effects modulate cell reproduction. For example, estrogenic compounds may inappropriately increase the growth and survival of estrogen-dependent cells and in this way increase the survival and proliferation of estrogen-dependent tumor cells. Insulin-like growth factor, a tyrosine kinase receptor-ligand, promotes cell growth. This pathway often alters gene transcription in a way that promotes proliferation.

Immortalization of cells can occur as a result of the insertion of viral DNA into the genome of the cell. The cells themselves are not immortal, but rather, their lineage can continue to divide many more times than would be allowed by normal telomere shortening. Telomeres are DNA repeat sequences at the tip of that chromosome that prevent DNA fraying and that are needed for DNA replication, but the final sequence cannot be copied by the replication proteins. Thus with each cell cycle, the telomere loses one repeat. This limits the number of times a cell can divide. Viruses also prevent cellular senescence and cell death by destroying pro-apoptosis proteins, allowing cells with mutations and cancer cells to survive. Some tumors promote the enzyme telomerase that can add telomere sequences to the chromosome and thus bypass limits of reproduction.

Alterations in nutrient supply can allow cancers to grow. Solid tumors are limited in size to about one cubic millimeter, unless they can develop their own blood supply. VEGF (vascular endothelial growth factor) and other vascular promoters are needed to sustain cancer growth and metastasis.

The first of the risk factors for cancer compiled by the NIH is the rate of stem cell division. This is similar, but not the same for everyone. Taller individuals have more cell divisions in their colonic stem cells as they have a slightly longer colon needed for a bigger body. However, they may be taller because they are more responsive to growth stimulation. Taller women have an increased risk of colon cancer. Patients with inflammatory bowel disease have increased cell turnover, and this doubles their risk of colon and rectal cancer. Chronic inflammatory conditions, where there is sustained damage, necessitates more stem cell divisions for repair of tissue damage, and thus, increases cancer risk.

A second mechanism causing cancer development is mutation. The typical DNA transcription error rate is enough to cause a large share of mutations. These are just "bad luck" occurring during DNA transcription, and there is little to do to avoid them, other than to avoid excess cell reproduction. There are also DNA errors caused by environmental mutagens including DNA adducts the cells are exposed to. Many carcinogens from smoking, diet, and the environment cause cancer by causing DNA transcription errors.

Another risk factor is DNA methylation. When DNA is methylated, it is bound more firmly to the histone proteins that it is wrapped around, and this protects the DNA from damage. Excessive methylation, however, may keep p53 and other regulatory proteins from being expressed, and thus lowers their activity. Like Goldilocks, we want our DNA methylation not to be too high or too low. Dietary deficiencies of some B vitamins may cause inadequate methylation.

The fourth risk factor is impaired DNA repair and culling of cells with irreparable damage. Young, proud stem cells are valiant and vain. They take good care of their health through frequent grooming and are robust and fit. They also will self-sacrifice if things go amiss. They can either self-destruct or more gently retire by transforming themselves into two, mere mortal daughter cells that have a normal lifespan and disappear.

Stem cells have a choice when they divide. They can bud-off a single daughter cell, and remain a stem cell capable of budding off daughter cells as frequently as every day. Or, the stem cell can retire, and just divide into two progenitor cell daughter cells. This starts a clock, as the two daughter cells, as progenitor cells, budding off terminal cells for a while but after a number of divisions they become terminal cells themselves.

There is also a third choice – stem cells can split into two stem cells. This is, of course, the most dangerous time to make mistakes as these errors become permanent mistakes transferred into daughter cells and accumulate in the stem cells with each division. Daughter cells, with mutations, can go rogue and become cancers.

When stem cells age, they stop cleaning up as well. Aged stem cells are at least as likely to make mistakes, and likely have accumulated errors from previous divisions. Old cells are more liable to suffer oxidative damage that can cause DNA damage and are less apt at finding and repairing DNA errors. They are also less likely to sacrifice themselves and undergo apoptosis. Older cells are more prone to giving rise to cancer.

As cells age, their health often declines. Healthy cells are better at autophagy, and thus better at replacing worn-out parts. The mitochondria are essential to the process of apoptosis and paraptosis. When the mitochondria get old, and lazy, not only does programmed cell death not occur efficiently, but the mitochondria start to leak free radicals that cause damage to proteins and to the DNA. This leads to the accumulation of errors that can cause cancer and decreases the chances that those cells self-destruct. Most aberrant cells do not have a single mutation or error; they have many. Most adult-onset cancer is sporadic and the result of not one, but several mutations that accumulate in a cell line with aging. Cancer is thus a disease of aging.

Sporadic cancer refers to those caused by new somatic mutations, rather than by mutations passed from parent to offspring. Even in breast cancer, where hereditary mutations such as BRCA1 and BRCA2 heap an extremely high risk of disease, inherited cancer genes account for only five to ten percent of cancers. Most cancer is from sporadic mutations.

Although a single mutation can "cause" cancer by setting the stage for cancer, it does this by opening the door for other mutations. Cancer cells typically have numerous mutations. If the gene for the protein p53 is damaged in a manner that defeats its activity, cells with other mutations can survive. The defective BRCA proteins impair DNA repair and allow the survival and reproduction of multiple mutations. Most of these mutations don't promote cancer and don't help it survive, but some do and can be enough.

One of the difficulties in treating cancer is that the cancer mutates and becomes resistant to the chemotherapy, and can come back as a more aggressive disease. A frightening aspect of cancer is that it is not a single entity. Cancer cells are clones from an original deviant cell, but this does not mean they are all the same. It is very common for cancers to have mutated and dysfunctional p53. This defect does not cause cells to have bizarre cancerous behavior, but rather it fails to stop cells with other mutations from multiplying. The same is true for BRCA1 and BRCA2 mutations. This makes it easy for clones of cells with defective p53 or BRCA to develop new mutations. Thus, the descendants of the first cancer cells can easily mutate, forming new clones. Some of these clones will be too defective to survive, but others may be more aggressive or more resistant to therapy. Smaller, less developed cancers usually have fewer mutations and are less resistant to cancer treatment.

This is also why it is so important for patients with cancer or with BRCA mutations to avoid mutagens and carcinogens. Cancer cells are many times more susceptible to mutagens and carcinogens than are normal cells. The more cancer cells present, the more likely that an additional mutation can transform a slowly growing cancer into an aggressive, invasive one.

Most genetic errors are of little consequence. They may affect genes that are not used for that cell, or just slow a metabolic process some. More consequential mutations can mess up cell function; they just are a waste of a cell, and they die and are replaced with a functioning cell. These runts may survive a normal span and then die a normal demise or function poorly enough that they eliminate themselves or get eliminated by the immune system. Others will immediately die because they fail a critical function. Since many of these cells are rapidly renewing cells, even if they can't make all the proteins they are supposed to, they are temporary and will soon be replaced.

It is a minority of DNA errors that cause cancer. Of 19,000 genes, there are less than 500 genes that when mutated are suspected of being cancer "driving" genes. Most of these genes are for proteins falling into one of five functional classes:[37]

- Proteins controlling cell signaling or proliferation
- Proteins for DNA repair or controlling the cell cycle
- Proteins involved in chromatin remodeling
- Proteins involved with mRNA processing.
- Proteins involved in cell adhesion

Errors that allow cells to proliferate, either by promoting cell growth directly or by failing to regulate growth obviously cause proliferation of the cancer cells. Most importantly in this group are defects that inhibit apoptosis or other forms of programmed cell death that would normally be eliminating aberrant cells.

Mutations that impair the DNA repair mechanism cause cancer by increasing the number of mutations. Cancer is rarely caused by a single mutation. Pediatric and hematologic cancers (leukemias and lymphomas) usually require at least two cancer-driving mutations, and most solid adult cancers require about nine cancer-driving mutations. Cancer cells in adults usually contain 30 to 60 mutations, with those from older individuals having more. Lung cancers in smokers often have 200 mutations, and colorectal cancers may have hundreds, but only a few of these mutations drive cancer,[38] the rest are luggage. The reason that there are many cancers is often that the DNA repair mechanism is failing due to a mutation.

Chromatin remodeling concerns the packing and storage of the DNA around histone proteins. Defects in this process can make DNA errors much more common. It can also cause problems by making it harder for the DNA sequence of a protective gene to be read.

Cell adhesion protein mutations can promote cancer growth. Normally cells stop growing when they sense that they have a full complement of neighbors, and will divide to fill an adjacent lot when they sense an open space. If a protein for sensing the presence of neighbors is broken, it can signal cell growth even when all the lots in the neighborhood are filled. Less frequently, genes for proteins involved in RNA processing may be dysfunctional, inhibiting the formation of protective proteins, such as proteins controlling proliferation and apoptosis.

These cancer-related genes contain about 100 million base pairs, but not every error in them causes cancer. Only several thousand mutations in specific areas of these genes cause cancer. Even then, the development of cancer almost always requires mutations in more than one oncogene.

Most of these mutations are not the result of any specific exposure to carcinogens, viral agents, UV or cosmic rays, or evil eye, but rather, just random bad luck that occurs as cells reproduce, and errors are made.

DNA mutations underlie the formation of cancer, but this is rarely enough to cause disease. Cells with mutations are made every day, and a number of these have mutations which could cause disease if the cells survive and reproduce. Fortunately, the cell's DNA repair mechanisms catch and repair most DNA errors.

The next line of defense against cancer is apoptosis and paraptosis. Cells are able to detect many DNA problems and are sensitive to delayed or aberrant cell division. If a delayed or aberrant cell division is detected in cells with intact apoptosis mechanisms, the cell self-destructs. This prevents the creation of mutant cell lineages. This is why mutations in genes that regulate gene transcription or repair and apoptosis are so dangerous. If aberrant cells with oncogenic mutations fail to self-destruct, they can continue to grow.

Additionally, DNA mutations that cause proteins to misfold can cause paraptosis. Protein folding is critical to protein function. Thus, most cells with significant mutations are eliminated. Most protein is fed directly from the ribosome into the endoplasmic reticulum where it is folded. It takes, on average, about 170 milliseconds for protein to fold, with an upper limit of 8 seconds.[39] Proteins that fail to fold correctly can accumulate, and this promotes paraptosis. This acts as a safeguard, helping to protect the cell from intracellular infections by viruses that can try to hijack the cells into making viral protein. If the viral protein does not interact correctly with the host's HSP proteins, which aid in the proper sequencing of the folding process, the cell will hit the self-destruct button, and thus, prevent the spread of the virus.

Another contributor to cancer causation is impaired immunity or immune diversion. The immune system likes to focus its energies on one type of target. It uses cytokines as signals for which type of immune cells to develop. Thus, if there is a bacterial infection, it signals the development of white blood cells appropriate for the tasks needed for killing bacterial pathogens and making the proper antibodies. If there is a parasitic infection, cytokine signals promote the development of basophils or eosinophils. Food allergies and IgG-mediated food sensitivities may cause chronic inflammation that diverts immune function. When the immune system is off hunting for worms, it is more likely to ignore emerging cancer cells. Other immune cells are used to fight viruses that are hijacking cells. Furthermore, just as older cells accumulate errors and don't clean up as well, an older immune system may not eliminate cancer cells readily as more spry ones do.

Since cancer cells are derived from host cells, they are often not easily recognizable as foreign terrorists. In paraptosis programmed cell death, the cell spills its misfolded proteins. This alerts the immune system so that other cells bearing these abnormal "foreign" proteins can be recognized by the immune cells. If the cancer makes mutated proteins that present on the outer surface of the cancer cell wall, they can be recognized by the immune system, and these cells targeted for destruction.

When there is an injury and cells are lost, new cells are needed to fill the gap. Normal cells will divide until they touch their neighbors on all sides. Some mutations keep the cell from recognizing that it has neighbors, so these mutations can cause the cells to continue replicating even when not needed.

The final cause on the list, *alteration in nutrient supply* is essential to the growth of solid tumors; without a dedicated vascular supply for nutrients, solid cancers cannot grow beyond about a few million cells or larger than about one cubic millimeter.

Autopsy studies of individuals killed in accidents or by other injuries often have microscopic cancers. In a study of women in their forties, 39% of them had at least one tiny, clinically undetectable breast cancer and nearly half of these had bilateral tumors,[40] yet only about 8% of women will ever be diagnosed with breast cancer. Over 24% of men in their fifties have microscopic prostate cancer, but most of these never advance. The lack of adequate blood supply limits the growth of these cancers. Most cancers never develop into clinical disease. They can remain dormant and harmless for life.[41]

A mutation that allows one of these tiny dormant cancers to promote the growth of new blood vessels can promote the growth of the cancer. Inflammation external to the cancer can also promote angiogenesis and the progression of tiny, dormant cancers into killers. (See PGE_2 in Figure 25-2 as a pro-angiogenesis factor.)

Summary

When a person gets cancer, they do so because something caused it. We are constantly replacing cells in our body. Cancers form when an error in the cell's function causes the cell to continue to reproduce. If the underlying cause of the cancer does not change, it is likely that more cancer cells will be formed and grow.

Even though we replace cells less rapidly during adulthood, our cells may accumulate and pass on errors over the years, like a game of telephone or Chinese whispers. This is one reason that the risk of cancers increases with age.

Adult-onset cancers typically have five to ten cancer-driving mutations in the same cell; it is very rare for an adult-onset cancer to be caused by a single mutation. It is not rare, however, for a cell that already has multiple mutations to become cancerous by adding one more mutation. Furthermore, additional mutations in a slowly growing tumor can turn it into a rapidly growing, aggressively spreading cancer.

If you, or someone you love, have had cancer, there was a reason. A metabolic environment that fosters the growth of cancer cells will continue to support cancer development and growth. If the person continues to be exposed to carcinogens, new cancers are likely to form, and existing cancers are likely to become more aggressive and dangerous.

7: Cancer Causation

Cancer is the second most common cause of death in the United States, a close second only to heart disease, and it likely will overtake heart disease as our number one killer in the coming years. Like heart disease and many other diseases, cancer is largely a lifestyle disease.

When I hear that word "lifestyle", I think of lifestyles of the rich and famous; or of Silicon Valley millionaires with mini-vineyards surrounding their hillside, multimillion-dollar homes overlooking San Francisco Bay.

But here, lifestyle refers to our repeated behaviors, not so much single chance occurrences. Cancer can be caused by walking in front of a death ray or a single, massive exposure as occurred in Hiroshima and Chernobyl; however, most cancer is caused by chronic repeated behavior. Lung cancer is not caused by a single polonium-laced, radioactive cigarette but by smoking a half million cigarettes over 35 years. Cancer is very often a choice, or more accurately, a long series of poor choices.

When epidemiologists talk about causality, they are talking about factors that increase the risk of disease. A risk factor that doubles the risk of the disease means that susceptible individuals exposed to that risk are twice as likely to get the disease. Usually, there are multiple risk factors for any disease, and usually no single risk factor or cause that is a necessary factor.

For heart disease, smoking, diabetes, high LDL cholesterol, lack of physical activity, and diets high in saturated fats are some of the risk factors. Some people have none of these but still, get the disease.

Attributable risk (AR) is a metric used to determine what percent of cases of a disease would be prevented if that risk factor was eliminated from a population. This can be thought of as a threshold effect. If one risk factor is eliminated, it may lower the risk in some individuals enough to prevent the disease, even though other risk factors are still present.

A concept that may seem odd in understanding disease risk is that when adding up the risk factors that explain a disease, they often add up to more than 100%. If you remember the fire triangle (Figure 7-1), it takes fuel, ignition heat, and oxygen to start and sustain a fire.

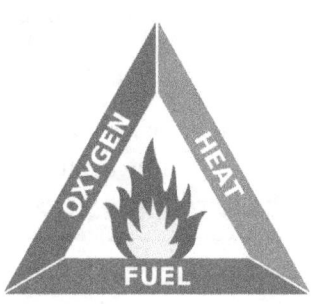

A 21% oxygen atmosphere is plenty for a roaring blaze, but more oxygen will assist the process. You can have all the O2 required from room air for a fire, but a leaky oxygen gas tank adds additional risk. Other oxidizers can also start and sustain fire. The fuel can also come from various sources or a mixture of sources. If the fire is deprived of O2, heat, or fuel, combustion stops. In the same way, diseases have more than one sufficient cause. When the causes of a given disease are summed, it can add up to well above 100 percent. Also just eliminating some causes may prevent cancer risk, even though other risks continue.

I provide this forewarning because, although 65 percent of the cancer-causing mutations are randomly occurring transcription errors, 90 to 95 percent of cancers have an environmental cause, and most of these can be controlled.

Cancers are similar. In cancer, there is a chain of causation, and if one step in the process is eliminated, that cancer may be prevented.

Cancer and cancer reoccurrence are preventable. Lifestyle changes can slow the progression of cancer, and at times even stop cancer growth. This may give the body's immune system a chance to attack and fight the cancer.

> **Note:** Nothing contained in this book should be interpreted as a recommendation to ignore, neglect or decline medical treatment for cancer. Great strides and improvements have been made in the medical treatment of cancer in recent years. The information given here is provided to decrease the probability of cancer development, to slow its growth and lower the chances of its return.
>
> The body's immune system eliminates most bacteria that enter body tissues without difficulty, but a major infection can be easily fatal without the use of antibiotics. Similarly, the immune system is usually successful at eliminating sporadic cancer cells or tiny clusters of cancer cells that develop in the body but has limited ability to destroy a large, rapidly growing cancer mass.
>
> It is important to understand that neither medical treatments, such as surgical removal of cancer, chemotherapy, nor dietary interventions are

> guarantees against cancer recurrence. They lower the odds.
>
> **Numbers:** Therapy that lowers the risk of an event from 30% to 15% cuts the risk in half. A decrease in risk of a deadly condition by 15% is a significant benefit; however, it is not a guarantee. Cutting the risk in half may also mean lowering it from two percent to one percent.

For an 85 years old person, with an average life expectancy of 6 years, a one percent difference in survival would be about 18 days of life, assuming the disease if present caused death in one year. Although not a direct comparison, *statistically*, if a therapy lowered the risk of death by one percent in similar patients, this is how many days of life might be added on average by the therapy. A five percent decline would multiply this number of days by five. When assessing the personal benefit of a treatment, diet, medical or other, the personal cost also needs to be weighed. If I were 85 years old and offered a treatment that made me feel ill for 6 weeks, with a probable increase of 18 days of survival, I would politely decline the generous offer. If I was offered a couple of extra months of life for restricting my diet to foods I hate and passing my days feeling hungry, I would decline. But if the diet gave me more energy, made me feel better, and tasted great, I'd go for it.

Some antibiotics fight infections by preventing the bacteria from reproducing; others block their metabolism, killing them. Even when using an antibiotic, the immune system helps the body defeat the bacteria. Some antibiotics do not kill bacteria, but only stop them from dividing long enough for the immune system to react. Also, most infections are biofilms – masses of bacteria protected by a slimy coat that the white blood cells have difficulty attacking.

If insufficient doses of antibiotics are used, or the antibiotic is not specific enough for the infection, the antibiotic may only kill or block the growth of some of the bacteria. Bacteria have frequent genetic alterations, and the ones that resist the antibiotic will grow, making the antibiotic ineffective in all subsequent generations of those resistant bacteria. This is especially true in patients with massive infections, where the number of disease-causing bacteria may be in the trillions, and in patients with impaired immunity. Bacterial infections that a healthy immune system might easily defeat can overcome a patient with an impaired immune system.

The situation is similar in cancer and chemotherapy. For many cancers, the healthier the immune system, the more likely that chemotherapy or other treatment will be able to control the disease by eliminating cancer cells – especially lone cells that have migrated away from the primary cancer. Another similarity to bacteria is that chemotherapy kills the most susceptible cancer cells most easily.

This leaves the more resistant cells, similar to how antibiotics can cause the selection for the most resistant bacteria. What this means is that the first course of chemotherapy is usually the most successful, and gives the longest lasting effects, as the cells that it does not kill tend to be those most resistant. A different antibiotic may kill the resistant infection, and a different chemotherapy may kill resistant cancer cells, but each time there is a higher risk of failure.

The immune system is best at killing single cancer cells, rather than attacking a large mass. The best time for a healthy immune system and dietary intervention to work is before the first cancer cell develops. The next best time is before a single cancer cell divides.

The science of epidemiology, which studies disease distribution in various populations, has identified major causes of cancer. If we can avoid the things that place us at risk, the risk factors, we can greatly reduce our chances of getting cancer.

If a person has developed cancer, if risk factors have not changed, it can be assumed that they are still at high risk of cancer, even if the original cancer is cured. If the situation under which cancer developed remains in place, why would a new cancer not be prone to develop? If a person's family members develop cancer, and they live in the same environment and have the same lifestyle and genetics, they are likely at similar risk of developing cancer. Thus, understanding risk factors, and changing those which can be changed, can help prevent cancer.

Some families are at very high risk of cancer. While these individuals may be at very high risk, inherited genes only explain about five, perhaps up to ten percent of all cancers. While these comprise only a small minority of cancer cases, these may be among the most destructive cancers as they can occur during youth. Genetically induced cancer risk reduction will be discussed in Chapter 8. Nevertheless, even in those with high genetic cancer risk, environmental factors greatly influence risk and survival.

Ninety to ninety-five percent of cancers are caused by environmental factors. The distribution of these causes is illustrated as a pie chart in Figure 7-2.

The hardest category to control may be "Other" environmental risk factors. This set of causes underlies the causation of 10 to 15 percent of cancers. These risks include exposures to (medical and other) ionizing radiation, including X-rays and gamma radiation, and excess UV radiation from the sun or tanning beds. It also includes workplace and environment exposure to chemicals such as pesticides, by-products of petroleum combustion, and heavy metals.

It includes indoor and outdoor air pollution. Additionally, some medications, especially those used for treating cancer, are carcinogenic.

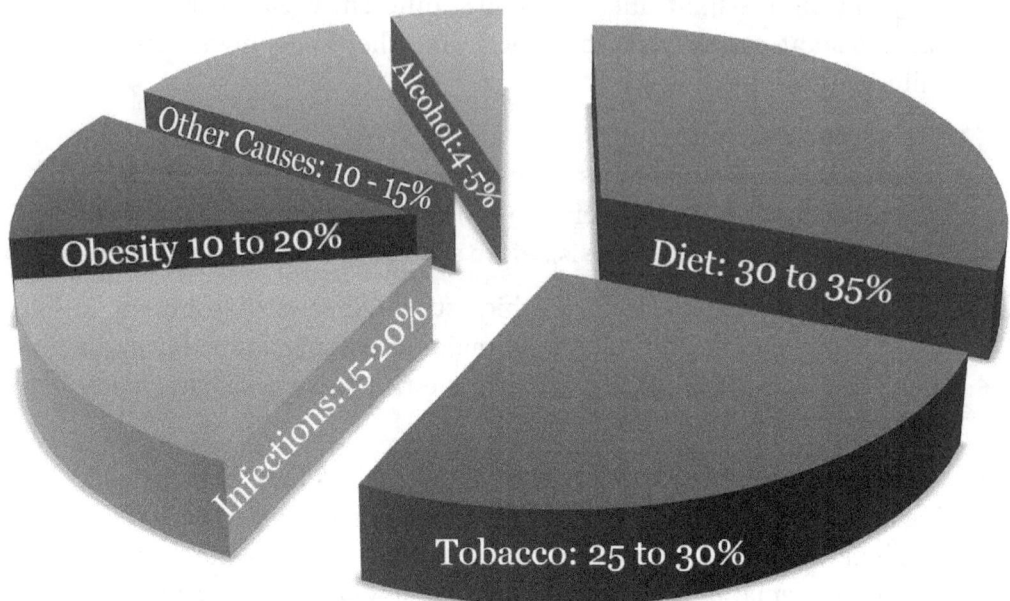

Figure 7-2: Major Modifiable Cancer Risk Factors[42]

The vast majority of environmental cancers are caused by the things that we put into our own mouths: food, tobacco, and alcohol.[42] These are the risk factors that will be discussed in most detail in chapters ahead. You may be stuck with your genetics, but you can change your diet and control the things that go into your and your child's mouth.

8: Hereditary Cancers

All cancers have genetic defects, but most of these mutations are not present in the germ cell lineage and are not heritable. Hereditary cancers require an inherited gene defect. These are rare; less than three in 1000 persons inherit a genetic mutation that imparts a large increase in cancer risk; nevertheless, these risks are large enough to cause three to ten percent of all cancers as they can impart very high risk.

There are a couple of dozen hereditary genetic syndromes associated with very high risk of cancer, and several of these are caused by more than one gene.[43] These are gene defects that are inherited from the parent's germline and passed to offspring generation to generation. Of our 19,000 genes, there about 450 genes that can drive cancer development. Many of these defects are incompatible with the birth of a normal, healthy child. Thus, the number of cancers caused by heritable genes is limited.

Growth regulation gene mutations that cause cancer are often incompatible with a developing fetus; thus, these are usually not heritable. Additionally, for a genetic defect to pass from one generation to the next, the person needs to live long enough to have children. The defective gene cannot be passed on if it prevents survival into adulthood long enough for the carrier to pass it on to their children. Other severe defects cause disabilities or deformities that decrease the chances that the individual will mate and have children.

Thus, most heritable cancer-causing mutations in phenotypically normal individuals do not directly cause cancer. Rather, most inherited cancer-causing mutations affect proteins that repair DNA errors or eliminate aberrant cells. These gene defects, rather than causing abnormal cell proliferation directly, allow the development and accumulation of cancer-causing errors by failing to stop them. Thus, the carriers of these genes can live into adulthood but are more susceptible to somatic mutations than other adults.

Eight percent of women in the general population develop breast cancer by the age of 70, but 65 percent of women who carry the "BRCA1 gene" develop this breast cancer by this age. Not only do these cancers increase the risk of cancer, they greatly increase the risk of early-onset and aggressive cancers. These "cancer risk" genes are also not responsible for just one type of cancer. Although named BReast CAncer gene 1, BRCA1 defects not only cause breast cancer, but also increase the risk of cancers of the ovary, fallopian tube and peritoneum in women, and increase the risk of melanoma in men and women. BRCA2 not only increases the risk of breast cancer in women, but it also increases the risk of breast cancer in men by as much as 65 times. BRCA2 causes 40 percent of all breast cancer in men in some populations.[44] BRCA2 also increases the risk of early-onset prostate cancer and pancreatic cancer.

Not to frighten you, but everyone has BRCA1 and BRCA2 genes. As previously explained, oncogenes, such as mutated BRCA1 and BRCA2, are genes that carry a mutation that prevents them from functioning normally. The normal BRCA1 and BRCA2 genes code for proteins that repair DNA breaks. BRCA1 also participates in metaphase checkpoint signaling, and thus prevents cells with DNA damage from dividing. These genes code for proteins that prevent cancer. It is when they are mutated and produce dysfunctional proteins, that they cannot do their jobs.

In recessive genetic disorders, the gene inherited from both parents must be defective. In the case of genes for metabolic enzymes, if one gene is functional and one dysfunctional, often enough of the functioning enzyme can be produced to get the job done. The disease may be very mild or not present at all with one functioning gene. In genetically dominant diseases, a defective gene from one parent is enough to cause the disease. Sometimes this is because one gene gets silenced – only one copy of the gene is used by the cell.

Cancer-causing gene defects usually act in a dominant manner. A defective gene only needs to be passed from one parent. Even though one gene produces normal proteins, the other one does not. Some cells may transcribe protein from one gene while the other cells code from the other. Cells may transcribe protein from both the good and mutated gene. The problem is that the damaged gene encodes for an ineffective protein. The protein is still produced, but it is like having a drunk driver behind the wheel. It does not get the job done, or worse, messes the job up, fails to perform the repair or inspection process and allows somatic mutations to survive.

If a defective BRCA1 protein allows a single, one-in-a-million cell with oncogenic, somatic mutations to divide, that cell can reproduce and reproduce every 24 hours until it becomes a cancer.

BRCA1 and BRCA2 are the most common heritable genes imparting breast cancer risk and account for a large portion of heritable breast cancer risk. Still, hereditary BRCA cancers combined account for less than four percent of all breast cancers.

BRCA1 and BCRA2 mutations do not in themselves induce cancer; they allow it by failing to stop it. It is other DNA defects that actually cause the uncontrolled growth and aberrant cell behavior. Thus, *avoiding other environmental carcinogens is even more important in individuals with altered BRCA genes.* Having a high-risk BRCA gene *multiples* the risk of several forms of cancer.

The prevalence of BRCA1 and BRCA2 mutilations varies by ethnic group. In the United States about 1% of African Americans have BRCA1 mutations and 3% have BRCA2 mutations. About 4% of Hispanics have BRCA1 mutations. Nine percent of those of Ashkenazi Jewish origin have BRCA1, but only 1% of these have BRCA2 mutations. Both are rare in Asian Americans. Other Caucasians have a 2% prevalence of each.

There is also not just one BRCA1 mutation. Over 25 different BRCA1 mutations have been identified, and most of these have been around for a very long time, each mutation coming down from a single ancestor. We know this, as most populations carry only certain BRCA1 mutations. The French Canadian mutation is distinct from the Greek BRCA1 mutation or the Italian one, the one found in the Northern Irish, or the one found among Spanish populations. In addition to germline mutations (those passed from parents to offspring), BRCA genes are also susceptible to sporadic mutations in the tissues, and thus, somatic mutations in these genes can also increase cancer risk. A BRCA mutation can arise in the tissue and cause cancer. These somatic mutations, however, are not passed on to a person's children as is the case for germ cell mutations.

Table 8-1 shows some heritable cancer-causing gene defects and their associated cancers. Table 8-2 shows gene mutations that cause cancer; however, most of these are somatic mutations rather than heritable cancers.

Retinoblastoma is an exception to the age of onset rule for heritable cancers, as this cancer affects very young children. As you will recall, the Rb protein prevents cells from prematurely moving from the G1 into the S phase of cell division. About 45 percent of retinoblastoma cases arise from inherited mutations, the rest being somatic mutations, most occurring during fetal development. With treatment, most children survive, although often without their vision. Survivors of this cancer have an increased risk of cancer later in life, largely due to exposure to radiation. This exposure mostly increases the risk of head and neck cancers, secondary to exposure during treatment.

Table 8-1: Heritable Cancer Genes[43, 47]

Gene	Cancer Site	Function and Syndrome
BRCA1	Female breast, ovary, prostate, melanoma	Double-stranded DNA repair
BRCA2[45]	Female breast, ovary Male breast, prostate	Single-stranded DNA repair
CDH1	Stomach, breast, colorectal, thyroid and ovarian cancer.	Cell adhesion glycoprotein; loss of function increases the risk of metastasis Hereditary diffuse gastric cancer: Cancer occurs as early as age 14, and mostly before age 40.
CHEK2	Sarcomas, breast cancer, brain tumors, prostate	Checkpoint kinase 2 Stabilizes p53 and activates BRCA1
HOXB13	Prostate cancer	Transcription factor
MSH2, MLH1, MSH6, PMS2	Colon, endometrium, stomach, small intestine, hepatobiliary, urinary tract, brain, skin, ovary	Lynch Syndrome (hereditary nonpolyposis colorectal cancer) accounts for about 4% of all colon cancer. It is caused by defects in one of several genes: MSH2 (60%), MLH1 (30%), MSH6 (7-10%) or other rare gene defects. These defects impair DNA mismatch repair, a proof-reading process for the newly synthesized DNA.
PTEN	Thyroid, breast, melanoma endometrium, acute lymphocytic leukemia	Cowden Syndrome, PTEN defect allows increased Akt activation.
RB1	Retinoblastoma, pineoblastoma, osteosarcoma, melanoma, leukemia, lymphoma	A malignant tumor of the retina with an average age of diagnosis at 15 months.
SMAD4	Pancreas, juvenile polyposis and colon cancer	Signal transduction proteins accumulate in the nucleus and regulate the transcription of target genes
STK11	Pancreas, testis, intestinal polyps STK11 is also known as LKB1	Activates AMPK and regulates cell polarity and functions as a tumor suppressor. Peutz-Jeghers syndrome
TP53 (p53)	Adrenocortical, basal cell, colon, pancreas, glioma, hepatic, nasopharyngeal, osteosarcoma, breast,	Li-Fraumeni syndrome; P53 is a tumor suppressor that promotes apoptosis of aberrant cells.

By their early 40's, a third of retinoblastoma patients treated with radiation have secondary cancers. Nevertheless, even those who undergo surgical removal of the eye, laser, or cryoablation of tumors have an excess of cancer; about 13% of those survivors have a secondary cancer by their early 40's. Much of this excess risk is for cancers of the bone, soft tissue sarcomas, and melanomas.[46]

Since cancer is caused by mutations, each individual's cancer has its own array of mutations. In genome analysis of 6800 human cancers, the most commonly mutated human cancer gene was TP53, which codes for the p53 protein. This protein activates DNA repair activity and can arrest the cell cycle at the G1/S checkpoint to give the cell more time to repair DNA errors before the synthesis of new DNA. It also promotes apoptosis if the cell spends too much time at the G1/S checkpoint or during cell division.

Mutations in the TP53 gene have been found in 32% of cancers, including 93% of ovarian cancers, 85% of small cell lung cancers, 80% of squamous cell lung cancers, 57% of colorectal cancers, half of low-grade gliomas, esophageal and bladder carcinomas, and pancreatic adenomas, and a third of all breast cancers. The second most common mutation is in the PIK3CA gene for the kinase enzyme that activates Akt and Raf and thereby promotes signaling for cell proliferation. Mutations in the PIK3CA gene are found in 11 percent of all cancers, including half of uterine endometrial cancers and 30% of breast cancers. Mutations in the KRAS gene are present in 86% of pancreatic adenomas and 45% of colorectal adenocarcinomas.[47] KRAS defects are not inherited but appear as somatic mutations. KRAS is a GTPase that acts as a molecular switch. When GTP levels are low, it signals the cessation of cell growth. Defective KRAS GTPase fails to remove GTP, and cells continue growth.

There is a wide variance in the diversity of cancer-causing genes for different types of cancer. For example, TP53 defects are present in 93 percent of ovarian cancers and BRAF gene defects are present in 56% of thyroid carcinomas, but the most common gene driving prostate cancer, SPOP, is only present in 9% of prostate cancers. Over 180 different cancer-driving genes have been found in breast carcinomas.

Knowing which genes are malfunctioning can allow targeted treatment with medications that affect particular defects. The diversity in driving gene in some cancers, however, makes this difficult. Genome testing of cancers will likely become routine in the next few years, and with it, more specific and successful targeting of the underlying defects causing the cancer.

Table 8-2: Common Gene Mutations for Various Cancers[47, 47]

Cancer Site	Common Gene Defects
Bladder Carcinoma BLCA	TP53 – 50%, ARID1A – 28%, KDM6A – 26%, MLL2 – 24%, MLL3 – 24%
Carcinoma of the Pancreas PAAD	KRAS – 86%, TP53 – 50%, SMAD4 – 19% MLL3 – 6% TGFBR2 – 5%
Prostate Cancer - PRCA	SPPO and TP53 – 9%, PTEN, and ATM – 5%
Uterine corpus endometrioid carcinoma – UCEC	PTEN – 62%, PIK3CA – 50% ARID1A and CTNNB1 – 29%, PT53 – 27%
Ovarian Cancer - OV	PT53 – 93%, NF1 – 4%, BRCA1 – 3% BRCA2 – 3%
Colorectal Adenocarcinoma CRAD	APC – 79%, TP53 – 57%, KRAS – 45%, PIK3CA –15%
Stomach Carcinoma - STCA	TP53 – 44%, ARID1A – 17%, PIK3CA – 15%, ACVR2A – 11%
Breast Cancer BRCA	TP53 – 33%, PIK3CA – 30%, GATA3 –9%, MLL3, CDH1 and MAP3K1 – 6%, NCOR1, MAP2K4, PTEN, and MACF1 – 3%, BRCA1 and BRCA2 < 2%
Thyroid carcinoma - TCA	BRAF – 57%, NRAS – 8%, HRAS – 4%
Renal Cell Carcinoma RCCC	VHL – 52%, PBRM1 – 33%, SETD2 – 12%, BAP1 – 9%
Small Cell Lung Cancer SCLA	TP53 – 85%, BR1 – 54%, ANK3 and EP300 – 10%, MNDA, ASPM, TAF1, and BCLAF1 – 9%

Screening

Presently, screening for heritable cancer genes is limited to high-risk individuals, with either a personal history of cancer or their family members. While all cancers are caused by genetic alterations, only a minority of cancers are heritable. Nevertheless, I advocate universal genetic profiling for disease risk susceptibility (not just for cancer). This would allow us to take steps to avoid the diseases we are at high risk of, avoid adverse reactions to medications that depend on genetically determined enzymes for their processing. It would provide information on which foods might help or hinder our health. If we know the diseases we are most susceptible to, we could avoid the risk factors and target screening more effectively. We could prevent transmission of genetic disease to our children. We would, at least, know what we were up against and then live according to how we wanted to approach life and its hurdles.

At this time, genetic testing is usually done too late and for too few. Women with a family history of early-onset breast cancer may be screened, but this only occurs after a family member has fallen victim to early onset breast cancer, and usually too late for her siblings to avoid the preventable risk factors that have their highest potency during puberty and adolescence. Clearly, women with fathers who have early-onset prostate cancer should be screened for BRCA mutations, as these women are at high risk. Men should be tested as well; not only are they at elevated cancer risk, but also risk passing the gene to their children.

Protective Surgery

The actress Angelina Jolie has a strong family history of breast cancer and carries the BRCA1 gene. She thus elected to undergo prophylactic surgery to lower her risk of breast cancer. In doing so, and by announcing it publically, she brought this treatment and the role of BRCA1 to the public eye.

Prophylactic mastectomy, which removes nearly all breast tissue, may be able to reduce a woman's risk of breast cancer by 97 percent. Premenopausal oophorectomy, the removal of the ovaries, reduces the risk of breast cancer by 50%. Removal of the ovaries and fallopian tubes almost completely eliminates the risk of cancer of those tissues.

An online decision tool for women with BRCA cancer mutations breast cancer shows the probabilities for different outcomes for women with BRCA1 and BRCA2 for various screening and prophylactic surgeries at different ages.

http://brcatool.stanford.edu/brca.html

For example, a woman with BRCA1 that does not have breast cancer screening or prophylactic surgery has only a 15% probability of surviving to age 70 without cancer. A woman with BRCA1 who has both prophylactic mastectomy and oophorectomy at age 35 has a 66% probability of surviving to age 70 without either breast or ovarian cancer.

Genetic Cancer Summary

Although all cancer is caused by genetic defects, only five to ten percent of cancers are caused by genes inherited from parents by their children. Most of these heritable cancer genes cause cancer by failing to eliminate sporadic mutations in other genes which can occur during life.

Even in individuals – no, especially in individuals – with heritable cancers genes, cancer risk can be mitigated by avoiding cancer risk factors. Heritable cancer genes multiply risk. Genetic screening should be done early so that individuals at exceptionally high risk for cancer can make lifestyle, screening, and medical choices that help best prevent cancer.

The same risk factors, tobacco, alcohol, infection, radiation exposure, obesity, and diet, apply to individuals with heritable cancer genes. All these risk factors act to multiply the individual's cancer risks.

9: Infectious Causes of Cancer

The devastating plague of smallpox was estimated to have killed 300 to 500 million persons during the 20th century. In 1967, in a single year, while I was being bullied by several of my seventh-grade classmates, smallpox killed two million people. Ten years later, it was eradicated; there have been no cases since. Smallpox was eradicated through a global vaccination program.

In 1977, there were a quarter of a million Americans living with paralysis from infection with viral poliomyelitis. This disease has been eradicated from the United States. Worldwide, there were 350,000 symptomatic cases of paralytic polio in 1988, however, through global vaccination efforts; by 2015 the number was down to 106 cases. Civil wars and the targeted assassinations of vaccination workers have prevented the complete eradication of this disease. As I write this in mid-2016, there have only been 22 cases of polio worldwide this year, with wild virus circulating only in Pakistan and Afghanistan. By the time you read this, the scourge of polio may have been eliminated from the world forever. Call me an optimist.

Table 9-1: Cancers Due to Infectious Agents

Cancer	Total Cases	Percent due to infection	Infection Caused	Infectious Agent Responsible
Stomach	870,000	90+	783,000+	Helicobacter pylori, EBV
Hepatic	750,000	77	577,500	Hepatitis B, Hepatitis C
Cervix	530,000	100	530,000	Human Papilloma Virus (HPV)
Lymphoma & Leukemia	459,000	20	91,800	Ebstein Barr Virus (HHV-4)
Nasophayrnx	84,000	88	73,920	Ebstein Barr Virus
Kaposi's sarcoma	43,000	100	43,000	Human Herpes Virus-8
Anus	27,000	88	23,760	HPV
Oropharynx	85,000	26	22,100	HPV
Vulva	27,000	43	11,610	HPV
Penis	22,000	50	11,000	HPV
Vagina	13,000	70	9,100	HPV

How great would it be if we had effective vaccines for cancer!? What if we could not only protect ourselves and our children from cancer but could expunge those cancers and the suffering they cause from the human population, never to return? It is great and we can! We already have vaccines that prevent certain cancers, and in the coming decades should have several more.

Infections are responsible for almost 18 percent of cancers worldwide (Table 9-1); amounting to two million new cancer cases each year, but the distribution is uneven. In developed areas, such as North America and Australia, infections account for about ten percent of all cancers. In China, they account for over a quarter of all cancers, and in Sub-Saharan Africa, infections are the cause of nearly a third of all cancers. Cancers are caused by some viral and bacterial infections as well as by certain parasites. Viruses take the lions' share, causing 12 percent or all human cancers (Table 9-2).[48]

Viral Causes of Cancer

Viruses have a very devious means of reproduction. Viruses enter the cell, often fooling the cell to carry the virus inside, like a Trojan horse. DNA viruses enter the nucleus where they induce the cell's DNA replication mechanism to make copies of the viral DNA. They may even insert their genetic code into the host cell's DNA. They then induce the cell to make replicas of the virus. RNA viruses are reproduced in the cell cytoplasm by the ribosomal protein production mechanism. The viruses use the cell to reproduce their genetic material, as well as viral surface proteins that appear on the cell's outer membrane. The viruses then bud off from the cell, taking some of the cell membrane lipids and the viral proteins with it, as illustrated in Figure 9-1.

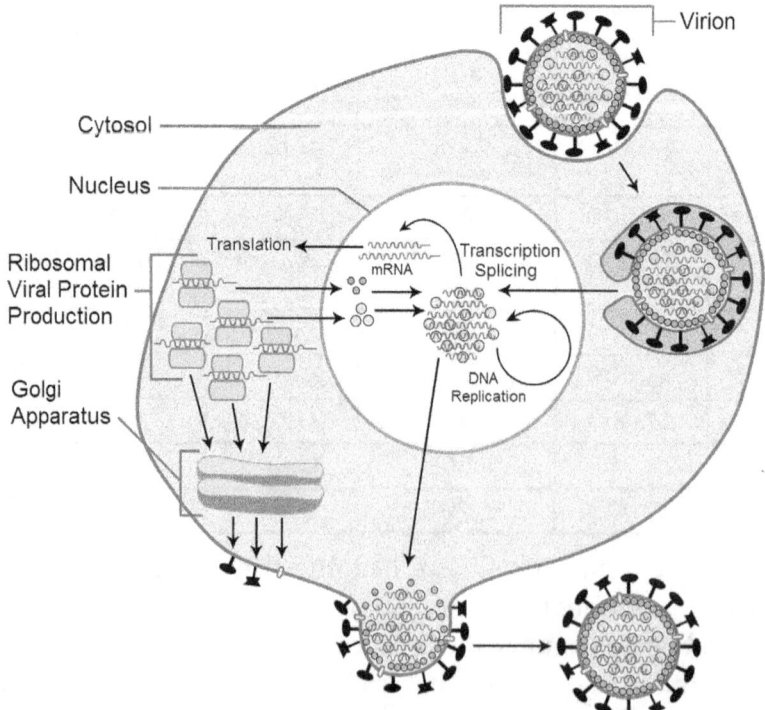

Figure 9-1: Viral reproduction[49]

A virus is a cell that has been turned into a viral bomb factory. In fact, the infected cell is the virus. Numerous new virions (infectious particles) bud off from the cell to infect other cells. Most viruses avoid killing their host cell; it is suicide. After commandeering a cell, they produce new crops of virions, like apples from a tree. Eventually, however, the production of virions can exhaust the cell. Having diverted its efforts from sustaining the cell to making viruses, the cell, unable to maintain its housekeeping activities, undergoes apoptosis. When this happens, macrophages come to clean up the cellular remnants, which include virions. The macrophages may then become infected themselves. This is one way the HIV spreads, as macrophages carry it to different parts of the body.

Table 9-2: Viral Agents Causing Cancer[50]

Virus	Cancers	Mechanisms
Human Papillomavirus Types 16, 18, 31, 33, 45, 52 and 58 (HPV)	Cervix, oropharynx and tonsil, vulva, vagina, anus, penis	Prevents apoptosis and direct mitogen
Hepatitis B Virus (HBV)	Hepatocellular and pancreatic cancers, multiple myeloma, Hodgkin lymphoma[51]	Inflammatory mitogen
Hepatitis C Virus (HCV)	Hepatocellular, pancreatic, non-Hodgkin lymphoma	Inflammatory and direct mitogen
Epstein-Barr virus (HHV-4)	Burkitt lymphoma, nasopharyngeal carcinoma, Hodgkin lymphoma Non-Hodgkin lymphoma, gastric	Direct carcinogen
Human Herpesvirus-8 (HHV-8)	Kaposi sarcoma, primary effusion lymphoma	Direct carcinogen
Human T-cell Lymphotropic Virus (HTLV-1)	Adult T-cell leukemia and lymphoma	Direct carcinogen
Human Immunodeficiency Virus (HIV-1)	Kaposi sarcoma, non-Hodgkin lymphoma, carcinoma of the cervix, anus, conjunctiva, MCC	Indirect carcinogen: Immune suppression allows other viruses to proliferate.
Merkel Cell Polyomavirus (MCV)	Merkel cell carcinoma (a rare and highly malignant skin cancer.)	Direct carcinogen

Some DNA viruses cause cancer by inserting their DNA into the host cell's DNA and causing the host cell to make proteins that favor the formation of cancers. Other viruses merely cause a ruckus. They induce inflammation and indirectly cause cancer by damaging cells and inducing their replacement. HIV causes cancer by impairing the immune system and thus allowing the proliferation of other cancers, especially those caused by other cancer-inducing viruses, such as Human Herpesvirus-8, the etiologic agent of Kaposi's sarcoma.

Viruses cause cancer both directly, by inducing oncogenes, and indirectly, by inducing inflammation. There are eight known human oncoviruses (Table 9-2).

Human Papillomavirus (HPV)

The most common viral infection that induces cancer in North America as well as in other parts of the globe is the Human Papillomavirus. There are about 150 strains of HPV, 40 or more of these infect the mucosa of the genitalia and are spread through sexual contact; at least a dozen are known carcinogens. The two most common carcinogenic strains of HPV are 16 and 18; these two strains are responsible for well over 80 percent of all cervical cancers. HPV-16 also causes rectal, penile, vaginal, and oral-pharyngeal cancers. Most HPV infections regress on their own and do not progress to cancer. Having a healthy nutritional status, perhaps particularly having adequate folate intake, lowers the risk of chronic HPV infection, and thus risk for cancer.

About ten percent of HPV cervical infections become chronic, and these may develop into cancer in situ. Pap smears are used to look for early superficial cancerous lesions (carcinoma in situ), which can then be killed by freezing the lesion or excised with a cone biopsy.

If not caught as a localized lesion, cervical cancer can progress and become invasive cancer with a high mortality. There are about 530,000 new cases of invasive cervical cancers worldwide each year, and about 270,000 deaths from this cancer.

HPV induces cancer by inserting its DNA into the DNA of the infected cell. One of the HPV viral DNA genes codes for the "E6-associated protein" (E6-AP). E6AP causes ubiquitination of the protein p53, which causes it to be targeted for degradation by proteasomes in the cell. P53 is a tumor suppressor gene that promotes apoptosis of tumor cells. The virus gains a survival advantage by eliminating the host cell's p53 protein and thereby preventing the destruction of the cell through apoptosis and increasing the survival of the cells the virus has infected. This does not directly cause the cancer-causing mutations, but rather prevents the destruction of aberrant cells, and promotes the survival of infected cells and the spread of the virus. It thus allows other mutations to survive. HPV also contains another gene, E7, that codes for the E7-associated protein that increases cell proliferation[52]. E7 is a mitogen that promotes cancer proliferation.

HPV is highly contagious and easily transmitted. It is sexually transmitted, and while only about 12 percent of women worldwide have antibodies to it, about 75–80% of sexually active Americans will be infected with HPV at some point in their lifetime. The CDC estimates that 79 million Americans are infected with the HPV virus and that there are 14 million new cases each year. About 360,000 of these individuals will develop ugly genital warts. Twenty-seven thousand HPV-associated invasive cancers are diagnosed in the United States each year.

HPV is a vaccine-preventable disease. Gardasil and Cervarix protect against HPV types 16 and 18. Gardasil also provides protection against HPV-6 and HPV-11 strains which are responsible for 90% of genital warts. An updated vaccine, Gardasil-9, approved by the FDA in December of 2014, adds protection against five more strains of HPV that are responsible for another 20 percent of cervical cancers. The new vaccine now provides protection against over 90 percent of cervical, vaginal, anal and penile cancers.

Gardasil was only approved by the FDA in 2006. In 2010, only 23 percent of girls had gotten even a single dose of the vaccine, and only 13 percent of girls had received the three recommended doses.

Nevertheless, those getting even a single dose decreased their risk of disease by more than 80 percent. In communities in which vaccination is common, the infection rate among all teens falls. This happens even among those who have not been vaccinated as the disease spreads less efficiently person to person.

Unfortunately, these vaccines are not effective against established HPV infection or cervical lesions. Thus, to effectively protect the individual, vaccination must be done prior to the onset of sexual activity. It is thus recommended that adolescents be vaccinated at age eleven or as soon as possible before the age of 18. There are no currently available anti-viral medications demonstrated to cure HPV.

A vaccine against cancer sounds like a no-brainer. Nevertheless, there has been considerable opposition to this vaccine (and vaccines in general). One of the arguments against HPV vaccination, its opponents contend, is that vaccination would promote sexual activity among adolescents. Under this logic, providing tetanus vaccination to children entering the seventh grade should be associated with an epidemic of 12-year-olds jumping on rusty nails.

Hepatitis C (HCV)

One of the most common and deadly virally induced cancers is hepatocellular carcinoma (HCC). HCC is caused by both the hepatitis B (HBV) and hepatitis C (HCV) viruses. Most of the carcinogenic effect is indirect; these diseases cause chronic liver inflammation. HCV additionally induces the production of mitogenic proteins that increase both hepatic cellular proliferation and cancer growth. In health, hepatocytes (liver cells) are replaced about once a year. During infections, the rate of hepatocyte replacement increases, and with it, the risk of malignant transformation multiplies, especially if there is exposure to other carcinogens.

Hepatitis C is the most common, chronic, blood-borne infection in the United States. It is most commonly transmitted through the use of a contaminated needle or from being born from a mother infected with the disease. Twenty-two thousand Americans are infected each year. Around 3.2 million Americans, a bit over one percent of the population, have chronic HCV infection. Worldwide, about three percent of the world's population has the disease. Today, 250 million people are living with HCV infection.

Egypt has the highest rate of HCV infection; in the year 2000, twenty percent of all individuals over the age of 30 had active HCV infections. This occurred in large part from an anti-Schistosoma campaign, in which reusable needles were not properly sterilized between patients. However, poor medical practices continue in Egypt, and 573,000 new infections occur there each year.[53]

Only about one in four persons infected with HCV develops immunity to it. According to the Centers for Disease Control and Prevention (CDC), 75 to 85 percent of those infected develop chronic hepatitis. The CDC recommends that all Americans born between 1945 and 1965 be tested for Hepatitis C, as well as any person exposed to illicit injected drug use or receiving transfusion products or organ transplants before 1992.[54] Between 50 and 90 percent of HIV positive persons that used illicit injected drugs have chronic HCV infection.

If left untreated, 60 to 70 percent of individuals with chronic HCV develop chronic liver disease, five to 20 percent will develop liver cirrhosis, and as many as five percent of these will die from either the liver cirrhosis or hepatocellular carcinoma. Hepatitis C also raises the risk of pancreatic cancer.[55] HCV kills more Americans than does HIV/AIDS.

There is not currently an available Hepatitis C vaccine, although several are in development. There is, however, medical treatment for the disease that is curative for about 90 percent of those treated. These new HCV treatments are simple; one pill a day for eight or twelve weeks cures the disease in as many as 93 percent of patients.

There are two sticking points. One is that there are six genotypes and several subtypes of HCV, and different strains respond to different medications, so genotype testing of the virus is required to give the appropriate treatment. The other snag is the pills for the 8 to 12-week treatment of HCV may cost as much as $1,125 – per day! The treatment cost may be as high as $94,500. The cost to treat every infected American would be (only) $244 billion. If a $244 billion price tag sounds like a bargain to you, you might just be right. The 350,000 Medicare recipients with HCV each cost Medicare three times as much as does the average Medicare patient. The average cost of a liver transplant was $577,100 in 2011, and if untreated, the virus returns and destroys the new liver. If Medicare were allowed to negotiate the price down, similar to the 44% discount obtained by the VA, it could lower the cost to one that actually cuts the cost of caring for chronic HCV disease.[56] Until then, the out-of-pocket cost for a Medicare recipient with Part D prescription coverage could be $7,000 for a single bottle of pills. Or one could take a vacation to India, where the cost ranges frome $153 to $615 for the course of treatment.[57]

Hepatitis B (HBV)

HBV also causes chronic hepatitis infection that can lead to liver cirrhosis and hepatocellular carcinoma. Persons with chronic HBV infection are more than 13 times more likely to develop HCC than those not infected. Individuals with a history of Hepatitis B infections also have a 60% higher risk of pancreatic cancer, and for those with active HBV infection, the risk is even higher.[58]

Similar to Hepatitis C, chronic HBV infection causes inflammation. This inflammation, and the cellular damage it creates, increases the replacement of hepatocytes, and this mitogenic drive increases cancer risk.

HBV is a common infection. About one-third of the 7 billion human residents of this planet have been infected with HBV at some point in their life, and more than 350 million persons worldwide are currently infected with HBV; 240 million have chronic HBV liver disease. Each year more than three-quarters of a million people die from this disease.

While less than one percent of the population in the United States and Western Europe are infected with HBV, it is a rampant plague in sub-Saharan Africa and East Asia, where five to ten percent of the population is chronically infected.

This disease is easily transmitted from mother to child at birth, person to person, or by blood products. While ninety percent of healthy adults recover from the virus, 80 to 89 percent of infants infected during the first year of life develop chronic HBV disease. A third to half of children aged one to six will develop chronic HBV if infected at this age. Twenty percent of the children who develop chronic hepatitis will die from liver cirrhosis or liver cancer.[59]

Children are commonly infected in lesser developed countries where the disease is endemic; three to five percent of children who are chronic carriers will develop cirrhosis, and some will develop hepatocellular carcinoma before reaching adulthood.

We have a vaccine that can prevent almost a million deaths a year. The HBV vaccine has been available since 1982. This vaccine is about 95 percent effective, effective enough to stop lateral transmission. Ninety-four countries, including the United States, now give the vaccine at birth. Two booster vaccines are needed in the following months. In countries where the vaccine is regularly used, the chronic disease rate in children has fallen to less than one percent. Vaccination against HBV should decrease the incidence of hepatocellular carcinoma over time.

Most children born in the United States after 1990 have been vaccinated, and these individuals are protected. Adults who have not been vaccinated remain at risk. About 20,000 Americans get infected with HBV each year, and the CDC estimates there are over one million Americans with chronic HPV. Adults at risk of HPV exposure (exposure to blood or needles) who have not been vaccinated should be.

Epstein-Barr Virus (EBV)

EBV is the virus that is perhaps best known for causing mononucleosis. It is a human herpes virus (HHV-4) and is easily transmitted through the oral transfer of saliva. Thus, it is a kissing disease, easily and is commonly acquired during adolescent snogging. It can also be transmitted by sharing cups or ice-cream cones. The virus is also present in the genital secretions of infected persons and can be transmitted from them.

By the age of forty, 90 to 95 percent of adults have antibodies to the virus as evidence of a previous EBV infection. In the United States, about half of all five-year-olds have antibodies to it.

Generally, primary EBV disease syndrome severity and duration correlate with the individual's age at the time of infection. Younger children usually have mild, insignificant illness from EBV. It may manifest with mild cold or flu-like symptoms or a sore throat. If one has to get the disease, this is usually the best time.

In adolescents, EBV usually causes mononucleosis. Here it causes fever lasting one to two weeks, sore throat, swollen lymph nodes, especially on the sides and back of the neck. It can cause abdominal pain, swelling of the spleen and liver, fatigue, and body aches that can last for several months. One risk of the disease is that while the spleen is enlarged, it can be ruptured easily by abdominal trauma. Thus, during active disease, adolescents may be advised to avoid contact sports and heavy lifting.

When adults are infected by EBV, they have less of the sore throat symptoms, and much more of the prolonged fevers, fatigue, malaise and body aches. In adults, the disease may last six months or longer. I got mine when I was in the Peace Corps at the age of 27. I was mostly bed-bound for a month, extremely fatigued for another, and then had episodic exhaustion for months. I would need to sit down and take rests along the way, walking up the hill to my Peace Corps village. I remember watching the sun go down, sitting along the trail less than a mile from my home, too exhausted to go on.

After having EBV infection..., well actually, there is no after the infection; it just sticks around. The viral genome hides out, lying dormant, in the nucleus of certain white blood cells, the B memory lymphocytes, in the bone marrow. The latent infections do not have active viral production and do not bud virions. But viral replication can be stimulated by specific activation of the B-cells, likely by certain unrelated infections, antigens or chemical compounds. This stimulus can cause a periodic viral proliferation with a brief infection affecting tissues such as the epithelial cells of the tonsils. It also causes the production of a new crop of virion particles. These show up in the saliva and can transmit the disease. In persons with a healthy immune system that recognizes and eliminates these virus cells, the infection is brief and inconsequential,[60] but transmittable. Ninety percent of adults carry EBV as a persistent infection, with periodic viremia. This means you.

EBV disease is held in check by natural killer (NK) cells, a type of white blood cells that attacks and destroys cells with active viral protein production. The NK cells recognize surface proteins that the virus causes to be present on the outer cell membrane as part of its reproductive endeavor. If there is a loss of NK cell competence during the active infection or with aging, there can be a massive expansion of the population of infected B lymphocytes. It is this huge number of infected cells that can give rise to EBV-associated cancers.[61]

The first cancer identified to be associated with EBV was Burkitt lymphoma, a disease most commonly occurring in African children. These children usually have a co-infection with malaria; however, this disease is also seen in patients with HIV infections. Not only is there immune dysregulation, but there is also immune activation with production of cytokines that increase the proliferation of lymphocytes. Burkitt lymphoma occurs when there is a mutation in the Myc gene. This gene helps regulate the expression of other genes. If pathologically activated, Myc can cause continuous cell proliferation. Burkitt lymphoma results from having the Myc gene transposed into the wrong part of the chromosome in a lymphocyte. Rather than being transcribed only during cellular reproduction, its protein is transcribed along with other proteins used in G0 and G1 cell activity. This creates a lineage of cells that continuously replicate, causing cancer.

EBV can infect mucosal cells of the oropharynx, B-Cells, T-cells, NK cells, and cells of the gastric mucosa. It can also cause cancers in all the cells it infects.

Cancers associated with EBV infection include:[62]

- Burkitt Lymphoma (cancer of the lymphatic system)
- Nasopharyngeal Carcinoma (cancer of the upper throat)
- Hodgkin Lymphoma and Non-Hodgkin Lymphoma
- T-cell Lymphomas
- Gastric Cancer (about 7 – 10 percent of cases)
- Leiomyosarcomas (smooth muscle cancer, such as in the uterus)

If that were not enough, infections with EBV can also cause meningitis, encephalitis, optic neuritis, swelling of the spinal cord, hemiplegia, and Guillain-Barré syndrome. EBV infection is associated with Parkinson's disease and more than doubles the risk for multiple sclerosis. Did I mention that EBV is also associated with pancreatitis, myocarditis, and interstitial lung disease?[62]

Although no vaccines for EBV are available, there is ongoing work to develop vaccines to prevent the infection, disease progression, and EBV-related cancers.[63] HHV-4 (EBV) should be a top target for vaccine development efforts.

Merkel-Cell Carcinoma

Merkel cell carcinoma is a rare, very aggressively malignant skin cancer caused by a widespread virus, the Merkel Cell Polyomavirus (MCV). There are about 1500 new cases of MCC in the U.S. each year. The disease was first described in 1972, and the virus causing it was discovered only in 2008. MCV infection is common. Forty-five percent of children have antibodies to MCV by age ten, 60% of young adults have antibodies by age 20, and 81 percent of those in their 60's have antibodies to it.[64] It is found in the saliva, respiratory secretions, skin, and stool, and appears easily transmitted. Most of us form antibodies to it that keep us safe. However, if immune defenses fail, the virus can embed itself into the DNA and cause mutations that give rise to cancer.

Merkel-cell tumors usually arise on sun-exposed skin and form a firm, flesh-colored, red or blue nodule, as seen in Figure 9-2. It typically is found among persons over the age of 65, and risk increases with age. Fair skinned individuals, especially those living in sunny climates, are at highest risk. Persons using immunosuppressant medications and others with impaired immune systems, such as HIV patients, and the elderly are also at higher risk. Early treatment, before metastasis, can be life-saving. This virus may also be involved in some other skin and lung cancers.

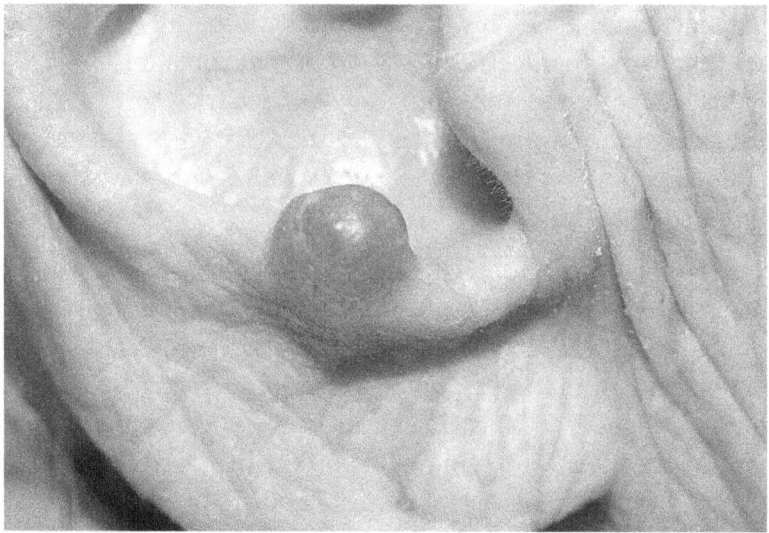

Figure 9-2: Merkel Cell Carcinoma on the earlobe of an elderly woman.[65]

Helicobacter Pylori

Helicobacter pylori are a species of bacteria that have adapted to live in the harsh, acidic environment of the human stomach. Most mammals harbor helicobacter bacilli. Pigs have *H. suis* living in their stomachs. Dolphins have *H. cetorum*; cheetahs have *H. acinonyx*. These bacteria have adapted to their mammalian hosts over the millennia. The species are specific to their host. Human infections are limited to transmission from other humans.

Less than ideal hygiene, especially during childhood, is associated with higher risk of infection. Most people become infected during the first five years of life. *H. pylori* are not commonly passed between adults, but rather mother to child, or between siblings. Before baby food came in a jar, mothers often prepared food for her infant by chewing the food and then passing it in a spoon to her infant. The more small children living in a home, the more likely it is for cross-contamination as they share food and other objects they may put into the mouth, to have unwashed hands, and be exposed to diapers. With better hygiene, infection rates have fallen, and if a girl does not contract *H. pylori* as a child, she is unlikely to transmit it to her children. With each generation living with indoor plumbing, fewer children are infected. Still, if untreated, an *H. pylori* infection acquired during childhood lasts a lifetime.

In the developing world, about 80 percent of the population still harbors *H. pylori*, having acquired it at a young age. Thus, infection rates in developing countries are about twice those found in developed countries. New infection among adults in developed countries is uncommon – less than half of one percent per year.

Helicobacter pylori, a bacterium, causes chronic inflammation in the stomach and is highly associated with peptic ulcer disease; however, most *H. pylori* infections are asymptomatic. About one in five persons with the infection develop gastritis or peptic ulcer disease. *H. pylori* are also highly associated with gastric cancer. Chronic infection with H. pylori imparts a one to two percent lifetime risk of gastric cancer.

Prior to the 1930's, stomach cancer was the most common cancer in the United States and elsewhere in the world. Prior to indoor plumbing, commercially prepared baby food, smaller family size, and the use of antibiotics, *H. pylori* infection was nearly universal in the human population. Gastric cancer is no longer one of the major cancers in the West but remains common in East Asia and South America. This infectious agent is responsible for 783,000 cases of gastric cancer each year. Infection with *H. pylori* accounts for over 80 percent of all gastric cancer, with another ten percent attributable to EBV infection[66]. Since they are both common chronic diseases, co-infection is also common, and they likely interact in the causation of severe gastritis in children[67], peptic ulcer disease, and gastric cancer.[68] *H. pylori* is the number-one cancer-causing pathogen in the world.

Unlike most bacteria, *H. pylori* tolerates stomach acid. This environment offers them an advantage; there is a lack of competition from other bacteria. Nevertheless, *H. pylori* don't really like high acidity. So they lower it. These bacteria make proteins that put tiny holes in the cell membranes of the stomach lining and inject a protein into these cells that create inflammation. This results in a moderation of the acid output of the stomach so that the stomach is acidic enough to keep most bacteria from growing but is a Goldilocks – just right acidity for *H. pylori* bacteria.

H. pylori and its homesteading activities cause inflammation of the stomach (gastritis) and peptic ulcers. The chronic drilling and inflammation eventually exhaust the acid-producing cells in the stomach, resulting in atrophic gastritis – the stomach loses its capacity to produce acid. With atrophic gastritis and loss of acidity, the body loses its ability to absorb vitamin B12 and certain minerals. It also impairs the ability to denature and digest protein. The chronic inflammation raises the risk of stomach cancer, and rates of this disease rise dramatically in the 7th or 8th decade.

H. pylori infection is an indirect carcinogen. It does not cause mutations, but rather creates chronic inflammation that causes gastric atrophy and a change in the structure of the mucosa lining the stomach, causing it to appear more like the cells lining the intestine. This atrophy, along with increased turnover in cells, and loss of nutrients, increases the risk of cancer. Eradication of *H. pylori* infection cuts cancer risk nearly by half, but only if treatment occurs prior to the development of atrophy.[69]

H. pylori infection can be detected by blood test, breath test, or stool sample, which is preferred by children everywhere. The stool test is also more accurate than blood tests for determining whether treatment has been effective. Certain antibiotics are effective for the eradication of *H. pylori,* although confirmation of cure is appropriate as treatment failure rates can be as high as 25 percent.

Barrett's Esophagus

With the fall in prevalence of H. pylori, stomach cancer incidence has and continues to fall. (See Figure 4-1). What could go wrong with that? GERD: Gastro-Esophageal Reflux Disease.

A side effect of the treatment of H. pylori is an increased incidence of GERD. *H. pylori* infection decreases stomach acid production and may additionally alter the function of the stomach and esophagus in other ways. When *H. pylori* infection is eradicated using antibiotics, more stomach acid enters the esophagus. The entry of stomach acid causes a burning sensation in the chest, experienced as heartburn.[70]

Heartburn is more than just a painful annoyance. Injury to the mucosal lining the esophagus can cause scarring and dysfunction of food transport in the esophagus. The exposure of the mucosa to acid causes metaplasia, a change from squamous cell epithelium that lines the esophagus, similar to the mucosa of the mouth to that more like that of the small intestine, which includes glandular cells. This condition is known as Barrett's esophagus.

The greatest risk of Barrett's metaplasia comes from tobacco use, especially chewing tobacco, and this is amplified when it is combined with alcohol consumption.

Not all patients with heartburn have Barrett's, and many patients with Barrett's don't have heartburn. Symptoms that accompany Barrett's include:

- Frequent and long-standing heartburn
- Pain under the sternum, especially the lower sternum
- Difficulty swallowing food
- Vomiting blood
- Weight loss because eating is painful

With Barrett's metaplasia, there is a great increase in risk for adenocarcinoma of the esophagus. About 80 percent of esophageal cancer is attributed to Barrett's metaplasia. Individuals with Barrett's esophagus have a 0.5% incidence of esophageal cancer each year. Being diagnosed with Barrett's at age 55 gives a one-in-seven lifetime risk of developing esophageal adenocarcinoma.[71]

Barrett's esophagus needs to be treated and monitored, as once established, it is a risk factor for esophageal cancer, even if it is no longer symptomatic.

Salmonella Typhi

Salmonella typhi, the bacteria that causes typhoid fever, can cause chronic infection in the gallbladder. Gallstones may be formed around these bacteria, which help maintain the infection. Individuals with chronic *S. typhi* infection are eight times more likely to develop gallbladder carcinoma and 200 times more likely to develop hepatobiliary carcinoma than those without the disease. The infection also slightly increases the risk of pancreas, colorectal and lung cancers.

S. typhi is one of many bacteria that can metabolize the primary bile acids used in digestion, cholic acid, and chenodeoxycholic acid, into the secondary bile acids lithocholic acid and deoxycholic acid. Both these secondary bile acids are known carcinogens. Primary bile acids promote apoptosis, but secondary bile acids inhibit it.

Salmonella also produces the enzyme glucuronidase. This enzyme may create conjugates with procarcinogens that form DNA adducts that cause mutagenesis.[72]

Since *S. typhi* infection in the gallbladder can greatly increase secondary bile acid concentration locally, this is where risk increases the most. The gallbladder, the bile duct, and pancreas are areas exposed to highly concentrated bile.

Although secondary bile acids are also formed by bacterial fermentation of bile in the cecum and colon, lithocholic acid has poor solubility, limiting the amount that is reabsorbed by the body. Thus, this bile acid is less dangerous when formed in the colon. Additionally, some bile acid becomes bound to dietary fiber in the intestine, preventing its reabsorption and damage. Lithocholic acid appears to be a more potent carcinogen than is the deoxycholic acid.

Other Bacterial Infections

Chronic infection that stimulates chronic inflammation may be sufficient to cause cancer. An example of this is chronic osteomyelitis.

When osteomyelitis occurs just below the skin, especially on the tibia of the lower leg, the chronic inflammation forms an ulcer and drainage tract. About one percent of these infections give rise to skin cancer, usually squamous cell carcinoma, but also to other forms of cancer, including basal cell carcinoma, fibrosarcoma, myeloma, angiosarcoma, and lymphoma can form. There is also often a mix of bacteria involved.

Mycobacterium tuberculosis, (TB) is associated with an increased risk of lung cancer and of Kaposi's sarcoma. The mechanism for this may be impaired underlying immunity or chronic inflammation. *Tropheryma whippelii*, the agent that causes Whipple's disease, is associated with lymphoma and gastric adenocarcinoma.

Having a history of *Chlamydophila pneumoniae* infection, a bacterium that causes community-acquired pneumonia, is associated with a forty-eight percent increase in risk of lung cancer. It is chronic infection and cell replacement caused by this agent that promotes lung cancer risk.[73] The related bacterium, *Chlamydia trachomatis,* has three forms, one that causes the chronic eye infection trachoma. This disease causes conjunctivitis that can cause blindness. It is a common infection in children in Africa where it is endemic. Rarely, it causes ocular lymphoma. Another form of *Chlamydia* is sexually transmitted and causes pelvic inflammatory disease, ectopic pregnancy, and urethritis. This agent is associated with chronic infection and associated with a very small increase in the risk of ovarian cancer.

In all these diseases the risk of cancer is associated with chronic infection, chronic inflammation, and increased cellular turnover.

Parasites and Cancer

There are a few parasites that are important causes of cancer; happily, these are rare in North America. One is malaria, as discussed above, as a co-infection of EBV in the causation of Burkitt lymphoma.

Another infection-associated cancer is caused by the parasitic flatworms that cause schistosomiasis. These parasites have a complex life cycle that involves freshwater snails as an intermediate host. There are seven species that infect humans, only one of which is present in the Americas.

While not endemic to continental North America, *Schistosoma* represents a major cause of disease in humans, infecting 200 million people. *Schistosoma mansoni* is endemic to the United States, as it is present in Puerto Rico. It is found in many areas of the Caribbean.

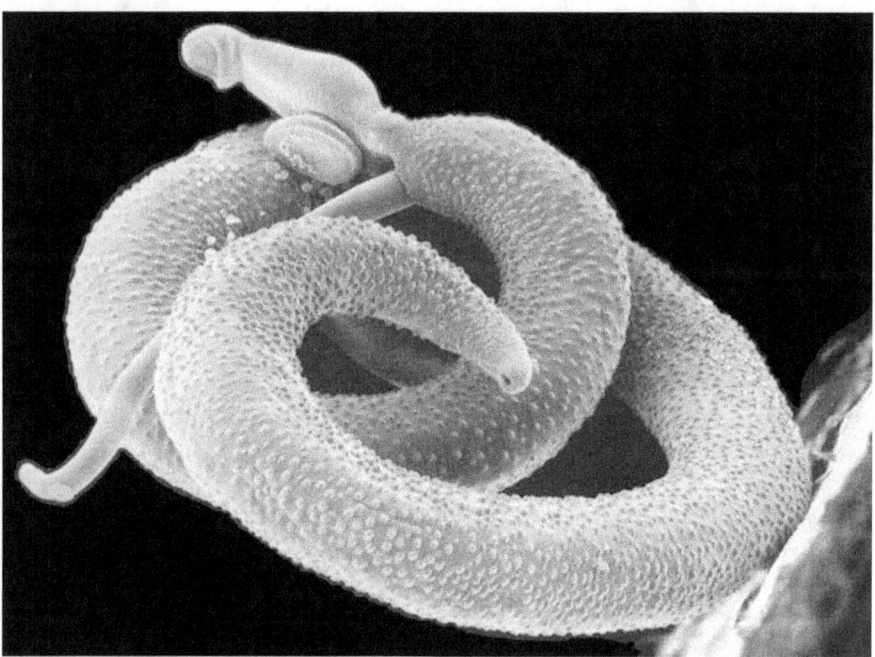

Figure 9-4: *Schistosoma* are monogamous and mate for life, as shown here, with the slender, smooth female within the male. Cute, aren't they?

Interestingly, it is not the bloodworm feeding on us that causes most of the disease. The worms evade an immune response by their mucous coat, antioxidant system, and other mechanisms. The disease is caused by the strong immune reaction to the parasite's eggs. The eggs get into the blood flow from the intestines into the liver where they cause fibrosis and can induce portal hypertension, and into the lungs where they also can cause fibrosis.

Some of these bloodworms live in the liver and intestines; these cause liver and colon cancer while other *Schistosoma* live in the kidneys and cause bladder cancer. Those that live in the intestines spread through feces, and those that live in the kidney are typically spread by little boys, peeing in ponds. It's amazing how parasites can capitalize on an inherent behavior of young boys. Oh, what fun it was to be young, in warm weather, with a place to swim!

The life cycle of this parasite (Figure 9-3) starts in humans when the infective cercaria, which are present in freshwater, penetrate the skin of someone wading, swimming or washing in a pond where the co-host, freshwater snails, live. The cercaria then make their way to the bloodstream and migrate to the liver. Here the parasite reaches adulthood, feeding on the liver and then moves to the intestines to lay eggs. The eggs are shed in the feces. If egg contaminated human feces makes its way into a pond, the eggs develop into miracidia that penetrate the foot of a snail. These mature in the snail and produce sporocysts that develop into cercaria. What could be simpler?

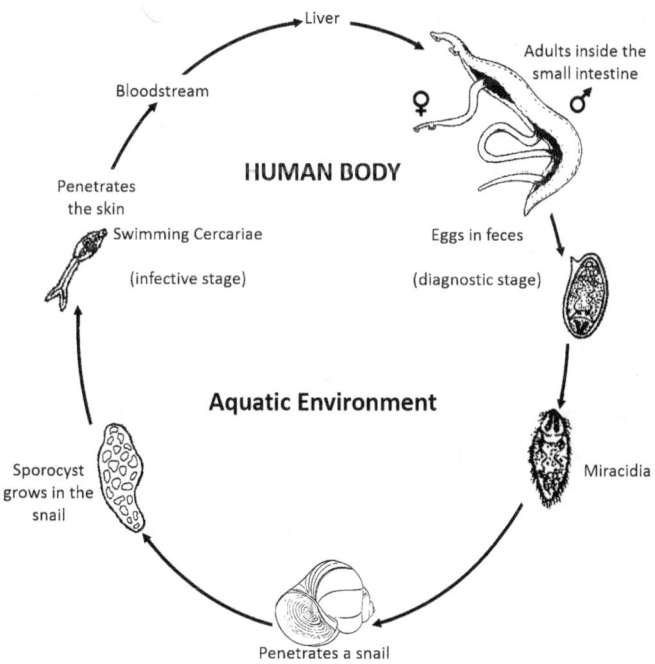

Figure 9-3: Life cycle of *Schistosoma haematobium*[74]

Schistosoma haematobium, bladder fluke, is found in Africa and the Middle East. Because it causes penile sores, it increases the transmissibility of HIV. This parasite increases the development of carcinoma of the bladder and cervical cancer. *Schistosoma mansoni* and *Schistosoma japonicum* live in the intestine and increase the risk of colorectal and liver cancers. It is our chronic immune response to these parasites that causes the production of oxygen and nitrogen radicals. The injury from chronic oxidative stress increases the risk of cancer. In *Schistosoma*-related bladder cancer, there is activation of H-ras and inactivation of p53 and Rb, and In *Schistosoma*-related colorectal cancer, there is also inactivation of p53.[72] Thus, the parasite, like HPV infections, helps ensure its reproduction by preventing apoptosis of its host cells.

Infection associated cancers are preventable. We have the vaccines and medications to eliminate most of them and the technology for developing vaccines against the rest. It is a matter of international will. We can protect ourselves and prevent suffering everywhere. It is not enough to vaccinate ourselves, as travel, migration, and international commerce circulate infectious agents, and can reintroduce them.

> Guinea Worm *(Dracunculus* – meaning little dragon) is a human parasite that can wrap around the nerves and blood vessels. The parasite's head emerges from the skin, unusually on the lower extremity, causing severe burning pain. This induces the victim to cool the burning in water, which allows the parasite to release 1000's of larvae, which enter the water, and restart the infection cycle. There are no medications to treat this parasite. Instead, when the parasite emerges from the skin, it is carefully extracted from the flesh by slowly winding it around a small stick, a process that can take days. Still, the pain may continue for months, making it difficult to walk. These worms can be a meter long and as thick as a fine spaghetti noodle.
>
> In 1986, when I was studying public health after medical school, there were an estimated 3.5 million persons plagued with Guinea worms. In 2015 there were 22 cases. Simple public health measures, such as filtering drinking water, will likely eliminate this disease before you read this book. We can end disease.

10: TOBACCO

Of all the causes of cancer in the United States of America, tobacco is among the most important, and most simple, but tobacco should get the shortest chapter. All one needs to know is simply and concisely: DON'T.

Twenty-five to thirty percent of all cancer in the United States is caused by tobacco exposure.

It is a statement of the obvious. Tobacco kills. Tobacco is not only a risk factor for at least fourteen types of cancer; it is a major cause of heart and vascular disease, including myocardial infarction and stroke. It is also the most significant cause of COPD (chronic obstructive pulmonary diseases), including chronic bronchitis and emphysema. Thus, tobacco is a major risk factor for the first, second and third most common causes of death in the United States. Around 443,000 people die each year in the United States from smoking tobacco, resulting in 5.1 million years of life lost.[75] That comes out to about eleven and a half years of life lost per smoker. Not only does smoking shorten the life of the smoker, it raises the risk of cancer and other diseases for those who live with them.

Table 10-1: Cancers linked to Smoking Tobacco

Oropharynx	Cervix	Breast
Larynx	Uterus	Esophagus
Lung	Vulva	Stomach
Kidney	Anus	Pancreas
Bladder	Penis	Renal Pelvis

Tobacco and tobacco smoke contain numerous carcinogens. Additionally, tobacco smoke promotes the activation of liver enzymes that convert pre-carcinogens into active carcinogens. Smokeless tobacco is carcinogenic without burning; it causes oral, pharyngeal, and esophageal cancers.[76] When associated with alcohol, smokeless tobacco promotes high-risk infection with HPV virus, associated with head and neck cancers.[77]

And smokers are not throwing away years from their old age; they are cutting years from their healthy productive middle years. It makes you want to ask a smoker if they would mind handing over some of those years they are trashing.

In fact, if one examines the 10 top causes of death in the United States, it can be seen that tobacco is a risk factor for each of them, including Alzheimer's disease and accidents, which are more common among smokers.

Table 10-2: Top 10 Causes of Death in the USA in 2014[78]

- ☠ Heart disease: 614,343 deaths
- ☠ Cancer: 591,699 deaths
- ☠ Chronic lower respiratory diseases: 147,101 deaths
- ☠ Accidents (unintentional injuries): 136,035 deaths
- ☠ Stroke (cerebrovascular diseases): 133,103 deaths
- ☠ Alzheimer's disease: 93,451 deaths
- ☠ Diabetes: 76,488 deaths
- ☠ Influenza and pneumonia: 55,227 deaths
- ☠ Nephritis, nephrotic syndrome, and nephrosis: 48,146 deaths
- ☠ Intentional self-harm (suicide): 42,773 deaths

If you would like to avoid the diseases listed in Tables 10-1 and 10-2, avoiding tobacco will help.

While tobacco is not a risk factor for developing diabetes, it is a risk factor for amputations and death among patients with diabetes. You might be surprised that smoking is a risk factor for accidental death. A meta-analysis of several separate studies found that smokers were 51 percent more likely to die of unintentional injuries than non-smokers and had a 35 percent higher risk than ex-smokers.[79]

Fun Fact: Tobacco is a unique plant in that it concentrates the radioactive element polonium-210 from extremely small amounts present in phosphate fertilizer. Because fertilizer is heavily employed in the intensive farming practices used in the U.S., American-grown tobacco has about three times as much Po-210 as does tobacco grown in developing countries. When tobacco is smoked, the Po-210 is deposited in the smoker's airways, where it undergoes radioactive decay, emitting radioactive alpha particles.[80] It has been estimated that a daily pack and a half habit exposes a smoker to the equivalent radiation of 300 chest X-rays per year. This radiation is a significant contributor to lung cancer.[81]

Tobacco is even a risk factor for suicide. A study done by researchers at Washington University found that when states increased taxes on tobacco, not only does the smoking rate decrease, but the suicide rate also falls about 10% for every dollar per pack in taxes.[82] Previous to this evidence, many assumed that the association between smoking and mental health was that the mental health issues promoted higher tobacco use; that depressed individuals and those with psychiatric illness smoked more as a form of self-medication. The fall in suicide rates following a decline in tobacco consumption indicates that smoking is a cause of depression, mental illness, and suicide.

If you think it takes years for tobacco to kill someone, consider its impact on babies. The Surgeon General's Report on Women and Smoking found that ten percent of all infant deaths are caused by the mother smoking during pregnancy[83]. Either parent smoking during pregnancy increases the risk of ADHD in the child,[84] and increases the risk of ear infections[85] and permanent hearing losses.[86] Just being exposed to second-hand smoke may be enough to cause a loss of hearing.[87] Children whose parents smoke are at increased risk of leukemia,[88] and even if they never smoke, children exposed to tobacco smoke are at increased risk of cancer as adults.[89] Women who have never smoked are estimated to have a 65% increased risk of premenopausal breast cancer if married to a smoker.[90]

It also does not take much time for declines in smoking to lower the risk of death. Communities that have banned indoor smoking have seen falls in myocardial infarction rates within days of the implementation of these rules.

The medical community has long known that smoking causes cancer, emphysema and heart disease. The Surgeon General made it the official position of the U.S. Public Health Service that cigarette smoking caused cancer in 1957. It took another seven years to come out of the closet with it. I remember seeing the Surgeon General on announcing it on TV while at my grandfather's house in 1964. My granddad, disabled from emphysema and watching from his easy-chair, put out his last cigarette.

Most people, however, do not quit smoking, do not lose weight, and do not sustain their diet or long-term physical activity. Even when interventions have been proven to decrease the risk of diabetes or to help weight loss, follow-up studies generally show that people return to their old habits after the active intervention program has ended.

Change can be hard, and our habits are reinforced by our environment, our economies and those around us; otherwise, we would not have adopted the behavior in the first place. Many of those who quit smoking relapse, most of those who lose weight regain it. Most exercise programs fizzle.

The goal needs to be sustainable change. We can do this. The way to end a bad habit is to replace it with an easier one, a tastier one, a less expensive one, a more convenient one.

If as a doctor, I just scare my patients but don't give them a way of attaining the needed remedy, all I have accomplished is add to their suffering. Have you ever had a boss that gives you tasks and responsibilities, but provides neither authority nor resources to complete the tasks? The result is often frustration and failure.

People can and do quit smoking. It is not easy. The key is to make quitting easier and make smoking harder. Here is a strategy for success in smoking cessation.

1. Break the habits that maintain the smoking behavior first, and work on the addictive element later. To break the habits, set some ground rules that make it less likely that habit cigarettes will be used without being driven by cravings.

- Rule 1: Make cigarettes less accessible. Encourage the smoker to agree to rules that allow them to keep smoking for the present, in preparation for quitting. If the cigarettes are kept in a cabinet, and the user has to go get one each time they want one, they will smoke less than if they are handy in a shirt pocket or purse.

- Rule 2: Smoking is only permitted outdoors. If they have to smoke outside, they will smoke less, and everyone, including the smoker, will be less exposed to second-hand smoke. This includes prohibiting smoking in a car, even if the windows are open.

- Rule 3: Disallow smoking while talking on the phone, or drinking coffee, beer or other beverages. Allow the coffee, allow the beer, and in the beginning, allow the cigarettes, but first, break the habits that reinforce the behaviors. Beer and cigarettes are allowed by this rule, but not at the same time.

Once the habit cigarettes are gone, most smokers will slow the number of cigarettes to about half a pack a day or less.

2. Now work on the addiction. Cut the smoking down by one cigarette per day until smoking only 5 cigarettes a day. Then quit. It is much easier to quit from 5 cigarettes a day than 40. Remind them that they will feel withdrawal symptoms for about 5 days, but assure them that you are confident in their ability to overcome this challenge.

- I know you can quit. If you are a smoker and have the tenacity and interest to read this book, then you most certainly have the grit and gumption required to quit and stay quit.

- Don't bother trying to quit – just quit. If you think you will give quitting a try, you are starting on the wrong foot, don't bother. Commit to it. Make a firm decision to quit. Even if you fail your first go, take what you have learned, and quit. If you "try" you will most likely fail.

- Remember that as you quit, that "Cigarette Satan" that will try to woo you back, saying that that just one cigarette will be OK; assuring you that you will be able to control it, and that one cigarette will fix your craving and relax you. Temptation will assure you that you can cheat *just a little bit*; just a half cigarette will be OK. This is the devil lying, tempting you. You will be tested but don't fall for it. The only way to outsmart the devil is not to give an inch.

- ϒ Medications may help with quitting smoking.

> Link: The state of Florida has a toll free number (1-877-U-CAN-NOW) to help with smoking cessation and free, face-to-face and online programs to help people quit, (www.TobaccoFreeFlorida.com) and may provide nicotine replacement therapy. Your state or local area may have similar programs.

Summary

Twenty-five to thirty percent of cancers in the developed world are caused by tobacco. Even after being diagnosed with invasive, incurable cancer, quitting tobacco use typically doubles survival time. *Thus, quitting tobacco may be as effective as chemotherapy treatment or radiation therapy* for extending the life of many cancer patients with tobacco-related cancers.[3]

Let me repeat:

Quitting tobacco may be as effective as chemotherapy or radiation treatment for extending the life of cancer patients with tobacco-related cancers.

Increasing cigarette taxes saves lives and deters young people from adopting a smoking addiction.

11: ALCOHOL

Although alcohol causes nowhere the risk of cancer as does tobacco, it gets a much more thorough discussion. Alcohol consumption can be a risk factor for cancer, but its effect is much more nuanced and complex than the outright murderer tobacco. Several cancers are clearly linked to consumption of alcohol; we have known that alcohol increases the risk of oropharyngeal cancers for over 100 years. Nevertheless, the mechanisms by which alcohol exerts its carcinogenic effects are not fully worked out, and the links between alcohol and cancer is especially complex with breast cancer. Alcohol is more often a co-carcinogen than a carcinogen. For most cancers, alcohol has accomplices, including tobacco and other carcinogens, infections, and poor nutrition.

In the United States, it is estimated that about 4.0 percent of cancers in men and 3.1 percent of cancers in women are attributed to alcohol.[91] In European countries, where alcohol consumption is higher than in the U.S., the attributable risk is two to three times higher.[92] In some countries, with very high consumption, over 20 percent of all cancer cases may be attributable to alcohol.

Table 11-1: Risk of Cancer Associated with Alcohol Use

Site of Cancer[93, 94]	RR of Heavy Alcohol Use*
Upper Aero-Digestive Tract (UADT)	
Cancers of the Oral Cavity	4.64
Pharyngeal Cancer	6.62
Laryngeal Cancer	2.62
Esophageal Cancer	1.2 – 3.35
Other Cancers	
Liver Cancer	1.4
Breast Cancer	1.55
Colon and Rectal Cancers	1.52
Endometrial Cancer	1.19
Prostate Cancer	1.24
Cancer of the CNS	1.35
Stomach	1.12
Pancreas Cancer	1.23

* Heavy consumption defined as more than 50 g/day or 64 ml of pure alcohol; 3.6 U.S. standard drinks a day. RR: Relative Risk.

Oral, Pharyngeal and Esophageal Cancers

The cancers most strongly attributable to alcohol are those in which alcohol has direct contact with the tissues. These are cancers of the mouth, tongue, upper airway, larynx, pharynx, and esophagus; these as a group are known as cancers of the upper airway and digestive tract (UADT).

UADT cancers are more common in men than women as it is more common for men to be heavy drinkers and use tobacco products heavily than it is for women.

Table 11-2: Signs and Symptoms of UADT Cancers

The key signs and symptoms of UADT cancers are sores or other problems that are persistent. Any of the following problems that last more than a month should be evaluated by a doctor:[95]

- A sore in the mouth that doesn't heal or that bleeds easily
- A patch of red or white skin in the mouth that won't go away
- A persistent lump or swelling in the neck
- A persistent sore throat
- Persistent hoarseness or a change in the voice
- Persistent pain in the neck, throat, or ears
- Bloody sputum
- Difficulty chewing, swallowing or moving the jaws or tongue
- Numbness in the tongue or other areas

Compared to non-smokers who consume an alcoholic beverage less than once a week, non-smokers who have 30 or more drinks* a week are nearly 6 times (Relative Risk (RR) = 5.8) more likely to develop an oral or pharyngeal cancer. Smokers who rarely drink, but who smoke 20 to 40 cigarettes a day have an RR of 1.9 for these cancers. Men who smoke and drink this much have an RR of 23.8! [96] These risk factors have an interaction which multiplies the risk. Women are at no less risk of oral and pharyngeal cancers if they consume this quantity of alcohol or smoke this heavily.

Individuals who consume large amounts of alcohol get a large number of calories from these beverages, often replacing other nutrients. A couple of rum and cokes does not form a balanced meal. Heavy drinkers with poorer nutrition, those with lower intake of fruits and vegetables, were three times more likely to develop

---

* See definition of drink size below. Herein, the U.S. standard of 0.6 fluid ounces of pure alcohol in a beverage is used as a "drink".

esophageal cancer than those consuming similar amounts of alcohol but eating well.[97]

Oral, pharyngeal, laryngeal and esophageal cancers are squamous cell carcinomas arising from the mucosal lining of these tissues, which are directly exposed to alcohol. Some alcohol is directly absorbed by the mucosa lining the UADT. One theory is that alcohol acts as a solvent and helps carry carcinogens, from tobacco or other sources, into the UADT mucosa where the carcinogens damage the DNA. Tobacco is a potent co-carcinogen for alcohol in this area of the body.

Table 11-3: In the United States, a Standard Drink contains 14.0 grams of ethanol, which is equivalent to 17.74 ml (rounded to 17.8 in use) or 0.6 fluid ounces of pure alcohol.

Beverage	Fluid Ounces	Drink	Alcohol (% by volume)
Beer	12 oz.	A Can	5%
Malt Liquor	8 oz.		7%
Wine	5 oz.	A Glass	12%
Fortified Wine	3 oz.	Glass*	16 – 18%
80-Proof Liquor	1.5 oz.	A Shot	40%

* Often served in a cordial or brandy glass

Table 11-4: The volume in a standard drink serving size differs between countries, and thus, there can be confusion when comparing alcohol consumption and studies of the effects of alcohol in different localities.

Countries	Grams/ ml Pure Alcohol Per Standard Drink
Austria	6 g / 7.62 ml
The UK and Iceland	8 g / 10.0 ml
Australia, France, Ireland, Italy, New Zealand Poland and Spain	10 g / 12.7 ml
Denmark and Finland	12 g / 15.2 ml
Canada	13.6 g / 17.24 ml
The United States and Portugal	14 g / 17.8 ml
Hungary, Sweden	17 g / 21.5 ml
Japan	19.75 / 25.0 ml

Note that the alcohol content is given in rounded numbers; red wine typically has an alcohol content of 12.3% and beers from just below three to six percent alcohol.

Acetaldehyde and Methanol

Alcohol is a risk factor for UADT and other cancers even in the absence of smoking or smokeless tobacco. It is not alcohol, but rather its metabolite, acetaldehyde, that is a carcinogen that damages DNA in the mucosa of the upper airway and upper digestive tract.

Figure 11-1 illustrates the enzymes used in the metabolism of alcohol: ethanol is enzymatically oxidized into acetaldehyde and then into acetate. Acetate is harmless, but acetaldehyde is not. The principal enzymes for metabolizing alcohol to acetaldehyde are alcohol dehydrogenases (ADH), cytochrome p450 2E1 (CYP2E1), and catalase (CAT). The ADH1 genes are expressed in many cells; p450 CYP2E1 is mostly expressed in the liver and catalase is most active in the brain. Acetaldehyde is metabolized by an aldehyde dehydrogenase (ALDH) to acetate.

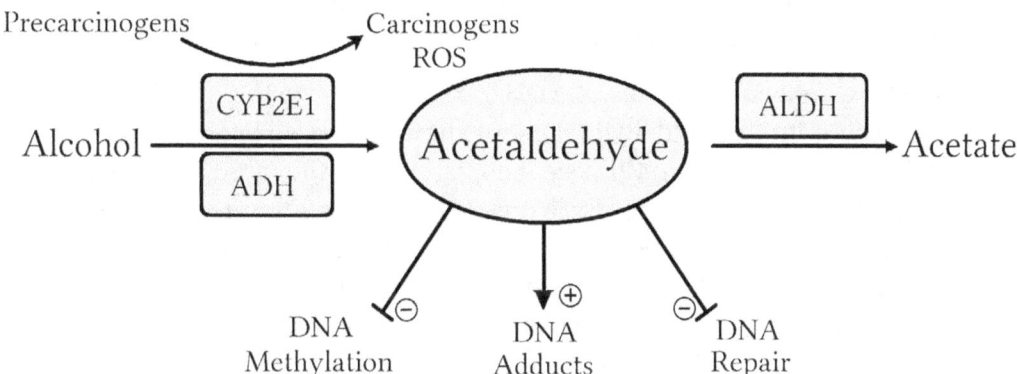

Figure 11-1: Alcohol Metabolism and Cancer Risk[98]

In the first step of alcohol metabolism, ethanol is converted to acetaldehyde, mostly by alcohol dehydrogenase (ADH) enzymes. ADH1B is the predominant form of ADH in the liver; other tissues have other ADH isoforms. Chronic heavy alcohol consumption induces the production of the cytochrome P450 enzyme 2E1 that also oxidizes ethanol into acetaldehyde.

In chronic alcoholics, up to 30% of the alcohol is metabolized by CYP2E1. The induction of CYP2E1 has negative consequences as this enzyme also avidly oxidizes many pre-carcinogens present in tobacco, the diet, and the environment into active carcinogens. CYP2E1 oxidation additionally produces reactive oxygen species that may contribute to cell damage and carcinogenesis. [98]

In the next step, acetaldehyde is further oxidized into harmless acetate (acetic acid) by one of the several forms of aldehyde dehydrogenase (ALDH).

It might seem that having robust enzymes that quickly break down alcohol would be advantageous. It may have the effect that a person can consume more alcohol without feeling drunk. This occurs in people with heavy alcohol consumption through the induction of CYP2E1. But this rapid oxidation of alcohol comes with a major drawback; it causes increased levels of acetaldehyde, a carcinogen. Additionally, not everyone processes alcohol at the same rate. There are several genetic alleles of ADH1B and ALDH that vary in enzymatic activity.

If alcohol is converted into acetaldehyde faster, then cells exposed to alcohol need to deal with greatly elevated levels of acetaldehyde, a toxin and carcinogen, and one of the factors causing hangovers. Either fast conversion of alcohol to acetaldehyde or slow metabolism of acetaldehyde to acetate can form an acetaldehyde trap and increase acetaldehyde levels. Individuals that oxidize ethanol into acetaldehyde rapidly or metabolize acetaldehyde slowly can build up dangerous levels of this toxin even when consuming what appear to be ordinarily tolerable amounts of alcohol.

There are genetic alleles of ADH1B that accelerate the metabolism of alcohol into acetaldehyde. One of these alleles, ADH1B 47Arg, is common in the Han Chinese people. When the 47Arg allele is inherited from both parents, it raises the conversion rate of alcohol to acetaldehyde by about 40 times. Individuals homozygous for ADH1B 47Arg that were classified as non-drinkers were 1.2 times more likely to develop esophageal cancer compared to persons with the more typical ADH1B 47His variant. Heavy drinkers that are homozygous for the 47Arg allele are 70 times more likely to develop, esophageal cancer than of persons who do not carry this variant and do not drink. This genetic variant traveled along the ancient Silk Road to the Middle East and is also found among the people of Turkey and Northern Iran.[99]

Once acetaldehyde has been formed, it needs to be detoxified by conversion into acetate by ALDH, primarily by the ALDH2 isoform. There is also allele variation in this gene. One of these, found mostly among Asians, is the ALDH2 Lys+ allele that slows acetaldehyde metabolism. Those homozygous for this variant metabolize acetaldehyde at about 8% of the normal rate. Most of these people avoid alcohol, as they easily get flushing, nausea, and hangovers from even small amounts of alcohol. Heterozygotes, having just one copy of the Lys+ allele, may be less fortunate; as they can drink, but doing so increases their risk of oropharyngeal, laryngeal, esophageal, gastric, colon, and lung cancers.[100]

> The Drug disulfiram (Antabuse) is used to treat alcoholism

> as it inhibits the enzyme ALDH and thus causes a buildup of acetaldehyde that is five to ten times higher than would normally occur. This produced very unpleasant effects that deter alcohol consumption.

The p450 enzymes are inducible, meaning that as the liver is exposed to alcohol, production of these enzymes increases.[101] Induction of CYP2E1 also increases acetaldehyde levels. In addition to this, when alcohol is metabolized by p450 CYP2E1 in the liver, free radicals are released, causing lipid peroxidation, damage to proteins, and inflammation. Among the lipid peroxides is 4-hydroxy-nonenal, another DNA adduct. The oxidative stress depletes the principal antioxidant of the liver, glutathione. Glutathione protects the mitochondria, nucleus, and cell organelles from oxidative damage.

Furthermore, induction of p450 CYP2E1 by alcohol may induce the biotransformation of procarcinogens into active carcinogens, as in the case of nitrosamine. Alcohol is not alone in this, as certain drugs, chemicals and solvents also induce p450 CYP2E1 activity.[102]

In a third and associated pathway, ethanol also alters DNA and histone methylation and acetylation. This affects how tightly the DNA strand is bound to the proteins that protect it when it is not in use. If it becomes more loosely bound, the genes are more easily transcribed but are more susceptible to breaks and more likely to suffer errors in the repair process. Methylation of DNA depends on the B vitamin folate as a coenzyme for transfer of single carbon units. Folate is required along with methionine for histone methylation.

Ethanol (or one of its metabolites) can impair normal methylation by impairing folate metabolism. Alcohol interferes with the enzyme methylenetetrahydrofolate reductase (MTHFR). This enzyme recycles folate, a B vitamin. Ethanol also alters the binding and transport of folate in the intestinal and kidneys, reducing the uptake of folate. Thus, alcohol can both worsen a deficiency of folate and impair folate activity.[103] Folate is also needed for the formation of purines for building the DNA.

Folate deficiency affects about ten percent of the world's population, making it, along with Vitamin D deficiency, the second most prevalent vitamin deficiency. The interaction with alcohol makes impairments of folate metabolism more severe and raises the risk of cancer.[104] While the RR for colorectal cancer for those drinking 50 grams of alcohol a day is 1.2 compared with abstainers, the RR is 7.4 for those consuming more than 20 grams of alcohol in association with low folate and methionine levels.[105] Impaired folate function has been documented in multiple forms of cancer, and this is further discussed in Chapter 26.

There are two common allelic forms MTHFR. About ten percent of the population has a single nucleotide replacement of thymine (T) in the 677th nucleotide position of the gene, rather than the usual cytosine (C). The MTHFR 677T variant breaks down more readily and is thus less active than the MTHFR C form. The MTHFR genotype impacts the effect of alcohol on folate metabolism. When a person with the MTHFR 677TT allele consumes more than two drinks a day, it decreases MTHFR activity by 70%, thereby increasing the risk of breast, prostate, UADT, and other cancers. Having the MTHFR 677TT allele increases the RR of pancreatic cancer 4.5 times among drinkers compared to non-drinkers.[106] The 677TT allele is associated with an 83% increased risk of post-menopausal breast cancer as compared to the CC form.[107]

Retinoic acid, a form of vitamin A, is also more quickly degraded by the enhanced CYP2E1 activity induced by heavy alcohol use. Low retinoic acid levels may enhance proliferation of poorly differentiated cells.[108]

Acetaldehyde inhibits DNA methylation and increases the risk of DNA damage. Acetaldehyde forms DNA adducts that can cause single-strand breaks in the DNA and cross-linking of the DNA. It also inhibits DNA repair.

In addition to that formed from alcohol by the metabolism, most alcoholic beverages contain acetaldehyde. While distilled spirits have the highest level, only small amounts are usually consumed. Beer generally has low acetaldehyde levels. At very low levels the flavor of acetaldehyde is not detectable; at moderate levels, between 120 to 500 mg/L, it provides pleasant fruity aromas to foods and wine. Higher levels, however, impart a flavor reminiscent of dry straw or rotten apples. Small amounts of acetaldehyde are found in apple juice, yogurt, cheese and butter. Beer usually has very low levels. Cider contains about 200 times the amount of acetaldehyde as vodka[109], and fermented stone fruit beverages also have very high levels. Levels in red wine can vary from tiny amounts to about 200 mg/L. White and sweet wines have about twice the acetaldehyde levels as do red wines.[110] The highest levels are found in fortified wines, especially brandy, and sherry, in which the acetaldehyde is considered a desirable flavor characteristic. Careful fermentation can make for much lower levels. Further creation of acetaldehyde occurs in wine as it oxidizes if old, poorly stored, or open, giving the wine a flat flavor.

Another source of acetaldehyde in the mouth comes from oral bacteria that process alcohol into acetaldehyde. It is not just the exposure of the mucosa to alcohol during drinking of the beverage, but also from exposure to absorbed alcohol. The level of alcohol reached in the saliva after drinking is higher than that of the blood.[111] Certain strains of oral bacteria convert alcohol from the saliva into acetaldehyde and malondialdehyde that bathes the mucosa. These aldehydes, produced by some Streptococcus species, increase bacterial attachment to the squamous cells of the mouth, pharynx, and esophagus, and promote these cells to produce an enzyme that facilitates infection with the HPV-16 virus. This is one of the same viruses that cause cervical cancer.[112] Thus, HPV-16, alcohol and poor oral hygiene all interact to increase the risk of head and neck cancer.

Although the levels of acetaldehyde present in alcoholic beverages or converted from alcohol by bacteria in the mouth, likely play a role in UADT cancers where the tissues are directly exposed, these levels are much lower than the levels created by enzymatic conversion of alcohol in the liver and other tissues. A standard three-ounce serving of sherry may contain as much as 50 mg of acetaldehyde, but the 14 grams of alcohol in this drink would be enzymatically oxidized to 13,000 mg of this carcinogen. Acetaldehyde is also present in tobacco and marijuana cigarette smoke.

In addition to alcohol and acetaldehyde, alcoholic beverages may contain small amounts of other toxic and pre-carcinogenic substances including methanol. This is especially true of less carefully and illegally produced fermented beverages.[113] Apples and stone fruits, such as peaches and plums, contain large amounts of pectin. Grapes contain smaller amounts. During fermentation, pectolytic enzymes increase the formation of methanol that the body metabolizes to the toxin and carcinogen formaldehyde.

Formaldehyde is also found in some alcoholic beverages as a breakdown product of methanol. High formaldehyde levels suggest high methanol formation in a beverage. Vodka and beer generally have undetectable levels of formaldehyde, while sake and tequila have high levels. Brandy and fruit spirits have intermediate levels of formaldehyde, and grape wines have lower levels.[114]

Pectinase is present and commercially produced from the fungus *Aspergillus niger*, (black mold, but not to be confused with the type that grows on water-damaged building materials). *Aspergillus niger* attacks grapes, onions, and peanuts after harvest. Some strains of this fungus produce the toxin and carcinogen Ochratoxin A. (Chapter 21). Thus, wine made from moldy fruit may have high methanol levels.

Commercially produced pectolytic enzymes are added during the fermentation of some wines to increase the release of terpenes that add flavor to white wines, such as Gewurztraminer and Moscato, Riesling and others. Less commonly, pectinase may be used during the production of red wines.[115] The strain of yeast used in fermentation also affects methanol production. High methanol content is suspected as one of the contributing factors of hangovers. Methanol toxicity acts in part by impairing DNA methylation. This is especially pronounced if folate (vitamin B9) levels are inadequate; adequate folate levels appear to prevent toxicity and DNA methylation from low levels of methanol.[116] Methanol toxicity may also be a risk factor for Alzheimer's disease.[117]

Liver Cancer and Alcohol

The liver is the principal metabolic site for alcohol, and here, it is a liver toxin and carcinogen. For cancers of the UADT, much of the damage is thought to be a result of acetaldehyde. The damage to the liver includes this, and also, injury from cytochrome CYP2E1 processing of alcohol and methanol as described above

Like many other tissues, the liver metabolizes alcohol into acetaldehyde using the enzymes ADH1B and ALDH2 but additionally the liver metabolizes alcohol using cytochrome P-450 2E1 (CYP2E1) and catalase.

As a toxin, alcohol damages hepatic cells. Alcohol causes oxidative damage that kills hepatocytes that then require replacement. As the number of healthy cells declines, the load of toxins is distributed among fewer hepatocytes, and fatty liver disease develops followed by cirrhosis. Recall that healthy cells are valiant and vain. They give up the ghost when they are exposed to excess oxidative stress, preventing the reproduction of cells with DNA damage. Alcohol causes DNA damage and increases the frequency of single-strand DNA breaks. Cancer cells induced by alcohol have been shown to have increased ADH activity, but not an increase in ALDH activity, causing higher levels of acetaldehyde to accumulate in these cells when exposed to alcohol. The chronic oxidative stress in the liver exerts a selection pressure favoring the survival and growth of hepatic progenitor clones that are more resistant to oxidative damage.[118] Unfortunately, this includes cells with other mutations.

Risk becomes greatly elevated with cirrhosis of the liver when replacement is dependent on fewer cells. Just increasing cell turnover, increases cancer risk. Acetaldehyde and formaldehyde form DNA adducts and promote DNA breakage and errors. Methanol, present in many alcoholic beverages, impairs folate metabolism and alters DNA methylation, causing changes gene transcription.[117]

Alcohol is a risk factor for hepatocellular carcinoma (HCC) and accounts for about 32 to 45 percent of all cases of this disease.[92] Similar to the effect of tobacco and alcohol for UADT cancers, the risk from alcohol alone is much smaller than when in concert with other carcinogens. Among very heavy drinkers (80 grams/day, about 6 drinks/day) the RR for HCC is 2.4. However, if the person has hepatitis B (HBV) or hepatitis C (HCV), the RR for heavy drinking is 53.9. Among those with the virus who do not drink, the RR is 19.1. The risk of HCC is also greatly elevated in diabetics who are heavy drinkers.

The metabolic activity of the liver exposed to high levels of alcohol may increase the risk for other cancers. Alcohol, as well as tobacco, and other toxins induce cytochrome p450 enzymes. This can increase the processing and conversion of pre-carcinogenic compounds into carcinogens that may enter the circulation and injure other organs. Additionally, when folate recycling is impaired in the liver, it depletes folate from the rest of the body.

Breast Cancer and Alcohol

Alcohol is a powerful risk factor for breast cancer. Like the epithelial cells of the oral mucosa, the breast epithelium makes the enzyme ADH and metabolizes alcohol into acetaldehyde that can accumulate in the breast tissue and form reactive oxygen species.[119] Alcohol metabolism in the liver induces the conversion of pre-carcinogens to carcinogens which may reach the breast, and folate depletion also affects the breast. Alcohol induction of CYP2E1 can alter sex hormonal levels.

Studies show that for every gram of alcohol consumption per day, the risk of breast cancer goes up by about one percent. One standard U.S. drink per day raises the risk by 14%.[120] Estimates using this dose-response to alcohol attribute a large portion of the alcohol-related breast cancer burden to women who are light drinkers (less than 1.4 drinks/day). This is because there are so many more women who drink moderately than heavily. Because breast cancer is the most common alcohol-associated cancer in women, it accounts for about two-thirds of all alcohol-related cancers in women. Among heavy drinkers, about half the cases of breast cancer could have been avoided by avoiding alcohol. Even among breast cancer patients who consume light to moderate amounts of alcohol, over a quarter of the cases could have been avoided.

Table 11-5: Alcohol-Related Breast Cancer Attributable Deaths

Alcohol Consumption	Light to Moderate Any to 20 g/day	Moderate 20 to 40 g/day	Heavy Over 40 g/day
Percent of alcohol-attributable cases	14.4 to 17.2	25.5 to 35.2	47.5 to 60.2

There have been over a hundred epidemiologic studies that show alcohol to be a risk factor for breast cancer. The demon, however, is in the details.

When we do epidemiologic studies, we group subjects into exposure groups and compare the rate of disease between the different groups. If a 130 pound woman has five ounces of red wine with dinner every evening, which is equivalent to about 98 grams of alcohol a week, should she be in an alcohol consumption group higher than a person who only drinks a couple of times a month on Friday nights, but gets staggering drunk, downing five drinks (70 grams of alcohol)?

The hard part in epidemiology is classifying people into the right group. Are we asking the right questions? Do they tell the truth about their alcohol consumption? Memories can change after 40 years and months of lying awake or crying into your beer and wondering "Why me?" Does the alcohol in red wine act differently than that in rum? Is there a difference if the alcohol is served with food, with a sweet beverage or dessert? Perhaps most importantly, how was the alcohol consumption distributed over time?

Much of the risk of breast cancer incurred by alcohol consumption may occur before or during breast maturation. It is difficult to ferret out how much cancer risk from alcohol occurs during breast development as opposed to risk from drinking as an adult, as most women who consume alcohol early in their youth continue, and continue to do so after their pregnancies. Alcohol is a risk factor for Benign Breast Disease (BBD), which is a major risk factor for breast cancer, and alcohol consumption between menarche and first full-term pregnancy has a higher correlation with breast cancer than does alcohol consumption after the first pregnancy. The alcohol-related risk of breast cancer is highest and may be mostly explained, by alcohol consumption prior to pregnancy-induced breast maturation, and via the induction of benign breast disease. The longer the interval between menarche and the first pregnancy, the higher the woman's risk. Women with a greater than a ten-year interval between menarche and the first pregnancy were at the highest risk, likely because they have more years of exposure to alcohol or other risk factors.[121]

Young people often indulge in binge drinking. When asked, about a quarter of college students will report having had a hangover within the previous seven days. The high-dose exposures that occur prior to breast maturation impart risk for BBD. It is also reasonable to expect that the timing during the breast/menstrual cycle when alcohol consumption occurs impacts risk. The highest risk would be expected to occur during the mid- and late- menstrual cycle when breast cells are proliferating under the influence of progesterone and thus, at highest risk of DNA damage. (See Figure 27-1)

Most of the risk for breast cancer from adult alcohol consumption appears to be limited to postmenopausal women consuming more than 7 drinks per week. The risk is particularly high in women who drink at least five days a week and drink six or more drinks in a single day at least once a month.[122] This suggests that maintaining high enzymatic activity in the liver, plus high alcohol doses, are the key to alcohol-induced breast cancer. Heavy drinkers metabolize alcohol about two-thirds more quickly than do light drinkers. This causes heavy drinkers to have higher concentrations of toxic metabolites and higher oxidative stress than would other drinkers from alcohol.

Individuals, who drink frequently, metabolize ethanol more quickly into acetaldehyde as a result of CYP2E1 induction and thus, create a more potent oxidative risk.

There is much weaker evidence for adult-premenopausal risk from alcohol. Ductal carcinoma is by far the most common type of breast cancer, followed by lobular and ductal-lobular carcinomas. Medullary, tubular, comedo, and mucinous breast cancers are much less common. Among postmenopausal women, the strongest alcohol-induced risk is for lobular and ductal-lobular carcinoma. Here, even moderate drinking may raise the risk by 30 to 40 percent. In contrast, consuming less than one drink per day does not increase the risk of ductal carcinoma of the breast in postmenopausal women. Drinking more than 7 drinks a week increases ductal carcinoma risk by about 20 percent.[123]

Thus, for premenopausal adult women (after childbearing or over the age of about 30) with mature breasts, consumption of one alcohol equivalent a day does not confer a significant risk of breast cancer. For most postmenopausal women, the risk of less than one drink a day also remains low. Nevertheless, as people age they may metabolize alcohol/acetaldehyde more slowly, and thus, the drink size should also decrease to keep blood alcohol levels as low as they would be in a younger person consuming one drink. Additionally, as people age, their nutritional status may suffer. Vitamin B12, which helps in folate metabolism, is often low in the elderly and folate metabolism may slow with age. Those who choose to consume alcohol should be careful to maintain good nutrition through a healthy diet.

In a study of nearly 10,000 women who had been treated for breast cancer and followed for an average of just over 10 years, consumption of alcohol did not significantly increase breast cancer recurrence or breast cancer mortality. There was, however, a nearly significant decrease in total *mortality* due to a decrease in cardiovascular deaths among women who drank alcohol. No difference in risk for estrogen receptor status was found for alcohol. A twenty percent increase in breast cancer recurrence risk was found for postmenopausal women who consumed higher levels of alcohol.[124]

Alcohol-associated risk also varies by breast cancer's estrogen receptor status. Alcohol use is associated with an 11% increase in risk for estrogen-receptor positive (ER+)/progesterone-receptor positive (PR+) cancers. Alcohol increases the risk of ER+PR– by 15%, for each additional drink consumed per day. There was, however, not an increase in risk of ER–/PR+ or ER–/PR– tumors,[120] other than for ER–/PR– cancers in women drinking more than 30 grams of alcohol, about two drinks, a day.[122]

Women (or men) who have been diagnosed with breast cancer should curtail alcohol use and avoid drinking more than one drink a day. They may have allelic variants that increase ADH activity or slow ALDH or reduce MTHFR activity, putting them at higher risk from alcohol. Women with a history of ER+, lobular, or ductal-lobular breast cancers should avoid alcohol completely.

Low Dose Alcohol and Cancer

High levels or extreme exposures can give big effects, and thus are easier to find. Table 11-1 shows the effect of alcohol on cancer risk among heavy drinkers. As discussed above, the risk for breast cancer-related to alcohol use appears most strongly during the span of time between menarche and a woman's first pregnancy and in postmenopausal women who drink most days and drink heavily enough to become drunk at least monthly. In both age groups, the risk is most closely related and likely limited, to binge drinking where blood alcohol levels are high.

Small effects are more difficult to perceive. It is harder to perceive risk with moderate or low levels of alcohol consumption. Most adults fall into the low consumption category. Few people who prize their health and plan for a long future are downing 5 or more drinks a day. Binge drinking is usually not an isolated behavior; its participants often also smoke, may ignore the need for sufficient restorative sleep, vigorous exercise, and a nutritious, balanced diet.

What I want to know, and suspect my readers are concerned with, is what level of alcohol use is without long-term, detrimental effects, or which may even provide health benefits.

Low Dose Alcohol and UADT Cancers

In cohort studies that follow groups of people, light alcohol consumption was not a risk factor for cancers of the upper airway and digestive tracts, but binge drinking was. Spirits impart a greater UADT cancer risk than an equivalent alcohol content of wine, probably because consumption of spirits is more closely associated with binge drinking. Most of the risk of UADT cancer occurs in smokers. [125, 126]

Squamous cell carcinoma of the esophageal is the cancer most strongly associated with alcohol use. Binge drinking should be avoided. The risk of light alcohol consumption, particularly of red wine, is low enough that in individuals with no other UADT cancer risks, there is not sufficient risk to avoid enjoying up to one drink a day. For those with other risk factors, alcohol should be avoided.

The most relevant risk factor is a history of UADT cancer. Among survivors, however, complete abstinence from alcohol and tobacco is recommended. Continued alcohol use in these individuals (more than 15 beers a week) increases the risk of a second UADT cancer by 3.8 times.[127] Complete abstinence from alcohol decreased the risk of death in patients with head and neck cancers by 38 percent.[128] Here the issue is not light use or alcohol as a risk factor, but the high risk of binge use in individuals who were former heavy abusers of tobacco and alcohol.

Other risk factors are a family history of UADT cancer, Barrett's Esophagus, or a history of leukoplakia. Individuals with these risk factors should avoid alcohol use. The risk of head and neck cancers may be lowered by good oral hygiene, including flossing or water-jet, good nutrition, and avoiding HPV infection.

Thermal Injury: Although green and black tea and coffee contain cancer-preventive compounds, they are also associated with esophageal cancer. It is not the tea, matte, or coffee that is carcinogenic, but rather the heat. These beverages are often served at temperatures between 70° and 90° C (158° to 194° F). In parts of Africa and Iran where

> consumption of very hot tea is common, cancer of the esophagus is the second and fourth most common cancer. Repeated burn injury and cell replacement promote cancer development and proliferation.[129] Water at 160° F causes scalding injury in less than 0.5 seconds. However, it takes about one to two seconds for liquid to transverse the esophagus in healthy young people but takes longer with aging.[130] The International Agency for Research on Cancer (IARC) classifies beverages consumed at temperatures above 65° C (149° F) a probable human carcinogen.[131] Liquids need to be limited to less than 60° C (140° F) to prevent thermal injury of the esophagus, and since foods can take over 12 seconds to take the trip, food can cause scalding injury to the esophagus at temperatures above 56° C (133° F).[132] Beverage and foods should not be served this hot.

Low Dose Alcohol and Breast Cancer

The main risk from alcohol for breast cancer is from binge drinking, especially before a woman's first pregnancy, while the breast is still developing. Alcohol consumption should be avoided completely until legal age, a time by which most of the breast growth has occurred. Heavy and binge drinking should be avoided. The breast is likely most sensitive during the mid- to late breast/menstrual cycle during and after ovulation when estrogen and progesterone are at their highest. (See Figure 32-1). Although many studies suggest that low-dose alcohol raises cancer risk by about 5 percent, it is probable that this risk can be attributed to infrequent, high dose alcohol especially during breast development and later in life, rather than risk emanating from frequent low dose consumption where BAC levels do not rise above 0.04 percent.

Women with a high risk of breast cancer should understand that alcohol multiplies breast cancer risk; this risk is especially high during adolescence. Young women with BRCA gene alterations should be especially cautious. Postmenopausal women with a history of breast cancer may lower their risk of reoccurrence by avoiding alcohol.

Low Dose Alcohol and Other Cancers

There is no statistical increase in risk for colorectal, liver, ovarian, or other cancers (excluding the oral cavity, pharynx, esophagus, and breast) from low-level alcohol consumption.[133],[134] As stated earlier, most, if not all of that risk is from binge drinking, especially in those who metabolize alcohol quickly. Much of the cancer risk arises when combined with other risk factors that multiply risk, such as tobacco use or infections, such as Hepatitis C.

Winemaking 101:[135]

To make wine, grapes are crushed, forming "must": grape juice with the pulp, skin, and seeds included. The winemaker determines how long the must sits before separating out the juice and adding the yeast. During this first stage, putrescine, cadaverine, and phenylethylamine can be formed by wild bacteria and wild yeast. Wine yeast is then added for the alcoholic fermentation, and low levels of ethylamine and phenylethylamine may be formed.

Next, the winemaker usually adds a *Lactobacillus* culture for malolactic fermentation. Grapes grown in cooler regions have higher levels of malic acid, which makes them tart, and gives the wine a green-apple flavor. The malolactic fermentation step turns some of the tart malic acid into the milder and more buttery tasting, lactic acid.

The malolactic fermentation process is the main mechanism of biogenic amine formation in wine, and especially of histamine, tyramine, and putrescine.[136] The strain of bacteria used has a large effect on the amount of bioamines produced. Thus, some wines have less biogenic amine content than others. Red wines often have high tyramine levels, and sake (rice wine), high histamine levels.[137]

Commercially cultured bacteria used in winemaking are usually selected to avoid strains of bacteria that produce high levels of biogenic amines. More traditional methods of winemaking, however, use wild yeast and wild bacteria that allow less control over the taste of the wine and the levels of bioamines formed in it. These biogenic amines can cause headaches in sensitive individuals. The variation in bioamine production by different bacterial strains partially explains why some wines will cause headaches much more so than others.

Pectolytic enzymes derived from *Aspergillus niger* may be added to the must to digest pectin in the fruit to release terpenes from the grape skin. The terpenes are flavor components. Pectolytic enzymes are often used for white wines. This process increases the methanol content of the wine, an undesirable side effect.

Sulfites are then added to stop the fermentation process before bottling, halting the further conversion of amino acids into bioamines. Without sulfites, fermentation would continue in the bottle, causing cloudiness, CO_2 production, and spoiling the wine's flavor.

Port wine is produced by adding distilled wine alcohol to the grape must, thereby stopping the fermentation process at a point where only about half of the grape sugars have been fermented into alcohol. This distillation increases the concentration of acetaldehyde and methanol in the wine. The port is then aged. This gives fortified wines a higher alcohol content.

Sweet wines are made by adding partially-fermented or unfermented grape juice to fully fermented wine.

WARNING: Alcohol is a toxin, and toxic amounts should be avoided. Even small amounts of alcohol should be considered toxic in children. Alcohol can also lead to dependence in many individuals. Alcohol is a teratogen and causes fetal alcohol syndrome and thus should be avoided in women who are or may be pregnant. Alcohol is a carcinogen at levels that cause intoxication.

Wine

While most alcoholic beverages are associated with obesity, at least in women, consumption of three to four ounces of wine a day is associated with a lower body mass index. Red wine contains phenolic compounds that are associated with health benefits, including lowered risk for cardiovascular disease.

Wine during Pregnancy

South African mothers of children with *partial* fetal alcohol syndrome reported drinking five drinks a week, but mostly on weekends, and then, three drinks at a time.[138] Partial fetal alcohol syndrome is a severe condition in which there are cranial deformities and large losses in IQ levels, associated with consuming sufficient alcohol to attain peak blood alcohol content of 0.102 during the third trimester, the time of highest susceptibility to damage.[139] This level of blood alcohol may be associated with disinhibition, impairment in reasoning and depth perception, staggering and slurring of the speech. Clearly, this level is toxic and not moderate intake. It is the peak alcohol level that appears to be most damaging to the unborn child.

One drink (5 ounces of wine) contains 0.6 ounces of alcohol; enough to raise the blood alcohol content to 0.045% for a 100-pound woman. Driving with this blood level or higher is considered "driving under the influence" in most countries. Children that had prenatal exposure to even light alcohol consumption (more than zero, but less than 0.3 ounces of alcohol a day [2.5 ounces of wine; half a drink]) are more than three times more likely to have elevated scores on externalizing behavior (aggressive and delinquent) and internalizing behavior (anxious/depressed and withdrawn) syndrome scales.[140] In utero exposure to alcohol increases the risk of breast cancer in animals.[141]

Alcohol up-regulates the expression of the inflammatory receptors TLR4 and TLR2 on microglia cells in the brain, activating an inflammatory response and inducing the production of inflammatory cytokines and reactive oxygen species. This causes apoptosis of neurons,[142] in a similar mechanism to that which promotes chronic inflammatory brain damage after traumatic brain injury. Alcohol also impedes production of nerve growth factors.

Resveratrol, found in red wine, can impede the inflammatory cascade initiated by TLR activation by inhibiting NF-κB activation.

Alcohol should be completely avoided during pregnancy. If a woman is pregnant and can feel the effects of alcohol – she has achieved levels toxic to the fetal brain. There is no benefit, and no justification, for exposing a child to severe, lifelong harm.

> Men: Paternal alcohol consumption prior to conception can have detrimental effects on the physical and mental development of offspring, even when there is no alcohol exposure during pregnancy. Alcohol reduces the activity of DNA methyltransferase enzymes, causing hypomethylation of DNA, and causing aberrant expression of normally silent genes in the sperm[143]. Paternal fetal alcohol syndrome not only affects the child's development, but also decreases the offspring's fertility, and may even affect subsequent generations.[144]
>
> It takes about 90 days for sperm to develop from stem cells. It is prudent for men planning on fathering a child to avoid more than limited alcohol intake (more than one drink on any day) for three months prior to expected conception.

> Marijuana
>
> Several studies have explored the risk of marijuana use on cancer. A review of these studies finds conflicting evidence for UADT and lung cancers. Associated risk may have been confounded by the use of, or interactions with alcohol, tobacco, or other risk modifiers. There is insufficient evidence to link marijuana to UADT cancer. Three studies on marijuana use and testicular cancer were consistent; smoking marijuana more than once a week doubles the risk of testicular cancer.
>
> Although there are only a limited number of well-performed studies on cancer in children born to mothers using marijuana during pregnancy, its use does appear to increase the risk of childhood cancer. Paternal prenatal marijuana use also appears to be a risk factor for childhood cancer. Neuroblastoma risk was elevated in children whose mothers smoked marijuana during pregnancy and risk increased with the frequency of use. Astrocytoma risk has also been found to be increased with maternal gestational exposure to marijuana. Several other childhood cancers have been associated with both maternal and paternal use of marijuana, including rhabdomyosarcoma and leukemias.[145] The relationship between testicular cancer and marijuana serves to strengthen the link between paternal use and childhood cancer. Even though limited, the data appear consistent enough to advise strongly against the use of marijuana during pregnancy in women and for men during the three months preceding a planned conception.

Safe Alcohol Consumption Limits

Most adults, outside of pregnancy, can consume some alcohol without significant risks of endangering their health. For women, this amount is equivalent to the amount of alcohol in one ounce of red wine for every 30 pounds of body weight. For men, it is one ounce of wine for every 25 pounds of body weight. Red wine has health benefits that, in most adults, lowers mortality rates when consumed in safe quantities (Table 11-6). Other forms of alcohol, such as beer and spirits, do not offer health benefits that outweigh their risks.

Table 11-6: Safe Limits for Adult Alcohol Consumption

	Upper Limit for Safe Wine Consumption* (Red Wine; 12% alc/vol.)	Est. Peak Blood Alcohol Content
Men	One fluid ounce /35 pounds body weight 1.9 ml wine / kg body weight	0.03
Women	One fluid ounce /41 pounds body weight 1.6 ml wine / kg body weight	0.03
	Upper Limit for Safe Wine Consumption (Red Wine; 12% alc/vol.)	
Men	One fluid ounce /25 pounds body weight 2.5 ml wine / kg body weight	0.04
Women	One fluid ounce /30 pounds body weight 2 ml wine / kg body weight	0.04
	Upper Limit for Safe Beer Consumption (Beer; 5% alc/vol.)	
Men	One fluid ounce /11 pounds body weight 6 ml beer/ kg body weight	0.04
Women	One fluid ounces /13 pounds body weight 5 ml beer/ kg body weight	0.04

*Based on Wingate calculation using average total body water estimates of 58% for men and 49% for women. Rounded to facilitate ease of usage.

A transient peak alcohol level below 0.04 percent is probably insufficient to cause mood disorders or other health problems in most adults. Outside of pregnancy, most adults can safely consume this level on a daily basis without significant risk. It takes about 3 hours to clear a blood alcohol level of 0.04% in healthy individuals without slow ALDK alleles.

The pleasant, Goldilocks spot for alcohol consumption to relax with a glass of wine with friends is a bit below a BAC of 0.04 percent. Unless you don't mind occasional social blunders and revealing secrets, you probably want to keep it under 0.04 percent, closer to 0.03, a level at which alcohol gives a sense of relaxed well-being. The amount of red wine required to achieve a peak BAC level between

0.03 and 0.04 imparts little, if any risk of cancer in most populations, and may decrease overall mortality.

There are no legal requirements nor health demands to consume alcohol. It is safe however to enjoy small amounts and even to get a buzz from it if you like the stuff. If you don't, there are many other great ways to lower cancer and cardiovascular risk and other places to get polyphenolic compounds from the diet. If you only drink because you want the effects rendered by higher doses, and a "safe" level of drinking is not your bailiwick, don't bother imbibing.

If you want to drink wine occasionally or even daily, the levels of red wine consumption that don't cause illness and that may decrease disease risk for most people are given above. Everyone who likes you will like you better if you keep your peak BAC below 0.04%, except the someone trying to get your secrets or into your secret places. At twice this level you will not even like yourself. Much higher than that, you will likely not remember. Those having difficulty controlling their alcohol intake should avoid it.

Alcohol as a Sexual Lubricant

Even in marital relationships, alcohol is often employed, especially by women, to lower sexual inhibition or reluctance. Alcohol, however, suppresses the release of oxytocin, which is normally released during gentle touch, physical intimacy, and orgasm. Alcohol prevents oxytocin-induced promotion of emotional bonding, the experience of intimacy, and romance. Use of alcohol during intimate contact can reduce the appetite for future sexual pairing and thus reinforce the requirement for alcohol as a sexual lubrication. Without oxytocin to reinforce bonding, sexual activity can become mechanical and can lead to the failure of intimacy.

Excuses for Enjoying Red Wine

Red wines (consumed in moderation: three or four ounces per day) contain antioxidant polyphenols, which appear to prevent the oxidative damage caused by alcohol. Thus, of various alcoholic beverages consumed, red wines stand out as having low chronic toxicity. Rats given red wine do not have accelerated lipofuscin in their brains, compared to control rats. In contrast, rats given an equivalent amount of distilled alcohol have accelerated lipofuscin accumulation.[146]

Red wines, particularly Pinot Noir, Cabernet Sauvignon, Merlot, Egiodola, and Syrah varietals, are high in polyphenols such as catechins.[147] Red port wine, however, does not provide this benefit.[148] This may be a result of the early termination of fermentation in making port wines, preventing the processing of polyphenols into bioactive, absorbable forms. Tannins are large polyphenolic molecules and are not absorbed; however, fermentation promotes their decomposition into smaller, absorbable phenolic compounds.

Port and other sweet wines do not offer health benefits. This may be due to higher acetaldehyde and methanol levels in fortified and sweet wines, or secondary to their higher content of sugars. In an animal model, alcohol with a sugar content equivalent to that of port wine was significantly more damaging to the neurons than was the same amount of alcohol consumed alone.[149] This suggests that red wine should be consumed on its own, (not with dessert) or consumed with a meal to cause slower absorption, helping to mitigate peak alcohol levels, compared with the same quantity consumed on an empty stomach.

Summary for Wine

1. Alcohol is toxic. Red wine in moderation can be consumed by most adults without increased risk of chronic disease and may provide health benefits, including lower risk of heart disease and obesity. Moderation means limiting intake to no more than one ounce of red wine per 30 pounds of ideal body weight day per. Other forms of alcohol cannot be justified by health benefits. Sweet wines and port should not be considered as having health benefits. Wine and other forms of alcohol should not be consumed with sweets or desserts as this may increase the toxicity of alcohol.

2. Wine can increase the risk of migraines and pseudoallergic reactions: Wine contains sulfites that some individuals react to. Wine, depending on its fermentation, may contain biogenic amines that trigger migraines or block the enzymes that break down biogenic amines. Alcohol can inhibit these enzymes. Wines from California, for example, usually use bacteria specifically cultured to avoid production of bioamines, and thus may not provoke pseudoallergic reactions as much as wines using wild bacteria, such as traditionally used in Portugal. Foods consumed with wine, such as aged cheeses or salami, may contain biogenic amines, and alcohol can decrease the ability of the body's enzymes to break down these compounds. Foods consumed with alcohol may interact and provoke migraines or other pseudoallergic reactions.

3. Alcohol is a teratogen and a carcinogen: Alcohol should not be consumed, even in moderation, during pregnancy to avoid risk of injury to the child. Men should avoid heavy drinking for three months prior to a planned conception.

Alcohol is also a carcinogen, and if health is a concern, consumption should not exceed one ounce of red wine per 30 pounds ideal body weight a day for most individuals. Some high-risk individuals should avoid alcohol completely. Some of the effects of alcohol are caused by an increased production of oxygen free radicals. Trimethylglycine (TMG; betaine) a vitamin-like compound found in vegetables, may attenuate this risk.[150]

4. Red wine contains healthful phenol compounds: True. However, the amount per serving is less than found in chocolate, tea, coffee, plums, beans and many other foods. There is no unique health advantage to drinking wine that is not available with other foods. If red wine is enjoyed, consumption of moderate amounts is reasonable for many adults.

Alcohol Risk Summary:

Heavy alcohol consumption is a risk for several cancers, (Table 11-1) but light alcohol consumption very rarely is. Light to moderate consumption, particularly of red wine, is associated with a lower overall mortality rate, mostly because of a decreased risk of cardiovascular disease. If you enjoy a glass of red wine, there is not a health reason to avoid it other than during pregnancy, history of alcoholism, or known genetic susceptibility. Safe amounts of alcohol consumption that are not associated with elevated cancer risks in the general population are given above in Table 11-6.

Most of the risk of cancer associated with alcohol intake is linked to drinking to intoxication and when alcohol exposure is combined with other risk factors, such as tobacco use or infection, such as HPV and hepatitis.

The risk of breast cancer from alcohol exposure may be greatest for young women whose breasts are still developing, prior to a first pregnancy. This risk, as for other cancers, is likely from episodes of heavy drinking when there is a buildup of toxic metabolites such as acetaldehyde from the alcoholic beverages.

The earlier the exposure to heavy alcohol use, the the higher the risk of alcoholism is. Preteen exposure to intoxication creates a risk of chronic alcoholism many times higher than exposure during during adolescence. Risk of developing alcoholism for those introduced to alcohol as adults (over the age of 28) is significantly lower.

Table 11-7: Effects of Various Blood Alcohol Concentration Levels[151]

BAC %	Mood and Emotion	Motor Control
.01 - .02	Average person appears normal	
.02 - .03	Mild euphoria and loss of shyness. Mild relaxation or lightheadedness.	Subtle loss of coordination and slowing of reaction times that can be detected with testing tools.
.03 - .04	Relaxation. Lowered social inhibitions. Emotions become more explicit. Mild loss of judgment; reasoning skills may be impaired. Slight body warmth.	Mild decline in tracking moving objects and decline in multitasking ability.
.04 - .06	Impaired judgment and self-control. Caution, reason, and memory are impaired. Emotions are intensified; often euphoric. Increases desire to drink more. More body warmth.	Impaired concentration. Slowing of reaction times. Coordination and alertness lowered. Increased risk of collisions if driving.
.06 - .08	Mood swings. Behavior exaggerated, talking louder. Loss of inhibitions, sense of invincibility. Risky behaviors are likely. Impaired judgment	Less alert. Reduced coordination, reduced response to emergency situations. Difficulty with steering and tracking moving objects. May have difficulty focusing eyes.
.08 - .10	Severely impaired judgment and underestimated impairment. Bad choices. Poor memory.	Drunk driving in all of the U.S. Poor balance and motor skills. Impaired perception.
.10 - .13	May become aggressive and belligerent. Thinking is slow. Loss of self-control.	Difficulty staying in lane and braking to avoid accidents. Slurred speech. Staggering gait. Decreased peripheral and night vision.
.13 - .15	Anxiety and restlessness. Judgment and perception are severely impaired.	Blurred vision, further loss of muscle control.
.15 - .20	Dysphoria, confusion, nausea.	Sloppy drunk. Falls.
.20 - .25	Vomiting and risk of choking on vomit. Blackouts are likely. If injured, unlikely to seek care.	Pass out zone. Inability to walk unassisted. Vision falls from 20/20 to 20/200; legally blind.
> .25	Lack of comprehension of surroundings. Risk of death from asphyxiation or other injury. Likely to pass out or be in a stupor.	Risk of severe injury or death from falls or other accidents and from asphyxiation.
> .30	Stupor, hard to awaken. Death is possible.	Coma likely, high risk of death. Half of all people die with a BAC of 0.40

12: OBESITY

Most cancer is caused by things we put into our mouths. Most of this consists of cigarettes and other forms of tobacco, alcohol, and food. In the United States, a country where infection-related cancers are less common than much of the world, perhaps half of all cancer cases are from food. For most non-smokers, food is the major cause of cancer. In the chapters ahead, food specifics will be discussed, but here, it will be just food excess and a bit of how and why.

In the United States, excess body fat is estimated to account for 14 percent of all cancer deaths in men and 20 percent of cancer deaths in women. Obesity is additionally a risk factor for adult-onset diabetes, stroke and heart disease. It is almost easier to list the cancers that have not been associated with adiposity than those that have been. A list of some of the cancers associated with excess body fat is given in Table 12-1.[42]

Table 12-1: Cancers Associated with Obesity

Esophageal Cancer	Cervical Cancer	Liver Cancer
Gastric Cancer	Endometrial Cancer	Pancreatic Cancer
Gallbladder Cancer	Ovarian Cancer	Renal Cancer
Colon Cancer	Uterine Cancer	Multiple Myeloma
Rectal Cancer	Breast Cancer	Non-Hodgkin's Lymphoma
Prostate Cancer		

Overweight and obesity can be lumped together with other cancers caused by things we put into our mouths, although it is not entirely true. Obesity is caused by more than just too many French fries, or too much food. It is not just too many calories in or too few calories out (insufficient physical activity); lack of sleep and inflammation are important causes of obesity. Nevertheless, diet has large effects on the waistline.

Defining Obesity

In 1960, the prevalence of obesity in U.S. adults was 13.4%. By the late 1970's, 15% of adults were obese. As of 2010, 36% of adults and 17% of adolescents in the United States are obese.[152] Just since 1980, the prevalence of obesity in the U.S. has more than tripled, an average overweight person has gotten progressively heavier, and the obese population is far more obese than it previously had been. Since obesity is a risk for cancer, this means we will see a rise in obesity-related cancers.

One standard measure of obesity is the BMI, the body mass index. This index uses the formula:

$$\text{Weight in Kg} \div \text{Height in Meters}^2$$

A BMI from 18 to 24 is considered healthy, and indeed, women are considered to be most attractive with a BMI of 20. Individuals with a BMI over 25 are considered overweight, and those with a BMI over 30 are considered obese. Thus, a 5' 5" tall person weighing 125 pounds has a BMI of 20. If the same person weighed 180, they would have a BMI of 30. This metric is often used in studies but has some problems. A 5' 10" tall man weighing 185 pounds has a BMI of 26 and be considered overweight, but could also be a very healthy and muscular athlete or bodybuilder.

When doctors discuss obesity, we recognize that not all obesity is created equally; it's like apples and oranges, or in this case, apples and pears. When some people gain weight, they collect it mostly in the belly (apples), and others, especially some women, gain it on the hips (pears). Two people can have the same height, weight, and body fat mass, but one has a belly circumference greater than their hip circumference, and the other may have the waist narrower than the hips. "Apple" fat and "pear" fat do not impart the same risks.

A more revealing metric of obesity is the waist-hip ratio (WHR) (Figure 12-1) which is calculated as:

$$\text{Waist Circumference} \div \text{Hip Circumference}$$

In studies of heart disease, the WHR is far better at predicting risk for myocardial infarction than is the BMI. In one large study, the WHR was three times more accurate at identifying risk.[153] Fat mass within the abdominal walls, where the fat surrounds the organs in the body, is a much better predictor of metabolic risk. This fat is associated with a higher risk of diabetes, heart disease, and cancer. Excess fat on the outside of the body and on the hips (subcutaneous fat) has much less if even a significant impact on health than the fat surrounding the organs (visceral fat).

If you can pinch it, the fat is subcutaneous. The WHR, or even just the circumference of the waist alone, is a better measure of metabolically active intra-abdominal fat. Metabolic disease risk is lower when the waist circumference is less than 94 cm (37 inches) in men and less than 80 cm (31.5) inches in women. Men with a waist circumference over 102 cm (40 inches) are three times more likely to have hypertension than those with a circumference less than 94 cm (37 inches).[154]

An elevated WHR is referred to as abdominal obesity. The World Health Organization defines abdominal obesity as a WHR over 0.85 for women (larger hips) and over 0.90 for men. Women are considered most attractive (and most fertile) in most cultures when they have a WHR of 0.7.

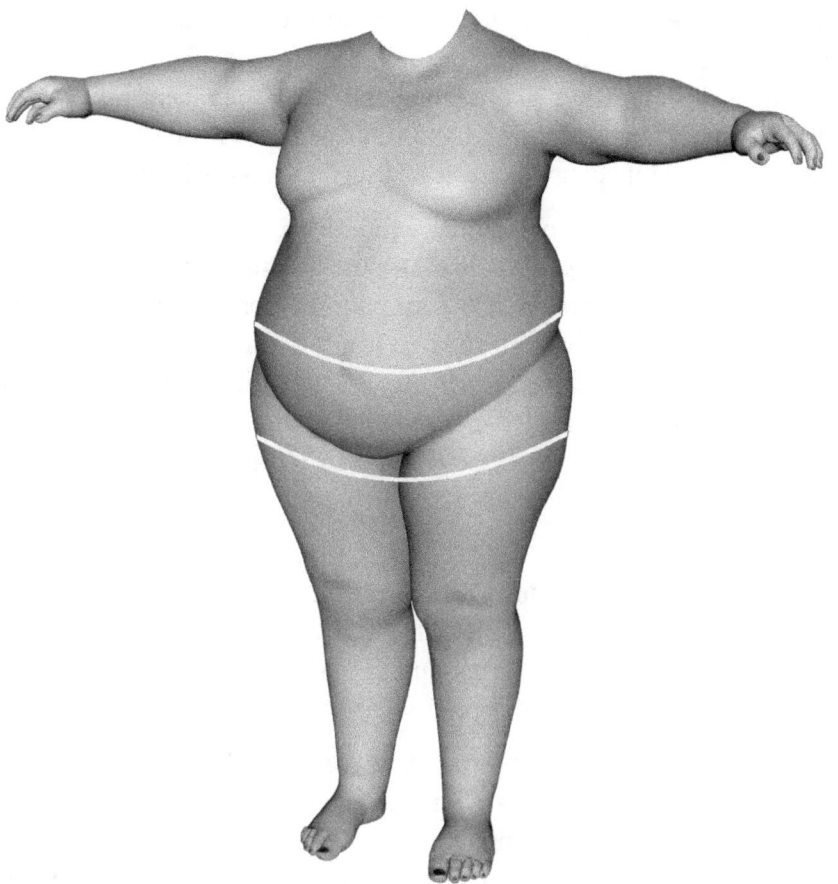

Figure 12-1: Waist-hip ratio

Different studies use different measures of obesity, so it can be difficult to compare their results. The most accurate measure for epidemiologic studies of obesity and disease risk might be to use abdominal MRI to quantify a visceral fat to ideal body mass ratio. A measuring tape, however, works very well.

Obesity and Breast Cancer

For *premenopausal* breast cancer, BMI has not been found to be a risk factor in most studies. WHR and waist circumference, however, are associated with premenopausal breast cancer. Compared with women with a waist less than 80 cm (31.5 inches), women with waists from 81 to 88 cm (31.9 to 34.6 inches) had a 56 percent increased risk of breast cancer.[155] In the Nurses' Health Study II, women in the top 20% for waist circumference were 2.75 times as likely to develop estrogen-receptor negative (ER-) breast cancer as were the 20 percent with the thinnest waists.[156]

As importantly, gaining weight is a risk factor for breast cancer mortality among these women. Women who are diagnosed with premenopausal breast cancer that gained more than 35 pounds since the age of twenty were twice as likely to die from breast cancer as those who gained less than 13 pounds. Overweight does not increase the chances of getting premenopausal breast cancer, but it does increase the chances of dying from it, as well as for death from other causes. It may not "cause" cancer as much as makes it grow.

Obesity has been consistently found to be a risk factor for developing *postmenopausal* breast cancer. The BMI at age twenty does not seem to have as much impact on postmenopausal breast cancer risk, but weight gain during adulthood does, and even more so, weight gain after the age of fifty. A 28 pound (12.7 kg) weight gain after the age of fifty nearly triples the risk of death from postmenopausal breast cancer[157]. Each 10 cm (4 inches) increase in waist circumference increases postmenopausal breast cancer risk by 13 percent.

Like other women, those women who are at increased breast cancer risk from having BRCA1 or BRCA2 mutations, have no increase in premenopausal risk due to obesity; however, weight gain does increase their postmenopausal cancer risk[158].

Weight loss in BRCA1 and BRCA2 mutation carriers does, however, lower risk. Women who were overweight at age eighteen, who lost more than 10 pounds of body weight between the ages of 18 and 30, lowered their risk of being diagnosed with breast cancer between the ages of 30 and 40 by a third. For those with a BRCA1 mutation, who are at very high risk of breast cancer, the risk was lowered by two-thirds. Two of three breast cancer diagnoses between the ages of 30 to 40 were avoided by a 10-pound weight loss!

In a study of breast cancer patients, patients with a WHR of 0.84 or greater had a 50% higher risk of death than thinner women.[159] In this study, BMI was not statistically predictive of mortality. This suggests that risk is associated with visceral fat.

Moreover, women who gain weight after the diagnosis of breast cancer had worse outcomes. In the Nurses' Health Study, women diagnosed with breast cancer that gained from 0.5 to 2.0 BMI points (an average of six pounds) had a 35 percent increase in death within the nine-year follow-up period. Those that gained more than two BMI points had an average 65 percent increased risk of death.[160]

How about diet and *weight loss* after the diagnosis of breast cancer? We know these women are still at risk of new cancers, but does losing weight lower the risk of death from cancer or prevent the development of new cancers?

The Nurses' Health Study also provides us with information on this. Only women with invasive breast cancer were included in this study; those whose cancers that were diagnosed and treated before it became invasive and those with metastatic disease were excluded. Those maintaining the "prudent diet," one low in fat and high in fruits and vegetables, did not have a reduction in breast cancer mortality.[161] In another study, dietary fat intake did not affect breast cancer survival, but those eating more protein had a higher survival – however, red meat was not helpful.[162]

Intentional weight loss has been demonstrated in several interventional trials of women with breast cancer.[163] As you can imagine, these individuals are motivated. No survival outcome is yet available from these studies. Nevertheless, the increased estrogen, insulin, and leptin, along with decreased sex hormone binding globulin (SHBG) concentrations seen in overweight women with breast cancer, factors thought to promote breast cancer recurrence, have been shown to respond to weight loss.[164]

Unintentional weight loss after a breast cancer diagnosis is associated with a 40% increase in mortality.[163] This finding almost certainly results from cachexia (wasting associated with disease). Cachexia is induced by leptin and cytokines such as TNF-α, IL-6, and interferon which result from the immune response to severe disease. It is cancer causing the weight loss, rather than the weight loss promoting cancer growth.

Pancreatic Cancer

Obesity and being overweight are risk factors for pancreatic cancer. A meta-analysis of over 800,000 individuals in various follow-up studies found that obese individuals (BMI over 30) were 47 percent more likely to develop pancreatic cancer. It also found that risk 30 percent higher among individuals who were overweight during early adulthood. Furthermore, in addition to the risk incurred from being overweight at a younger age, there was an increased risk of pancreatic cancer for those gaining more than 5 BMI points, with a 40 percent increase in risk for those gaining 10 BMI points.[165] It is central obesity that is most strongly associated with pancreatic cancer risks. Waist circumference and WHR were both associated with risk, with a seven percent increase in risk for every 10 cm (four inches) in waist circumference.[166]

Prostate Cancer and Obesity

Being obese or overweight is a risk factors for prostate cancer. Men with a BMI of 27.5 were at a 44% increased risk compared to men with a BMI of 22.5.[167]

Obesity at the time of prostatectomy, the surgical removal of the prostate for the treatment of prostate cancer, is associated with a higher risk of cancer recurrence. Furthermore, weight gain around the time of diagnosis also increases the risk of recurrence. Men who gained more than 2.2 kg (@ 5 pounds) during the 5 years prior to or one year after prostatectomy had nearly twice the risk of prostate cancer recurrence, while men who had intentional weight loss had reduced risk of cancer recurrence.[168] This suggests that the mechanisms causing and maintaining obesity may be as or more important than that fat itself. Gaining one pound of body mass per year nearly doubles prostate cancer recurrence. The same factors that are fueling fat accumulation are fueling cancer growth.

Even after the diagnosis of prostate cancer, intentional weight loss appears to lower the risk of recurrence.

Prostate cancer shares several risk factors with metabolic syndrome, a major risk factor for Type 2 diabetes and cardiovascular disease. Metabolic syndrome is the combination of obesity, impaired glucose tolerance, hyperinsulinemia, elevated cholesterol and triglyceride levels, and inflammation. Metabolic syndrome is associated with unhealthy dietary habits and caloric excess, lack of physical activity, and poor quality sleep.

When the fat cells get full, they become lazy and less responsive to insulin. This is called insulin resistance. Insulin helps regulate blood sugar by increasing the uptake of blood sugar (glucose) by the muscles and other tissues. Insulin is the hormone that tells fat cells to consume glucose and turn it into fat. Insulin resistance impedes glucose uptake from the blood, and thus raises the blood sugar level; the pancreas responds by increasing insulin output. This increases the blood insulin level causing hyperinsulinemia, and other metabolic disturbances. As the fat cells get more numerous (they divide when they get too big) and more resistant, the pancreas has to continually work harder, but eventually it can't keep up, and gets burned-out. When the insulin output of the pancreas can no longer drive the blood sugar level down to a normal level, type 2 diabetes occurs.

High insulin levels and high blood sugar may both be causes of cancer. High blood sugar levels are pro-inflammatory and help activate NF-κB. High fructose levels are likely even more inflammatory, as excess fructose can only be stored as fat.

Insulin also acts as a growth hormone; it signals the availability of energy resources for cell growth. Insulin-like Growth Factor-1 (IGF-1) is another growth factor whose level increases in metabolic syndrome. These growth factors signal cells with growth factor receptors for these hormones to grow (multiply). Unfortunately, these growth receptors are present on cancer cells, and it makes them grow too.

Obesity and high-fat diets are also often accompanied by leptin resistance. Leptin is a regulatory hormone produced by fat cells (adipocytes). When the fat cells have a full tank, leptin inhibits hunger and increases the utilization of fat to fuel the body's energy needs. When the fat content of adipocytes falls, leptin levels fall, causing increased hunger. Leptin acts as a slow-acting, long-term regulator of hunger to help regulate body fat content.

Obese individuals and those eating a high-fat diet, however, stop responding normally to leptin. They become leptin resistant. Even though leptin levels should suppress the appetite and promote the utilization of fat for fuel, the body stops responding to it normally.

Diets high in fructose also cause leptin resistance[169]. A high fructose diet induces the production of the inflammatory cytokine Tumor Necrosis Factor-alpha (TNF-α).[170] This cytokine causes leptin and insulin resistance in the hypothalamus, fat cells, and muscle cells.[171, 172] In older animals with leptin resistance, any diet will cause increased feeding and obesity.[173]

Sleep

Sleep deprivation also increases insulin and leptin resistance. Not only that, sleep deprivation increases ghrelin, a hormone that increases appetite. Ghrelin is released from the GI tract when blood sugar levels fall. It promotes the selection of food indulgences: sweets and foods with high palatability, including those high in saturated fats, which tend to be associated with obesity. Ghrelin not only increases cravings for comfort foods but, since it acts through dopamine reward pathways in the brain, it also increases the desire for alcohol and other substances of abuse.[174] [175]

Sleep deprivation is a cause of obesity. A meta-analysis of 45 studies including over a half a million subjects from around the world found that children who sleep less than ten hours a day are 1.89 times as likely to be obese than children who get more sleep, and adults who get less than six hours sleep are about 1.55 times as likely to be obese than adults who get more than six hours of sleep.[176]

Sleep deprivation, including sleep disturbances from sleep apnea, such as in heavy snorers, increases insulin and leptin resistance and inflammation. Since obesity promotes snoring and poor quality sleep, and sleep deficits promote leptin and insulin resistance that promote obesity, there is a vicious cycle of sleep deprivation and obesity. Sleep deprivation also causes increased levels of several inflammatory cytokines, including IL-1β and IL-6,[177] which are risk factors for cancer.

Just as with hepatitis B, schistosomiasis, or chronic osteomyelitis, chronic inflammation raises the risk of cancer. Obesity is an inflammatory condition, and chronic inflammation is a risk for many cancers. High-fat diets can cause increased inflammation and induce the production of the inflammatory cytokines IL-1β and TNF-α in the gastrointestinal system.[178]

Inflammation causes oxidative stress and increases the risk of DNA errors. Certain inflammatory signals prevent apoptosis of compromised cells that later give rise to cancer. Inflammatory signals can also divert the immune system away from surveillance against mutant cells. The immune system likes to fight its wars on a single front. When it equips itself to fight parasites, it will be less prepared to battle bacterial infections or mutant domestic terrorist cells. Inflammatory signals can divert the immune system's attention away from the elimination of tumor cells.

In addition to elevated insulin levels, obesity is also associated with higher levels of the hormone IGF-1 (Insulin-like Growth Factor). IGF-1, as the name says, is a growth hormone. IGF-1 may work synergistically with other hormones, such as androgens and estrogens, and growth factors to further promote cell proliferation. IGF-1 and IGF-2 help us grow tall and strong; we need growth hormones when we are young and growing, but not so much when we have passed our twenties and are done growing. The problem is that IGF-1 helps cancer cells grow. This may explain why tall women are at higher risk for breast and other cancers.[158] Insulin and IGF-1 both exert mitogenic effects, stimulating cell proliferation and inhibiting apoptosis of cancer cells.[179]

Avoiding Obesity Lowers the Risk of Cancer

If weight loss was easy, only sumo wrestlers would be fat. Very few people want to be obese. I made a promise earlier in this book not to waste your time and energy with therapies suited only to saints and warriors.

Take a look around; a third of the U.S. population is overweight or obese. Seventy years of dieting advice, telling people to count and restrict calories, has not worked. This will not change tomorrow. The only guarantee caloric restriction can give you is that it will make you hungry, miserable, and irritable, and then, any weight loss will be temporary. It is a well-tested strategy that has failed consistently. In the piggy bank theory of thermodynamics, there are calories in and calories burned. Too many in, and they get stored as fat. Too few burned, they sit and collect. While true, it does not explain why people consume excess calories.

There are 3500 Calories in a pound of fat. If a person or animal consumes 10 extra Calories a day for a year, that would add 3650 calories, just over a pound's worth. Over 20 years, those 10 calories a day would add 21 pounds of body weight; not an unusual weight gain between the ages of 20 and 40. But how does the body regulate appetite so closely that less than one mouthful of food difference can make a 20-pound weight gain? For tens of thousands of years, humans did not get middle age central obesity. Before the 1960's, most people could get buried in the suit they got married in. The body has redundant systems to maintain energy homeostasis. We probably need to mess up several of these systems to become obese.

Some of the reasons for weight gain include excess fructose, hydrogenated fats, televisions, and less physical activity. Fructose, sleep deprivation, and less physical activity all support chronic inflammation which causes subtle, or not so subtle increases in appetite. In Table 13-1, you may notice that watching television has a significantly lower metabolic cost than does sitting at a desk or reading. Additionally, many people spend their hours watching TV as a recreational activity, often munching on fattening snacks. Even if this time was spent socializing, just talking with friends, the metabolic expenditure difference would be much higher than 10 calories a day. A 70 kg man quietly sitting at a desk doing paperwork burns 35 Calories an hour more than he does watching television. Additionally, television is a common sleep sucker; many people exchange sleep time for TV time, fall into a poor quality sleep with the TV going, and delay sleep onset as a result of the light from TV.

One hour of TV a day, much less than our national average, reduces caloric expenditures enough to add three pounds of fat a year, as compared to sitting and reading for that hour.

Metabolic Syndrome

Metabolic syndrome describes the common cluster of metabolic disorders including visceral obesity, hypertension, hyperlipidemia, elevated uric acid, systemic inflammation, and insulin resistance that puts people at high risk for type 2 diabetes, cardiovascular disease, stroke, gout, and by the way, hepatocellular, colorectal, breast,[180] prostate,[181] pancreatic,[182] and other cancers.

Disease risk reduction should not focus on obesity or weight loss, but rather on the inflammatory and metabolic disturbances that cause obesity. Obesity and weight gain are red flags that a metabolic disturbance that raises cancer risk is present. It is this underlying problem that should be addressed. If the underlying problem is resolved, weight loss will likely follow. This requires that inflammatory cytokines, insulin, blood sugar, leptin, and IGF-1 levels be normalized. Insulin and leptin resistance need to be reversed.

The more than doubling of liver cancer rates among the obese appears to be mediated by the inflammatory cytokines IL-6 and TNF.[183] These cytokines also promote other cancers. Insulin-like growth factor 1 (IGF-1) is also elevated in metabolic syndrome, and it promotes cell proliferation and survival by inhibiting apoptosis, via activation of phosphatidylinositol 3-kinase (PI3K)/Akt signaling pathway.[180]

The accumulation of fat surrounding the viscera is associated with insulin and leptin resistance and chronically elevated IL-6 levels. When blood samples of veins draining the viscera are collected from obese patients during surgery, the IL-6 level is 50% higher than it is from their peripheral blood and leptin levels are lower.[184] What would happen if a large portion of this fat was surgically removed? This experiment has actually been done and results published by at least five research groups. In these studies, obese patients underwent gastric bypass surgery, and some patients were randomly selected for additional resection of intra-abdominal fat. In each of these studies, there were no significant differences in adipose cytokine level or insulin sensitivity after removal of the fat.[185][186][187]

These negative results strongly suggest that it is not the abdominal fat or obesity that is the risk factor for diabetes, heart disease, metabolic and inflammatory disease, and cancer. Rather, the processes that stimulate fat accumulation and boost obesity cause these diseases. Obesity is a result of the same risk factors that cause these diseases. Visceral obesity is associated with elevated risk of cancer but does not cause it. It is the process that counts. If a severely obese person loses weight over a few weeks, they remain severely obese, but their inflammatory profiles improve dramatically.[188] The opposite occurs during weight gain.

Fructose

Fructose is a sugar found in fruit. It also makes up half the weight and half the calories of table sugar (sucrose), with glucose comprising the other half. Until the Caribbean colonialization and its sugarcane plantations, humans did not consume much fructose. Even the old breeds of apple trees, such as those sold by Johnny Appleseed, bore tart, cider apples with much lower fructose content than modern varieties bred for sweetness.

Nowadays, it is not uncommon for people to consume 20 percent of their daily caloric intake as fructose. Fructose, like other nutrients, is mainly metabolized in the liver as it is absorbed directly from the intestine, although fructose is absorbed somewhat more slowly. In the liver, fructose is used to replenish glycogen stores. Problems, however, occur when the amount of fructose in a meal exceeds the amount the liver utilizes. Blood fructose levels are generally about one-tenth those of blood glucose levels after a meal that contains equal parts of glucose and fructose. Other than the fructose that enters the bloodstream, most of the excess fructose in the liver is converted to glucose or lactose. These can be used for fuel by other organs and tissues. About 7 percent is converted to glycerol, which can form the backbone for fats or be used as fuels, and about one percent can be converted into fatty acids.[189]

In the hypothalamus, the area of the brain that controls hunger, glucose oxidation promotes the formation of the energy transfer molecule, ATP. Plentiful ATP inhibits the enzyme AMPK, and this, in turn, allows malonyl-CoA to be formed. In the hypothalamus, malonyl-CoA causes a fall in the production of the pro-hunger hormones NPY and AgRP and a rise in the hormones α-MSH and CART that decrease hunger. Thus, after eating, glucose from the meal decreases hunger hormones and provides satiation.

Fructose is metabolized differently in the brain than in most other tissues. The hypothalamus lacks the enzyme phosphofructose kinase-1, forcing an alternate metabolic pathway for fructose oxidation that depletes ATP and activates AMPK. Thus, in the hypothalamus, fructose increases appetite by depleting ATP and thereby shifting the production of hormones to those cause hunger and suppressing those that provide satiation.[190]

Fructose is sweeter than glucose, making it more pleasant. The pancreas does not release insulin in response to it. It is absorbed slightly more slowly from the intestine. A small fraction of fructose that exceeds the immediate needs of the liver is turned into fat. Fructose decreases and delays satiation. Remember, it only takes 10 extra calories of Calories of food a day, less than a small spoonful to add a pound of fat to the body a year. How many bites can get added to a meal, when satiation is delayed by a couple of minutes?

When there is excess fructose, in the liver it can deplete ATP, and this promotes the formation of uric acid. Elevated uric acid levels cause mitochondrial oxidative stress not just in the liver where they form, but also in other tissues. Uric acid causes the mitochondria to export citrate that is then converted to fat. Additionally, the formation of uric acid from fructose increases the activity of the enzyme AMPD, which inhibits AMPK. Inhibition of AMPK prevents the cell from utilizing fat as a fuel, thus causing fat accumulation.[191]

Uric acid is a multiple bad actor. When elevated, it increases oxidative stress. Uric acid stimulates MAPK, ERK, AP-1, and NF-κB and thereby TNF-α and IL-6. It raises c-reative protein (CRP) production that increases inflammation. It also stimulates appetite by decreasing adiponectin and ghrelin, and it may promote leptin resistance. It can also impair the homeostatic sleep drive.[192] Elevation of uric acid thus pushes towards inflammation and survival and proliferation of cancer cells. Many of the pro-obesity and pro-cancer effects of fructose are mediated by uric acid.

> Many whole fruits, especially oranges and berries, contain phenolic compounds, including luteolin, kaempferol, quercetin, and myricetin have been found to inhibit xanthine oxidase, the enzyme that processes the last two steps in uric acid production.[193] These phenolic compounds also prevent the formation of superoxide radicals by xanthine oxidase. Cherries have been used as a folk remedy for the prevention of gout; its efficacy is likely based on these actions. The phenolic compounds present in many fruits may mitigate the production of uric acid.

Rats fed a high fructose diet develop fatty liver, insulin resistance, hypertriglyceridemia (high blood fat levels), and elevated blood pressure, whereas rats fed the same caloric intake of glucose or starch do not. Even when there is no overall excess caloric intake, diets high in fructose intake cause uric acid production with stimulation of inflammatory mediators and inflammatory injury to the pancreatic islets cells responsible for the formation and release of insulin.[194] In humans, consumption of beverages high in fructose causes accumulation of visceral fat and of fat in the liver and muscles.[195] Consumption of high fructose beverages can raise uric acid levels within an hour.[196] Just as elevated blood glucose levels cause organ damage, high blood fructose levels cause the degradation of ATP in the liver and the formation of uric acid. This occurs when intake exceeds the amounts that can be quickly utilized.

It is the peak levels of fructose after meals that elevates triglycerides and uric acid.[197] The effect is much stronger for large doses of rapidly absorbed forms of fructose, such as those from fruit juice or sweetened beverages.

High levels of fructose intake can induce metabolic syndrome with elevations in uric acid and blood pressure, insulin resistance, hepatic lipid accumulation of fat and hyperlipidemia in only two weeks.[198] Lots of fructose is great if you are a bear, and want to put on a nice insulating coat of fat in preparation for a long, cold, winter hibernation. It's not so great for the rest of us. Consuming a high-fat diet can promote leptin resistance within four weeks.

Summary: Preventing Obesity and its Risks

Remember that obesity is not a personality defect. Calorie restriction diets only succeed at making people hungry. They do not cause sustained weight loss and do not treat the underlying causes of appetite imbalances. Obesity is a metabolic, not a moral disease. Willpower will not overcome this disease. However, educated lifestyle choices that help correct abnormal hunger signaling from the brain may be helpful.

- Avoid high-fat diets. (For the skinny, read Chapter 25)
- Avoid high intake of beer. It's called a beer belly for a reason.
- Avoid sweet beverages.
- Limit fructose intake.
- Get sufficient sleep.
- Engage in vigorous exercise.

Limit fructose intake to less than 10 percent of the ideal dietary caloric intake. This limits fructose to three Calories per kg of ideal body weight (IBW) a day.[199] Here are IBW formulas for adults over five feet tall:

> Males: IBW = 50 kg + 2.3 kg for each inch over 5 feet.
> Females: IBW = 45 kg + 2.3 kg for each inch over 5 feet.

Thus, a 5' 4" tall woman has an ideal body weight of 54.2 kg (119.5 lbs), and a recommended daily fructose limit of 163 Calories, equivalent to about 40.5 grams of fructose.

Individuals with metabolic syndrome or a waist circumference more than 94 cm (37 inches) for men or more than 80 cm (31.5) inches for women should limit their fructose intake to two Calories per kilogram of IBW.

One level teaspoon of table sugar (sucrose) contains two grams (8 Calories) of fructose, and a heaping teaspoon contains about three grams of fructose. A typical 20 oz. soft drink contains about 36 grams of fructose, nearing the recommended daily limit for a 5' 4" tall woman. This is roughly the amount of fructose found in three apples, 5 bananas, or nine cups of strawberries. Apples have been bred for sweetness and are higher in fructose than most other fruits. Apple juice has similar fructose content to that of soda pop. Apple juice is not a health food. It causes obesity, even in infants.

Nutrients from beverages are absorbed more quickly than from solid foods, raising peak glucose and fructose levels higher, and increasing insulin output. Avoid sweet beverages, especially those with high levels of fructose, such as fruit juices and soda pop.

Eating whole fruits is different from drinking fruit juice. Whole fruits contain fiber and are digested more slowly than juices and soda pop are. This slows their digestion, helps prevent a rapid rise in blood fructose levels that raise uric acid levels, and slows the return of hunger.

> Individuals with metabolic syndrome, gout, obesity or type 2 diabetes, and attempting to lower IGF-1 levels because of cancer may benefit by substituting table sugar with dextrose. Dextrose is pure glucose, and raises blood sugar, but does not contain fructose. It is about 75% as sweet as sucrose, and thus more is needed for sweetening, and recipes, especially for baking, usually need to be modified for its use. It should give quicker satiety than fructose. Dextrose can be purchased at beer brewing stores or online.

Get plenty of quality sleep. Insufficient sleep stimulates the release of ghrelin, a hormone that increases the appetite for soft, palatable, high-caloric foods that are easy to overeat. A typical adult, healthy sleeper needs eight hours in bed and 7.5 hours of sleep each night to get sufficient sleep. If an adult needs more than nine hours of sleep a night to feel well rested, they most likely have poor quality sleep and should be assessed by a doctor familiar with sleep disturbances.

Exercise: Read the following chapter. Much of the cancer-related risk associated with obesity can be prevented with the right kind of exercise.

13: Exercise

Leisure time may seem like a good way to recuperate from cancer, but patients with colorectal cancer who had more than six hours of leisure time a day to sit and relax and recuperate (likely watching TV) had a 27 percent increase in mortality.[200] Who would have guessed?

In contrast, female colorectal cancer patients who engaged in more than 18 MET-hours of physical activity per week (4.5 hours of brisk walking) had a 61 percent decline in cancer mortality as compared to women who did less than 3 MET-hours of activity. Increasing activity levels after the diagnosis was also associated with a 52 percent decline in colorectal cancer deaths and a 49 percent decline in all deaths.[201] In a study of men with colorectal cancer, the findings were similar, except that men required 27 MET-hours of activity to achieve a 50% decline in cancer deaths.

> What is a MET? A MET is a metabolic equivalent of the energy consumed while one is awake and at rest. Walking at slow pace doubles the body's use of energy and oxygen consumption; thus slow walking uses about 2 METs per hour. A standard MET is one kilocalorie (kcal) per kilogram of body mass per hour. Table 13-1 shows the typical MET costs of various activities. During sleep, we burn about 0.92 METs. Thus, a sedentary, 70 kg man, sleeping 8 hours a day, would burn 515 kcal during sleep and 1120 during wakefulness, for a total of 1635 kcal a day.
>
> This standard was based on healthy non-obese young people. Older and heavier persons use slightly more energy per kilogram of body weight to perform the same activities.[202]
>
> A kcal is called a Calorie or Cal by nutritionists. A physiologist's kcal is 1000 (lower case c) calories or cal, just to clear up that confusion.

Women in the highest quartile of exercise, after the diagnosis of breast cancer, also have an about 50 percent decrease in mortality. The level of exercise prior to the diagnosis is only associated with a 23 percent decrease in mortality. For every 10 METs of exercise per week breast cancer patients did after their diagnosis breast cancer, mortality fell by 16 percent, and total mortality fell by 24 percent.[203]

If a physically active person develops cancer, it indicates that their level of activity was insufficient to overcome their other risks. Increasing activity after the diagnosis of colorectal cancer lowers the risk of death from the disease.

Table 13-1: Activity Metabolic Equivalents[204]

Physical Activity	METS
Sleep	0.92
Watching television	1
Sitting in church	1.3
Working at a desk	1.5
Cooking	2
Washing dishes	2
Walking 1.7 mph (2.7 km/h) on level ground	2.3
Shopping	2.3
Typical indoor work in education, hospitality, health services, where person is active in light activities	2.5
Mowing lawn with a riding mower	2.5
Walking, level surface 2.5 mph (4 km/h)	3
Vacuuming	3.3
Walking level surface 3.0 mph (4.8 km/h) (20 min/mile)	3.5
Mopping	3.5
Typical construction, logging, and mining work	3.9
Bicycling < 10 mph (16 km/h) leisurely for pleasure	4
Gardening	4
Walking firm, level surface 3.5 mph (5.6 km/h) (17 min/mile)	4.3
Mowing lawn, pushing a power mower	4.5
Dancing	4.8
Walking firm, level surface 4 mph (15 min/mile)	5
Golf; walking and pulling clubs	5.3
Stationary bike, 100 watts	5.5
Playing basketball	6
Jogging 4 mph (15 min/mile) (6.4 km/h)	6
Mowing lawn, pushing an unpowered mower	6
Hiking, cross country	6
Tennis	7.3
Walking firm, level surface 5 mph (12 min/mile)	8.3
Running 5 mph (12 min/mile) (8 km/h)	8.3
Running 6 mph (10 min/mile) (9.7 km/h)	9.8
Playing soccer	10
Running 7 mph (8.6 min/mile) (11.3 km/h)	11
Running 8 mph (7.5 min/mile) (12.9 km/h)	11.8
Running 9 mph (6.7 min/mile) (15.5 km/h)	12.8
Running 10 mph (6 min/mile) (16 km/h)	14.5
Running 12 mph (5 min/mile) (19.3 km/h)	19
Running 14 mph (4.3 min mile) (22.5 km/h)	23

Many studies of exercise and cancer have suggested that there is a benefit from exercise but fail to achieve statistical significance. Are we asking the right questions when it comes to exercise? Most studies have looked at METs of exercise per week. One may take 14 hours of leisurely strolls (3 × 14 = 42 METs) or play soccer for 4 hours a week (10 × 4) and burn about 40 METs. But, even when we are not exercising, we still have to breathe. If you calculate exercise METs as METs above baseline, for example, above working at a desk (1.5 METS), these calculations yeild 1.5 × 14 = 21 for the walking and 4 × 8.5 = 34 for the soccer cited above. The first calculation would tell about theamount of calories burned per week; if total calorie use was sufficient to explain the difference in cancer, this would be enough. If the exercise intensity needed to reduce cancer progression has a higher threshold, the difference between these two exercises may be even greater.

Physical activity has been found to decrease the risk of cancer progression in men with prostate cancer. Men who, after the diagnosis of prostate cancer, walked on average more than 3 miles a day (a brisk walk, more quickly than 3 mph) had a 66 percent decline in cancer recurrence. While even moderate physical activity was found to lower total mortality rate in men after the diagnosis of prostate cancer, *non-vigorous activity was not associated with a decline in prostate cancer progression.* Non-vigorous exercise, even one and a half hours a day, 10.5 hours a week, did not slow or stop prostate cancer progression. Walking, even when walking more than an hour each day, did not reduce the risk of cancer progression in men with localized prostate cancer if the pace was less than 3 mph. Five hours of vigorous physical exercise a week appears to be three times more effective in lowering prostate cancer death than 15 hours of non-vigorous exercise. Even the weak effect in men doing 15 hours of non-vigorous may have been from the occasional hill or staircase they encountered that pushed their normal routine to a higher level. Men who walked 3 or more hours a week at a quicker pace than 3 mph had a nearly 50 percent reduction in cancer progression.[205] [206]

Let me reiterate: In men with prostate cancer, moderate levels of non-vigorous exercise decrease the risk of death due to heart disease and other causes but decrease neither cancer progression nor the risk of cancer death. The intensity of exercise required to put a dent in cancer is probably limited to exercise performed at levels of above 3 METs per hour. Below this level, there seems to be minimal if any benefit.

If you just went for a walk and took any more than an hour to walk three miles, get back out there and do it right! You need to do it in less than 50 minutes! Vigorous exercise, 6 METs per hour or higher, is even more efficient at decreasing the risk of cancer.

The baseline MET threshold required to drive a reduction of cancer progression is likely at least 3 METS per hour. The 14 hours of walking per week, discussed above, may give close to zero MET hours above the threshold effect while the four hours of soccer may produce 28 MET hours above baseline.

Tennis, biking, rowing, and running are all vigorous exercises. Hiking through fields and hillsides is as well. If you want to increase the MET level, add a backpack and some hills to climb. Choose the exercises you enjoy! Golf may be pleasant, but it is not vigorous exercise, especially if you have a caddy and a golf cart.

Vigorous exercise gets you breathing harder. You may be able to carry on a conversation, but you will need to catch your breath between phrases. If you are not getting your heart and respiratory rate up, you are not effectively reducing cancer risk.

How Does Exercise Work?

At the beginning of the book, I promised to make things easy. But to do that I need to make things complicated first. Here, by easy, I mean accessible. Who has time to do 15 hours of exercise a week? How many of us have the time or energy to do five hours of vigorous exercise a week as adults? What if 9 minutes a week were enough? Could you commit to that? To achieve the most benefit from the least physical work, one needs to understand how to get the most benefit from our exercise.

There are several reasons that exercise fights cancer.

Exercise does a lot more than just burning calories that might otherwise be stored as fat. It actually helps prevent obesity.

Insulin and IGF-1 become elevated in obesity, and these hormones enhance tumor growth and inhibit apoptosis. Men in the highest quartile for endogenous insulin production were 2.4 times more likely to die from prostate cancer as compared to men in the lowest quartile. Exercise improves insulin sensitivity found with visceral obesity, lowers insulin and IGF-1 levels, and also increases IGF-binding protein-1 that decreases IGF-1 activity.

Exercise also causes a transient elevation of inflammatory cytokines, including IL-6 and TNF-α.[207] TNF-α can help to trigger apoptosis. IL-6 can either promote or impede apoptosis depending on its level, interactions with other cytokines, and cell activity. IL-6 is pro-inflammatory, and increased levels are seen in many inflammatory conditions as well as in obesity. During exercise, IL-6 can increase 100-fold.[208] But following exercise, an acute, very high IL-6 level is followed by the sustained reduction in IL-6 levels. IL-6 promotes cell proliferation and inhibits apoptosis of prostate and other cancer cells in cell cultures.[206]

Additionally, exercise increases adiponectin levels that promote apoptosis. Among men with prostate cancer, those with the highest adiponectin levels had a 61 percent lower risk of dying from prostate cancer as compared to men with lower levels.[206]

When serum from the blood of 60-year-old men who participated in exercise was added to prostate cancer cell cultures, it doubled the p53 content in the cells, slowed the tumor cell growth and increased apoptosis by 3.7 times in comparison to serum from sedentary men.[209]

Physical activity also helps activate the immune system. In breast cancer, exercise was associated with improved function of natural killer cells, cells that attack cancer.[203]

Exercise also promotes the culling of old, worn-out mitochondria (mitophagy), and development of more vigorous ones. Exercise promotes the turnover of aging intracellular proteins and organelles (autophagy), renewing the machinery of the cell. Young, healthy mitochondria produce fewer oxygen and nitrogen radicals that damage cell proteins, in contrast to leaky old geezers. They are thus less likely to promote the intracellular oxidative damage to the DNA that causes cancer. Old, poorly functioning mitochondria are a central cause of cellular senescence and the aging process.

Healthy cells with efficient mitochondria depend on oxidative respiration for energy rather than inefficient glycolysis. Tumor cells mainly depend on glycolysis for energy as this allows growth of tumor cells in low oxygen environments. It may not be the vibrant, healthy mitochondria that slow cancer progression, but rather factors that promote healthy mitochondria also promote elimination of cancer cells.

Go Slow! Several new terms are being introduced. Don't worry. You don't need to memorize or understand all the details here; just focus on ATP, AMPK and p53 and how they interact with other molecules. Get familiar with the concept of glycolysis, and ATP, AMPK, and p53, as they will be important for understanding cancer development and prevention and treatment in coming chapters. It may take a couple of readings to understand this and see where it is going. Take it slowly.

ATP: The cell's energy source molecule. All work done by the cell, building new chemical compounds and protein, transport of molecules against a gradient, movement, is powered by ATP. ATP is like electricity running all the electrical devices in your home; you can use solar, wind, or gas generators, but they run off electricity. We get energy from carbohydrates, fats, and protein, but use them to generate ATP.

AMPK: AMP-activated protein kinase. This protein acts as a bookkeeper that lets the cell know when it has resources for adding a new bedroom, or when it is broke and needs to hold a garage sale to pay the light bill. When activated, AMPK halts the building of the extra proteins and lipids needed for forming a new daughter or sister cell and begins recycling older proteins and using lipids for fuel. Several of AMPK's recycling activities are mediated by p53.

P53: The p53 protein accumulates in the cell during phases of growth. If too much p53 accumulates before that phase is completed, it indicates that the cell has stalled out because of a problem, often because of DNA replication problems. During cell division excess p53 causes the cell to trigger the programmed cell death mechanism, as it is safer to destroy the cell than to create a new line of cells with DNA errors.

Glycolysis: The first steps in converting the energy in glucose to ATP.

Within a few weeks of consuming a high fat or high-fructose diet, the body develops insulin and leptin resistance, and becomes resistant to utilizing fat for energy. Exercise training reverses that, and improves insulin sensitivity quickly, followed by improved leptin sensitivity after a couple of weeks. Leptin promotes AMPK activity and increases utilization of fats as fuel for muscles. Energy consumption during and following exercise consumes ATP and converts it to AMP. AMP activates AMPK. Additionally, exercise causes an influx of calcium in the muscle and the generation of reactive oxygen species (ROS).

- ATP depletion activates AMPK
- Calcium influx activates CaMKII, which co-activates AMPK
- ROS activates p38 MAPK

P53 is a central regulator for many aspects of organelle and cell survival. The cell makes p53 continuously and breaks it down at about the same rate. AMPK and p38 MAPK are kinase enzymes that phosphorylate p53; this stabilizes it, preventing its destruction, and activates it. P53 promotes the transcription of genes that induce cell component recycling through autophagy and mitophagy in healthy G_0 and G1 phase cells. After exercise, p53 forms a complex with a mitochondrial growth factor (Tfam) and mitochondrial DNA (mtDNA). In mice, after exercise and recovery, there is a marked increase in mRNA for PGC-1α, NFR-1, and Tfam. Mice bred with dysfunctional p53 do not have this response to exercise.[210] If p53 formation is blocked, there is no renewal of mitochondria, and minimal if any response to exercise training.

P53 promotes a shift from glycolysis towards using lipids as a fuel for the cell. Reduced p53 function is associated with insulin resistance, reduced longevity, and tumor development.[211] Recall that dysfunctional p53 is the most prevalent gene error found in cancer cells. P53 promotes apoptosis of compromised cells at three checkpoints during cellular mitosis.

So far, p53 looks like the lynchpin for the impact of exercise on muscle cells. But how would activation of p53 and its movement into the nucleus of a muscle cell affect independent cancer cells that are not getting a workout helping one zip around a tennis court?

The most important things that happen during exercise have to do with how fuel (especially glucose) gets turned into energy during vigorous exercise and that brings us to Biochem 102.

Cellular Energetics Simplified

When the cell uses glucose and other sugars, fat, alcohol, or proteins for energy, it does this via the production of ATP. ATP then powers the machinery of the cell to do its work. Starch and glycogen are composed of chains of glucose molecules that are broken down into glucose and used for energy.

The conversion of glucose or other sugars to ATP goes through three sequential processes: glycolysis in the cytosol of the cell, followed by the citric acid cycle and then oxidative phosphorylation (OP) in the mitochondria. For each molecule of glucose, this process yields a net production of 30 molecules of ATP.

The first step is glycolysis (glyco-lysis: glucose-cutting). During this process, glucose is metabolized into two molecules of pyruvate. Glycolysis is an anaerobic process that does not use oxygen. For every molecule of glucose, glycolysis yields two molecules of ATP, pyruvate, NADH and H+.

Pyruvate is transported into the mitochondria. Here it is converted into acetate that binds to Coenzyme A, forming acetyl–CoA and yielding a molecule of NADH in the process. Fatty acids are also transported into the mitochondria where, through a process called beta-oxidation, each pair of carbon molecules in the fatty acid generates an acetate molecule to form acetyl-CoA. Amino acids can also be metabolized for use in the citric acid cycle via conversion to acetate.

Acetyl-CoA converts oxaloacetate into citric acid. In the citric acid cycle, the molecules from acetate are decomposed into carbon dioxide and water, and oxaloacetate is reformed. This process generates three molecules of NADH and one of FADH. The citric acid cycle does not directly produce ATP but provides NADH and FADH for oxidative phosphorylation by the mitochondria.

Pyruvate can also be converted to oxaloacetate, but although this increases the throughput of energy production during times of high energy demands, pyruvate that is converted into oxaloacetate itself does produce ATP.

NADH and FADH are intermediates in oxidative phosphorylation in the mitochondria for the generation of ATP. This process requires oxygen. NADH and FADH cannot be converted to ATP without oxygen. This is aerobic respiration.

The two ATP molecules formed during glycolysis only yield about seven percent of the energy available from glucose. Nevertheless, glycolysis provides this energy very quickly, about 100 times faster than oxidative phosphorylation. As a bonus, glycolysis produces ATP without requiring oxygen. Glucose is the only cellular fuel that can produce ATP without oxygen.

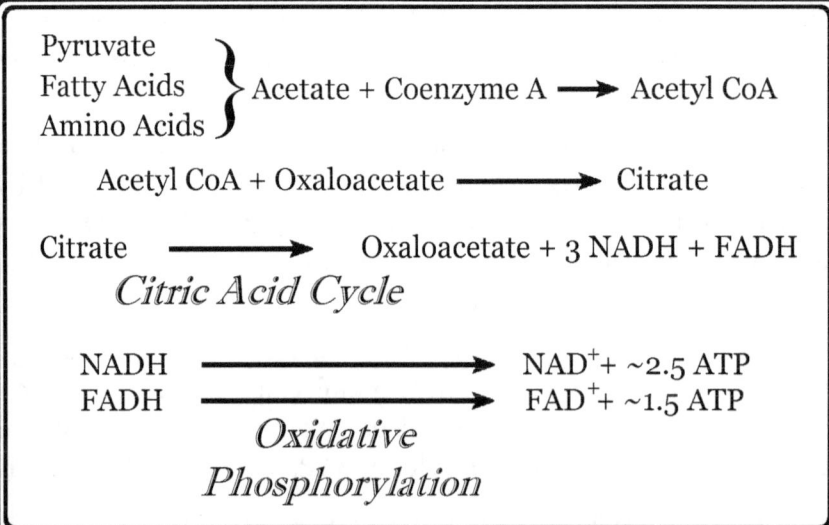

Figure 11-2: Glycolysis

Anoxic generation of ATP through glycolysis may be inefficient, but nevertheless is a very effective means of energy production for short-term, intense exercise. It provides a burst of ATP that can fuel muscular contractions for 10 seconds to 2 minutes. It is the dominant energy source

> for only the first 10 to 30 seconds during a maximal muscular effort. Fight or flight; you need to get it done quickly.
>
> During intense exercise, glucose is broken down by glycolysis into pyruvate. Due to the speed of glycolysis compared to oxidative phosphorylation and creation of oxygen deficits during intense muscular activity, pyruvate, NADH and H⁺ are produced much more quickly than they can be consumed. If left to accumulate in the cell, they inhibit the enzymes of glycolysis. Thus, the cell converts them to lactate.
>
> $$\text{Pyruvate} + \text{NADH} + \text{H}^+ \rightarrow \text{Lactate} + \text{NAD}^+$$
>
> Lactate is then transported out of the muscle cells, and into the bloodstream. During exercise, lactate levels can rise up to 100 times their normal resting levels. Lactate is taken up by other cells, especially the heart and brain, which quickly reverse this process, and convert lactate back to pyruvate that can be used in the citric acid cycle.

During *intense* exercise, muscles use glycolysis but produce more pyruvate than they can utilize. This results from its very rapid creation and perhaps in much lesser part because of limitations in the delivery of oxygen to the muscles. The muscle needs to get rid of the excess pyruvate, or it will inhibit glycolysis. Thus, during vigorous exercise, the muscles export excess lactate into the bloodstream. During intense exercise, serum lactate levels can increase from 0.5 - 2 mmol/L to over 20 mmol/L.

During intense exercise, adrenaline shifts blood flow from the intestines and kidneys to the muscles, heart, eyes, and brain. Lactate is a favorite fuel for our immortal cells. Lactic acid is the principal fuel for the heart muscle cells and neurons during exercise when glucose can be quickly and precipitously exhausted. Lactate easily crosses the blood-brain barrier and is one of, if not the brain's favorite fuel. The retinal pigment epithelial cells also use lactate as fuel.[212] The eyes and brain need more energy during exercise to quickly process and coordinate movement. Lactate is the main source of energy for the heart, eyes, and brain during vigorous exercise.

Lactate is more than just fuel; it is a signaling molecule. Similar to the response of muscles after intense exercise, in the brain, lactate causes an increase in PGC-1α, and this is associated with an increased expression of mitochondrial DNA.[213] When lactate is used as an energy source, production of hydrogen peroxide (H_2O_2) by mitochondria increases. This induces the expression of hundreds of genes, many involved in energy metabolism and several with mitochondrial reproduction.[214] Thus, exercise not only increases ROS production in non-muscle tissue but also increases the creation of new proteins for mitochondria. The positive effect exercise has on the brain is mediated, in large part, by lactate.

During intense exercise, the muscles become energy depleted. In the following hours they recover. Within the first couple of minutes of exercise, glucose is depleted. If available, the muscles will then use glucose stored in the form of glycogen. When glycogen is depleted or unavailable, the muscles burn fats for use as energy.

Exercise increases AMPK activity that activates the enzymes that convert triglycerides (fats) into glycerol and fatty acids. The muscles also use glycogen or fat during the post-exercise recovery period. If glycogen stores are low, fat is used during recovery. In the unfed state, free fatty acids levels remain elevated for several hours after intense exercise. The fatty acids are converted to energy through the citric acid cycle in the liver, with β-hydroxybutyrate (β-OHB) as a by-product. β-OHB is another fuel for the brain. β-OHB is a class 1 histone deacetylase (HDAC) inhibitor that prevents cancer by increasing p53 expression,[215] and improves cognition and memory by promoting production of BDNF, a neurotrophic growth factor in the hippocampus area of the brain.[216] β-OHB, as a class one HDAC inhibitor, can help reprogram maladaptive epigenetic binding of DNA to histones that occurs with aging and increases cancer risk.

Cell stress, malnutrition, and aging can cause aberrant binding of DNA to their histones that increase or decrease the expression of gene clusters. Epigenetic imprinting can pass from one cell to its daughter cells, and thus pass on the adaptive or maladaptive gene expression. Several foods compounds that have anticarcinogenic properties are Class I HDAC inhibitors.[217]

Table 13-2: Epigenetic Reset Factors

N-3 fatty acids EPA and DHA	Promote reversal of hypermethylation [218]
EGCG (green tea) Sulforaphane (cruciferous veggies)	HDAC and DNA methyltransferase inhibitors[217]
Butyrate (cheese, butter, dietary fiber. Diallyl sulfide (garlic) Resveratrol (red grapes and berries) Piceatannol (red wine, black grapes) Isoliquiritigenin (licorice root)	Histone deacetylase inhibitors[219, 220] These mostly inhibit Class I HDAC enzymes (HDAC1, HDAC2, HDAC3, and HDAC8), however, piceatannol and isoliquiritigenin inhibit multiple HDAC enzymes. Resveratrol also activates SIRT1.
β-hydroxybutyrate (exercise)	HDAC2 and HDAC3 inhibitors[216]
Melatonin	Inhibits DNA methyltransferase[221]
Curcumin (turmeric)	Inhibits histone acetyltransferase.

Thus, intense exercise results in elevated lactose levels that the brain and heart use during intense exercise; during recovery, fatty acids and β-OHB are available as fuels after glucose (and glycogen) depletion. β-OHB stimulates p53 activation and expression in the muscle and other cells of the body, including the brain. The effect of p53 activity and its downstream products in these cells from lactate and β-OHB are sufficient to be cytoprotective by repairing cell organelles, or it can promote apoptosis in aberrant cells.[215, 222] Cancer cells love glucose and use glycolysis as their principal source of energy. Since glycolysis does not require oxygen, it allows cancer cells to grow even before new blood vessels have grown to supply it. Intensive exercise robs cancer cells of glucose, making life hard on them.

Putting it to Use

Now that we have an inkling of the mechanism by which exercise decreases the proliferation of cancer, we can hack exercise to do this more efficiently. The evidence supports p53 as a central mediator of the protective effects of exercise. Upstream of p53 are glucose depletion, AMPK, p38 MAPK activation, and oxidative stress. Downstream are PGC-1α and mitochondrial biogenesis along with the induction of hundreds of different proteins and the potential for apoptosis in cells with DNA errors or other health issues.

Cancer develops slowly, and exercise trials for cancer outcome require many years to get sufficient follow-up. Athletes, however, seem willing to try all sorts of things to get better performance. Thus, exercise trials with mitochondrial biogenesis can serve as a quick proxy for the type of exercise likely to be effective in preventing cancer progression.

Studies have determined that brief, intense exercise is much more effective in stimulating mitochondrial biogenesis than is sustained, low-level exercise. The most efficient exercise for renewal of mitochondria appears to be sprints or Wingate exercises: repeated brief bouts of intense exercise, lasting only 30 to 60 seconds, followed by a three- to five-minute recovery period, and then repeating the intense muscular effort. This is just what would be expected from intense, anaerobic glycolysis, glucose depletion, and production of excess pyruvate and lactate.

In a study using one minute, "all-out" efforts followed by 75 seconds of low-intensity recovery exercise, there was a significant increase in SIRT1 and PGC-1α, which was associated with an increase in mitochondrial biogenesis.[223] In one study, a sprint interval training (SIT) group had more training benefit and equivalent mitochondrial enzyme production than did the endurance training (ET) group, even though the ET group did 10.5 hours of training and the SIT did only 2.5 hours of total training time a week. In this study, the SIT group expended only about one-tenth as many calories during the exercise as did the ET group. The ET group increased their training until they were riding a stationary bicycle for 120 minutes per session at 65% of their maximal cardiac output, and the SIT group did six repetitions of 30-second maximal output followed by 4 minutes of light cycle or rest.[224] In this SIT workout, there were six cycles of 30 second all-out sprints interspersed with four minutes of cool down, three times a week. This requires only 9 minutes of intense exercise per week! Other studies have repeated these results.[225] [226] SIT exercise training has also been demonstrated to improve mitochondrial function in the liver,[227] indicating that the benefits of SIT exercise effect are not limited to skeletal muscles.

> Indoor SIT training is usually done on a stationary bicycle, as it is well adapted to maximal efforts as the person pedaling sets the pace and can control the workload. Most treadmills are not well adapted, as the speed is set and does not respond to the person's effort. Outdoors or on track, SIT training can be done running.

SIT exercise for efficiently increasing lactate should begin with a warm-up period, followed by repeated bouts of intense exercise, interspaced with low-intensity exercise recovery periods.

Fasting prior to and for 3 hours after exercise nearly doubled the levels of p53 in the muscles immediately after exercise and raised levels more than two and a half times at three hours after exercising when compared to exercising in a fed state or eating in the hours following exercise.[211] Do not load carbs if you want to grow your muscles or get anti-cancer effects from exercise. Intense, glycogen-depleting exercise increases the production of βOHB and induction of p53 and its downstream compounds.

A small amount of caffeine (one cup of black coffee without sugar) before exercise may increase the liberation and utilization of fat as fuel. Other than the coffee or tea, intensive exercise should be performed on an empty stomach to encourage the burning of fat as fuel, as this is the source of βOHB production. Avoiding eating for three hours after exercise sustains βOHB production.

> Warnings: Sprint Interval Training is not appropriate for many people, especially for those with heart conditions, at risk of heart disease, arrhythmias, or lung disease. SIT should only be done in persons acclimated to cardiac endurance training or currently engaging in strenuous sports, such as singles tennis, basketball, or jogging. Consult your physician before engaging in any

vigorous exercise training program. It is often appropriate, especially for older persons, to begin exercise training under the care of a physician in a cardiovascular or pulmonary exercise rehab program. Since most cancer occurs in older people, most cancer patients would need a physician's evaluation and exercise training prior to attempting SIT.

Individuals who have not been actively engaging in vigorous exercise should start with a comfortable exercise load that increases their respiratory and heart rates moderately and gradually increase their workout intensity and duration to an appropriate target exercise load over three to four months, working out three times a week, and allowing a day after vigorous exercise for recovery.

While caffeine may increase the metabolic utilization of fats, high doses of caffeine are associated with an increased risk of cardiac arrhythmias in persons susceptible to them. The risk of arrhythmia, however, may actually be from sleep deprivation from associated with caffeine use rather than being the direct effect of caffeine. Nevertheless, an abundance of caution suggests that persons at high risk of arrhythmias should avoid large amounts of caffeine prior to vigorous exercise.

Exercise Target Levels for Rehab:

Exercise target levels can be derived from the estimated maximum heart rate:[228]

Step 1: Calculate the person's maximal heart rate as:

HR_{max} = 209 − (0.716 × age) (men)

HR_{max} = 209 − (0.804 × age) (women)

Step 2: Calculate the target heart rate range for vigorous physical activity as 70 to 85% of the maximal heart rate. E.g.: For a 60-year-old woman:

HR_{max} = 209 − (0.804 × age) = 209 − (0.804 × 60) = 160.76

Vigorous workout target lower heart rate = 160.76 × .70 = 113

Vigorous workout target upper heart rate = 160.76 × .85 = 137

Thus, for a 60-year-old woman, the target heart rate range during vigorous exercise would be to maintain a heart rate between 113 and 137 beats per minute for the duration of the exercise. A person that has not been involved in vigorous physical activity should work up to this level over three to four months, starting with exercise in the 50 to 60 percent of maximal heart rate range, and gradually increasing intensity and duration over 12 to 16 weeks.

The results from SIT training help us understand the mechanisms by which exercise prevents cancer progression. SIT exercise, however, is not for everyone. On a personal note, I occasionally do sprint interval training to boost my exercise capacity. Nevertheless, I enjoy other forms of exercise more. While SIT exercise is effective and saves time, for me, it is just not as much fun as other forms of exercise. I also backed off from it because I was losing more weight than I preferred. Nevertheless, I often work a sprint or two into my other exercise activities.

When walking for exercise (minimum 3.5 mph), jogging, or biking, try to find a place that has hills that can substitute for sprints by increasing your workload. Alternatively, throw a few "sprints" into your walk with a few flights of stairs. If it doesn't take your breath away, it's unlikely to stress your metabolism sufficiently to raise your lactate and β-OHB levels. As individuals train and become more adapted to a higher exercise load, they may need to increase the workout level to maintain the same effects.

> It is a long-standing myth that lactose build-up from exercise causes muscle aches. It is not true. Delayed onset muscle soreness (DOMS) that can appear 24 to 72 hours after exercise is caused by microscopic tears in the myofilaments within the muscle cells. DOMS can be avoided by increasing exercise workload slowly, by not more than 10% each sequential workout day.

If they aren't enjoying it, most people quickly fall off the exercise wagon. Find an activity you enjoy. People who exercise alone are much less likely to maintain their exercise routines. Make exercise fun by making it a time to spend with a friend. Successes in maintaining exercise routines are more than doubled by enjoying the activity and doing it with a friend or as part of a group.[229] Share your exercise routine, where you are running or playing, as a time to engage with a companion. Having a scheduled time with a companion makes the exercise harder to blow off, and helps keep us on schedule. The word compete comes from the Latin; to seek together. Having a friend to compete alongside with helps us succeed.

If exercise is just a work-out that you don't enjoy and never expect to enjoy, you can just accept then, that it is work, but worth the effort. The less you enjoy exercise, the better a deal SIT becomes. SIT training on an exercise bike may be appropriate for you. You can sprint through commercials and do light cycling during your favorite TV program.

If You Can't Exercise, Take a Bath

You want easy? Well, here it is for the ill, the infirm, the indulgent and indolent or incapacitated. Here is how to get at least some of the benefits of exercise without hardly trying.

Hot baths have some of the same beneficial metabolic effects as does exercise. The hormones, cytokines, and metabolic products resulting from elevated body temperature from a hot bath are similar to those occurring from vigorous exercise. Hot baths increase blood levels of IL-6, epinephrine and norepinephrine release, growth hormone, cortisol, G-CSF,[230] HSP72,[231] 3-hydroxybutyrate, and lactic acid.[232] Epinephrine release should promote lactate utilization.[233] Using a cold clamp (cool baths during experimental exercise conditions, or swimming in cool water during exercise, prevents many of these beneficial effects of exercise. Thus, swimming may not provide the anti-cancer benefits of other intensive exercises.

Hot baths have many beneficial effects paralleling those of intense exercise, but without the work. The core body temperature needs to increase to about 99.5° to 101.3°F (37.5° to 38.5° C).[230] This can be done in a hot bath, hot tub, or sauna. Hot baths also help to improve glucose tolerance [234] and increase insulin sensitivity in type 2 diabetics.[235] This action is apparently mediated by normalization in the production of HSP72 in these patients. A study using a hot tub water temperature of 100° to 105.8° F (37.8°C to 41.0°C) for 30 minutes a day found improved blood sugar levels and weight loss in insulin-dependent diabetics.[236] Hot baths have also been found to be one of the most effective non-pharmacologic treatments of fibromyalgia.[237]

In exercise, if you are not breathing hard, you are likely not getting anticancer benefits. In bathing, a sweaty head is a sign that the body is responding to the heat.

Warnings: Test the bathwater temperature with a thermometer to make sure it is in the appropriate range and never over 43.0° C (111° F). Small children can be burned at bath temperatures that are tolerated by adults. The elderly and persons with poor circulation may also be injured more easily. Persons with heart conditions may not tolerate hot baths or saunas.

Hot baths and saunas cause vasodilatation and can precipitate a fall in blood pressure. The last time I went to a hot spring, I nearly fainted when I got out of the water. It can happen to anyone. Be sure to hydrate before a long, hot bath. If water is consumed just before or during a hot bath, it should be warm to avoid cooling the body.

Additive Effects

Fasting anyone? Fasting should be no work at all, and it also increases the production of the β-OHB. Certainly, fasting prior to and for three hours after exercise will increase its efficacy for burning fat and promotes p53 production. Fasting is further discussed in Chapter 37.

How about eating? That should be much more fun. Several flavonoids found in plant-based foods have been found to induce p53 activity and autophagy. The flavonoids resveratrol, quercetin, luteolin, and kaempferol are among those that have been demonstrated to induce autophagy.[238] Flavonoids and other phenolic compounds are discussed in more detail in following chapters.

Combinations of exercise, hot baths, fasting or flavonoids may increase the efficacy of these modalities to cancer prevention.

Exercise Summary

Exercise can prevent metabolic changes that increase cancer risk and cancer progression. Relaxing, romantic walks on the beach may be great for the heart, but will not slow cancer. It appears that only vigorous exercise provides these benefits. If exercise does not get the heart pumping and get one short of breath, it is unlikely to prevent cancer growth. For the weak, infirm or indulgent, soaking in a hot bath, between 100° to 105.8° F, for 30 minutes a day may have similar effects on cancer as exercise does.

14: Diet and Cancer

Lung cancer is mostly caused by smoking; gastric cancer by a chronic *H. pylori* infection; and cervical cancer by HPV infection. While about 90% of these cancers are linked to a specific cause, even with these cancers, nutrition plays a role. For example, women with the HPV virus that have lower levels of the B vitamin folate in their blood have been found to be four times more likely to develop cervical dysplasia,[239] and nine times more likely to develop high-grade or invasive cervical cancer.[240]

The general consensus of researchers is that dietary factors explain about 35 percent of all cancers in the United States. As many as 70% of colorectal and prostate cancers, and half of all breast, endometrial, pancreatic, gallbladder, and urinary cancers are linked to dietary factors.[241, 242] Even the risk of malignant melanoma, a deadly skin cancer is greatly affected by diet.[243]

Before you get too excited, let me 'splain something: diet epidemiology is treacherous and difficult. There have been hundreds, probably thousands, of diet-and-cancer association studies. The association between cancer cells and diet doesn't give up its secrets easily, and an answer extracted by torturing data doesn't mean you are going to get the truth.

Is there an interaction between different foods? Do combinations of certain foods affect risk? Can you remember what you ate for lunch a week ago Thursday? What was the serving size? Now try what you ate twenty years ago.

When cancer (or the lack of cancer) is affected by diet, it is a long slow process. If a man is diagnosed with prostate cancer at age 70, does what he ate two years ago give a reliable association of what causes cancer risk, or does one need to go back to what he ate when he was 14? Does what he ate last year tell much about what he was eating 50 years ago? Are study subjects even reliable witnesses, or do they fudge the data so that they appear less self-indulgent or more self-controlled?

Even when scientists have a good idea about what people actually eat, it is not easy. The Adventist Health Study 2 took diet histories of 89,000 Seventh Day Adventists. Vegans ate more nuts and seeds than did the vegetarians, and vegetarians ate more nuts and seeds than did meat eaters. But the vegans also ate more avocados, legumes, fruits and vegetables, and no meat or dairy; they added less fat and consumed far fewer sweets, less coffee, soda, and alcohol.[244] People don't eat single foods in isolation. It is comparatively easy to look at a single food and assess its relation to disease risk; it is extremely difficult, however, to discern the effect of a single nutrient or chemical compound from a dietary soup containing hundreds of foods with thousands of chemical compounds.

Adding to the mess is genetics. In most ways, we are more alike than we are different. However, there are many polymorphisms that modify our metabolism. Remember how different alleles affect the metabolism of alcohol? About 10 percent of people of European descent have an allele for the enzyme that recycles folate (MTHFR) that is less stable, and thus less active.[245] Women with the less stable allele of MTHFR are 23 times more likely to develop cervical intraepithelial neoplasia.[246] This risk appears to be mitigated, however, if they have a folate levels in the upper half of the "normal" range. Thus, a diet that provides adequate folate for some people is inadequate for others and puts these individuals at higher risk for stroke, heart disease, and cancer.

What if it is not only the number of servings of vegetables that is important but the variety of various nutrients? What if the soil they are grown in makes a difference? Does cooking those veggies into a pasty submission make a difference from eating them raw? There are hundreds of food ingredients, and these are processed and combined into thousands of different food items. There are more variables than people.

People are not lab rats, all with the same genetics, that allow scientists to place populations on the same diet and exercise routine, and then alter the amount of one foodstuff at a time to see if it changes the outcome 45 years down the road. Scientists have often spent millions of dollars and most of their career doing long-term follow-up studies on diet, only to find they asked the wrong question. It's brutal out there.

Very often, scientists have examined the effect of an individual nutrient on cancer. Does carotene or vitamin E make a difference? Several studies found that diets high in beta-carotene are associated with lower risk of colon cancer. So then, scientists spend over 20 years performing randomized cancer prevention trials involving thousands of people, giving half the study population beta-carotene to see how effective it was in preventing cancer. Dang! It increased cancer risk!!! When supplementation with antioxidant vitamin E was studied for its effect on cancer, it generally has been found to provide no benefit,[247] or to increase the risk of cancer and risk of death from other causes.[248]

What went wrong? Beta-carotene is not a food; it is a substance found in many plants that is converted to vitamin A in the body. Vitamin A acts as a growth hormone, and growth hormones cause cells to grow, including cancer cells. Foods high in beta-carotene are usually high in fiber, minerals such as magnesium and boron, and compounds such as PQQ, lutein, and zeaxanthin and bioflavonoids. Perhaps one or more of these, or one or more of hundreds of other substances that are also found in the same foods that are high in beta-carotene, lowered the cancer risk. It may not have been beta-carotene at all.

For the studies of vitamin E, it seems that scientists, including the National Academy of Science, chose the wrong form of vitamin E. The α-tocopherol form of vitamin E, that is generally used, actually depletes vitamin K and other forms of vitamin E from the body. In lab animals at least, some forms of vitamin K and some of the non-α-tocopherol forms of vitamin E appear to lower cancer risk, while α-tocopherol may increase risk. (See Figure 20.1)

Populations that eat more fruits and vegetables have fewer cancers. But maybe it is not what they eat, but rather what they don't eat. Perhaps the reason for lower cancer incidence is that people who eat lots of veggies also eat more fruit or eat less meat, or less fat, or just fewer calories. Adding complexity, people with the unhealthy lifestyle habits that increase cancer risk (smoking, drinking, sloth and staying up late) may be less interested in or can't afford to eat vegetables. Smoking alters the perception of taste and smell, and likely alters food choices. We cannot judge guilt by association. Even when an exposure is associated with cancer risk, it does not guarantee that the factor caused the risk. When exposure is associated with lowered risk, it does not mean that it prevents the risk either.

What if beta-carotene lowers the risk of cancer development when a person is young (likely) but increases the risk of tumor growth after carcinogenesis when it, after conversion to vitamin A promotes growth? What if the anti-carcinogenic substances are destroyed by cooking? How about mixing different foods; does that have an effect on cancer risk? Does cooking time and temperature affect the carcinogenic risk of food? (Yes, yes and yes.)

All these factors make the study of diet and cancer a formidable, arduous, and tricky task. Scientists cannot keep people in cages for 50 years to feed them and see what causes cancer. Mice are easier to keep caged, and with their short lifespan, can reveal answers in months. But will it apply to humans? It is unlikely that a single study could reveal the effect of a single food on a single form of cancer within a single population. It takes looking at thousands of studies to start putting the pieces together. It has taken a long time, but we are putting the puzzle together, and it is starting to make sense.

Diet has a great impact on the occurrence of cancer, but this relationship has been a conundrum. The following chapters will explain a substantial portion of this puzzle. I will start by giving you a clue: mostly, the foods you eat are not nearly as important in the prevention and development of cancer as when they are eaten it and how they are prepared. How's that for an enigma?

15: Meat and Heat

Meat is a great source of nutrients. It can also be an excellent source of carcinogens; however, it does not have to be. Diets high in meat are associated with an increase in cancer risk, especially for certain types of cancers. So, if you would like to lower your cancer risk, you can become a vegan. Or you can slice your meats thinner.

There are many reasons to be vegetarian, or at least to decrease meat consumption. Perhaps you just can't look Bambi in the eye and think, "Oooh, what a tasty, savory burger you would be, my dear!" Or, perhaps you realize that feedlots have enormous negative consequences for the human environment, even if ignoring the plight of animals that live there. But if you enjoy meat, and wish to avoid carcinogens while continuing to eat it, this can be done. And the following chapters explain why and what to do.

> Some may consider vegetarianism after learning that the overuse of antibiotics in feedlots and chicken houses causes antibiotic resistance and the generation of MRSA (methicillin resistant *Staph. aureus*). Unless you work in a hospital, the most likely place you will come face-to-face with multidrug-resistant *Staphylococcus aureus* may be the meat you bring home from the grocer. Over half of the raw meat you bring into your home is contaminated with *Staph. aureus*. About five percent of meat tested is contaminated with MRSA.[249][250] Seventy-eight percent of raw beef liver is contaminated with *Campylobacter*, and most isolates are multidrug resistant,[251] similar to the 67% percent contamination rate of chicken livers and gizzards.[252] These bacteria are a leading cause of foodborne disease, and they can trigger the onset of irritable bowel syndrome and other disease conditions.
>
> What You Can Do: Bag meat you purchase separately from other items. Any liquid in the package should be drained *before* putting it in your refrigerator, and meat should be stored separately from any foods that may be eaten raw. Clean your food preparation area, tools, and hands after handling raw meat to avoid contaminating other foods that may be eaten uncooked. To be safe, handle all raw meat as if it were contaminated with antibiotic-resistant *Staphylococcus aureus* or other disease-causing bacteria.

Multiple studies indicate that consumption of red meat is associated with increased risk of cancer, including colorectal[253] and breast cancers in adults[254] and brain cancer in children. The good news for carnivores is that meat is not carcinogenic until the cook makes it so. The way that meat is prepared is the major determinant of whether it causes cancer.

There are five principal pathways by which meat causes cancer. Three of these are the result of chemical changes that occur during the heating of organic materials.

1. Burning organic material, including food, wood, coal, tobacco, and petroleum products, causes the formation of polycyclic aromatic hydrocarbons (PAH) such as benzo[a] pyrene, some of which are carcinogens (Chapter 16).

2. When meat is cooked at high temperatures, creatinine, amino acids, and certain sugars are transformed into heterocyclic amines (HCAs) that the body metabolizes into mutagenic DNA adducts. These are among the most potent dietary carcinogens and are discussed in Chapter 17.

3. Processed and preserved meats contain nitrites that when heated, form N-nitrosyl compounds (NNC) which increase the risk of stomach, colon, rectal and brain cancers. NNC may also be formed in (and eliminated from) other non-meat foods, and are the subject of Chapter 18.

4. Meat is an excellent source of iron. It is so good that it can increase the risk of cancer in some people. This risk will be discussed in Chapter 20.

5. Most commercially available red meat is from animals fed a feedlot diet dominated by corn. Since the fatty acids in corn are essentially all n-6 fats, animals fed corn have a predominance of n-6 fatty acids in their tissues. Grass-fed animals have a lower n6:n3 ratio, as grass has more n-3 fatty acids than corn does. N-6 fatty acids are converted into pro-inflammatory eicosanoids that promote cancer. Meanwhile, n-3 fatty acids are converted into eicosanoids that decrease inflammation and the risk of heart disease, stroke, and cancer.[135] When the human diet contains copious quantities of meat from corn-fed, feedlot animals, or other high n-6 foods, the human body also will have cell membranes loaded with n-6 fatty acids. Fish from cold water have mostly n-3 fatty acids. Fats from fish appear to decrease the risk of colon cancer. Diets high in n-6 fats or with high n6:n3 ratios are associated with higher prostate and bowel cancer risk.[255, 256] This role of fats in cancer risk will be further discussed in Chapter 25.

16: Percivall Pott and the Flue of Death

During the 18th century, coal was commonly used to heat homes in London and other urban areas. With time, coal-tar creosote would build up inside the chimney flues. This creosote was composed mostly of volatile, cyclic hydrocarbons, including benzenes, toluene, xylenes, and polycyclic aromatic hydrocarbons formed and released as the coal is heated. Chimney flues are designed to create a draft to carry smoke out of the building efficiently; however, as the smoke rises through the chimney, it can cool and condense on the inner surface of the flue, just as moisture in the air condenses on a cold glass window. Over a single season, a layer of creosote tars can build up and be an inch thick or more around the inside of the chimney flue, impeding airflow, and causing smoke to back up into the home. But more treacherously, these tars are flammable, with a flash point only around 75°C (167°F). If these materials ignited from the hot gasses from the stove, it could cause a dangerous chimney fire. Compounding the risk, during summer months, when the chimney is not used, birds may build a nest in a flue, adding tinder. Prior to the 1990's, when better-insulated flues were mandated by building codes, a quarter of U.S. home fires were caused by chimney fires from the ignition of wood creosote.

A flue 9 × 14 inches was a standard size during the 18th century; however, they were sometimes half this area. Since they needed to be cleaned, young boys, often from orphanages or workhouses, were conscripted for this task, starting at the age of six. They were small enough to climb into and up the flues, cleaning them as they climbed through. If the chimney was particularly narrow, they worked naked so that they could more easily move within the tight spaces. It was obviously a dangerous and filthy job. The boys sometimes got stuck, suffocated, or burned to death. There were also longer-term consequences of this employment.

In 1775, Sir Percivall Pott, a British surgeon, described a high incidence of invasive, scrotal cancer in chimney sweeps as they reached their late teens or early twenties. He suggested that the repeated exposure to soot from coal-burning stoves was to blame. This was the first cancer identified as having an environmental cause, the first known carcinogen. A century and a half later, benzo[a]pyrene, a polyaromatic hydrocarbon (PAH) that resulted from the burning of coal, was found to be a mutagen and carcinogen.

Professional chimney sweeps in Europe still have a high risk of occupation-related cancers.[257]

In the body, benzo[a]pyrene is oxidized by the cytochrome P450 enzyme CYP1A1 and then by epoxide hydrolase to benzo[a]pyrene-7,8-dihydrodiol-9,10-epoxide, a molecule that binds to DNA. (Don't worry, I won't test on this). This epoxide covalently binds to DNA forming adducts that can cause a guanine to thymine substitution in the p53 gene. This benzo[a]pyrene adduct prevents the normal transcription of the TP53 gene,[258] preventing p53's activities, including autophagy during lean times and apoptosis in cells with mutations. This DNA adduct can thus allow cells with DNA damage to replicate.

DNA adducts adhere to the DNA strand and cause errors, breaks, or substitutions in the DNA during replication when the cell divides. If breaks are not repaired correctly by DNA repair mechanisms, mutations result. If the adduct causes a substitution error, it may change the behavior of the protein that the gene codes for. These substitution errors can be transcribed into subsequent generations of cells.

Some mutations do not cause problems and go unnoticed. Others cause the cell to function poorly or die. Dying eliminates the problem, along with the cell. If the cell was an irreplaceable neuron, well, you just got dumber, but you'll survive. If the mutation occurs in a critical area of a gene that controls growth, it may cause cancer; and you may not survive.

Benzo[a]pyrene is just one of numerous pre-carcinogens present in smoke, including coal and tobacco smoke. Benzo[a]pyrene is also present in the smoke from flame-broiled, barbecued and grilled beef, as well as in fried chicken. Luckily, cytochrome CYP1A1 in the mucosal cells that line the intestine prevents most benzo[a]pyrene from being absorbed into the body, and this very effectively prevents cancer risk from most food-related benzo[a]pyrene exposure.[259] This is in stark contrast to benzo[a]pyrene inhaled into the lungs or skin, which is absorbed, as in the case of the chimney sweeps.

Like benzo[a]pyrene, most environmental and food carcinogens are pre-carcinogenic compounds that are metabolized into DNA adducts. Often, this conversion is a two- or three-step enzymatic process that begins with oxidation of the pre-carcinogen by a cytochrome p450 oxidase enzyme.

Polycyclic Aromatic Hydrocarbons (PAH)

PAH are formed during the incomplete burning of organic materials, including both biomass and fossil fuels, when heated to temperatures over 200° C (392° F). Over 100 PAH have been identified, and they are of concern as several of these compounds are carcinogens. PAH can form when various foods, especially fats, are burned. This can occur when meat is grilled, and the drippings fall on hot coals. The food can be coated with PAH from the smoke that precipitates on the meat or on other food being grilled. PAH are also found in air pollution from coal-powered power plants, vehicle exhaust, and tobacco and wood smoke. Benzo[a]pyrene is found in cigarette smoke and was the first PAH found to be carcinogenic. Fifteen PAH compounds are known carcinogens. PAH are found in foods cooked at temperatures which cause charring, oil refined at high temperatures (peanut, soy, corn oils), and in smoked foods[317] as well as in air pollution.

Children of women exposed to higher levels of PAH from air pollution during pregnancy had verbal IQ scores about five points lower at age five than less heavily exposed children[260]. Prenatal exposure is also associated with lower birth weight[261]. Dietary benzo[a]pyrene increases intestinal inflammation and may increase the risk of type 2 diabetes in those consuming a high-fat diet.[262]

The risks of cancer from food sources of PAH have been difficult to evaluate, in part, because of lack of biologic markers. In experimental animals, tumors caused by exposure to PAH generally occur in the area of exposure. The most likely increase in cancer risk from PAH associated with food is lung cancer from inhalation of smoke and volatiles formed during cooking at high temperatures and during barbecuing. A vented hood fan should be used while cooking at high temperatures indoors or the cooking should be done outside.

Other than perhaps occupational exposure from cooking smoke, most of the exposure to PAH in developed countries is from exposure to tobacco smoke and air pollution.[263] About half of the world' households cook over biomass, including wood, dried dung, grass, and agricultural residues, and much of this cooking is done indoors, creating health hazards of respiratory infections and emphysema, especially for women and female children in developing countries.[264] Even in these populations, studies of risk associated with smoke inhalation have attributed the risk of cancer to use of coal as a fuel or to smoking tobacco,[265] rather than to wood smoke.

Carcinogenic polycyclic hydrocarbons are created by overheating and charring of meat, smoke from meat drippings, and from charring or burning of other foods, especially those high in fat.

PAH from food can cause cancer, but the risk is much more from inhalation smoke and vapors during the preparation of the foods than from swallowing them. Thus, the risk is more to the cook than the consumer of PAH-containing food. Much higher cancer risk from eating meat cooked at high temperatures from other DNA adducts formed compounds in meat, including heterocyclic amines (HCAs) and nitrosamines (NNCs).

Summary

Polycyclic hydrocarbons (PAH) are carcinogens created during the burning of organic materials. When food is charred or fats are burned, PAH are created. PAH exposure from food-borne PAH in a normal diet is very unlikely to create cancer risk, as the intestinal mucosal cells prevent these compounds from being absorbed. Exposure of carcinogenic PAH to the skin or lungs, from exposure to tars and smoke, however, increases the risk of cancer.

17: Heterocyclic Amines

The premier food carcinogens are the HCAs, heterocyclic amines. Epidemiologic studies link HCA consumption with cancers of the breast, prostate, colon, rectum, pancreas, lung, esophagus, and stomach. Breast cancer is associated with consumption of well-done meat.[266] The risk of colonic polyps is higher among individuals who consume red meat cooked at temperatures that cause high production of HCAs.[267,268]

There are about 15 to 20 HCAs that are suspected human pre-carcinogens. HCAs contain a six-atom ring with five atoms of carbon (C) and one of nitrogen (N). HCAs are formed during the heating of creatine or creatinine in the presence of an amino acid, a reducing sugar, and water, which are all present in muscle. But not all HCAs are dangerous. In fact, the two HCAs illustrated below are the B vitamins niacin (left) and pyridoxine (right). In the stick figures, as used in the illustrations below, biochemists use shorthand and do not mark C's for the carbon atoms that are at ends of the sticks that represent covalent bonds.

Figure 17-1: The HCA niacin and pyridoxine

At least 17 HCAs can be produced during the cooking of muscle tissue. Many of these are mutagenic, and at least four of these are *amino imidazo aza-arenes* (AIA), which are human carcinogens:

2-amino-3,4-dimethylimidazo[4,5-*f*] quinoline (MeIQ)

2-amino-3,8-dimethylimidazo[4,5-*f*] quinoxaline (MeIQx)

2-amino-3-methylimidazo[4,5-*f*] quinoline (IQ)

2-amino-1-methyl-6-phenyl-imidazo[4,5-*b*] pyridine (PhIP)

MeIQ, MeIQx, and IQ are many times more carcinogenic than benzo[*a*]pyrene, more than 20 times more potent carcinogens than aflatoxin (Chapter 21), and about 100 times more potent than PhIP.

Like benzo[*a*]pyrene, AIAs are actually pre-carcinogens; they require metabolic activation to do their dirty work. First, in the liver, the cytochrome p450 CYP1A2 enzyme oxidizes the AIA into N-hydroxy AIA. CYP1A1 and some other p450 enzymes can also perform this step.

In a second step, the enzymes N-acetyltransferase (NAT-1 or NAT-2) convert N-hydroxy AIA into a highly reactive N-acetoxy ester that spontaneously hydrolyzes into an aryl nitrenium ion. These reactive ions form DNA adducts.[269] As an alternative second step, however, N-hydroxy AIA can be biotransformed by the enzyme glutathione S-transferase (GST), or one of several other cytosolic enzymes: prolyl-tRNA synthetase, sulfotransferase (*SULT*), or phosphorylase (Figure 17-2). This second step of AIA metabolism determines the compound's potential to bind to DNA and act as a carcinogen.

The human population has significant genetic diversity in how we metabolize AIA compounds. Individuals with certain polymorphisms of the enzymes that metabolize HCA (*NAT1, NAT2, GSTM1/T1,* and *SULT1A1*) can have increased or decreased risk for carcinogenesis from exposure to HCA AIA compounds. Those with fast-acting CYP1A1, NAT1, and NAT2 genotypes are at increased risk of cancer from exposure to AIA. Those individuals that metabolize the AIA via GST more quickly have lower cancer risk, as glutathione S-transferase binds the N-hydroxy AIA to glutathione, forming a conjugate that can be easily eliminated in the urine.

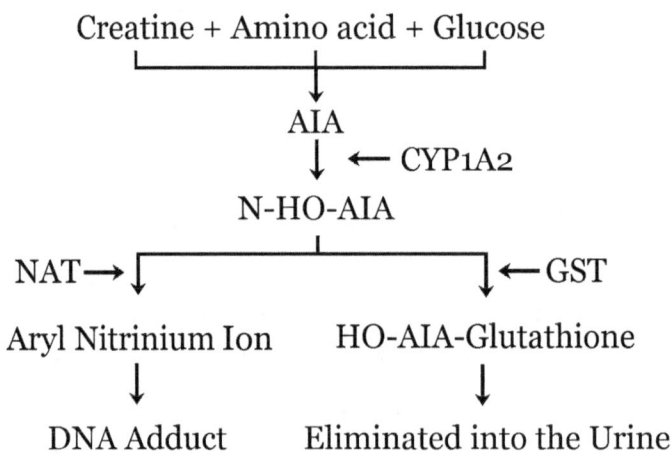

Figure 17-1: AIA metabolism

The increased risk of colorectal cancer associated with HCA from meat cooked at high temperatures is greater in individuals with fast-acetylating alleles of NAT. Fast acetylators may also be at increased risk of colorectal cancer from smoking tobacco.[270]

Cigarette smoking causes cancer in various organs, not just in the lungs that are directly exposed. HCAs increase cancer risk from smoking through its induction of the p450 enzymes CYP1A1 and CYP1A2 in the liver, thus increasing the metabolism of AIA into N-HO-AIA in the liver (Figure 17-1). These pre-carcinogens that are then distributed throughout the body.[271, 272, 273] Individuals with a polymorphism of easily inducible CYP1A1 are at much greater risk of lung cancer than other smokers.

Rodents fed a diet with HCAs developed cancers in several organs, including the colon, breast, and prostate. One HCA produced hepatomas in monkeys. The cells from these cancers exhibited alteration of the genes for several proteins, including APC, β-catenin, and Ha-ras, all proteins involved in cell growth regulation.[274]

In a study including women with and without breast cancer, a test meal was given with a known content of AIA. Several hours later, their urine was tested for AIA metabolites. Higher levels of carcinogenic metabolites were found in the women with breast cancer. These women apparently absorb and/or metabolize these compounds more actively.[275] Colorectal, breast, prostate, and pancreatic cancers are those most clearly linked to HCA consumption from meat.[273, 276, 277] Red meat consumption is a risk factor for adenocarcinoma and squamous cell carcinoma of the lung, *even among individuals who have never smoked.*[278]

Dietary-caused cancers occurring during middle age or later often result from exposure to carcinogens during adolescence or even earlier. The Nurses' Health Study found that red meat consumption during adolescence was tied to a 43% increase in the risk of premenopausal breast cancer.[279] There was a 22% increase in risk for each serving of meat consumed per day during adolescence. The association was greatest in well-done and fried meats. The risk was not as high for meat consumed later, during early adulthood. The risk of breast cancer is highest during breast development. Similarly, it should be expected that cancer risk imparted by meat is most potent when consumed during periods of growth.

> CAUTION!
>
> Carcinogenic HCA compounds can be found in the breast milk of rats fed meat cooked at high temperatures, and DNA adducts of these carcinogens are found in the organs of their pups.[280] Carcinogenic HCAs are also found in human breast milk.[281] More dangerously, carcinogenic HCAs cross the placenta, and their DNA adducts can be found in the organs of preborn infant primates.[282]
>
> During fetal life and infancy, animals are at greatly increased risk of mutation because of the high rate of cell division during growth. Mice exposed to carcinogenic HCA in the first days of life form liver cancers at middle age from HCA doses that are a minuscule fraction of the chronic exposure dose required to cause cancer in adult mice. The

carcinogenic dose for neonatal mice was one *five-thousandth to one ten-thousandth* the dose required to cause cancer in an adult mouse. [283]

Most of the eggs in a woman's ovaries are formed during her fetal life; before she was born. Thus, exposure to DNA adducts during pregnancy that results in a female offspring can potentially cause mutations that do not appear until the following generation. For males, sperm stem cells develop during early adolescence. Thus, these are times of high risk for induction of mutations that can later become cancer. These may cause germline mutations that can be passed down multiple generations.

Pregnancy, infancy, and adolescence are periods when mutagens and carcinogens should be vigilantly avoided. And not just by women. It takes 60 days for sperm to form from their stem cells. Those who plan to be fathers should be especially careful to avoid exposure to mutagens and carcinogens during the two months prior to conception. PAH forms DNA-adducts in sperm and decreases the number of normal sperm.[284] Men with insufficient seminal fluid vitamin C levels frequently have DNA damage in their sperm.[285] Heavy alcohol exposure can cause DNA methylation in the sperm, and these changes can affect the offspring. Male rats fed a high-fat diet prior to breeding impart a propensity to pancreatic β-cell dysfunction in their daughters, and thus, risk of obesity and diabetes, while their low-fat-consuming brethren do not.[286]

Creation and Prevention of Carcinogenic HCA

HCA compounds are formed in foods containing creatine or creatinine, an amino acid, a reducing sugar, and water heated to temperatures high enough to break covalent bonds. This results in reactive substrates that can form HCAs. HCA mutagenesis can be avoided by:

❖ Avoiding HCA-AIA formation during food preparation.

❖ Avoiding the biotransformation of AIA from precarcinogens into carcinogens.

❖ Consuming foods that help prevent or reverse the damage (Chapters 23 and 24).

Avoiding HCA Formation

Substrate Source: Creatine or creatinine in muscle tissue, along with free amino acids, makes meat an excellent source of substrates for the formation of HCA. Muscle contains about 95% of the body's creatine; lower amounts are present in the brain, intestinal and brown adipose tissue, and germ cells. Very low levels are found in the lungs, spleen, kidney, liver, and white adipose tissue. Shellfish and shrimp have insignificant creatine content. In invertebrates, such as shrimp, shellfish, and snails, creatinine is limited to sperm cells.

Most other high-protein foods, such as milk, cheese, beans, tofu, or other plant proteins, do not contain creatine and produce insignificant amounts of mutagenic compounds except during charring, and these are not HCA products. Egg yolks, however, do contain creatine and can produce HCA when cooked at high temperatures. [287] Meat sauces and meat and fish stocks, extracts, and gravies are often very potent sources of mutagenic HCA. Organ meats that are low in creatine, such as liver and kidney, produce very low amounts of HCA during cooking. And as would be expected, HCAs are not formed during the cooking of shellfish, milk, or plant products.

The type of HCA formed also depends on the amino acid that the HCA is formed from. Threonine, glycine, lysine, and serine are the amino acids that form the most mutagenic HCAs.

Grinding meat macerates and disrupts the muscle cells. This allows creatine, amino acids, and sugars to leak from far more cells than would be exposed during the cooking of an intact, sliced section of meat. Grinding meat greatly increases the substrates available for HCA formation. A single three-ounce ground beef patty may contain 14 times more HCA than the typical American adult average intake of 500 ng of HCA. The average adult intake is 8 ng/kg body weight per day.

Americans love eating hamburger, mostly as sandwiches in a bun, but also as meatloaf, meatballs, Sloppy Joes, and other concoctions. Over 40 percent of the beef in the U.S. is consumed as ground beef. Since ground beef is less expensive, lower income families tend to consume an even higher percentage of their meat as ground beef. Of great concern is that young people are those most likely to consume large quantities of ground meats that may be laden with home-cooked carcinogens during a developmental period when they are most susceptible to carcinogens. The average American teenage boy consumes 50 pounds of ground beef a year. Teenage girls eat less beef but still consume over half of the beef they eat as hamburger.[288]

Cooking Temperature: The principal factor determining the production of mutagens and carcinogens in meat is the cooking temperature. The total HCA content in cooked meat or fish can range from less than 0.1 ng/g to over 300 ng/g in flame-grilled chicken breast, depending on cooking temperature. In most studies, the highest association for meat consumption with cancer is for red meats; however, this may reflect how frequently ground beef is eaten in comparison to flame-grilled fish or fowl.[289] Charcoal-grilling, pan-frying, or deep-frying chicken or duck produces very high HCA levels.[290]

The first step in the formation of HCAs is the conversion of creatine to creatinine, which occurs more rapidly at high cooking temperatures.[291] Most of the HCAs in cooked food are formed in the first 6 minutes of cooking and are formed on the surface exposed to the heat. HCAs are also released as volatiles or smoke with further cooking. The amount of HCA formed plateaus as the available substrates are used up.

Under usual cooking conditions, HCAs do not form below the boiling temperature, 100°C (212°F). The amount of HCA formed in food quickly rises with temperatures over 150°C (302°F). The amount of HCA formed is about 3 times higher for foods cooked at 200°C compared to those cooked at 160°C. There is another three-fold increase in HCA formation at 250°C (482°F) compared to the amounts formed when the meat is cooked 200°C. This occurs even when meat is cooked to the same internal temperature. Since the center of a piece of meat is heated by conduction, higher cooking temperatures do not greatly reduce cooking times.[294]

HCAs can form at boiling temperatures if the conditions are right. High levels of HCAs were formed in an experiment where ground lamb was stewed for six hours in a mix of seasonings including oyster sauce, soy sauce, monosodium glutamate, and sugar.[292] This process provided high concentrations of creatine, free amino acids, reducing sugars, and water and allowed sufficient time for the reactions to complete. When meat is boiled, most of the HCA formed is released into the broth rather than being present in the meat.

Cooking in water limits the cooking temperature of the food to the boiling point; this limits the formation of HCA. Baking and roasting, which heat foods through indirect convection, do not reach high temperatures unless allowed to overcook and dry out. If the meat dries out, the temperature can rise, and HCA can form; however, if charring does not occur, levels usually remain low. Similarly, microwave cooking will not form HCA unless the meat is overcooked and dries out. Cooking techniques that heat food through radiation, such as broiling or roasting, or conduction, such as grilling or frying, heat the surface of the meat to very high temperatures. They thus lead to increased production of mutagenic HCA.

The effect of cooking temperature and technique are summarized in table 17-1.

Table 17-1: HCA Formation and Cooking Method

Method[293]	Temp °C	Temp °F	HCA formation[135]
Stewing, Simmering	70 – 80	158 - 194	None
Boiling	100	212	Low levels with long cooking times; more HCA will be in the water than in the meat.
Pressure cooking, in water	100 – 120	212 – 248	None (high humidity)
Microwave	≤100	≤212	None, as long as the meat is not allowed to dry out.
Sauté in water-based sauce	≤120	≤248	None or very low, as long as not allowed to dry out.
Baking, Roasting*	100	212	Usually, low to intermediate levels
Pan Fry – Sauté in oil	175 – 225	350 – 450	Intermediate production
Recommended Deep fat frying	150 – 175	300 – 350	Intermediate production
Typical Deep fat frying	190 – 240	374 – 464	High amounts that increase with temperature
Grilling	200 – 260	392 – 500	High amounts that increase with temperature
Charcoal Grill, Barbeque	230 – 270	466 – 518	High amounts that increase with temperature. Adds PAH risks and risks from volatiles
Flame Grill, Sear	≥430	≥806	Very high amounts; intended to char meat

*Note: Although baking and roasting use temperatures considerably above 100° C, these methods heat by indirect convection, so that the temperature of the meat being cooked is limited to the evaporation temperature of the moisture in the meat, and thus does not rise above boiling temperatures so long as the meat does not dry out.

When preparing a whole turkey in the oven, it is common to bake it covered and to finish the baking by roasting the bird, uncovered, at a higher temperature for the last 15 to 20 minutes of cooking to brown the skin. This browning greatly increases HCA formation. The HCAs are principally confined to the skin, and to the pan drippings.

One objective in cooking meat is to kill bacteria that may be present, especially on the surface of the meat, or within the meat in the case of hamburger or ground meat (Table 17-2). Hamburger, for example, cooked at a grill temperature of 160°C (320°F), turning the patty once a minute, produces low HCA levels. In a study of HCA formation during the preparation of hamburger patties, it took 8 minutes to cook 1.5 cm (5/8th inch) thick patties to an internal temperature of 70°C (158°F). Increasing the grill temperature from 160°C (320°F) to 200°C (392°F) had very little effect on cooking time but tripled HCA formation.[294]

Table 17-2: FDA Recommended Minimum Cooking Temperatures[295]

Meat	Temperature	
Fish	63° C	145° F
Steaks and Roasts	63° C	145° F
Ground Beef	71° C	160° F
Pork	71° C	160° F
Poultry	74° C	165° F

The typical temperature recommended by professional chefs for frying foods to obtain optimal flavor, appearance, and texture is 365° F (185° C). At this temperature, there is relatively little HCA formation. These temperatures, however, are easily exceeded when cooking in oils with high smoke-point temperatures, such as corn, soy, or canola oil. The high-smoke point is what gives these oils their advantage; they withstand higher temperatures, and food can be crisped more quickly. Nevertheless, cooking time does not change significantly. A higher frying temperature tends to overcook the outer layer before the center can be sufficiently heated to kill bacteria and cook the meat.

Creation of smoke and frying at high temperatures creates volatiles that contain HCAs and other carcinogenic compounds, such as PAH. Inhalation of these compounds increases the risk of lung cancer. When frying or grilling meat indoors, a vent should be used to avoid the inhalation of these volatiles. Smoked fish and meat can have high levels of PAH, which are mutagenic and carcinogenic.[296,297]

When cooking at high temperatures, HCA can also become aerosolized, exposing cooks to airborne carcinogens. Fried bacon produces especially high levels.[298] Baked, roasted, and microwave-cooked meat appears to impart little risk while fried, grilled, and well-done meat does. Different meats may favor the formation of different carcinogenic HCAs, but beef, pork, chicken, eggs, and fish all will form pro-carcinogenic HCA compounds when cooked at high temperatures.

Water content: HCAs are more efficiently formed when the moisture level in meat has fallen. Non-enzymatic browning reactions, called Maillard reactions, are formed most efficiently at water activity levels between 0.6 and 0.7. This is a point where much of the water has been lost from the meat and fish, and the water content is similar to dried fruit. Cooking procedures that minimize water loss can limit the production of HCA. This can be as simple as covering meat while sautéing it so that it cooks in its own steam, or by adding enough moisture to keep the meat from drying. Only very low levels of HCA are formed while cooking fish until it has lost over 50 percent of its weight through loss of moisture. If fish is cooked for the same length of time and at the same temperature, uncovered baking that allows drying of the fish produces five times as much HCA as does covered, steamed fish, a method that prevents moisture loss. *Poaching and stewing meats minimize the formation of mutagens.*

Reducing Sugars: HCA production is dependent on the presence of reducing sugars. Creatinine binding with amino acids is facilitated in the presence of a reducing sugar at about half the molar concentration of the creatinine or the amino acid. Beef, for example, contains glucose at about 0.07 percent. HCA conversion is most efficient when the reducing sugars (glucose, fructose, lactose and ribose) are present at about 0.15 percent (weight of monosaccharide/weight meat). Adding 0.08 percent glucose doubles the production of HCA. This would be equivalent to adding a third of a gram of glucose per pound of meat. Cooking meat with wine, which contains reducing sugars (about 1 gram/liter in red wine, 1.3 grams/liter white wines), can increase the production of HCA from 60 to 80 percent when wine is added to ground beef.[299] Cooking a steak marinated in a commercial honey barbecue sauce increased the level of HCA by as much as four times,[300] likely because of the reducing sugars present in corn syrup. Table sugar (sucrose) is not a reducing sugar and does not have this effect. Ribose is present in nucleic acids in the cell, and the free ribose content of meat increases with very long cooking times.

At higher concentrations, glucose and other reducing sugars reduce the formation of carcinogenic AIA compounds. At 0.67 percent (w/w), glucose and fructose decrease the production of HCA by about 50%.[299] This would be equivalent to adding 6 grams of glucose per kilogram, or 2.7 grams of glucose per pound of ground beef.

The addition of cornstarch to ground beef (15 grams/kg or 7 grams/pound) also reduces the mutagenicity of cooked hamburgers,[308] perhaps by retaining the meat juices internally and preventing their exposure to the heat of the pan.

Onions have enough sugar (about 14 to 20 grams of reducing sugars per pound) to influence the formation of HCA in beef. Adding a minimum of a half-pound of finely minced onion or 1/3-pound sweet onion to one pound of ground beef decreases the formation of HCA;[308] however, adding small amounts of onion (one tablespoon minced onion or onion juice or less, per pound of ground beef), could be expected to increase the formation of HCA.

Processing: Freezing meat, especially in home freezers that are not cold enough for flash freezing, causes the formation of large ice crystals that rupture the muscle cells. With commercial freezers, the temperatures are low enough that the ice crystals form more quickly, are smaller, and less likely to rupture the cells. Ruptured muscle cells leak creatine, amino acids, and glucose, and during cooking, raise the amount of substrates for the formation of HCA. Thawing and refreezing meat increases the amount of substrates available for HCA production.

Processing, such as mechanical tenderization or grinding beef to make ground beef for hamburgers, ruptures or cuts large numbers of cells, greatly increasing the availability of creatinine and amino acids for forming carcinogenic HCA.

HCA production can be greatly diminished by removing extracellular water from the meat, along with the HCA substrates. This can be accomplished by microwaving ground meat in its ready-to-cook form (i.e., a hamburger patty) for one-and-a-half to three minutes and discarding the juice which separates prior to grilling the meat. A three-minute microwave pretreatment of hamburger patties has been demonstrated to reduce the HCA content after grilling at 250°C by nearly 90 percent and decrease mutagenicity by over 95%. Replacing these juices to the hamburger before grilling restored the formation of HCA.[301] Cuts of meat, or meat which has been diced prior to cooking, may be rinsed in water or soaked in a marinade that is then discarded, and the meat patted dry to remove surface substrates for HCA production.

Love the sizzle? Many cooks use the back of a spatula to express the juices from a burger while it's grilling to get a rush of sizzle, steam, smoke, and smell. This is a very efficient means of HCA production and volatilization.

The availability of extracellular HCA substrates explains why gravies, stock, extracts, and pan residues can have extremely high

HCA contents.[302] Gravy can be made from liver or other organs low in creatine to give lower HCA content gravy.

Marinades: When cooking meat, the surfaces are browned, and this is where the HCAs are produced. With hamburger meat, HCA inhibitors can be mixed into the meat before cooking. When cooking non-ground beef, the inhibitors cannot be mixed in as easily. Marinating the meat, however, can greatly reduce the production of HCA.[303] Both beer and red wine decrease the formation of most HCA, although they may increase the concentration of others.[304] Beer does not contain reducing sugars, and thus, and does not raise HCA production. Beer also has less effect on the flavor of the cooked meat.[305]

In a test of HCA formation using marinades, a liquid for the marinade made from water, soy oil, and vinegar did not lower the production of HCA when grilling steaks. Adding salt and table sugar to the marinade liquid reduced the formation of HCA by half. With the addition of herbs and spices, the production of HCA content in the grilled steak was lowered by as much as 88 percent. Garlic inhibits the formation of HCA. The herbs used included oregano, rosemary, and thyme, and which are high in antioxidant phenolic compounds including carnosic acid, carnosol, and rosmarinic acid.[306] An effective HCA-preventive marinade can be made from 30 percent sweet red onion, 30 percent garlic, 15 percent lemon or lime juice.[307]

Antioxidants: Antioxidants can prevent the formation of HCAs. Ascorbic acid (vitamin C) added at 3 grams/kg of ground beef also decreases the production of HCA by 50 percent.[308] At this level, it has little if any noticeable effect on flavor. Many other phenolic antioxidants have also been shown to prevent the formation of HCA. Different antioxidants may act differently to prevent the formation of different HCA.[309] The vitamin E content in vegetable oil was found to be inversely associated with HCA formation.[310]

Biotransformation

As previously discussed, smoking tobacco increases the biotransformation of HCA by the CYP enzymes in the liver, and enhances the metabolism of AIA for the formation of DNA adducts that can cause cancer in multiple organs. Androgens induce the transcription of NAT1, which may explain why many cancers are more common in men.[311] Other compounds increase the transformation of AIA into compounds that are easily excreted from the body.

Cruciferous vegetables (CV) contain isothiocyanate compounds that induce the production and activity of the enzyme glutathione S-transferase (GST). As illustrated in Figure 17-1, GST metabolizes N-hydroxylated AIA into conjugated compounds that are easily excreted into the urine. Thus, GST competes with NAT for the metabolism of N-hydroxylated HCA and lowers cancer risk by helping detoxify the AIA and ridding them from the body before they can be transformed into mutagens.

Freezing of boiling CV can prevent the formation of the active compounds that induce GST and other protective enzymes. These vegetables should be eaten lightly steamed or raw to receive the most anti-carcinogenic benefit from them. CV needs to be consumed prior to HCA exposure, so that the protective enzymes are already induced and present to shift metabolism of the compounds from NAT to GST pathways. Further details are given in Chapter 24.

Antioxidant phenolic compounds also prevent HCA-related carcinogenesis. Treatment of hepatic cells with several phenolic compounds has been shown to attenuate the mutagenic effect of HCA. The phenolic compound epigallocatechin gallate, found in black and green tea, prevents DNA binding with N-acetoxy-PhIP and the formation of PhIP-DNA adducts.[312] Cellular changes induced by HCA in hepatocytes were 75 to 90 percent eliminated by post-treatment with the phenolic compounds vanillin, coumarin, and caffeine.[313]

Once-in-a-While

Eating an occasional charbroiled hamburger should be OK, so long as it is not done frequently, right?

Well, actually, not. An occasional dose of hundreds or thousands of nanograms of HCA or other large doses of mutagens is a very effective way of surpassing protein "interference," detoxification pathways, and other natural defenses. Low-level exposures are much easier to detoxify, and the body adapts by up-regulating the enzymes that process these toxins. Also, these are not a cumulative poison with a threshold; they are more like Russian roulette, where even though the risk may be small, any exposure that escapes the natural defenses and reaches the nucleus and forms DNA adducts, cause risk for carcinogenic mutations.

The occasional high dose is especially of concern during growth, when great numbers of cells are susceptible to mutagenic injury.

Safer Burgers

Ground beef needs to reach a higher core temperature to kill bacteria than does steak. Grinding hamburger mixes bacteria throughout the meat and thus, requires enough cooking time to allow heat to transfer into the center of the patty or meatball. Cooking hamburger meat to an internal temperature of 160°F (71°C) or to 155°F (68°C) for at least 15 seconds kills the bacteria of concern.[295]

The grill or skillet temperature should be set to 320°F (160°C)[314] and no higher than 356°F (180°C). Heat has to be transferred to the center by conduction, and this takes time. A higher temperature has little effect on how long it takes to heat the center but increases the formation of carcinogens. A grill temperature over 212°F (100°C) gives the hamburger its outer crust.

Meat needs to be completely thawed to cook properly. Fish or meat that has been incompletely thawed is much more likely to be overcooked on the outside and raw in the center, resulting in HCA on the outside and live bacteria inside

Hamburger patties should ideally be about 6/10th to ¾ inch (1.5 - 2.0 cm) thick to be juicy, but no thicker to cook well

Do not use the spatula to press the juice out of a hamburger; it dries out the patty and creates more carcinogens. Mixing two levels teaspoons of cornstarch into a pound of ground beef will help retain fluid inside and decrease HCA formation during cooking. Other techniques for reducing HCA formation are given earlier in this chapter.

Flipping the patty once a minute, will cook it more quickly and evenly and avoid HCA formation.

Expect it to take 9 to 12 minutes to cook the hamburger, depending on its thickness. A brown center does not guarantee that a safe temperature has been reached during cooking.[295]

Summary

Heterocyclic Amines (HCA) are carcinogens created when meat is cooked at high temperatures. The HCA are some of the most potent and important dietary carcinogens. They can be avoided by cooking meat more carefully and avoiding overheating of meat. This chapter discussed techniques and temperatures for the safe preparation of meat so that HCA formation is minimized.

Hamburger and other ground meats are an especially rich source of carcinogenic HCA. Extra caution should be used in their preparation. The HCA are such potent carcinogens that I recommend that cancer patients avoid the consumption of hamburger or other ground meats.

18: N-Nitrosyl Compounds

In addition to cancer risk from HCA, processed meats are associated with additional risk for some cancers. This risk appears to be associated with the formation of N-nitrosyl compounds (NNCs). N-nitrosyl compounds are also abbreviated as NOC in the literature.

NNCs are formed during preparation and digestion of red meat, processed meats, and in certain other foods. Cured meats are a major source of dietary NNC. Hot dogs, sausages, bacon, lunch meats, and processed ham contain nitrates and nitrites that are additives used to preserve the meat's color. In the stomach's acidic environment, nitrite (NO_2^-) from cured meat can combine with amines and amides derived from foods and form NNCs. Curing, drying, and smoking meats, processes used to prevent oxidation of fatty acids in food, can cause amines or amides to form in the meat that can then be nitrosated.

NNCs can form under various conditions. Nitrite ions, in an acidic environment, such as the stomach, become protonated and form nitrous acid. The nitrous acid then splits into an ON^+ ion and water. This ion can then bind to a nitrogen atom in an amine, such as an amino acid, and form an NNC. Secondary amines, such as biogenic diamines formed during the fermentation of certain amino acids, can also form NNCs when heated. Diamines, such as putrescine and cadaverine, as their names imply, may be present in meat that is less than fresh. The acidic environment of the stomach mostly produces nitrosothiol compounds.[315]

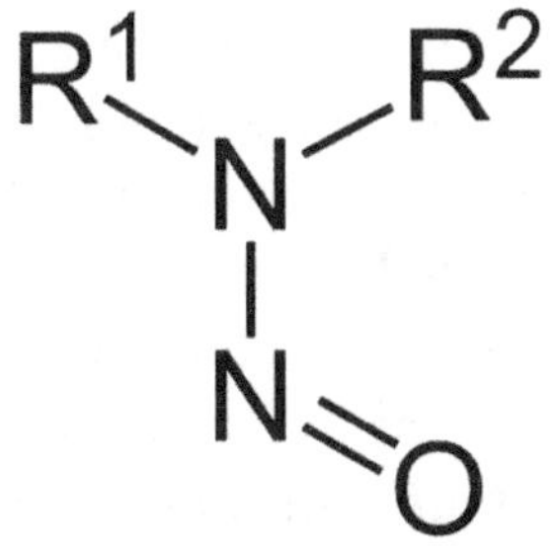

$$R^1\underset{\underset{N=O}{|}}{\overset{}{N}}R^2$$

Figure 18-1: General Structure of a Nitrosamine

Many NNC compounds, including nitrosamine, are known carcinogens. Of about 120 N-nitroso compounds tested, about 80 percent have carcinogenic activity. Cigarette smoke contains 13 different carcinogenic nitrosamines.[316] While most NNCs are carcinogenic, there is a wide diversity in their potency; the exposure dose that causes cancer in 50% of test animals for one NNC may be 3000 times lower than the dose required by another NNC to do the same damage.[349] Thus, the food source for the NNCs and conditions under which they form may have a tremendous influence on their carcinogenic potential.

Nitrates (NO_3^-) are present in many foods, including vegetables. Nitrates, however, do not form NNCs; it is nitrites that do. Nevertheless, many bacteria transform nitrates into nitrites. Thus, many foods that have been fermented, and foods with spoilage, may have their nitrates converted into nitrites. Then, in the acidic environment of the stomach, nitrites can interact with amino acids in the meal and form NNCs.

USDA now requires adding 550 parts per million of either sodium ascorbate or sodium erythorbate to bacon to lower levels of NNC, in addition to restricting the use of added nitrites. Reducing agents, such as vitamin C, Vitamin E, and certain phenolic compounds, prevent the creation of nitrites.

Some green vegetables also contain significant amounts of nitrates and some nitrites.[317] Since these fresh vegetables also contain antioxidants, these nitrites do not readily form NNCs.

Nitrosamines are created from bioamines, which are formed by many bacteria from amino acids and nitrates in food. Thus, spoilage or fermentation greatly increases their formation. Further transformation occurs during heating, especially at higher temperatures (frying), and in the stomach, where the compounds are exposed to acid.

Fermented and salted vegetables are associated with risk of cancer. Pickled vegetables are frequently consumed in China and are associated with increased cancer risk, specifically for esophageal[318] and gastric cancers. Pickling is the process of bacterial fermentation of food in salt brine or vinegar for preservation. It is the brine/fermentation process rather than the vinegar process that is associated with increased cancer risk. Pickled vegetable consumption has been found to increase gastric cancer risk by 50% and more than double the risk of esophageal cancer.[319] [320] Koreans who consume higher amounts of kimchi, spicy fermented cabbage, have a 57% increase in the risk of stomach cancer. Those consuming higher levels of fermented soybean paste have a 62 percent increase in risk while non-fermented alliums (onions and garlic) and non-fermented seafood lowered risk by 30 and 34 percent.[321]

While many bacteria do convert nitrates to nitrites, it is likely that contamination with fungal molds (e.g., Fusarium) promotes the formation of NNC. These fungi are common plant pathogens and saprophytes that contaminate crops, so it is easy for them to find their way into the pickling process. To complicate the picture, some species of these fungi produce carcinogenic mycotoxins, such as fumonisin B1.[322] Thus, the carcinogenic link to pickled vegetable consumption may be due to NNCs, the presence of mycotoxins, or a combination of these and other factors.

Food created from meat byproducts, such as hot dogs, sausage, or fish cakes, are more likely to have unintentional bacterial growth and fermentation which can supply polyamines. These products usually have nitrates added as preservatives to retain their color. Thus, processed meats have multiple sources of NNC precursors for delivering high amounts of NNCs.

Polyamines in foods can also be converted into carcinogenic NNC, such as N-nitroso-pyrrolidine and N-nitroso-piperidine, during cooking. This occurs, especially in fatty foods such as bacon, when exposed to high cooking temperatures. Putrescine and cadaverine are present in decaying fish and meat and in aged cheeses. NNC can also be formed from spermidine that is present in fresh meat when heated at higher cooking temperatures[323]. Aged cheeses are usually not cooked at high temperatures, and thus are not a common risk factor. Fermented, salted, and dried seafood can have very high NNC levels.[324] Pickled fish, as consumed in China, are associated with increased risk for nasal-pharyngeal carcinoma.

Processed meats are a risk factor for cancer. Processed meats form more, and a wider variety of NNC than do red meats.[325] In the Nurses' Health Study II 7-year follow-up, overall consumption of processed meats during adolescence was not associated with premenopausal breast cancer; however, hot dogs were.[326] If bologna is eaten uncooked, little if any NNC should form. If the baloney or hotdogs are cooked at high temperatures, NNCs easily form.

When nitrite-cured bacon was fried in a skillet at either 171°C (338°F) or 206 °C (402 °F), 11 ng/g of NNC were formed. When the bacon was cooked in a microwave, and not allowed to dry out, no NNC were formed.[327] In another study, bacon fried at boiling temperature, 100 °C (212 °F), or at 135 °C (275 °F) did not form NNC, but when fried at 177 °C (350 °F) for 6 minutes or at 204°C (400 °F) for 4 minutes (medium well-done), nitrosamines were found.[328] Allowing bacon to "fry-out" can increase NNC content by 10 times.[329]

Since many foods contain small amounts of nitrites, including fruits and fresh vegetables, the average nitrite intake for an adult is about one microgram per day. A few foods, however, have very high levels that cause concern. A food of great concern is salted fish, which contains levels between 20 and 373 micrograms per kilogram.[330] This high level in salted fish is likely secondary to spoilage and bacterial growth during drying as well as impurities in the salt used to dry the fish.[331] Other foods high in NNC are salted and cured pork, with levels of 3.6-490 micrograms/kg after frying.[332] Frying bacon increases the NNC content; after cooking it can have levels from 10 to 100 micrograms/kg; as much as 10 micrograms in a single serving. Some German beers have levels between 5 and 70 micrograms of NNC per liter.[333] These beers derive their nitrites from malt. The nitrites originate from microbial activity during the drying of sprouted barley. Enjoying Oktoberfest could expose one to hundreds of micrograms of NNC in a single day.

NNCs are metabolized by the cytochrome p450 enzymes CYP1A1 and CYP2E1 and then by glutathione S-transferase and aldehyde dehydrogenase. Various alleles of these enzymes influence the carcinogenic potential of NNC for the individual. Those with slower p450 metabolism and faster GST conjugation were at higher risk of stomach cancer.[321] This suggests that NNCs that are not oxidized, and endure to become water soluble, increase the risk of stomach cancer.

NNCs form adducts with DNA causing alkylation-induced mutations. Certain NNCs have been shown to induce G to A (guanine to adenine) mutations in the ras gene in exfoliated colonocytes,[334] the cells that line the colon. O(6)-alkyl-guanine is the major carcinogenic lesion in DNA, induced by alkylating mutagens. The DNA repair protein O(6)-methylguanine-DNA methyltransferase (MGMT) repairs these mutations, removing this DNA adduct. The liver contains MGMT mRNA levels 30 times higher than other tissues, and thus, it can be presumed to be the major area exposed to these mutagens.

Meta-analysis studies of red or processed meat consumption reveal either no or very low-risk associations with kidney,[335] breast,[336] ovarian,[337] and prostate[338] cancers. NNC exposure from red or processed meat does not appear to be associated with bladder cancer.[339] An increased risk from the consumption of processed meat has been found in stomach,[340] colon, and rectal cancers.[341] NNCs are also associated with risk of esophageal cancer.[318] This suggests that NNC act as a carcinogen locally on mucosa, but has much lower risk of causing systemic mutations than do HCA because the liver can process the NNC toxins and repair DNA damage caused by NNC.

NNCs, however, do cause non-mucosal cancer. They are a significant risk factor for cancers of the brain. About 12 percent of adults do not express the enzyme MGMT in their brain. These individuals are 4.5 times more likely to develop brain tumors.[342]

There is a wide range of MGMT activity in the brain; individuals with lower MGMT activity may also be at increased risk.

There is another population at high risk: preborn infants. MGMT expression develops along with fetal maturity. At six to eight weeks post conception, only 25% of fetuses express MGMT in the brain. By 15 to 19 weeks of development, 88% of fetuses have MGMT production in the brain.[343] Thus, NNC exposure during pregnancy is a risk for brain cancer, and the fetus is at highest risk during the first half of pregnancy. This likely explains the pathway for how hot dog consumption during pregnancy increases the risk of brain tumors in children.

An international study of maternal diet during pregnancy and risk of childhood brain tumor was revealing; not only did it show foods whose consumption was associated with elevated risk of childhood brain cancers, but it also showed foods which lowered the risks. Children of mothers who consumed higher levels of cured meats during pregnancy had a 50 percent higher rate of brain cancer, while the consumption of other meats was not significantly associated with risk. Higher consumption of eggs and dairy products was associated with a 20 percent increase in risk. Consumption of higher amounts of fresh fish during pregnancy was associated with a 30 percent reduction in risk of brain cancer in children, yellow-orange vegetables with a 20 percent decrease in risk, and higher intake of grain, with a ten percent decrease in risk. Cruciferous or green leafy vegetables, fruits, and caffeinated beverages during pregnancy did not have significant effects on risk of brain cancer for children in this population.[344]

In studies of adults, higher intake of yellow-orange vegetables was associated with a 30 to 40 percent decreased risk for glioma brain tumors; the decreased risk was associated with carotenoid consumption.[345] In a Chinese study of brain cancer and diet, brain cancer risk was inversely associated with consumption of fresh fish, fresh vegetables - especially Chinese cabbage, onions, fresh fruit, and poultry. The risk was increased with salted vegetables and salted fish consumption.[346]

The levels of nitrosamines present in foods have been declining over the past four decades, as a result of a lowering the concentration of nitrite used for food preservation and better control in the preparation of malt for making beer.[347]

Although the amount of nitrates and nitrites added to processed meats has fallen over time,[348] consumption of processed meats should still be minimized. Processed, smoked and preserved meat consumption should be avoided in individuals at high risk for colon and rectal cancers, and the consumption of yellow-orange vegetables encouraged to decrease the risk from NNC. Helicobacter pylori infection is a risk factor for stomach cancer, and thus, should be treated. Ascorbic acid (vitamin C) inhibits the formation of most nitrosamines and shifts NNC production to forms that are less carcinogenic; thus, it is used in the processing of meats to decrease NNC creation. The phenolic compounds gallate, tannic acid, and vitamin E prevent nitrosamine formation.[349] In lab animals, a low calcium diet resulted in very high NNC levels among animals fed cured meat, as measured in their feces; a high calcium diet resulted in much lower fecal NNCs levels.[350] Dietary soy has also been found to decrease the content of NNC in the stool.[351]

Pregnant women should be advised to avoid processed and smoked meats and fish, and be encouraged to eat fresh fish and yellow-orange vegetables to decrease the risk of brain cancer in their children.

Summary

NNC are carcinogens, but mostly for the mucosal or skin surfaces that are directly exposed to it. Thus, dietary NNCs are risk factors for cancers of the esophagus, stomach, and large colorectum. NNC are present in tobacco smoke and are carcinogens for the lung. The temperatures needed to form NNC are lower than those required to form HCA. Frying processed meats at 171°C (338°F), a typical frying temperature, readily creates carcinogenic NNC.

The enzyme MGMT detoxifies NNC and protects most tissues from NNC carcinogenesis, other than the mucosa and lungs that are directly exposed. All young fetuses and about one in eight children and adults fail to make the enzyme MGMT in the brain, putting them at greater risk for NNC-induced brain cancer. Since NNC are also produced in the stomach, it is prudent to completely avoid processed meat consumption during pregnancy. Genome testing may be used to identify those that do not make MGMT in the brain.

If hot dogs are eaten, they should be boiled. Frying or grilling them creates carcinogens. A method for cooking bacon that avoids overheating and NNC formation is given below. This method may be used to heat hot dogs and other processed meats. Lunch meats that are made to be eaten without being reheated are safest unheated. Individuals with high risk for esophageal, stomach, colorectal or brain cancers because of personal or family history or other risks would be prudent to avoid the consumption of processed meats. NNC are particularly dangerous carcinogens for the fetal brain. Pregnant women should thus avoid eating hot dogs or other cooked processed meats.

Salted fish and salt-pickled vegetables, both common in Asian cuisine, are often high in NNC and are associated with cancer risk due to fungal and bacterial fermentation. Beer may also be high in NNC from the unintentional fermentation of barley during its drying process.

Better Bacon

To prevent NNC and HCA formation, cook bacon in the microwave:

Lay three or four sheets of paper towels on a plate. Next, lay strips of bacon on the paper towels, avoiding overlapping the strips, so that the bacon is laid out as a single layer. Place a paper towel over the bacon to prevent splattering. Try a microwave cooking time of four minutes for small microwave units and 3:30 minutes in larger units. Since different microwave ovens have different power ratings, adjust cooking time as needed. The bacon should be cooked but not dried out or crispy. Allowing the bacon or other meats to dry out and harden in a microwave will greatly increase NNC and HCA formation.

Much of the excess fat will be absorbed and discarded with the paper towels. Risk of the paper towels being ignited in the microwave can be lowered by trimming off corners of the towels hanging over plate edges.

Oyster sauce and soy sauce often contain the carcinogen 3-MCPD. 3-MCPD is formed when protein hydrolysis is achieved using hydrochloric acid and heat to break proteins into amino acids. 3-MCPD is metabolized into glycidol, a genotoxic an animal carcinogen, and a suspect human carcinogen.[352] 3-MCPD and glycidol are found in processed refined vegetable oils, especially refined palm oils, while unrefined virgin oils, by in large, contain undetectable concentrations of 3-MCPD and glycidol.[353] Glycidol and 3-MCPD are formed during deodorization of the oils at high temperatures. In 2015, seven of seven brands of infant formula were found to contain 3-MCPD esters.[354]

These are a technological problem, rather than one inherent in the refining of vegetable oils, as alternative vegetable oil processing protocols have been demonstrated to lower MCPD levels to 5% of that formed during typical industrial production.[355] Similarly, with soy and oyster sauces, natural fermentation of soy and non-HCl protein hydrolysis of oyster sauces do not cause 3-MCPD formation. These, however, are slower and more expensive means of producing these products.

19: Maillard and other Heat Reaction Products

The Maillard reaction, (pronounced "my-YAR" in your best French accent) is a non-enzymatic, browning reaction occurring in foods during cooking. It can occur at room temperature, but occurs most efficiently and rapidly at temperatures from 140° to 165° C (284° to 329° F). (Enzymatic browning is what happens to apples when cut open and exposed to air.)

The first steps in the Maillard reaction appear to be similar to the formation of HCA; in the presence of heat and water, reducing sugars cause non-enzymatic glycation (addition of a sugar) of amino acids. An essential difference with HCA formation, however, is that neither creatine nor creatinine is involved. The Maillard reaction forms an unstable glycosylamine that spontaneously degrades into numerous other compounds.

If you enjoy the aromas and flavors of fresh-baked, golden brown bread; roasted coffee; crispy French-fried potatoes; lush, gooey dulce con leche; roasted nuts; chocolate; or toasted marshmallows; you are enjoying the aromas and flavors of Maillard reactants.

Just about now you are thinking about abandoning this book. I can see it in your eyes. Yes, those are some of my favorite things, too. Please, just trust me here; the good news is on its way. Just as the B vitamins niacin and pyridoxine are HCA compounds, and do not cause cancer, not all Maillard reactants in food are bad for your health. In fact, as will be detailed in Chapter 23, many prevent cancer! Now that I've gotten you to stay for the moment, let's start with the bad news. I assure you, the good news is worth waiting for.

Maillard reactions don't just occur on the stove; they happen in the body. When these reactions occur, they are known as Advanced Glycation End-products (AGEs): sugar or other small carbohydrate molecules become non-enzymatically bound to proteins. These are not functional glycoproteins, but rather dysfunctional glycosylated proteins. AGEs formed in the body are associated with diabetes, and have been implicated in several diseases of aging, including Alzheimer's disease, stroke, and cardiovascular disease. Hemoglobin A1c, used as a blood test for diabetes control because its level rises with blood sugar, is an AGE. AGEs can cause cross-linking of proteins, reduce muscle function, and cause cell stress. A well-documented result of AGEs is their association with the development of cataracts. Glucosepane is an AGE that crosslinks collagen and collects as we age, causing cataracts and wrinkling of the skin. Some AGEs promote oxidation stress. An apt acronym, AGEs cause aging.

The body can eliminate most of the AGEs that it makes through the kidneys. In diabetics, however, the copious quantities of AGEs damages the kidneys. As the kidney is progressively injured by the disease, renal function is degraded. These products accumulate and accelerate kidney damage.

The formation of AGEs and their negative effects can be prevented by a healthy diet and a healthy anti-oxidative status. (See Chapter 23 on Stress Response). Diets high in natural phenols help prevent damage from AGEs. In fact, diets containing certain Maillard reactants also help eliminate and destroy endogenous AGEs. Most of the AGEs that are detrimental to health are ones created within the body; having elevated blood sugar greatly contributes to this.

Maillard reactants formed during cooking, in general, are much less likely to be problematic than those created in the body. When these compounds are ingested and absorbed, most are easily eliminated by the kidneys.

A few Maillard reactants are animal carcinogens and suspect human carcinogens. The one that has been most studied is acrylamide. Acrylamide is present in many toasted foods, especially in French fries and potato chips, as potatoes have high levels of available asparagine, the amino acid precursor of acrylamide. Acrylamide is easily absorbed through the skin; industrial exposures can be 100 times higher than exposure from heavy consumption of toasted foods. Smoking cigarettes is a major exposure to acrylamide; smokers have acrylamide blood levels three times higher than non-smokers.[356] The average American dietary intake of acrylamide is 1 μg per kg body weight per day, and those consuming high amounts may consume four μg/kg body weight/day. Smokers have a far higher consumption as each cigarette exposes them to 1.1 to 3.3 μg of acrylamide.[357]

Acrylamide is oxidized in the body by CYP2E1 to glycidamide. Glycidamide is a more potent DNA adduct than acrylamide, and it causes sister chromatid exchanges[358] and DNA adducts in TP53 gene that codes for p53.[359]

Nevertheless, even among smokers, the acrylamide level does not appear to be a risk factor for lung cancer. And while there have been multiple epidemiologic studies assessing cancer risk from dietary acrylamide, no such risk has been found.[360, 361, 362]

There is concern that sperm cells are uniquely susceptible, and glycinamide-induced gene damage may pass across generations.[363]

Acrylamide and glycidamide also form adducts with hemoglobin in the blood, as well as with many other proteins, damaging them. These proteins likely run interference and shield the DNA from damage from acrylamide at glycidamide levels likely to be found from acrylamide in the diet. This does not vindicate acrylamide from being genotoxic; the damage even to proteins can cause aging of the cells and acrylamide is a suspected neurologic toxin.

Temperatures above 120° C (248° F) promote the formation of acrylamide, and longer cooking times and higher temperatures increase its production. Raising the frying temperature from 170° C to 190° C (338° F to 374° F) increased acrylamide content of potato chips by five times.[364] Frying at 150° C gives even lower levels than does 170° C. Acrylamide production peaks at the temperature of 190° C; at higher temperatures, it begins to break down by pyrolysis into other compounds, although these may be just as toxic.

Most of the acrylamide is formed at the surface during frying; fried potatoes with a higher surface-to-volume area have higher acrylamide content. Shoestring potatoes have a higher surface area, and acrylamide content, than do potato wedges. Pan frying, where only one surface at a time is cooked, also creates lower acrylamide levels than does deep fat frying. Microwave cooking of potatoes very efficiently creates acrylamide. This may result from the rapid heating from within affecting the entire mass of the potato, rather than just heating the surface as occurs with other forms of cooking.[365]

> Potatoes are best stored between 8° - 12° C (46° and 54° F). When potatoes are stored in commercial cold storage or in a refrigerator, the starches begin to turn into sugars. This low-temperature sweetening is especially pronounced at normal refrigerator temperatures between 2 and 4°C (36 and 40°F). This also causes potatoes to darken when cooked. Potatoes get chilling damage at 36°F (2°C) or below. Freezing causes potatoes to become watery after cooking. When potatoes are purchased from a grocer, they should have been allowed to recover from cold storage for two to four weeks, for the sugars to become starch again. This takes about 2 weeks at 18° C (65° F) or 4 weeks at 10° C (50° F).[366]
>
> Gold-fleshed potatoes are naturally sweeter and can be stored in the refrigerator without browning.

When potatoes are stored at cold temperatures, below 8° C (46° F), the amount of reducing sugars available increases. It is these sugars, fructose and glucose, rather than asparagine that are the limiting substrates in acrylamide formation in potatoes. Identically cooked potatoes had 40 times higher acrylamide levels after storing potatoes at 2°C (36°F) than when stored at 18°C (64°F) for four weeks.[367] Since gold fleshed potatoes have higher sugar content, they should not be used for frying, or cooked in a microwave if acrylamide is to be avoided.

Lower acrylamide levels can be achieved by first blanching or soaking the potatoes in water before frying, as it removes much of the freely available reducing sugars present on the cut surface of the potatoes.[368] Considerably more effective, is soaking the potatoes in a 0.15 molar solution of acetic acid solution at room temperature for 60 minutes. This lowers acrylamide production by 90%.[369]

A 0.15 molar acetic acid solution is geeky even for me. It is equivalent to one cup of table vinegar (5% acetic acid) in a quart of water. Citric acid, in the form of citrus juice, can also be used as a solution to remove reducing sugars from potatoes. The acid causes protonation of the asparagine and impedes the Maillard reaction and acrylamide formation.

Sweet potatoes and plantains also form acrylamide when fried. As plantains ripen, even more sugar is present. Some of the same techniques used to lower acrylamide formation in potatoes work as well in sweet potatoes and plantains as they do with potatoes: rinsing and blanching, soaking in acetic or citric acid (vinegar or lemon juice), and lowering the frying temperature. Sweet potatoes and ripening plantains have much higher sugar and lower asparagines contents than do white potatoes, thus in these foods, asparagine is likely the limiting acrylamide-forming substrate.[370][371]

The color intensity of fried potatoes and chips is highly correlated with acrylamide content; the darker the color, the higher the content.[367] Darker fries should be avoided. When deep fat frying, the fried food gets darker as the same oil is repeatedly used. This likely results from the accumulation of substrates, asparagine and reducing sugars, in the oil with its repeated use.

The level of acrylamide present in a typical diet is probably not sufficient to act as a carcinogen of concern. This may be because they attach to hemoglobin in the blood or other proteins, thus protecting the DNA. The principal health outcome that has been documented from dietary acrylamide, at levels typically consumed in the Western diet, is increased insulin sensitivity and decreased insulin production.[357]

It will be seen in Chapter 23 that several Maillard reactants formed during food preparation are important dietary anticarcinogens. In stark contrast to the heat-induced browning and HCA formation in foods containing creatine (meats and eggs), many pleasantly flavored Maillard browning compounds provide health benefits. So go ahead and enjoy them.

One caution, however, is for individuals with diabetes and poor renal function. In these persons, the kidneys may have difficulty removing endogenous AGEs. For these people, dietary AGEs, especially toxic ones such as acrylamide and glycidamide may add to the burden of renal AGE elimination, and increase their accumulation and harm to the body.

Pyrolysis

At temperatures above those that cause Maillard reactants, food begins to pyrolyze. In pyrolysis, food compounds begin to decompose without oxygen. When sugar is pyrolyzed at temperatures above 170 °C (338 °F), it forms a caramel. If pyrolysis continues, the result is char.

Pyrolysis occurs after the water in the material has steamed off, allowing the temperature of the material to rise above the boiling point. As long as water is present, pyrolysis does not occur.

> In a pressure cooker, with adequate water, or with long cooking times, some proteins hydrolyze, breaking up into primary proteins, and when protein hydrolysis occurs, the proteins decompose into smaller chains of amino acids and freeing some individual amino acids. These shorter chains of amino acids are less likely to cause immune response and are easier to digest, and can add to the flavor of the food. The amino acids, however, do not decompose. In a pressure cooker, there should be no charring unless there is inadequate water or poor distribution of the water so that the food can overheat.

Usually, during cooking, only the outer layer of food that dries out becomes pyrolyzed. Wood charcoal is made by pyrolysis of wood until it becomes char.

Pyrolysis of lipids, such as oils and waxes in foods, also occurs at high cooking temperatures. The pyrolysis temperature for different compounds depends on the lipid and fatty acid mixture of the triglyceride. Saturated fats produce more acrolein than do unsaturated fats. The pyrolysis temperature of fat is about the same as its smoke temperature and is just below its ignition temperature. Butter has a much lower browning temperature, (about 150° C - 302° F), as it contains milk proteins that brown more easily. Smoke temperatures of some common cooking oils are given in Table 19-1.

Table 19-1: Smoke Temperatures for Some Common Cooking Oils[295]

Type of Fat	Degrees F	Degrees C	18:2 trans fat %
Unrefined canola oil	225	107	
Butter	302	150	0
Extra virgin olive oil	320	160	0
Coconut oil	351	177	0
Refined canola oil	400	204	0.365
Virgin olive oil	420	216	0
Refined corn oil	450	232	0.286
Refined soy oil	450 - 495	232 - 257	0.53
Refined sunflower oil	440 - 450	227 - 232	
Refined safflower oil	450 - 510	232 - 266	
Extra light olive oil	468	242	

Acrolein

When fat is pyrolyzed, it forms solid and volatile tars, that make cause a sticky coating on walls and surfaces in the kitchen and in the lungs. One of the common compounds formed is the volatile toxin and irritant acrolein.

When fat is heated to around 180° C (357° F) or higher, triglycerides decompose into fatty acids and glycerol. The hotter the temperature, the more rapidly this occurs. Heating corn oil to 300° C (572° F) for two hours produces ten times as much acrolein as does heating it to 280° C (536° F). Acrolein volatilizes and continues to be produced as long as heating continues. Some acrolein is absorbed by the foods being cooked.

Canola oil, in spite of having a smoke temperature similar to that of corn oil, produces more acrolein at 240° C (464° F) than corn oil does at 300° C (572° F). Although olive oil has a significantly lower smoke temperature than does canola oil, canola oil pyrolyzes at a lower temperature and produces much higher levels of acrolein than does olive oil at 180° C, and this difference is even more pronounced at 240° C.[372]

Acrolein is commonly found in French fries and other foods fried at high temperatures. It is also one of the most abundant non-carcinogenic toxins in tobacco smoke. While acrolein forms DNA adducts *in vivo*, extensive testing has not shown it to be a carcinogen,[373] perhaps because the body is capable of efficiently conjugating it to glutathione, and eliminating it into the urine. Acrolein also easily forms protein adducts, and thus, it may preferentially bind to proteins, sparing DNA. This does not spare us from injury. While acrolein is not a carcinogen, it is an irritant, mutagen, and cytotoxin. It can cause damage and aging of the cells. It depletes glutathione, activates oxidative stress and AP1 signaling, causes endoplasmic reticulum stress, disrupts mitochondrial integrity and function, and promotes cell death through apoptosis.[374] Wow! It sounds like it might make a decent chemotherapy agent, but nothing you want for supper.

Acrolein has been implicated in cellular injury responsible for Alzheimer's disease, cardiomyopathy, vascular disease, diabetes mellitus, neurologic injury, liver toxicity, and nephrotoxicity.[375] Consumption of fried foods should be limited, but if frying is done, there are ways to decrease the formation of aldehydes such as acrolein.

The recommended deep fat frying temperature for ideal culinary results (ignoring health) is 185° C (365° F). Thus, there is little reason to use higher temperatures, although higher temperatures are often used. Oil with a smoke point above this temperature must be used to avoid fire hazards and other risks. Canola oil produces many times higher amounts of acrolein and other products of pyrolysis than olive or corn oils. Other oils should be tested and characterized to find those that produce the lowest amounts of acrolein and other toxic products. Canola oil should not be used for frying, and its use should be limited to unrefined (expeller) canola oil as a salad oil. In kitchens where frying is done, the stove and fryer should be hooded. A fan should be used to vent the volatiles created during cooking to avoid inhalation of these toxic compounds.

Cooking Eggs

Meat and eggs cooked at appropriate temperatures give the best culinary results and with minimal HCA formation. The ideal open skillet or griddle temperature for cooking an egg is 120 C° (248 F°), a temperature at which water in the butter will sizzle, but at which the butter does not brown. Hamburger, for example, cooked at a grill temperature of 160°C (320°F), turning the patty once a minute, produces low HCA levels.

Heterocyclic Amines (HCA) are potent carcinogens that are formed when meat, fish, or eggs are cooked at high temperatures. These carcinogens are especially dangerous during growth and development, and can cause cancer in multiple organs (Chapter 17). Hamburger is exceptionally susceptible to HCA formation

The various proteins in eggs coagulate between 63°C (145° F) and 80°C (176° F). Cooking at higher temperatures makes the egg tough and unpleasant. When eggs are cooked, the heat causes the proteins in the egg to denature (unwind) and then condense into solids. Egg yolks solidify at about 70°C (158°F) and whites become firm at around 80°C (180°F). Note that both these temperatures are well below the boiling point of water.[293]

A temperature of 160°F (71°C) kills bacteria that may contaminate eggs and cause illness. A soft-boiled egg or an egg with a runny center has not been heated sufficiently to solidify the yolk proteins or to kill bacteria which may be present. Pregnant women, infants, and other immune-compromised individuals should avoid soft-boiled eggs or eggs cooked with a runny yolk. Cracked, but otherwise good eggs should only be used for making baked foods, to avoid risk from *Salmonella*.

The ideal open skillet or griddle temperature for cooking an egg is 120°C (248°F), a temperature at which water in butter will sizzle, but at which the butter does not brown. At these temperatures, HCA should not be formed unless the eggs are allowed to overcook.

Butter is about 16% water, and thus when it reaches a simmering temperature of about 85°C (185°F), tiny bubbles begin to form. Butter is an excellent indicator revealing when the cooking pan is the perfect temperature for cooking eggs. Big bubbles in the butter indicate that the temperature is over the boiling point and too hot for cooking eggs. Smoking butter indicates that the pan is over 150°C (302°F), and much too hot for cooking eggs. A perfect omelet is tender, yellow and without browning or lacing.

When cooking eggs, there is little reason to heat eggs much hotter than the temperature required for killing *salmonella*. Temperatures over 82°C (180°F) will make the egg firmer, but with higher temperatures, eggs become tough and rubbery. Brown lacing on a cooked egg shows that it was either cooked too long or at too high a temperature. Egg yolks contain creatine that is converted into carcinogenic HCA if cooked at high temperatures. Browned egg yolk or a browned omelet may indicate the formation of carcinogenic heterocyclic amine compounds. Browning of the yolk or lacing during cooking indicates the eggs have been overheated. Your mouth is not the best place to recycle overcooked eggs.

Hard-cooked eggs, aka, "Hard-boiled eggs," are much more enjoyable if not hard and not boiled. Cooking eggs in boiling water makes them rubbery, sulfurous, and more likely for the yolk to turn green. Hard-cooked eggs are better cooked at a bubbleless simmer, a temperature between 80° C and 85° C (176° - 185° F) at sea level for the best culinary results.

Place two to two-and-a-half inches (5 to 7 cm) of water into a medium-

> sized saucepan. It should be at least deep enough to cover the eggs by half an inch. Heat the water until it just begins to simmer. Eggs that have been allowed to warm to room temperature, or warmed for a few minutes in warm water, are less likely to crack when placed in hot water. Using a large spoon gently introduce eggs into the hot water. Adjust the heat if needed to avoid boiling. Allow the eggs to cook at a low simmer for five to six minutes for soft-yolked eggs. For hard-cooked eggs, turn off the heat at six minutes, and let the water and eggs sit for 10 minutes, before removing the eggs from the water. The yolk should be a solid golden yellow.[295]

Cooking delicious eggs takes less heat and more patience. Using eggs that have been allowed to warm to room temperature will give better results as they will cook more evenly without overcooking the outside of the egg.

Summary

Acrylamide is a toxin produced via a Maillard reaction, present in fried potatoes and cigarette smoke. Acrolein is a product of pyrolysis of fats that occurs from frying oils, especially at high temperatures. Acrolein is also present in cigarette smoke. Although neither of these compounds is associated with cancer at levels likely to be found in a typical diet, both are toxic and promote aging.

Most of the health risks from acrylamide and acrolein arise from inhalation of fumes or from industrial exposure to the skin. Exposure to these toxins can be avoided by lowering frying temperatures, and use of an exhaust vent. Acrolein formation increases with the repetitive use of the oil for frying, as its substrates accumulate. Canola oil is very prone to the formation of acrolein, even at low frying temperatures.

Maillard reactions that occur in gently roasted nuts, garlic, coffee, and toast do not pose a health risk, and may act to stimulate anti-carcinogenic immune mechanisms. This is discussed in Chapter 23.

20: Red Meats and Iron

Red meats are much richer in heme than are white meats. Heme is an iron-containing molecule present in hemoglobin in blood and myoglobin in meat that transports oxygen. Myoglobin is the pigment that gives meat its red color when it is raw and its brown color when the iron is oxidized during cooking. Diving mammals, such as whales and seals, have high levels of myoglobin in their muscles. Heme is also present in cytochrome and helps in the production of ATP for cellular energy.

Nitrites can bind to this iron and prevent its oxidation and thus, preserve the red color; and therefore they are used in processed meats to give them the appearance of freshness. Meat sold in sealed plastic packaging, such as sliced lunch meats and bacon are often packaged in a carbon monoxide environment that prevents spoilage.[376] As an added advantage to the vendors, the carbon monoxide also binds to the myoglobin, giving it a pink color that consumers associate with freshness.

Although NNCs are formed in the preparation of white meat and fish, the products of this transformation have low mutagenicity,[377] and are not associated with increased risk of colorectal cancer. The presence of heme in the colon may favor the formation of nitrosyl-heme or nitrosyl-iron, but, these are not carcinogens. Sodium ascorbate (vitamin C) also favors the formation of nitrosyl-heme and nitrosyl-iron.

Heme may play a role in carcinogenesis due rather to heme-induced lipid peroxidation in the colon.[378] Freed heme can produce reactive hydroxyl radicals that cause cell damage. Heme promotes the formation of aldehydes in the colon that are genotoxic to the cells of the colonic mucosa.[379] This, however, is probably not a major reason that red meat consumption increases cancer risk.

Heme is an important and well-absorbed source of iron. For most individuals, the heme content in a quarter pound of red meat provides a healthy daily source of dietary iron. But things can go awry. Normally, heme is absorbed in the small intestine by specific heme transporters. The HFE protein helps mediate iron transport and absorption into the body. Hemochromatosis is an autosomal recessive genetic disease caused by mutations in the HFE gene. These mutations can increase iron uptake.

Since it is a recessive disease, it is mostly homozygous individuals, those who have inherited causative HFE alleles from both parents, who are at risk of overt disease. In the U.S., about one in ten persons is a carrier for this condition. Thus, as the result of random mating, about one in one hundred persons have the double recessive trait for risk of the disease. There are two common mutant alleles, HFE C282Y and HFE H63D. The risk of disease, additionally, is also affected by the combination of alleles inherited. Even with two high activity alleles, only about one in ten homozygotes develop symptomatic disease.

Humans are not the only ones at risk of hemochromatosis. For our not-so-distant relative, the black rhino, the condition is normal. In their native diet, iron is scarce. Avid uptake and retention of iron provides these animals a survival advantage. However, when you drop one of these big boys into a zoo and put them on a diet with an iron content fit for other large animals, they become iron overloaded and get the disease hemochromatosis.[380]

The carrier state of the HFE mutant allele may thus give humans having it an advantage, helping them avoid iron deficiency and anemia. People with the normal allele, absorb about 8 to 10 percent of the iron they consume. Homozygotes for the altered HFE alleles may absorb four times this amount and become iron overloaded. Iron overload can also occur in heterozygous, carrying just one of these alleles. Excess iron causes oxidative stress. Organ injury, caused by an iron overload in hemochromatosis, can cause fatigue, infertility, arthritis, liver cirrhosis, heart disease, and diabetes. Overt disease requires very high iron loads.

Hemochromatosis also increases the risk of cancer but increased cancer risk can be seen at much lower iron levels. Homozygotes for the HFE C282Y allele have a 2-fold higher risk of breast cancer, a 70 percent increased risk for colorectal cancer, and 360 percent higher risk for hepatocellular carcinoma. HFE C282Y carriers have a ten percent increase in cancer risk.[381] The HFE H63D allele also increases cancer risk; homozygotes for HFE H63D have about a 45% increase in risk of cancer, and the heterozygotes, who carry one altered copy and one normal copy, are 11 percent more likely to develop cancer. The HFE H63D allele does not appear to be associated with breast cancer but is associated with pancreatic and other cancers.[382]

Because red meat is such a good source of heme and heme is an easily absorbed iron, red meat is a risk factor for cancer in individuals who carry HFE alterations. Unless you have a parent or sib with hemochromatosis, it is unlikely that you would know that you carry one of these alleles unless you have genetic testing, or been found to have iron overload with serum ferritin and TIBC (total iron binding capacity) testing - yet another reason for universal genome testing. A ferritin level over 200 ng/mL in women and 300 ng/mL in men or 200 ng/mL in women suggests the presence of hemochromatosis. The ideal range for serum ferritin is 50 to 150 ng/mL.

Individuals with risk for iron overload should limit the amount of red meat they consume. Bluefin tuna should also be considered a red meat as it is also high in heme. Meat is not the only source of iron or the only risk factor in these individuals. Heavy alcohol consumption also increases iron absorption. Multivitamins with iron should not be used except for the treatment of iron deficiency.

The treatment for iron overload is blood donation as this removes iron from the body. Each pint of blood donated lowers the serum ferritin level by about 30 ng/ml. Other than bleeding, the body does not get rid of iron easily. Menstruation puts women at a lower risk of iron overload, but also of anemia. Vitamin C reduces iron and makes it more easily absorbed.

Summary

About ten percent of Americans carry a gene for but are asymptomatic for hemochromatosis. This allows them to absorb iron more easily. Red meat is a very good source of iron. So good, that it can cause an iron overload that causes an about ten percent increase in risk for liver and breast cancers. A person who has inherited the gene from both parents may have more than a doubling of the risk of certain cancers. Individuals with blood ferritin levels greater than 150 ng/ml may consider curtailing their intake of red meat. Ferritin levels greater than 200 ng/mL in women and 300 ng/mL in men merits genetic testing for the disease, curtailing the intake of red meat. Phlebotomy (removal of blood) is generally recommended for ferritin levels greater than 1000 ng/mL.

Patients with liver disease including liver cancer, and with iron overload, should be treated to maintain a ferritin level under 200 ng/ml.

21: Fungal Toxins

Aflatoxin and other Mycotoxins

Most people are aware that some mushrooms are deadly poisonous. Many people avoid even touching wild mushrooms because of this. While certain mushrooms are famously toxic, not many people die from them. There are, however, other more insidious, hidden fungal toxins that kill large numbers of people each year. It is estimated that as many as 155,000 people die from liver cancer each from exposure to just one of these hidden toxins.[383]

Aflatoxins are fungal toxins produced by several species of Aspergillus. These molds live in the soil and help break down decaying vegetable matter. When plants are stressed from drought, water-soaked soils, insect damage, or are poorly adapted to the climate or soil where they are grown, the plant's defenses are weakened. This allows these molds to flourish. These molds can also grow on harvested foods that are stored in warm, humid conditions. In many less-developed areas of the world, grain is often stored in dirt-floored rooms or other less-than-ideal conditions. Improperly stored grain can easily support the growth of molds, and such grain can easily be contaminated with fungal toxins.

Two of the food crops most commonly affected by *Aspergillus* and contaminated with aflatoxin are peanuts, which are affected while still in the ground, and corn that is affected post-harvest. Other crops that may be affected include cereals (wheat, rice, sorghum, and millet), oil seed plants (soybean, sunflower, cotton, and coconut), tree nuts, ginger, peppers (the vegetables, rather than peppercorns), dried figs, vine dried fruits, and spices.[384] Aflatoxin is so common in peanuts that in spite of the use of advanced farming practices to prevent it, aflatoxin is present in trace amounts in almost all peanut butter sold in the United States.

The FDA sets a limit on the aflatoxin content of foods that may be sold.[385] In a study performed in Texas, the foods associated with the highest aflatoxin intake were rice, corn tortillas, and tree nuts; however, not peanut butter or other corn products.[386] The levels encountered in the tortillas tested were high enough to impart risks and be of concern.

While aflatoxin toxicity is not thought to be a major carcinogen in the United States, about 5.2 billion of the 7.3 billion people on earth are exposed to significant amounts of aflatoxins, especially those living in warm climates and areas where food harvest and storage methods do not prevent *Aspergillus* contamination.[387]

Aflatoxins are acute toxins with high case-fatality rates, usually associated with consumption of corn that has molded. Many outbreaks of acute aflatoxin toxicity have occurred in India and Africa. Acute toxicity can result in liver necrosis. Chronic, lower-level toxin exposure can result in liver cirrhosis. This toxin crosses the placenta and is associated growth retardation of children in countries where significant amounts of aflatoxin are found in food.[388] These toxins appear more potent and deadly to poorly nourished individuals.

The dangers caused by fungal toxin exposure are growing with global climate change that supports conditions favoring the robust growth of these molds. *Aspergillus flavus,* a species which produces aflatoxin, prefers dryer climates and grows well in the Great Plains. In the year 2012, it caused nearly $200 million in losses from acute toxicity deaths of farm animals in the U.S. Aflatoxin contamination also forced a nationwide pet food recall, but not before many companion animals were killed.[389]

Claiming a far greater death toll than it does as an acute poison, aflatoxin is a potent carcinogen. It causes DNA alkylation adducts, resulting in liver cancer. Aflatoxin adducts cause mutations in the p53 gene,[390] a gene which signals for apoptosis, and which helps prevent cells with DNA errors from reproducing. Thus, aflatoxin adducts promote cancer development by preventing p53-induced apoptosis.

Individuals exposed to aflatoxin are 3.4 times more likely to develop hepatocellular carcinoma (HCC). Aflatoxin can cause HCC by itself but is even more dangerous as a co-carcinogen with hepatitis B (HBV) infection. The presence of hepatitis B surface antigens in the blood, evidence of ongoing HBV disease, increases the risk of HCC by about 7.3 times. Individuals who have HBV surface antigens *and* who are exposed to aflatoxins have nearly 60 times the risk of developing HCC as individuals with neither of these risk factors.[391] HBV infection raises the rate of hepatocyte replacement, and the mycotoxin forms a DNA adduct that causes a loss of p53 function. This creates a perfect storm with more cells are dividing and much less protection from DNA errors. This interaction amplifies the risk of HCC. In the United States, the HBV infection rate is fairly low, as is the intake of aflatoxin. In Southeast Asia and parts of Africa, this deadly combination is common.

Hepatitis C can also cause hepatocellular carcinoma, but does not appear to interact with aflatoxin. Aflatoxin induced HCC is common in China,[392] Taiwan,[393] Mexico, and many other regions. In China, HBV infection is endemic. It is estimated that nearly a quarter of the

782,000 new cases of HCC each year worldwide, are attributable to aflatoxin exposure.[394] [395] Aflatoxin adducts leave molecular traces that can be detected in HCC tumors. Aflatoxin adducts were found in 6 percent of HCC cases in Japan,[396] a country with low levels of exposure to these toxins. In a very small study, about five percent of HCC cases in the U.S. were associated with aflatoxin exposure.[397]

While aflatoxin is the best studied and most well known of the fungal carcinogens, it is not the only one common in food. Three hundred to four hundred mycotoxins have been identified, but only about a dozen are recognized as causing a significant burden of animal and human disease. Fungi are chemical factories. They make many B vitamins, vitamin D2, and penicillin. They also produce alcohol, LSD, and many other toxins. In addition to aflatoxin, two other mycotoxins that appear in the human food supply have been identified as probable carcinogens.

Ochratoxin A is found in foods contaminated by several *Aspergillus* species. Ochratoxin A is an acute toxin that damages the kidneys, liver, and the immune system, and is a suspected carcinogen, particularly for the urinary tract. This toxin may be responsible for sporadic epidemic outbreaks of kidney disease.

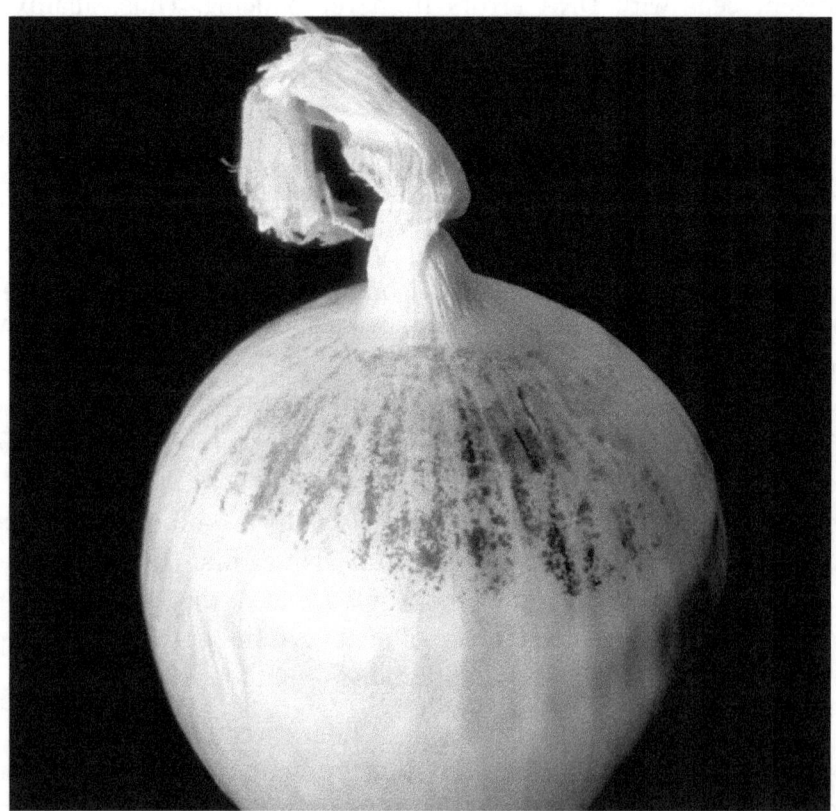

Figure 21-1: Onion with *Aspergillus niger* growth[398]

Ochratoxin A toxin can often be obtained at your local grocer on onions, shallots, and garlic, as well as in cereals, coffee, dried fruit, and red wine. If contaminated foods are eaten, it passes into milk, including human milk.

The black fruiting bodies of *Aspergillus niger* can be seen in the outer layer of the onion in Figure 21-1. Note additionally, the softening and depression around the middle of the onion that is caused by digestion of pectin in the onion. Some, but not all strains of *Aspergillus niger* produce the toxin and carcinogen ochratoxin A. Peeling away the black fruiting bodies on outer layers does not remove the fungus that has invaded the inside layers of the onion. The fruiting bodies are like mushrooms growing out of a log; the fungus is everywhere in the log, the mushrooms are just the fruiting bodies you can see. The toxin is everywhere the fungus grows.

There are over fifty species of *Fusarium* fungi that produce toxins, and their toxins, the fumonisins, are not a single chemical class of toxins, but a diverse set of toxins that includes trichothecene and T-2 mycotoxins. Fumonisin B is a neurotoxin that has economic importance for its effect on agriculture. In a five-year span in the 1990's, during weather that was wetter than usual, losses to wheat and barley from *Fusarium* fungal contamination totaled more than three billion dollars. *Fusarium* also grows on corn and other grains. This fungus and its toxins are neurotoxic to farm animals that are fed contaminated grain and cause losses of livestock. It is also an acute toxin that can cause abdominal pain, diarrhea, liver, and kidney damage. In Russia during the 1930's, *Fusarium*-contaminated grain that was baked into bread led to several outbreaks of acute toxicity. Sixty percent of those affected died, resulting in the deaths of 100,000 persons.

Fumonisin B1, unlike aflatoxin, does not cause DNA adducts and is not genotoxic. Fumonisin B1 acts as a toxin by blocking the enzyme ceramide synthase, (Figure 1, Appendix B) which promotes the formation of sphingosine-1-phosphate (S1P). S1P supports growth and repair and also supports the growth of tumor cells. Fumonisin B is also a teratogen that causes neural tube defects, such as anencephaly in humans (in which the fetus forms without a brain).[388]

Fumonisin B is a suspected carcinogen for esophageal cancer in various parts of the world, including within the United States.[399] Mostly, fumonisin B consumption is associated with moldy corn. However, fumonisin B and other *Fusarium* toxins are found on other crops, and as well, in brine-pickled foods (including fish) where *Fusarium* participate in the fermentation process.

Lessons in Cancer Prevention

Green tea polyphenols have been shown to reduce biomarkers of aflatoxins by over 40%.[400] Black tea polyphenols have also been shown to inhibit DNA adduct formation, by lowering the activity of CYP1A1 and CYP1A2.[401]

Lycopene, one of the several antioxidant carotenoids found in vegetables, also shifts the metabolism of aflatoxin B1, reducing the formation of aflatoxin DNA-adducts to a less toxic metabolite (aflatoxin M1) that is excreted in the urine.[402] However, tomato purée has a more vigorous anti-mutagenic effect in mice exposed to aflatoxin B1 than did pure lycopene.[403] In another study, two other carotenoids, canthaxanthin, and astaxanthin were more effective than lycopene at shifting aflatoxin B1 metabolism to aflatoxin M1 and in preventing DNA adducts and tumor formation. Beta-carotene, the precursor of vitamin A, had no effect.[404]

Dietary chlorophyll, found in green leaves, is highly effective in reducing hepatic DNA adducts in rats exposed to dietary aflatoxin B1 and helps prevent the development of premalignant tumors in the liver and colon. Here the mechanism is different and preferable to that for tea and tomatoes. Chlorophyll binds to aflatoxin in the diet and prevents it from being absorbed into the body.[405]

Thus, green tea polyphenols, (well, perhaps only epigallocatechin-3-gallate) certain carotenoid compounds, (but not beta-carotene) and chlorophyll can prevent aflatoxin B1 induced cancers. Since chlorophyll, carotenoids, and green tea polyphenols act through different mechanisms, a diet containing a combination of these would be expected to provide even more comprehensive protection.

But before you run off to your corner NSC (Nutritional Supplement Center) and load up on green tea polyphenols, chlorophyll and astaxanthin capsules to undo the damage, consider the timing in the mechanisms of these agents. Chlorophyll needs to be in the same meal as the toxin to prevent its absorption. If you have a contaminated corn tortilla for breakfast, a noontime spinach salad will be too late to prevent the aflatoxin absorption. And since carotenoids act by inducing the P450 enzymes, they need to be consumed a day or so prior to exposure to be up and running when the toxin is absorbed to assist in its metabolism. Consuming these compounds after exposure to aflatoxin would be like putting on a Kevlar vest after a gunfight to treat the wounds.

The best bet is to avoid exposure to these and other carcinogens and to have healthy, sustainable eating habits.

Summary for Fungal Toxins

Obviously, fungal toxins should be avoided. The toxins cannot be seen and are rarely measured. It is hard to assess the impact on cancer risk caused by fungal toxins that may be present in food. Many have not been studied.

Mold-contaminated foods should be discarded; they are not fit for animals as they are at just as much risk from these toxins as we are. Just cutting away the fruiting body that makes visible spores does not remove the mold that is typically growing throughout the contaminated food, nor does it remove the toxins. A handful of mold-contaminated corn kernels contains sufficient toxins to make a truckload of corn illegal to sell into interstate commerce.

The correlation between aflatoxin urinary metabolites and intake of corn tortillas, rice, and tree nuts suggests that the FDA may need to reassess monitoring of aflatoxins for these in foods in the U.S. Aflatoxins are just one of at least several fungal toxins found in food that cause human disease.

Green tea may help prevent aflatoxin-DNA adduct formation.

Although improperly stored grain is the typical culprit, fruits and vegetables are also hosts to these fungi. Dried figs, prunes, apricots, and raisins can be contaminated. Don't eat or allow children to eat fruit or vegetables that show signs of mold. While this is painting molds as being toxic with a very wide brush, even though most molds do not produce carcinogens, why take a risk on moldy food that would taste bad anyway?

> Aflatoxins fluoresce bright greenish-yellow under UV light.[384]

Not all fungi are toxic or carcinogenic. Some food molds, such as those in blue and gorgonzola cheese, are non-toxic. Many mushrooms are non-toxic, flavorful and nutritious, and at least several types of mushrooms have anti-carcinogenic properties. At least 20 different types of mushrooms are currently under study as potential cancer treatments for their antitumor, antioxidant, and immune-stimulating properties. Several of these are culinary mushrooms including shiitake, white button mushrooms, maitake, and lion's mane mushrooms.[406]

22: Ionizing Radiation

Notice: Although this chapter is concerned with ionizing radiation as a cause of cancer, it is dropped dead middle in the diet section. The reason this chapter is placed here is because understanding risk from radiation reveals much about cancer risk from the diet.

In 1945 two atomic bombs exploded in the skies over Hiroshima and Nagasaki, Japan, killing about 200,000 people. Those close to the blast were incinerated, and many more died from burns and acute radiation sickness. About 280,000 people, mostly those who were more than two kilometers away from the blasts, survived but were exposed to radiation, about 50,000 of these were exposed to dangerous amounts of radiation.

The radiation dose of these survivors ranged from 5 mSv (0.005 Sieverts) to over 5000 mSv (5 Sv). Five mSv is about twice the average exposure from background radiation due to cosmic radiation, radon, and the natural environment that the average American is exposed to over a year's time. It is about half the dose received from a CT scan of the colon (10 mSv). Five Sv is an extreme dose, typical of those who were less than 2.5 km from the blasts. An acute 5 SV dose is usually fatal, even with medical treatment. Radiation exposure dose declines by half for every 200 meters further from the bomb's detonation. Thus, if the dose was 5 Sv at 2.5 km, it would have been 156 mSv at 3.5 km.

Radiation can cause burns and damage protein and has sufficient energy to break the molecular bonds in DNA. The breaks can usually be repaired, but errors may occur during the repair process, especially if there are multiple breaks in the same cell. This DNA damage can prevent the cell from reproducing or cause mutations that keep the cell from functioning properly or that can lead to cancer. Cells that are in the S or M phases of cell growth (Chapter 5) are those most susceptible to radiation injury. This is why radiation therapy is used to kill cancer cells; they are frequently dividing and thus are at higher risk of being injured by radiation than is normal tissue.

About two years after the A-bomb detonations, there was an increased incidence of acute leukemia among the survivors exposed to radiation. The incidence of leukemia peaked about 6 years after the blast. Those within a mile of the blast were at highest risk, and children had the highest rates of leukemia.

Radiation exposure from the A-bombs also elevated the risk of lymphoma; however, with this disease, the lag time was longer, with the peak more than 10 years after the incident. Those with the highest radiation dose had the highest risk of lymphoma, but even those exposed to 100 to 200 mSv were at elevated risk.[407]

It took even longer for cancer risk from the A-bomb radiation exposure to manifest as solid tumors. As with leukemia, the greatest risk was for individuals exposed as children. Among those exposed as children under the age of six, the risk of developing a solid cancer (non-white blood cell cancer) by the age of 55 was 56 times higher than expected. The increased risk was limited to those with an exposure dose greater than 200 mSv, and the risk, compared to those with minimal exposure, increased with age. This indicates that for most of these cancers, the average time span between this single exposure to radiation and the manifestation of the cancer was over 25 years.[408]

Other than those treated for cancer with radiation therapy, few of us will ever be exposed to 200mSv during a year, much less in a single dose. Is there evidence of cancer risk from a lower, single dose of radiation?

The risk of cancer following radiation exposure from the A-bombs and from other sources has a linear relationship from 200 to 4000 mSv. Above this, there are few survivors. It is widely assumed that there is very low cancer risk at low doses of radiation. Nevertheless, a study of the effects of low radiation from the A-bomb exposures shows cancer risk even in those exposed to less than 20 mSv. The peak incident of cancers occurred after a delay of 11.9 years for stomach and pancreas cancers, 13.6 years for lung cancer, and 23.7 years for chronic leukemia. (Note: although they are both cancers of white blood cells, acute leukemia, which is mostly seen in children, and chronic leukemia that mostly occurs in the elderly, are different diseases.) The lag time between exposure and diagnoses was 36 to 42 years after low dose radiation exposure for hepatic cancer and over 36 years for urinary cancer.[409] [410] The latency period for solid cancer risk may be as long as 65 years after exposure for those exposed to these atomic blasts.[411]

Another observation of the cancer risk from A-bomb exposure in Japan was that the distribution of cancers by the organ of origin was similar to the background distribution of cancers unrelated to radiation exposure. Low dose radiation amplified the risk of cancers that were already most common. In the second half of the 20th century, stomach cancer was the most common cancer in Japan, as well as the most cancer common among A-bomb survivors.

Radiation exposure among those later infected with HCV increased the risk of HCC by 58 times for every 1 Sv of exposure. HCV infection on its own raises HCC risk by 5.7, while 1 Sv of radiation exposure alone only doubled HCC risk.[412]

On this graphic from the Department of Energy each bar, from bottom to top, raises the radiation dose by a factor of ten. Notice that radiation therapy for cancer has a dosage ten times higher than a lethal dose of radiation; however, it is narrowly focused to destroy tissue in the target area.

The radiation exposure from the A-bombs tells us a lot about cancer risk. It was a single exposure, and it raised lifetime risk of cancer among survivors, even when the dose of radiation was no higher than that of a CAT scan.

We also saw that exposure imparts more risk to children than to adults. Radiation risk is highest during cell growth, and children and adolescents are growing; more of their cells are dividing at any giving moment. If there is exposure during cell division, particularly during the S or M phases, the risk of mutation is higher.

We also saw that risk increased most for cancers already common in the population. A-bomb radiation increased the risk of stomach, liver, and lung cancer more than it did for breast cancer. These were the same cancers most prevalent in the unexposed Japanese population during the second half of the 20th century. Radiation exposure increases the risk of cancers the population is most at risk for. As noted above, having HCV infection with exposure to radiation multiplied the risk of hepatic cancer several times more than exposure to either of these risks alone. Breast cancer was not greatly increased, as breast cancer was not common in the exposed population.

There are long lag times and great variance of lag time between the exposure causing cancer and its manifestation. Different cancers had different lag times between the exposure and disease. Some cancers took 40 years after an initiating cancer-driving mutation to manifest as cancer.

How does this relate to cancer risk from the diet?

- ☢ Ionizing radiation causes breaks in the DNA that causes mutagenesis. It can take over 30 years for cancer to manifest. If the diet contains mutagens, or if substances in the diet prevent the action of mutagens, as chlorophyll and astaxanthin do, then these factors may be in play ten to 40 years before the onset of cancer.

- ☢ Studying the diet in the ten years leading up to prostate, breast, or other solid cancer may not help explain what caused cancer, and may only be relevant if the person eats the same foods as they did at the time of the mutations. It would not give clues to some moldy grain resulting from an unusually wet season years ago, or a burned steak or overcooked campfire hotdog as a boy scout.

- Since most mutagens in food are not part of the meal plan, it is unlikely that anyone knows when or with which meal he or she was exposed to a carcinogen unless they become acutely ill from the exposure.

- Children were those most susceptible to radiation risk from the bombs. This is because they are growing most quickly and have more cells dividing at any time. This is true for carcinogens in food as well.

- Most cancers are not caused by a single mutation, but a single mutation in a system that normally repairs DNA or that eliminates aberrant cells can allow subsequent mutations to aggregate over time, and thereby cause cancer.

Radiation Therapy in Cancer Treatment

In the chart from the Department of Energy, it can be seen that the dose of radiation used in radiotherapy for cancer is higher than the acutely toxic dose. Whole body exposure to 10 Sv of radiation is sufficient to kill pretty much everyone, even with expert medical care. Four Sv kills about 50% of persons if not treated. The total dose range for radiotherapy starts at 10 Sv.

How can that make any sense? In radiotherapy, the radiation is focused like a flashlight on the areas being treated. It is not the whole body being treated. As much as possible, exposure of tissues sensitive to radiation is avoided. Also, the radiation is spread over several treatments.

Why doesn't radiotherapy cause cancer? Well, actually, it does. Radiation is mostly used as palliative therapy to shrink tumors, thus providing pain relief or improved function. A tumor in the airways of the lung can prevent airflow and increase the risk of pneumonia that can kill the patient more quickly than cancer might. Bone tumors can be terribly painful, and may be shrunk with radiation. Most radiotherapy is not used to cure cancer, but to slow it down or shrink it. And similar to the Japanese exposed to the A-bomb, the first cancer to appear is leukemia. Five years after treatment with radiotherapy for breast cancer, women have eight times the usual rate of leukemia.

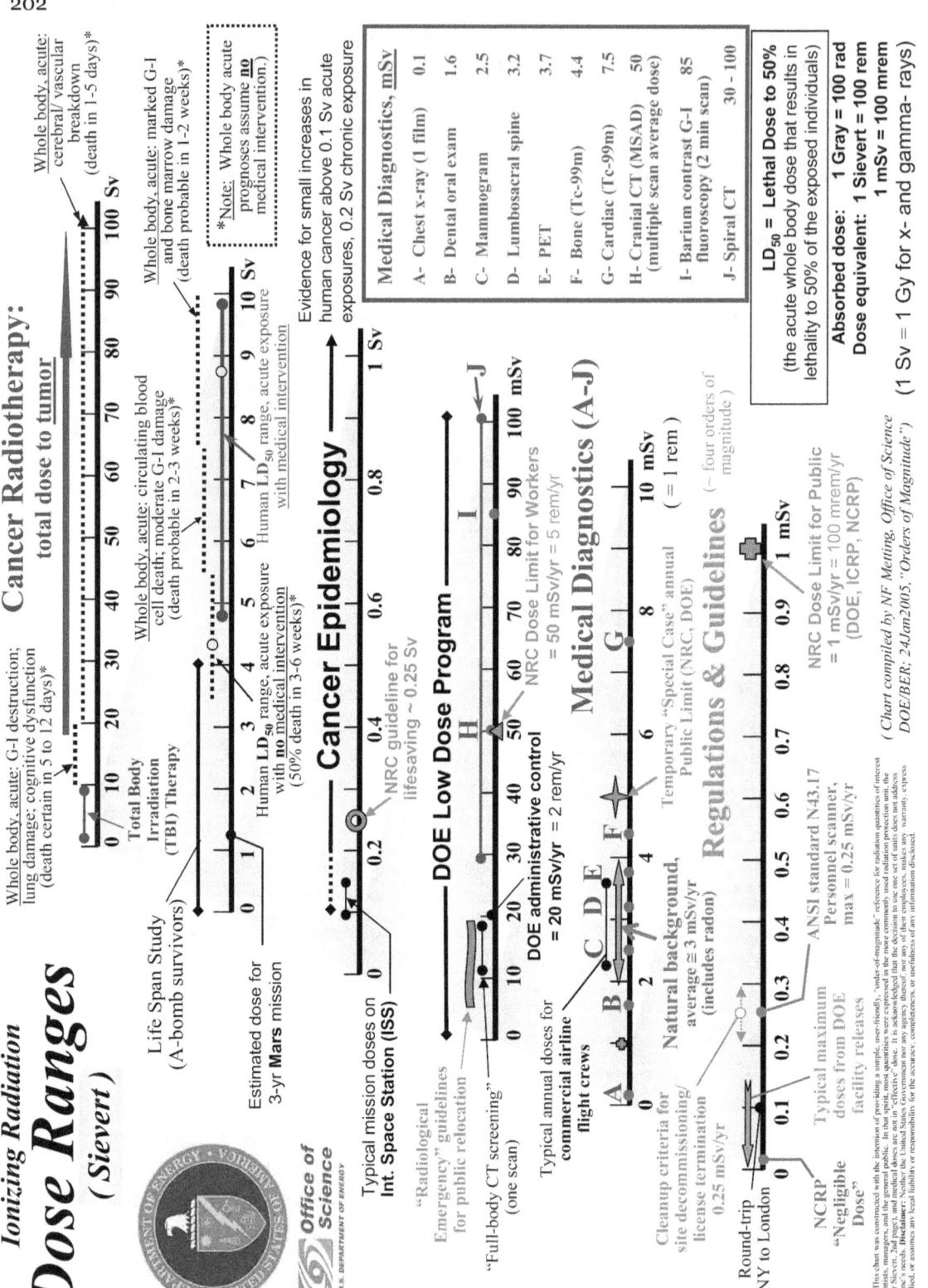

Figure 22-1: On this graphic from the Department of Energy each bar, from bottom to top, raises the radiation dose by a factor of ten. Notice that radiation therapy for cancer has a dosage ten times higher than a lethal dose of radiation; however, it is narrowly focused to destroy tissue in the target area.

To put this risk in perspective, the risk was three cases of leukemia per thousand patients compared to one case per 2400 women not treated with radiation.[413] This risk is small compared to the benefits in terms of quality and quantity of life. The risk of solid cancers was also slightly elevated, but would likely increase considerably if the patient lives another 30 years or more. Since most cancer patients are older, the risk of cancer resulting from radiation therapy does not outweigh the benefits this treatment can provide them. In this population, there is a 45% increase in the risk of solid cancers in the 13 years of follow-up after radiotherapy. This was equivalent to one extra case in 1,000 breast cancer patients, and risk was lower in older women. After 15 years there was an excess of five new cancer cases per thousand persons treated with radiotherapy.[414]

The risk of post-radiotherapy cancer is considerably higher for survivors of testicular cancer, as this is a young man's disease. Those treated with radiotherapy have a 90 percent increase in the risk of a solid cancer during the 10 years after treatment, and risk increases for at least the next 35 years. Similar to the Japanese A-bomb survivors, the younger the age at exposure, the higher the risk of a secondary cancer. In young men treated with radiation for seminoma, 36% of those surviving will develop a new solid cancer within the next 35 years, nearly twice that of the general population. Still, a treatment that gives a good chance of survival, with a risk of another battle, is far preferable than not surviving. Chemotherapy imparts nearly as much risk as does radiation therapy, and the combination of chemo and radiotherapy nearly triple risk of cancer in these patient's future.[415]

X-rays: Timing is Everything

During adolescence, pneumonia is a risk factor for breast cancer, not because of the disease, but because of the diagnostic X-rays.[416]

A set of chest X-rays give about 6 mSv exposure, and may be repeated if follow-up films are done. Mammogram gives a 13-mSv exposure. Each bitewing dental X-ray gives about 0.4-mSv exposure. Digital dental X-rays give lower doses than film X-rays.

Women with BRCA alterations are exquisitely sensitive to radiation exposure. Any diagnostic radiation exposure to women with BRCA1 alterations before the age of 30 (including mammography) nearly triples their risk of breast cancer.

A single mammogram may raise the risk of breast cancer by 50% for a young woman with the BRCA2 alteration. Before the age of 20, the risks are even greater. After giving birth, or after the age of 30 for women who don't, women with BRCA1/2 mutations are at considerably lower additional risk from exposure to X-rays.[417] Screening mammography and even diagnostic mammography is inappropriate in women under the age of thirty. MRI mammography should be used if a study is needed. MRI studies do not use X-rays. CT scans create much higher exposure to radiation than do simple X-rays. An X-ray of the pelvis gives a 70-mSv exposure; a CT of pelvis gives 1000-mSv (a 1-Sv exposure).

Why is there so much risk from a radiation exposure similar to the annual exposure of background radiation? Timing. Firstly, the risk is greater if the exposure occurs during growth when cells are rapidly dividing and at the highest risk. Secondly, the radiation exposure is concentrated into a flash lasting less than a second and focused on the one part of the body being imaged. Rather than creating a rare break in the DNA strand that is easy to repair, multiple breaks can occur simultaneously.

Imagine you have a magnetic tape such as video or cassette tape (remember those?) that breaks in one spot. It is easy to patch the two ends together and fix it. However, if the tape gets cut into dozens of pieces at the same time, what are the chances of blindly patching them back together in the original sequence?

X-rays should only be performed when clearly needed for medical decision making. Will an X-ray change the treatment plan for a clinically apparent pneumonia? Usually not in a young person where no other underlying disease is suspected. If an X-ray will not change a treatment plan, it should be avoided, especially in children and during puberty and adolescence. Dental panoramic X-rays should be avoided; their main purpose is to garner income for the dental practice. My children's dental charts were boldly marked "No Panoramas" on the cover to avoid unnecessary exposure to radiation. Shielding aprons should be used to protect the neck (thyroid gland) and body from X-rays for areas not being imaged.

Any X-rays that are needed, other than for emergency treatment, should be scheduled during a young woman's menstrual period, a time when few breast, ovary, and uterine cells are dividing. If X-rays are required for non-emergency purposes, they should be scheduled for the first 8 days of the menstrual cycle when risk is at its lowest, counting the first day of bleeding as day one.

If you are 80 years old, there is little risk. Fewer cells are dividing, and it is unlikely that you will live long enough for X-ray exposure from diagnostic X-rays to catch up with you. (Sorry for pointing that out).

UV Radiation

Ultraviolet (UV) radiation exposure, especially UV-B, causes damage to the DNA of the cells in the skin and can cause skin cancer. UV-C can also cause DNA damage, but penetrates less deeply than UV-B, and thus is less damaging. UV-A damages the collagen and elastin fibers in the skin but mostly causes aging and wrinkling.

I grew up in California and spent my summers outdoors in the sun, back when sunscreen was a thick white coat of zinc-oxide paste used almost exclusively to protect the noses of swimming pool lifeguards. My face was covered with freckles, and until my mid-twenties, I don't think a summer went by during which my nose was in a constant state of peeling from June through September from repeated sunburns. At age 26, I had a precancerous lesion removed from my face and started using the strongest sunscreen (SPF-15) available at the time.

Most of us get most of our lifetime's sun exposure and solar damage when we are young and carefree, and when we are not thinking about how the sun exposure is going to affect how we might look at age 40 or 64, or the possibility that we might one day develop skin cancer.

Put sunscreen on small children you care for and make sure your kids get into the habit of using sunscreen. Wear sunscreen, a hat, and sunglasses if you are going to be in the sun for more than 15 minutes. Stay away from tanning beds.

That is just about all I have to say on the topic UV radiation and skin cancer, other than if you want to make vitamin D by sun exposure, take off your shirt for 15 minutes or expose your legs. They will likely not get that much sun exposure during adulthood. Protect the face, neck, arms and upper chest, as those are the areas where sun damage takes its greatest toll.

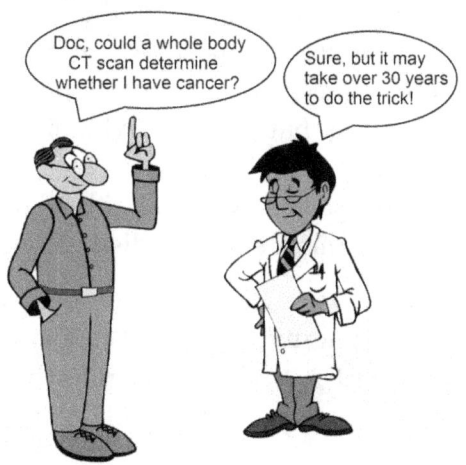

23: STRESS RESPONSE ELEMENTS

"The dose makes the poison."

~ Paracelsus

I am not saying that everything you know is wrong. But, numerous, large, well-conducted human trials using antioxidant vitamins to prevent cancer have had consistent and disastrous findings; supplementing antioxidant vitamins increases the risk of cancer and taking these vitamins after the diagnosis of cancer worsens the outcome.

In a randomized trial for the prevention of prostate cancer, 35,000 men were tested for and found not to have any signs of prostate cancer. Half of these men were given 400 IU of vitamin E a day for 7 to 12 years. The men who received vitamin E during the study had a 17% increase in cancer over those who received the placebo; about 1.6 cases per thousand person-years. Those taking selenium supplements in this study had a 9% increase incidence of prostate cancer.[418] In a meta-analysis of sixty-seven prevention studies using antioxidants involving over 230,000 patients, vitamin A increased mortality by 16%; β-carotene increased mortality by 7% and vitamin E increased mortality by 4%. Supplementation with vitamin C did not affect mortality,[419] but remember that the body limits the intestinal absorption of this vitamin.

In 18 blinded clinical trials including 46,000 patients, those taking synthetic vitamin E had no change in mortality rates, but those taking natural vitamin E had a 13 percent increase in mortality.[420] In a placebo-controlled randomized trial for the prevention of prostate cancer, folic acid supplement or a placebo was given over a ten-year follow-up period. Those who received the folic acid had a 9.7% probability of being diagnosed with prostate cancer during the follow-up period while only 3.3% of the placebo group was diagnosed with the disease. In this study, t*aking folic acid tripled the risk of prostate cancer.* Nevertheless, individuals who had higher serum folate levels but were not vitamin users at baseline were less likely to get prostate cancer.[421] Thus, dietary folate was preventative but taking folate as a folic acid supplement increased cancer risk. (Reasons for this are further discussed in Chapter 26).

And just FYI: women in a 22-year follow-up who took mineral supplements of zinc, magnesium, iron, and copper had a 3.0%, 3.6%, 3.9%, and 18% increased risk of death, respectively. Only calcium was associated with a decrease in mortality in this population, by 3.8%.[422]

Furthermore, pretty much every food that has been found to lower cancer risk in large epidemiologic studies does so, not because the food contains antioxidants, but rather because the food contains compounds that the cell sees as a toxin. Yes, toxins. So what is going on? This and the next chapter explain how some oxidative stressors help prevent aging and cancer, and how we can use this for better health and cancer prevention and management.

When the liver cell finds itself in possession of unwanted, lipophilic compounds, it tries to rid itself of the unwelcome guests. These may be medications, bilirubin, or just endogenous hormones the liver does not want. They also may be heterocyclic amines (HCA), fungal toxins, or other nefarious xenobiotic compounds.

Xenobiotics are foreign molecular compounds that have biologic functions. Most biologically relevant xenobiotics are lipid soluble, and thus, can slip unaided, directly into the cell across the lipid membrane. Once inside the cell, the compound can interact with intracellular elements and influence various cell processes.

The export of unwanted compounds from the liver has three steps or phases. The first phase of action is attacking the compound by oxidizing it. This action often alters the biological function of the compound, often stopping its activity; however, in other cases, it can make the compound more active. The second phase reaction is conjugation; now that there is an oxidative "hot spot" on the molecule, the compound can be linked to an antioxidant molecule, such as glutathione. This process, a sort of shotgun wedding, converts the lipophilic compound into one that is water-soluble by conjugating it with a water-soluble antioxidant. The third step is transporting the conjugated compound across the lipid membrane and dumping it into the trash: into the bile stream and headed for the feces or moved into the bloodstream so that it can be eliminated by the kidneys into the urine.

In the first step of elimination, the unwanted compound is oxidized by a cytochrome p450 enzyme. A medically important genetic difference between people is that we have different alleles of the p450 enzymes, and this affects the metabolism of many xenobiotics. We have many CYP p450 enzymes, and different ones are capable of interacting with and oxidizing different compounds.

Certain medications and food substances are metabolized differently in different people, according to the activity of p450 enzyme alleles inherited from their folks. Thus, a medication that needs to be metabolized into an active compound may work well for one person, but have low efficacy for someone else who does not have p450 enzymes that process that compound well. Conversely, a person that rapidly activates a medication may get a brief, intense response. Other medications may be metabolized so slowly that a drug accumulates and becomes toxic. These changes in metabolism can also occur if another xenobiotic impedes or enhances the specific p450 enzymes that process the medication.

Thus, medications that affect the p450 enzymes can cause drug-to-drug interactions. I used to collect pens as souvenirs from pharmaceutical companies that had names of drugs withdrawn from the market for this and other reasons; Posicor, Seldane, Vioxx, Baycol, Rezulin, Hismanol, Propulsid... For example, Posicor was removed from the market as it strongly inhibited CYP3A4 and CYP2D6, leading to drug interactions. Inhibiting a CYP450 enzyme can cause toxic levels of certain medicines to accumulate rather than being metabolized and eliminated, and the patient gets a toxic overdose. In other cases, it can prevent a medication from being activated, and the patient, in effect, goes untreated.

> CYP3A4 is highly expressed in the liver and intestinal mucosa and is among the most important enzymes for the activation and elimination of drugs and toxins. About 50 percent of commonly prescribed medications are metabolized by CYP3A4. Grapefruit, star fruit, and pomegranates contain substances that can inhibit CYP3A4 activity. Grapefruit can do this so potently that its consumption can raise drug levels for three to seven days, easily to toxic levels, and has caused fatal drug interactions.
>
> In the late 1990's, a woman in her thirties walked into my office complaining of palpitations and fainting spells. An electrocardiogram revealed *Torsades de Pointes* dysrhythmia. She is the only person I have ever seen with this potentially fatal dysrhythmia that could stand. She was using the medication mibefradil (Posicor) for blood pressure and had been eating grapefruit from the tree in her backyard.

The second phase of hepatic detox of xenobiotics and other compounds is conjugation. The enzyme GST binds reduced glutathione (GSH) to these oxidized compounds. The enzymes NQO1 and UGT also conjugate certain oxidized products. Normally, glutathione is present in the cells in a ratio of about 1000-to-1 of reduced glutathione to oxidized glutathione (GS:SH), so normally, there is plenty of GSH present. Still, this detoxification process is costly, with a loss of amino acids and antioxidants from the body.[423]

In the third phase of detoxification, the conjugate is carried across the lipid membrane for dumping. This is done by the ABCC2 protein. Interestingly, several antiviral medications inhibit the action of this protein.

Many of the compounds we think of as carcinogens are not actually carcinogens until the body activates them, via cytochrome P450, into oxidized lipids that can have a pernicious affinity for forming DNA-adducts that give rise to mutations. This process is especially prone to occur if phase one, P450 oxidation, proceeds at a rate faster than phase two, conjugation. In this case, the oxidized lipid products are created faster than they can be neutralized and prepared for export. As their concentration builds in the cytosol, it becomes more likely that the compound migrates into the nucleus where it is most dangerous.

Fortunately, we have a backup system that helps the cell protect itself from these nasty compounds.

Nfr2 is a small protein that spends its brief existence in the cytoplasm of the cell. Nrf2's half-life is only 20 minutes; it takes only this much time for Nrf2 to get tagged for ubiquitination, get taken up by proteasomes, and recycled into individual amino acids for reuse. However, electrophilic or oxidative stress, such as that from phase one compounds, can stop and reverse the ubiquitination of Nrf2, allowing it to survive, and find its way into the nucleus.

Nrf2 is a transcription factor for the Antioxidant Response Element (ARE), a section of DNA that codes for antioxidant enzymes. After entering the nucleus, Nrf2 induces the transcription of many antioxidant and cytoprotective proteins. During fair intracellular weather, not much Nrf2 enters the nucleus, as there is little need for and very sparse transcription of ARE proteins.

Nrf2 is detained in the cytosol by the protein KEAP1. KEAP1 keeps Nrf2 on a collar so that it cannot migrate to the nucleus. A second protein, (Cullin 3) binds to KEAP1 and ubiquitinates Nrf2, marking it for destruction. Within minutes, ubiquitinated Nrf2 is recycled back into its component amino acids for reuse.

KEAP1 is an oxidative stress sensor protein. It has 25 exposed sulfur-containing cysteine units that are easily oxidized or disrupted by electrophilic stress. When this stress occurs, it causes a conformational change in the KEAP1 protein that allows the release of Nrf2 from KEAP1. This prevents Cullin 3 from ubiquitination of Nrf2 and prevents its destruction. Nrf2, now freed, can migrate into the nucleus where it promotes the transcription of ARE-mRNA for antioxidant enzymes and cytoprotective proteins.

Included among the ARE proteins (Table 23-1) are enzymes that increase the production of the antioxidant glutathione and the enzyme glutathione S-transferase (GST) that conjugates glutathione with oxidized xenobiotics. But the ARE proteins do much more than just quench free radicals. The ARE proteins increase phase two and phase three detoxification, increasing conjugation and export of these compounds, protecting the cells from oxidative injury, aiding in detoxification and protecting the cell from mutagenic injury. The induction of ARE by Nrf2 occurs when KEAP1 senses an increase in oxidative stress. It is a great system, and it helps prevent cancer.

So here comes the surprise. Many of the vegetables that help prevent cancer do so, not because they are filled with vitamins, antioxidants, or fairy dust, but rather because they contain toxins.

Plants make various toxins that dissuade insects, worms, and other beasties from eating them; however, in some cases, these toxins are the reason we like to eat them. We like the way they taste. For example, the pungent flavors in capers and mustard deter insects, but we enjoy those flavors. After consumption of the toxins, the body responds by increasing the production of enzymes and other proteins that help metabolize and eliminate toxins from the body.

This may be a case of *hormesis*, a surprising biological phenomenon in which a toxin can have health benefits when given in low doses. In numerous experiments, when progressive doses are used to find the threshold for toxicity of a substance, it has been observed that the plant, animal, or fungus that is given very low doses of *some toxins* has a better outcome and longer survival than those receiving a zero dose of the toxin.[424] This low dose protects the animal from the damage caused by the toxin. It seems to be a crazy and unpalatable idea, and until recently, it was rejected by much of the scientific community.

I was never impressed by Nietzsche's "What doesn't kill us makes us stronger." Personally, I would avoid health advice from anyone dying with dementia and psychosis at the age of 56. Nevertheless, small amounts of certain stressors do help us adapt to them.

This appears to be true for many toxins that do their dirty work by way of oxidative stress. The intracellular oxidative stress response by way of the KEAP1/Nrf2 → ARE pathway can at times restore balance to the cell and eliminate the oxidative threat, and prevent DNA damage from other toxins.

While the small amounts of these toxins found in commonly eaten foods can promote a healthy hormesis, a high dose of these toxins may give a classic toxic response and cause end-organ damage. Thus, loading up on these salubrious, natural compounds from food in the form of supplements that exceed what one is likely to get in foods may not be such a great idea.

Table 23-1: Antioxidant Response Element (ARE) Proteins[425]

ARE Genes	Functions
GCL and GCLM	Glutamate Cysteine Ligase and the Glutamate-cysteine ligase regulatory subunit are enzymes that work together on the rate-limiting step in the synthesis of glutathione, the body's most important antioxidant system.
SOD	Superoxide dismutase converts oxygen radicals into normal O2 and hydrogen peroxide that can then be reduced by glutathione.
TXNRD1 and SRXN1	Thioredoxin and sulfiredoxin reductase repair oxidized disulfide bonds
NQO1	NAD(P)H dehydrogenase (quinone 1) detoxifies reactive quinones that cause oxidative stress and redox cycling.
GST	Glutathione S-transferase creates antioxidant conjugates with toxins so that they can be removed from the body, generally in the urine
UGT	UDP-glucuronosyltransferase catalyzes glucuronic acid conjugates, to help transport toxins into the bile or urine for elimination from the body
HMOX1	Heme oxygenase breaks down heme from hemoglobin and produces a molecule of carbon monoxide that acts as an anti-inflammatory signal. HMOX1 is thought to protect the organs from damage from oxidative stress during injury and sepsis.
ABCC2	This ABC protein binds and transports negatively charged metabolic waste across cell membranes into the renal tubule or bile canaliculi for disposal.

Also, I would add to the rules of engagement that some toxins accumulate in the body, such as heavy metals. Even though they may provide a hormesis benefit at very low doses, they should be avoided. The oxidative impact of arsenic at low levels increases Nrf2 and induces ARE transcription,[426] but what is the long-term outcome? Low dose cadmium, a known human carcinogen, has been shown to decrease certain tumors in rats but increase other tumor types.

Additionally, the toxic threshold may vary considerably among adults, depending upon their genetic alleles for the relevant enzymes involved in the detoxification process. Furthermore, ARE optimization of conjugation may increase biotransformation of certain compounds into more toxic ones.

And please, don't forget that fetuses, babies, and children are different. There may be no toxic threshold for some toxins during development. Low doses of alcohol may decrease the risk of heart disease, and do not appear to raise the risk of cancer, or may lower risk of some cancers, but the safe dose of alcohol for a fetus is zero.

KEAP1, the stress-sensing protein and jailor for Nrf2, releases Nrf2 when it senses intracellular stress. Stress induction of KEAP1 does not necessarily correspond to the genotoxicity of the substance. Thus, some substances that are of low toxicity or that are non-genotoxic can induce the survival and nuclear accumulation of Nrf2 and transcription of ARE without causing significant harm. Among these pseudo-toxic or minimally toxic compounds are several Maillard compounds, such as those present in coffee and chocolate, as well as many dietary phyto-phenolic compounds, such as those found in capers and green tea. Theobromine in chocolate, however, is clearly toxic enough for a chocolate binge to cause an overdose that manifests as severe neurologic dysfunction.

Nrf2 is not the only stress response transcription factor; NF-κB and AP-1 are others. NF-κB, rather than inducing ARE, induces the transcription of a set of pro-inflammatory genes, and rather than being held in check by KEAP1, NF-κB is held in the cytosol by being bound to the protein IκBα.

NF-κB promotes cell survival and immune defense when the body is under attack. NF-κB is a transcription factor for proinflammatory cytokines such as IL-1β; chemokines that attract immune cells; for the enzyme COX2 that makes prostaglandin E2 (PGE2), an inflammatory signaling molecule; and for TNF-α. NF-κB promotes the growth and survival of white blood cells to defend against infection and draws them to the area of inflammation. Thus, NF-κB helps defend the body against attack and helps us fight infection.

Chronic activation of NF-κB also promotes Alzheimer's disease, arthritis, asthma, and atherosclerosis, just to begin the alphabet of the chronic inflammatory diseases it participates in.[427] And when it comes to cancer, NF-κB is not our ally. NF-κB activation may be one of the principal mechanisms by which chronic inflammation promotes the development of cancer.

NF-κB is normally quiescent and inactive, bound to IκBα. IκBα can be phosphorylated by the enzyme IκB kinase (IKK), causing NF-κB to release from the IκBα:NF-κB complex. NF-κB is then free to enter the nucleus and induce the transcription of multiple inflammatory proteins.

NF-κB prevents apoptosis, in part, via the induction of COX2 and its production of PGE2. PGE2 has pro-proliferative activities via EP receptors and the downstream inhibition of BAX expression and increased expression of Bcl-2.[428] BAX promotes, and Bcl-2 prevents the formation of pores in the mitochondria that trigger apoptosis. The COX2 inhibitor, celecoxib, a medication used for arthritis pain, blocks PGE2 formation, and sensitizes hepatocarcinoma and lymphoma and cells to apoptosis, promoting programmed cell death.[429] [430]

Many compounds promote the activation of IKK through downstream activation of specific cell membrane receptors and thereby activate NF-κB. These include Toll-like Receptors, such as TLR2 and TLR4, Fas (TNF) receptors and RTK, including IGF-1 receptors. Activation of IGF-1 receptors promotes growth and survival and down-regulated apoptosis, in part, by downstream activation of NF-κB by Akt and ERK.

> ### Receptors for Tyrosine Kinase
>
> On the outer surface of the cell, there are protein signaling receptors for growth factors, hormones, and cytokines. Humans make fifty-eight different RTK (Receptor Tyrosine Kinases) surface receptors. The signaling proteins for RTKs usually have two or more identical binding sites so that they can bind two RTKs. When two matching RTKs attach to the signaling ligand, the RTKs are brought into close proximity to each other and can "dimerized". When two receptor proteins join, and the intracellular ends of the new protein complex dimerize, it activates a tyrosine kinase enzyme. This enzyme activity generally promotes cell division and survival.
>
> There are about 20 classes of RTKs. They include cell surface receptors for IGF (insulin-like growth factor), VEGF (vascular endothelial growth factor), endothelial GF, tissue GF-α, ErbB (epidermal growth factor), c-KIT, and fibroblast GF; all of which have been have been implicated in various cancers, as these ligands and ligand receptors are in involved with cell growth. The RTK ERBB2 (HER2), for example, is over-expressed in as many as 30% of breast, gastric, and salivary duct cancers.
>
> Several monoclonal antibodies (Mab) drugs block specific RTKs: cetuximab (Erbitux), trastuzumab (Herceptin), and rituximab (Rituxan) are used in the treatment of cancer as they block the activity of these receptors. Several small molecule drugs also target the RTKs, binding to and *inhib*iting them. These include afat<u>inib</u>, brigat<u>inib</u>, and motes<u>anib</u>.

TNF-α is a signaling ligand that, by activation of Fas receptors, can either stimulate inflammation and cell survival or apoptosis, largely depending on the activity of IKK. If IKK activates NF-κB, TNF-α promotes survival and inflammation; if not, TNF-α moves the cell towards apoptosis by activating caspases.

Toll-like Receptors (TLRs) are membrane receptors that recognize and are activated by PAMPs, pathogen-associated molecular patterns. TLRs allow cells to recognize the presence of many pathogens by identifying certain compounds commonly present in the cell wall or flagella of bacteria. This allows cells to respond, and via the response, to signal other cells of the presence of the threat. This response is largely mediated by NF-κB and the production of IL-1β, PGE2, and TNF-α.

The TLR2 receptor recognizes lipoteichoic from the cell walls of gram-positive bacteria. The TLR4 receptor is activated by lipopolysaccharides (LPS) present in the cell wall of gram-negative bacteria. Thus, a chronic bacterial infection can stimulate chronic NF-κB activation and inflammation. TLR4 and TLR2 are also activated by microbial compounds from protozoa including malaria and *Schistosoma*, fungi such as *Candida*, and several viral proteins. Chronic infection thus promotes chronic inflammation through TLR activation of IKK and NF-κB. Alcohol and opiates also stimulate TLR4. Recall that chronic bacterial and protozoan infections and chronic alcohol exposure cause cancer (Chapters 9 and 13). TLR4 also activates survival via Akt activation.

TLR9 responds to CpG-oligodeoxynucleotides, small segments of single-stranded DNA that are common in microbes. TLR 9 is only expressed on B-cell lymphocytes, precursor cells for plasma cells that make antibodies for fighting infections. Such stimulus from chronic infection might thus promote the malignancies of the B-cells, such as Hodgkin lymphoma, or multiple myeloma when these immune cells fail to clear an infection.

TLRs are primarily expressed on immune cells but are also present on some solid tumor cells, such as breast cancer cells. Thus, the TLR activators are most likely to stimulate NF-κB activity in immune cells. TNF receptors are found on the outer surface membranes of nucleated cells as are RTK (receptors for tyrosine kinase). Thus, ligands for these are more likely to promote the proliferation and survival of solid tumors. Oxidative stress and ultraviolet radiation also promote NF-κB activity.

If the intracellular milieu exceeds the capacity of Nrf2 to settle things down, oxidative stress and stress signaling molecules can trigger IKK activity that promotes inflammation. NF-κB activity inhibits that of Nrf2. Thus, if the level of intracellular oxidative stress signaling exceeds a certain tipping point, an inflammatory response begins that also down-regulates antioxidant response to oxidative stress. This makes sense, as the cells use H_2O_2 and other oxidants to fight infection during the inflammatory response.

When an oxidative stress gets out of hand, it can promote the AP-1, Activator Protein-1 early response transcription factor. AP-1 is a heterodimer formed from the pairing of two different proteins, each from one of four protein families. AP-1 and its component proteins are stimulated in response to certain cytokines, growth factors, viral and bacterial infections, tumor promoters, stress signaling, high levels of oxidative stress, or UV radiation. After pairing, AP-1 can enter the nucleus and induce the transcription of proteins that control cellular differentiation and proliferation or apoptosis.

Since AP-1 can be formed by pairing of several different proteins, there are actually many different AP-1 proteins, and they can have different effects. One common AP-1 pairing is comprised of the proteins c-Fos and c-Jun.

C-Fos is a growth regulator that increases the expression of cyclin D1, which helps move cells into the S phase of mitosis. C-Fos can be stimulated by growth factors and cytokines. It helps promote angiogenesis when there is tissue hypoxia. It is also stimulated by neural activity. As a growth promoter, c-Fos can contribute to the growth of cancers. Over-expression of c-Fos in cancer cells is associated with high-grade lesions that have a poor prognosis.

Another AP-1 protein is c-Jun. The activity of c-Jun is modified by its phosphorylation which occurs as the response to stress. C-Jun also regulates the transcription of cyclin D1 and decreases the presence of p53 and p21. Thus, it promotes the cell cycle and inhibits apoptosis. Increased c-Jun is associated with angiogenesis and cancer proliferation. The anti-apoptosis effect may be especially pronounced in the presence of NF-κB activation.

AP-1 can signal tumor growth or cellular senescence and apoptosis depending on factors including the upstream signaling for AP-1 activation, which proteins AP-1 is composed of; the level of oxidative stress and other intracellular signals; and energy availability for cell growth.

Thus, it can be understood that there are three tiers of oxidative stress, described here and in Table 23-2:[431]

1. Low-level stress triggers the Nrf2 → ARE Pathway that prevents oxidative damage.
2. Moderate stress signals for NF-κB transcription of inflammatory mediators and supports cell survival and replication.
3. High oxidative stress signals AP-1 transcription leading to apoptosis of the cell or cancer promotion.

Table 23-2: Cellular Stress Responses

Low-Level Oxidative Stress	Moderate Oxidative Stress	High Oxidative Stress
Nrf2 → ARE	NF-κB → Inflammatory Response	Activator Protein-1 (AP-1)
Induction of antioxidant enzymes and increased conjugation and elimination of xenobiotics. Prevents cancer by helping to eliminate potential mutagens from the body.	Inflammatory mediators can increase the risk of carcinogenesis by inhibiting the ARE response and by increasing the production of ROS and RNS that can damage the DNA.	AP-1 can induce the transcription of Cyclin D1, promoting proliferation, angiogenesis, and tumor growth. Alternatively, AP-1 can signal cellular apoptosis depending on the upstream signaling and other intracellular factors.

Either Nrf2 or NF-κB may be activated, or neither may be, but rarely both are, as they inhibit each other. AP-1 activation can occur with either NF-κB or Nrf2. AP-1 activation with NF-κB promotes cell proliferation, which is good when it rapidly promotes the development of white blood cells for fighting an infection, but a drag when it spurs the growth of cancer cells. When AP-1 is activated, and NF-κB is inhibited, AP-1 is more likely to signal apoptosis.

Stress Response and Cruciferous Vegetables

Sulforaphane (SPH), a compound present in many cruciferous vegetables (CV) such as broccoli, is a direct activator of KEAP1. Sulforaphane thus promotes the release of Nrf2, and in doing so, induces the production of proteins that conjugate and the elimination of mutagenic heterocyclic amines (HCA) and many other xenobiotics. However, if cells are pretreated with the antioxidant N-acetyl cysteine, the induction of ARE via Nrf2 does not occur.[432] SPH also induces autophagy through the induction of ERK activation. If the cell has too much antioxidant activity, the autophagy does not occur.[433] The autophagy and the renewal of cellular components are dependent on oxidative stress induced by SPH! Thus, it can be seen that antioxidant vitamins may inhibit the activation of KEAP1 and Nrf2. CV and their impact on apoptosis are discussed in 24.

Stress Response and Garlic

When garlic is injured by munching insects, or otherwise has its cells damaged by crushing, chopping, chewing, and mincing, an enzyme is released from damaged vacuoles in the cell that converts cysteine sulfoxides contained in the cytosol into allicin. Allicin instantly decomposes into diallyl sulfide (DAS) and other compounds. DAS activates Nrf2 and thus, ARE. DAS also activates the Constitutive Androstane Receptor (CAR) that stimulates the transcription of several enzymes involved in endobiotic and xenobiotic metabolism, including several p450 oxidases, sulfotransferases, and glutathione-S-transferases. DAS also inhibits IκBα phosphorylation and translocation of NF-κB to the nucleus.[434] Thus, diallyl sulfide not only increases phase 1 and phase 2 metabolism of endo- and xenobiotics, it also inhibits the transcription of pro-inflammatory mediators. This effect is likely limited to raw, or gently heated, garlic (Chapter 24).

Stress Response and Coffee

Rats drinking 2 ml (about half a teaspoon) of coffee daily have 130 percent higher cytosolic Nrf2 levels and a 25% increased antioxidant capacity of the liver.[435] A single dose of coffee can raise the level of phase (ARE) enzymes by 20% within an hour.[436] Not only does coffee protect the liver from cancer, but it is also associated with lower rates of depression, type 2 diabetes, and Alzheimer's disease.

When coffee is roasted, a Maillard browning reaction occurs in which trigonelline, a natural compound in coffee that is also found in peas, oats, and potatoes, decomposes into N-methyl pyridinium (NMP). Additionally, as coffee is roasted, the antioxidant, chlorogenic acid, is destroyed.

NMP from dark roasted coffee stimulates the KEAP1 release of Nrf2. Additionally, dark roasted coffee inhibits NF-κB activity by more than 80% and thus lowers the inflammatory response.[437] Dark roasted coffee has been found to decrease the number of spontaneous DNA strand breaks (measured in white blood cells) by 27 percent in a group of healthy men.[438] Darker roasts of coffee contain higher amounts of NMP and are more effective in stimulating the release of Nrf2 and ARE enzyme transcription than are lighter roasts of coffee. Coffee that has not been toasted does not contain NMP and is not effective in stimulating Nrf2. *Coffea arabica* has more trigonelline than does *Coffea robusta*.

In a trial, dark roasted coffee rich in NMP was found to lead to a significant weight loss while light roasted coffee did not. The dark roast was also associated with higher vitamin E levels and higher glutathione levels.[439] Dark roasted coffee also stimulates less gastric acid than does dark roasted coffee,[440] just FYI.

The transcription of Nrf2 appears to respond to positive feedback so that more of the Nrf2 protein is made available when the cell is under stress. Coffee not only affects the activation of Nrf2, but it also affects the amount of Nrf2 transcribed, although this may be secondary to compounds other than NMP in coffee.

The response to NMP in coffee is modified by genetics. There are several common polymorphisms of Nrf2, with three common, single nucleotide variants in the promoter region relevant to inducing ARE proteins. For most Nrf2 polymorphisms, coffee consumption increases ARE transcription by at least 50 percent. For one of the Nrf2 polymorphisms (-653A/G) the response is higher but for another, (-651G/A), found in about 20 percent of the studied population, ARE response to coffee is significantly muted.[441] Thus, about one in five persons has very little Nrf2 response to the NMP in coffee or other foods. Oh, genetics, what sayeth my genome?

Similar to coffee, when bread is baked or toasted, the Maillard reaction creates pronyl-lysine. Consumption of bread crust and malt increases transcription of antioxidant enzymes and raises the level of vitamin E in the blood, indicating that it is being destroyed at a lower rate.[442] Feeding bread crust prevented the formation of premalignant lesions in the colon of rats exposed to the carcinogen dimethylhydrazine.[443]

Maillard reaction products appear to fool the immune defense system. In Chapter 19, the Maillard reactions were described as being similar to the formation of HCA, where a reducing sugar was bound to an amino acid; however, Maillard reactions lack the creatine present in meats and eggs. KEAP1 responds to NMP and similar Maillard reactants as if they were genotoxic compounds, even though they have low toxicity. By stimulation of the ARE, the body becomes much more efficient at nabbing the real bad guys when they appear.

Stress Response and Phenolic Compounds

Various food compounds induce Nrf2 transcription, and there is also genetic diversity in these responses. Blackberry extract has also been found to up-regulate Nrf2 activity.[444] Oleacein, a phenolic compound in olive oil, has been found to activate Nrf2 transcription.[445] Several other phenolic compounds such oleocanthal and hydroxytyrosol, present in olive oil downregulate NF-κB. A higher concentration of most of these compounds can be found in green olives than in the extra virgin olive oil.[446]

Some food compounds, such as DAS in garlic, both induce Nrf2 and downregulate NF-κB.[447] Anthocyanins are plant pigments that give purple, blue, or red colors to plants depending on their pH. These pigments also induce Nrf2 and downregulate NF-κB. Anthocyanins in purple sweet potatoes[448], black currants[449], blueberries, and blackberries increase Nrf2 while inhibiting NF-κB.[450]

Ursolic acid and naringenin have been found to prevent hepatotoxicity and fibrosis caused by oxidative stress through the induction of Nrf2 → ARE signaling.[451][452] Ursolic acid is present in apples, especially the peels, basil, bilberries, cranberries, peppermint, rosemary, oregano, thyme, and prunes. Naringenin may additionally inhibit NF-κB. Naringenin is present in citrus fruit. Some flavonoid compounds down-regulate NF-κB without affecting Nrf2.

In the coming years, we will likely all have access to our personal list of genetic alleles, and the interaction of these polymorphisms to various foods will be much better characterized. As this occurs, we will be better able to select which foods best help us prevent disease and which to avoid; which medications to use and which are likely to cause problems.

Without other knowledge, the most appropriate strategy is to consume a mixture of foods known to help most individuals avoid oxidative and inflammatory injury. Dark roasted coffee, chocolate, cruciferous vegetables containing sulforaphane, allium vegetables, and berries and vegetables containing anthocyanins increase Nrf2 activation and may decrease NF-κB activation. Diets rich in flavonoid compounds decrease NF-κB activity.

Nrf2 protects cells from mutation from DNA adducts and oxidative stress. BRCA1 prevents cancer and helps protect cells from injury in part by inducing Nrf2. Mice with deficient BRCA1, similar to that of individuals with BRCA1 mutations, have low levels of Nrf2-induced antioxidant enzymes.[453] Sulforaphane, (SPH) and the phenolic compound resveratrol induce Nrf2 transcriptional activity, reduce ROS levels and reduce DNA damage from benzo[a]pyrene in BRCA1 deficient animals.[454] Thus, one of the reasons that BRCA1 mutations induce cancer is because they impair Nrf2 reactivity to oxidative stress and genotoxins. Although they may not restore this activity to normal levels, food compounds that increase Nrf2 activity in normal individuals also do so for those with BRCA1 mutations; thus, for aberrant BRCA1 carriers, they provide an even more needed salutary effect for cancer prevention.

Proteasome inhibitors (PIs) are drugs that block the action of proteasomes, protein complexes that break down proteins. These drugs are used in the treatment of multiple myelomas, a form of white blood cell cancer, and are under investigation for use in other cancers. PIs promote apoptosis by slowing the breakdown of p53 and other pro-apoptotic factors, but also by preventing the breakdown of Nrf2 and IkB kinase. IkB kinase inhibits the activation of NF-κB. Thus, PIs augment Nrf2 and ARE transcription and reduce NF-κB and the transcription of pro-inflammatory mediators.

Agents that augment Nrf2 and inhibit NF-κB not only help prevent oxidative injury and DNA damage, they can also promote apoptosis of injured and aberrant cells.

Summary

The stress response elements, Nrf2, NF-κB, and AP-1, are essential transcription factors that determine how the cell will respond to intracellular stress. Nrf2 activation protects the cell from oxidative and DNA damage that can cause cancer and helps the body protect itself and eliminate toxins, including genotoxic compounds.

Most of the foods that have been found to lower cancer risk in population studies contain compounds that activate Nrf2 → ARE (Antioxidant Response Element) transcription, and/or decrease the activation of the NF-κB proinflammatory response element. ARE promotes the transcription of proteins that help protect the body from oxidative injury and promote the detoxification of genotoxins, and other xenobiotics (Table 18-1 above). The foods that stimulate this response contain compounds that are "pseudo-toxins" that the cell recognizes as dangerous; however, they have low, or no toxicity at the levels found in the food. These foods include cruciferous vegetables, garlic and other members of the allium family, and certain toasted vegetable products, such as dark-roasted coffee, and bread. And don't forget the blueberries, blackberries, and black currents that also provide these benefits.

The efficacy of various foods in providing benefit via Nrf2 activation varies according to an individual's genetics. Most adults have a salutary response to coffee, but about 20% of the population has little Nrf2 response to coffee. Different people respond differently to cruciferous vegetables. BRCA1 mutations, in part, increase cancer risk by failing to promote the production of Nrf2. Consumption of foods that stimulate Nrf2 activation can help lower cancer risk for carriers of these mutations.

Antioxidant vitamin supplementation has consistently been found to increase cancer risk in human trials. The antioxidants may prevent the activation of Nrf2, thus preventing the transcription of the ARE antioxidant enzymes and detoxification and elimination of genotoxins.

24: Garlic, Broccoli, and Mustards

Cruciferous vegetables (CV) stand out among vegetables for their anti-carcinogenic potential. These vegetables from the mustard family have a four-petal flower that forms a cross shape and thus are called cruciferous, from the Latin for cross-bearing. Most of the cruciferous vegetables we eat are from the *Brassica* genus, but there are a few closely related vegetables that can also be grouped with them for their anti-carcinogenic potential.

These vegetables do not contain a single chemical entity that prevents cancer, but rather, several. In this section, I would like to provide a clear and simple overview of the actions of these compounds and give guidance as to how to use them to your best advantage. Sadly, having read ahead, I can tell you that your abecedarian fell short of the simplicity goal. At least he tried to make it entertaining.

Glucosinolates are compounds found in *Brassica* vegetables. When an insect chews on the plant, it ruptures vesicles within the cell that contain the enzyme myrosinase. The release of myrosinase and its commingling with glucosinolates in the cytosol causes the removal of a glucose molecule from the glucosinolate and converts it into an isothiocyanate (ITC). The ITC have pungent flavors, recognizable in horseradish, mustard, watercress, capers, and other *Brassica* vegetables. Not only do insects eschew the pungent flavor, but ITCs also make them sick. The ITCs are too toxic even for the plants that make them, which is why they keep the enzyme myrosinase in a separate container to avoid activating the toxin. We are interested in the ITC because they have anti-carcinogenic properties.

Glucoraphanin is one of the glucosinolates compounds. It deters insects from feeding on these plants. Myrosinase splits glucoraphanin into glucose plus an ITC, *raphanin* or *sulforaphane*. Raphanin has antibiotic and antiviral properties, but was judged too toxic for clinical use in the 1940's. There has been no medical research published on raphanin since the 1960's, so not much is known about it. Sulforaphane is a natural pesticide, which is the reason that broccoli bothers to make it. Sulforaphane has antimicrobial and anti-carcinogenic properties, which is a reason that you might consider eating it.

Another glucosinolate is sinigrin. Sinigrin, present in mustard seed and several other CV, is broken down by myrosinase into glucose and allyl isothiocyanate. Allyl isothiocyanate is bactericidal, insecticidal, and nematicidal (kills worms). Most animals don't enjoy its flavor and avoid eating it.

- Glucoraphanin –› glucose + raphanin or sulforaphane (SFN)
- Sinigrin –› glucose + allyl isothiocyanate (AITH)
- Glucotropaeolin –› glucose + benzyl isothiocyanate (BITC)
- Gluconasturtiin –› glucose + phenethyl isothiocyanate (PEITC)
- Glucobrassicin –› glucose + thiocyanate + indole-3-carbinol (I3C)

Glucosinolate	Source
Glucoraphanin → Sulforaphane	Broccoli, cauliflower, Brussels sprouts, cabbages. Lesser amounts in bok choy, kale, collards, Chinese broccoli, broccoli raab, kohlrabi, mustard, turnip, radish, arugula, and watercress.
Sinigrin → Allyl isothiocyanate	Mustard Seed, radish, horseradish, wasabi, and Brussels sprouts
Glucotropaeolin → Benzyl isothiocyanate	Garden nasturtium (*Tropaeolum majus*)
Gluconasturtiin → Phenethyl isothiocyanate	Watercress, horseradish
Glucobrassicin → indole-3-carbinol	Broccoli, cabbage, cauliflower, Brussels sprouts, collard greens and kale

The glucosinolate, glucobrassicin, is converted to glucose plus an unstable intermediary ITC that spontaneously converts into thiocyanate and indole-3-carbinol. *Indole-3-carbinol* (I3C) is the subject of considerable research for its anti-carcinogenic, anti-atherogenic, and anti-oxidant effects.

Now, just to keep things simple, the anticarcinogenic compound I3C, likely promotes cancer growth. I3C induces P450 CYP1B1 activity and increases the production of 4-hydroxyestrogen, a known carcinogen that promotes breast and prostate cancers. This effect may be amplified in smokers. I3C supplements are likely not a great idea.

When the small amount of I3C, that is likely to be found in food meets the stomach acid, it is quickly condensed into dimers or trimers, or it can bind with ascorbic acid (vitamin C). Even if stomach acid is not present, most of the I3C from food is quickly condensed, mostly into the I3C dimer (3,3'-diindolylmethane (DIM), and to a lesser amount, the linear trimer (LTR).

DIM, in contrast to I3C, suppresses the cytochrome p450 CYP1B1. I3C also induces CYP3A4, while DIM does not. It is most likely that it is DIM, not I3C that has anti-carcinogenic effects.[455] The I3C *metabolites* shift the production of estrogens to forms that are less favorable for estrogen-responsive tumor growth.[456] They also suppress NF-κB activation;[457] and stimulate the cell cycle regulatory proteins p15, p21, and p27; and down-regulate Bcl-2 and Bcl-xL, thereby, arresting tumor growth and promoting apoptosis.

DIM appears to act as an androgen receptor antagonist and inhibits the translocation of these receptors to the nucleus of prostate cancer cells, stopping their action. DIM downregulates prostate-specific antigen (PSA). PSA is a glycoprotein that promotes proliferation, migration, and metastasis of prostate cancer cells.[458] Thus, PSA is more than just a marker of prostate cancer risk; it is a prostate cancer risk factor and growth promoter. Isothiocyanates SFN, BITC, and especially PEITC, found in watercress, suppress the CXCR4 chemokine receptor in prostate cancer cells, and thus, also decrease prostate cancer cell survival and migration.[459]

CV compounds induce the enzyme glutathione S-transferase (GST) via Nrf2. From the discussion in Chapter 17, you will recall that GST conjugates *N*-hydroxylated AIA making it water soluble so that it is easily excreted in the urine, rather than being metabolized by NAT and converted into carcinogenic DNA adducts.

Sulforaphane appears to be isothiocyanate that most actively induces GST activity. Sulforaphane may also act as an anti-carcinogen by inducing the production of pro-apoptotic proteins in the cell,[460] and by protecting the mitochondria from oxidative stress through the induction of glutathione peroxidase/reductase enzymes.[461] Sulforaphane is not only an anti-carcinogen; it is cardioprotective,[462] lowers LDL-cholesterol, and has anti-inflammatory effects.[463]

Consumption of broccoli, Brussels sprouts, cabbage, mustard, watercress, rocket, arugula and other CVs has been associated with decreased risk of many types of cancer. Most studies find about a 20 percent reduction in the rate of various cancers among people consuming higher, rather than lower, amounts of cruciferous vegetables. These results, however, are influenced by genetics. For example, people consuming higher amounts of CVs have a 26% reduction in lung cancer incidence. Individuals with inactive GST enzymes received twice the reduction in risk as those with the active enzyme allele.[464] Similarly, consuming CVs decreased the risk for colorectal neoplasms to a greater extent for individuals with inactive alleles for GST T1.[465] Women with the GST_{P1} Val/Val genotype have an increased risk of breast cancer. For these women, consumption of turnips and Chinese cabbage cuts the risk of breast cancer by a third while it had little effect in reducing breast cancer among women with the GST_{P1} Ile/Ile genotype.[466]

There are 22 recognized human GST enzymes, and they are expressed in different amounts in different tissues. Their general function is to detoxify xenobiotics as well as some endogenously produced nonpolar (lipid soluble) toxins. The GST enzymes link a glutathione molecule to a hot spot on the toxin that would otherwise avidly bind to nucleic acids (DNA and RNA) or to intracellular proteins, forming adducts. Such adducts can incapacitate proteins and RNA and may cause mutations when DNA adducts are formed. Conjugation of the xenobiotic with glutathione prevents this, makes the compound water soluble, and aids in the transport of the conjugate from the cell.

Eleven percent of European Americans and 23% of African-Americans are homozygous for the GST_{P1} variant with reduced glutathione S-transferase activity, and about 20 percent of Americans *have an inactive variant of the GST_{T1} gene.*[467] *About half of Americans of European descent and 28 percent of African Americans have the GST_{M1} genotype that provides no enzyme activity.* Individuals with the impaired GST genotypes are at higher risk of cancer from exposure to potentially genotoxic compounds, such as HCA from meat cooked at high temperatures. It is these individuals, with inactive GST activity, in whom cruciferous vegetables give the greatest reduction in cancer risk.[464]

Sulforaphane acts via the KEAP1 release of Nrf2. By activating the ARE (Table 18-1), it induces various GST enzymes that provide benefits mostly to those with an inactive GST alleles, likely by activating other forms of GST, as well NQO1, UGT, and other ARE enzymes that take over for the crippled GST's role in detoxification. Thus, the detox effects of ITC are especially beneficial for individuals who have impaired GST alleles, and may offer only marginal benefits to those with normal ones.

GSTs are only one family of several cytoprotective proteins that are induced by ARE. Cruciferous vegetables not only decrease the mutagenicity of HCA and other toxins but decrease oxidative stress via Nrf2 activation and suppression of NF-κB. These effects are likely shared by everyone.

Not only have the cruciferous vegetables been found to lower cancer risk, but they also lower the risk of heart disease. The mechanism for this is different from that for preventing DNA damage or for improving DNA repair.

When higher doses of SPH are consumed, it increases the induction of the gene for the enzyme PAPOLG (poly(A) polymerase gamma).[468] After PAPOLG has been transcribed, the polymerase enzyme leaves the cytosol and enters the mitochondria. While the mitochondrion has its own DNA, its DNA only has enough space to code for about 31 genes, far fewer than it needs to do its housekeeping and other functions. Most of the proteins the mitochondria in our bodies use are actually human proteins coded in our genes. PAPOLG is one of these; it is the sole polymerase enzyme responsible for DNA synthesis in the mitochondria.[469] Without this enzyme, the mitochondria are kaput. With more of this enzyme available, the mitochondria can renew themselves more efficiently.

For most individuals, consumption of vegetables high in glucoraphanin slows the aging process by promoting mitochondrial renewal and improving the metabolism of lipids. Sulforaphane was found to ameliorate the cognitive dysfunction in an animal model of Alzheimer's disease.[470] Mitochondrial renewal and the anti-free-radical effect from this and ARE protein expression, prevent the formation of oxidative products that damage and age the cells.

The GST_{M1} and GST_{P1} enzymes also prevent activation of JNK and its downstream signaling that results from oxidative stress. GST_{M1} binds ASK1 (apoptosis signal-regulating kinase) and GST_{P1} binds to c-Jun N-terminal kinase 1 (JNK1), preventing their activation. These enzymes promote chemotherapeutic resistance through their protection from oxidative stress and by preventing the activation of the MAPK → c-Jun.[471] C-Jun can form a dimer with c-Fos to form AP-1. As discussed in Chapter 23, AP-1 is a transcriptional factor that induces gene expression in response to stressors including cytokines, growth factors, and intracellular infections. C-Jun:c-Fos AP-1 can promote cell growth and differentiation or apoptosis depending on what else is going on in the cell. When growth is stimulated, AP-1 can promote cancer proliferation; in other circumstances and under other influences, it can promote apoptosis. Under the influence of NF-κB, c-Jun:c-Fos AP-1 promotes growth and proliferation.

Allyl isothiocyanate (AITC) induces G2/M arrest and caspase 9 and caspase 3 activities in glioma and prostate cancer cells, promoting apoptosis; however, it does not do this in normal cells.[472] [473] Sulforaphane (SFN) promotes apoptosis of lung cancer cells, inhibiting histone deacetylase and arrests the cell cycle in the S phase.[474] SFN can also induce G2/M phase arrest; activate caspases 3, 8, and 9 activities; up-regulate BAX, BID, and Fas; and down-regulate the anti-apoptotic protein Bcl-x; thus promoting apoptosis in leukemia cells.[475] (Figure 36-1) SFN promotes the arrest of the cell cycle; increases JNK activity while inhibiting NF-κB, depletes glutathione; and promotes activation of caspase 8 and 9, thus promoting caspase 3 and the activation of apoptotic proteins, all promoting apoptosis.[476] PEITC induces apoptosis via ROS-mediated JNK activation and the upregulation of DR4 and DR5. Additionally, PEITC treatment significantly increased TRAIL-induced apoptosis in glioma and oral cancer cells.[477][478] DIM also sensitizes cancer cells to TRAIL.[479] PEITC has been shown to inhibit proliferation and promote apoptosis of glioma, lung, ovarian and leukemia cells.[480]

Even more remarkable than promoting apoptosis in cancer cells, the ITC compounds from cruciferous vegetables do so selectively while protecting normal cells.[481][482] This may offer normal cells protection from injury from chemotherapy. As a result of ARE expression induced by SFN, there is increased expression of heme oxygenase-1. (HMOX-1) This prevents the creation of ROS during treatment with doxorubicin that at least in vitro, protects cardiac stem cells from doxorubicin-induced oxidative stress and cell death.[483] Preconditioning with SFN 24-hours prior to an ischemic insult has also been demonstrated to protect the blood-brain barrier and decrease neurologic injury from an induced stroke.[484] The flavonoid curcumin has a similar protective effect.[485]

Furthermore, the ITCs have been found to sensitize several lines of cancer cells to chemotherapy. ITCs enhance ER+ breast cancer cells to 4-hydroxytamoxifen.[486] PEITC has been shown to reverse cisplatin resistance in biliary tract cancer cells,[487] potentiates the anti-carcinogenic effect of doxorubicin on hepatocarcinoma cells,[488] and enhances adriamycin-induced apoptosis of osteosarcoma cells.[489]

Thus, the ITCs

- ❖ prevent cancer,
- ❖ selectively promote apoptotic programmed cell death of cancer cells,
- ❖ protect normal cells from apoptosis,
- ❖ protect non-cancerous cells from chemotherapy, and
- ❖ enhance the anticarcinogenic effects of chemotherapy.

Cruciferous vegetables hold great promise for cancer prevention, as well as for the prevention of other diseases of aging.[490] Yes great promise, but sometimes they are a bit short on delivery. Several observational dietary intake studies find only weak and often statistically insignificant associations with cruciferous vegetable intake and reduced cancer risk.[491] This is typically the case for European studies, whereas American studies have been considerably stronger.[492]

The reason for this difference has been suggested to result from differences in "post-harvest processing." SFN and other ITC are a fragile lot.

Remember that ITCs are not actually present in these cruciferous vegetables; it is rather their precursors. ITC are formed when glucosinolates are acted upon by the enzyme myrosinase that is present in vesicles within the cells of the plant. In intact vegetable tissues, these two compounds are separated and only mixed when the cells are crushed, and the vesicles are broken. The purpose of the isothiocyanates is to act as pesticides; so activation only occurs when the plant cell is damaged, as when munched upon by an insect, rabbit, or human. Enzymatic hydrolysis of glucoraphanin occurs with the cellular disruption that occurs with chewing, cutting, gentle heating, and juicing, wherein the enzyme myrosinase and glucoraphanin can mix.[493] Even then, most of the ITC may be converted to inactive forms, such as sulforaphane nitrile.

Freezing CV greatly diminishes the production of ITCs. Furthermore, heating a cruciferous vegetable to over 70°C (158°F) inactivates myrosinase completely and thereby greatly diminishes the amount of isothiocyanate produced.[494][495] Sulforaphane and other ITCs are also heat-labile. SFN is stable at 50°C (122°F) but destroyed at 90°C (194°F).[496] Fully cooked or boiled cruciferous vegetables have insignificant levels of ITCs and have lost their anti-carcinogenic activity. Most of the CV consumed by people is prepared in a way that nullifies its benefits. Lightly steaming CV appears to increase the availability of ITC.

If cruciferous vegetables are briefly heated to 60°C (140°F) and then crushed (chewed) or liquefied into juice, the amount of sulforaphane produced is greatly increased.[497] A person derives more anti-aging and anticarcinogenic benefits from eating a single sprig of raw broccoli than a pound of boiled broccoli. This may be why cauliflower, which is often eaten raw, has been found in population studies to provide more benefit than broccoli. If myrosinase is inactivated, small amounts of glucosinolates from CV may be converted to ITCs by bacteria in the gut that produce myrosinase, and they can then absorbed as dithiocarbamates.[498]

Plants that have the myrosinase-glucosinolate defense system include cruciferous vegetables from the mustard family, which includes purple cabbage, red cabbage, and broccoli inflorescences. Some closely related plants, including radishes, watercress, garden cress, daikon, and wasabi, are also rich in glucoraphanin.[499] Radishes, radish seed sprouts, and watercress contain glucoraphanin.[500] One advantage of these is that they are usually eaten raw. Radish seedlings and watercress have pleasant spicy flavors.

> The health benefits of cruciferous vegetables can be maximized by eating them raw. They can also be juiced, preferably after heating them to 60°C (140°F). The juice can then be cooled for later consumption. To prepare cruciferous vegetables for eating cooked, they should be very lightly heated to an internal temperature of 60°C (140°F) and eaten while still warm to maximize sulforaphane availability.
>
> Thus, broccoli or other CV can be:
>
> - Heated in 60°C (140°F) water for 10 minutes
> - Broken into florets and steamed above boiling water for 3 minutes
> - Very briefly microwaved, just until the color darkens slightly.
>
>   Garlic may also lose its anti-carcinogenic potency when overcooks, and likely has its maximal potency when consumed raw, even if in small amounts.

Fresh cruciferous vegetables are recommended over frozen ones. Canning of CV would expose them to sterilizing temperatures destroying their anticarcinogenic compounds. Snacking on raw cauliflower, broccoli, cabbage (salad or coleslaw), radishes, or CV seed sprouts is a way to ensure that the ITC will be available and not destroyed by heating. Juicing CV can also provide ITC.

Seed sprouts of cruciferous vegetables, for example from broccoli, radish, and mustard seeds have very high glucosinolate contents; having 20 to 50 times as much as ITC as the mature harvested plants. Only a small amount is required to stimulate Nrf2-induced anticarcinogenic protection. Additionally, these are usually eaten raw.

How much and how often do I need to force this stuff down my gizzard?

Eating one or more servings of cauliflower a week decreases the risk of developing prostate cancer in men by over 50% compared to those men eating it less than once a month. One or more servings of broccoli a week decreased prostate cancer risk by 45% compared to men eating it less than once a month[501]. It does not appear to require high doses.

Even more compelling is that the consumption of cruciferous vegetables decreases cancer progression. In a study of men diagnosed with prostate cancer, those in the highest quartile of cruciferous vegetable consumption had a 59% decrease in cancer progression.[502] Those in the highest quartile were consuming broccoli about 3 times a week, or cabbage or cauliflower once a week, compared to the lowest quartile, who reported no CV intake.

Eating two to three servings of properly prepared, fresh CV a week (not boiled broccoli or Brussels sprouts rendered into a paste) is probably sufficient to provide anti-aging and anticancer effects. The most important thing is to make sure that the serving has anti-carcinogenic potential. These studies suggest that large or frequent doses of ITC are not required. Remember these compounds are seen by the body as toxins, and respond through hormesis, rather than as a pharmaceutical type, dose-response effect. A small dose two or three times a week may be more effective than large daily doses. There is no evidence of toxicity from eating the small doses of ITC that is encountered eating CV a few times a week. Moderate doses appear to be safe over the short-term,[503] but we have no published human studies on the effect long-term or mega doses of ITC that could be ingested with ITC supplements.

Garlic and other Allium

Garlic, onions and related *Allium* species, like CV, are rich in sulfur compounds, thiosulfinates in the case of *allium*, which are activated by an enzyme upon injury to its tissues. And like CV, garlic activates Nrf2 and the ARE. Garlic prevents cancer, by inhibiting activation of CYP1A1 and CYP1A2, enzymes that transform HCA to active carcinogens. It is antineoplastic; it promotes apoptosis of cancer cells by arresting the cell cycle at the G2/M checkpoint. Furthermore, it protects the liver from many toxins including the carcinogen aflatoxin, and the chemotherapy drug doxorubicin.[504][505] Garlic has been called, and may be, the most anticarcinogenic food. Garlic appears to both protect animals from cancer chemotherapy medications,[506] and may even enhance the efficacy of some chemo medications.[507]

The principal compound thought to be responsible for garlic's health effect is allium. About one percent of the weight of garlic is composed of allyl-thiosulfinates (ATS), and about 80% of these are the compound alliin. Upon crushing and rupture of the cell walls in the bulb, the enzyme alliinase is released and converts alliin to allicin. Although allicin may be present in the food, it does not reach the bloodstream. Allicin is reactive and is converted into several other compounds, mostly diallyl sulfides (DAS), and lesser amounts of allyl methyl sulfides, diallyl trisulfides (DATS), ajoene, and other compounds. Other ATS in *allium* are converted to S-allyl-cysteine (SAC) and S-allyl-mercaptocysteine (SAMC), other compounds.

Most research points to SAC and SAMC as the important anticancer compounds in garlic.[508] SAC has been shown to bind to estrogen, progesterone, androgen, and glucocorticoid receptors and inhibit their activity.[509] DATS, however, has been demonstrated to inhibit cell cycle progression and decrease mTOR, EGFR, VEGF, Bcl-2. Ajoene inhibits the proliferation of breast and colon cancer cells and induced apoptosis in human leukemia cells.[510] Consuming the food, rather than isolated garlic extracts supplies a wide range of anti-carcinogenic substances.

In a study of lung cancer, men consuming *raw garlic* two or more times a week decreased lung cancer among smokers by nearly one-half. The average amount of raw garlic consumed for this anti-cancer benefit was 30 grams, just over one ounce per week, about half the weight of a medium-sized head of garlic. Even those consuming only around 9 grams per week, about three good sized cloves of raw garlic a week had significantly reduced cancer risk.[511]

In a study of the efficacy of garlic on cancer, mice were implanted with sarcoma cells. The mice were then treated with extracts from fresh garlic or garlic leaves or extracts that had been heated in a microwave oven or boiled. Fresh garlic and its leaves prevented cancer growth, but heating reduced the effects dramatically.[512]

Studies of garlic for its anti-thrombotic or anti-hypertensive effects or its inhibition of LDL-cholesterol uptake by macrophages that reduce the risk of heart disease may or may not help in understanding its role in cancer. Nevertheless, most of the literature on the effect of cooked vs. raw garlic and other *allium* vegetables have studied their antiplatelet activity (APA), which can easily be tested in the lab (*in vitro*). The APA appears to be related to the presence of allicin, and thus, the APA is likely a helpful indicator of ATS activity or its loss of activity.

Steaming raw, quartered onions for one minute raises their internal temperature to 44° C (111° F) and decreases the APA by 18 percent as compared to raw onions. Steaming the onions for 3 minutes raised their internal temperature to 66° C (151° F) and reduced APA by 85%. By six minutes, platelet aggregation *increased* over baseline. Thus, 66°C is sufficient to inactive alliinase.[513] Garlic has APA activity about 13 times higher than does onions. Boiling or heating intact garlic in an oven set to at 200°C °F for 6 minutes completely inhibits APA activity. Crushing garlic (or onions) prior to heating allows alliinase to convert alliin into allicin prior to heating. This extends the APA resistance to heat, but still, APA activity is completely lost in crushed garlic exposed to boiling temperatures in less than 10 minutes. [514, 515] Thus, it is not just alliinase that is denatured by heat, but allicin is also lost.

At refrigerator temperatures (4°C – 39° F) allicin has a half-life of about one year, meaning that it loses half it activity in that much time. At room temperature (23° C - 73.4° F), the half-life of allicin is nine days. At 37 C (98.6 F is it 27 hours, and at 42° C (108°F) it is under 17 hours.[516] Extrapolating from this data, the half-life of allicin is estimated to be about 3.5 hours at 50° C (122° F) , 43 minutes at 60° C (140° F), less than about 9 minutes at 70° C (158° F) , under two minutes at 80°C (176° F), and less than 4 seconds at 90° C (194°F).

To obtain the health and anticancer benefits of garlic, it apparently needs to be consumed raw or very gently heated. Chopped onions can be added uncooked to salads and other dishes. When garlic is wanted to flavor a cooked food, it can be added, as crushed or finely minced fresh garlic, after the meal is cooked, just before serving, when the food temperature has fallen below 60° C. Recall from Chapter 11 that foods should be served at a temperature below 56° C (133° F) to prevent thermal injury and risk of esophageal cancer. Uncooked garlic has a stronger flavor and thus the amount needed for flavoring will be lowered. Swallowing garlic whole is not helpful, as alliinase is degraded by stomach acids, the allium must be crushed by chewing.

> Salsa verde, which is made with green tomatoes, quickly degrades allicin. It is also degraded by mango chutney.[505] Ah, another mystery.

Dry powdered garlic contains active alliin and alliinase and is stable at room temperature for months. The alliin in dry garlic powder is converted to allicin within seconds of hydration. Thus, adding garlic powder to a moist dish that is ready to serve is another way to deliver garlic's health benefits. During drying there is a loss of activity, so even though two-thirds of the weight of fresh garlic has been removed as water, so a similar weight of dry powder garlic as fresh garlic is needed to provide the same health benefits.[517] A level ¼-teaspoon of dry garlic powder weighs about 1 gram.

> CAUTION: While the low doses of garlic that are likely to be consumed as part of a healthy diet prevent liver toxicity, high doses may have toxicity. Chronic exposure to rats to garlic doses, converted to metabolically equivalent doses for humans,[518] found that 40 mg/kg body weight of garlic a day increased ARE enzymes. At 50 mg/kg, there was decreased spermatogenesis. Such growth inhibition is OK for cancer patients, but might not be helpful for children or pregnant women. At doses equivalent to 80 mg/kg for humans, the rats had a

decrease in ARE enzymes and lung and liver damage.[504] Forty mg/kg would be equivalent to two grams of raw garlic or garlic powder a day for a 50 kg (110-pound) woman. Garlic and onions may be toxic to dogs and cats, with some breeds being highly sensitive. Thus, extrapolating garlic toxicity doses from rats may be misleading. Although humans tolerate much higher doses of garlic, 40 mg/kg a day of raw or powdered garlic is a reasonable dose for increasing ARE for those wishing to avoid cancer. Higher doses, similar to those consumed by men who avoided lung cancer (thirty grams a week) would be appropriate for those with cancer.

Water extracts from garlic, such as those in Aged Garlic Extracts (AGE) have much lower toxicity than oil extracts, and thus, these would be recommended if higher doses are wanted. AGE are rich in SAC and do not give a garlic breath odor, but they do not provide all of the benefits of fresh garlic in cancer prevention. Garlic oil extracts are not recommended as they may be more toxic and do not contain SAC.

Allergic reactions to garlic are not rare and can be triggered by topical use on the skin, as sometimes used for acne. Many garlic capsules fail to hydrate and to activate the alliinase and thus are ineffective.

Summary

Eating broccoli, cauliflower or another cruciferous vegetable two to three times a week can lower the incidence of cancer by twenty percent or more. These vegetables are effective when eaten raw, or lightly heated, but the beneficial properties are lost by freezing and or boiling them. Consumption of these vegetables not only prevents cancer but also decreases the incidence of cancer progression. There is some human evidence, and considerable in vitro evidence that CVs are effective for a wide range of cancers. The same appears true for garlic and other allium vegetables.

The ITC compounds from cruciferous vegetables and ATS compounds from allium, not only prevent cancer, but they also induce the death of cancer cells by apoptosis. Furthermore, there is mounting evidence that they can enhance the efficacy of chemotherapy while protecting normal tissues from injury from the chemotherapy agents. It likely does not require consumption of large "doses" of these compounds to be effective. ITC and ATS compounds appear similarly activate Nrf2 and other pathways. Thus they can be used in place of each other, or used in conjunction. Doubling up on ITC and ATS, where their activity overlaps and they share mechanisms of action, is unlikely to add to their anti-carcinogenic efficacy. Some pathways are not shared, and thus there is likely benefit from consuming both.

The plant cells of CV and allium need to be disrupted by crushing, chewing or other means prior to reaching the stomach for their activating enzymes to mix with their substrates and form the active ITC and ATS compounds that provide anticarcinogenic effects. Both stomach acid and heat inactivate these enzymes.

Even after ITC and ATS compounds are formed, heat can quickly destroy them. Heating of cruciferous vegetables, such as broccoli, and allium vegetables, such as garlic, to temperatures above 60°C (140°F), causes rapid breakdown of the activating enzymes and prevents the formation of ITC and ATS from their precursors. They should not be heated to temperatures of more than 60°C (140°F) and then, only for short periods to prevent the inactivation of these compounds.

> ### WATERCRESS JUICE
>
> Watercress provides high levels of PEITC, an ITC with anticarcinogenic properties. Here is a distinctive juice with a refreshing bite from the book A Taste of Paradise,[295] made with watercress. (Used with permission.) It is used as a folk remedy in the Caribbean to treat colds and the flu.
>
> Ingredients:
>
> ½ cup of watercress leaves and stems
> 1 cup orange juice (chilled)
> 1 - 2 tablespoons sugar
>
> PREPARATION: Place the orange juice, watercress and sugar in a blender and liquefy for one minute at high speed. Serve directly or over ice.

25: FATS

If you consume the typical American diet, 70 percent of the nitrogen-based amino acids and 70 percent of the carbon in your organic mass came from corn. A substantial percentage of the remaining 30 percent of the nitrogen and carbon coming from the atmosphere into your diet and supporting your life came from the fixation of CO_2 and nitrogen from the atmosphere by soybeans. Sounds ridiculous, doesn't it. You may have never tasted edamame (soybeans). I have, and I have no desire to try them again, and surely you protest, 80 percent or more of your diet does not consist of corn and soybeans.

It is not just corn on the cob, corn flakes, corn chips, and tortillas, hominy, cornbread, or corn pudding you put in your mouth. The corn syrup that sweetens our drinks and that is widely used in processed food contributes a significant amount of calories. Some may be taken in the form of corn-based alcohol or corn oil. The largest intake of corn-based carbon may actually be through animals. Corn makes up nearly 90% of the feed given to cattle in feedlots. Most of the beef eaten in the United States is composed of amino acids and fats derived from corn. Corn is the major feed for chickens, and thus for eggs. While milk cows eat other things, their diet is often supplemented with corn. Pigs are fed a diet rich in corn. In a similar manner, perhaps 10% of the amino acids in the American diet come from soybeans. Remember, animals cannot make amino acids. The ones in our food came largely from corn and soy, even if first processed through other animals.

We can make fat. However, like essential amino acids, there are essential polyunsaturated fatty acids animals can't produce. The essential fatty acids have two unsaturated bonds: in α-linoleic acid, these bonds are 3 and 6 carbons from the tip of the molecule and in linoleic acid, they are 6 and 9 carbons from the tip. We have enzymes that can add carbons to the other end of the fatty acid molecule to make them longer, and we add double-carbon bonds, but not at the tip. Thus, our diet and our bodies have several different polyunsaturated fatty acids, some that have the first double bond at the third carbon from the end, n-3 fats and some with the first double bond at the n-6 position, and these are not interconvertible. Since they are at the end of the fatty acid chain, they are often called "omega-3" or "omega-6" fats, as Omega is the last letter of the Greek alphabet. And this is where having corn as our major source of these fatty acids gets us into trouble. Corn contains almost no n-3 fats. Since cows and chickens, like us, cannot make n-3 or n-6 fats, they are dependent on the ones in their diets.

Algae growing in cool water usually are rich in n-3 fats, so fish, like other animals, are rich in the polyunsaturated fats they eat. Big fish eating little fish eating these algae are usually rich in n-3 fats. Catfish raised in a pond, being fed corn, are still going to have mostly n-6 fats in their tissues.

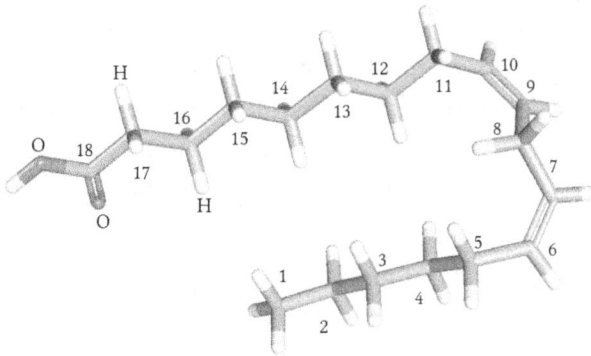

Figure 25-1: Linoleic acid, showing double bonds at n-6 and n-9

Table 25-1: Ratio of n6 to n3 Fats in Meats[519]

	Standard Corn Fed N-6 to N-3 Ratio	Grass Fed or Free Range N-6 to N-3 Ratio
Lean Beef	10.5 to 1	3.8 to 1
Bacon (Pork)	21.1 to 1	
Chicken Breast	14.6 to 1	
Chicken Eggs	15.5 to 1	1.3 to 1
Lamb		2.2 to 1
Elk		2.8 to 1
Whole Cow's Milk		1.57 to 1

If a high n-6 to n-3 ratio is unhealthy, then why are corn fed animals healthy? Don't ask. Calves are kept in feedlots only about five months, as they start getting sick after 6 months and even at five months have pathogenic bacterial overgrowth in their intestines. Chickens are harvested for meat around the age of three months. Both are kept on antibiotics.

When you think of fat in cows, chickens, and salmon, you may think of visible fat under the skin that can be trimmed away from the meat. However, fats are a major component of the cell membrane and other cellular structures present in the muscle in the form of phospholipids and other membrane components. These cannot be trimmed away.

The enzyme phospholipase A2 induces the release of long-chain polyunsaturated fatty acids from phospholipids and triglycerides in the cell membranes. When the n-6 fatty acid, arachidonic acid, is released from the membrane, it is converted into inflammatory eicosanoids, prostaglandins, and leukotrienes. The enzymes PTGS1 and PTGS2, (prostaglandin-endoperoxide synthase 1 and 2) more commonly also known as cyclooxygenase 1 and 2 (COX) convert arachidonic acid into the pro-inflammatory signaling compound prostaglandin E2 (PGE_2). Aspirin, ibuprofen, and naproxen decrease pain, inflammation, and fever by blocking the enzymes COX1 and COX2, thus preventing the formation of PGE_2. Conversely, n-3 fatty acids, such as those common in cold water fish are converted to non-inflammatory eicosanoids. Individuals with diets that have a high ratio of n-6 to n-3 fats thus have cell membranes with high n-6:n-3 ratios, and have stronger and more sustained inflammatory responses.

Non-steroidal anti-inflammatory drugs decrease the risks for cancer of the esophagus, stomach, colon, and several other solid tumors. In a study of patients with Lynch syndrome, which puts patients at very high risk of colorectal cancer, 600 mg of aspirin daily for two years decreased the risk of colon cancer by 59 percent at four-and-a-half years of follow-up.[520] In a study using the COX2 inhibitor, celecoxib, in patients with a history of colonic adenomas, risk of recurrence after three years of treatment was reduced by a third in those taking 200 mg twice a day and by 45% in those taking 400 mg twice a day.[521] About 20 percent of patients, however, had serious side effects from the use of celecoxib, which makes the risk associated with the use of this medication higher than its benefits except in those patients at the highest risk of colon cancer death.

The anti-carcinogenic effects mediated through the action of aspirin and celecoxib occur in part by the inhibition of the enzyme, cyclooxygenase and its formation of PGE_2, although they also have other anti-carcinogenic mechanisms. PGE_2 acts as a cancer promoter by increasing angiogenesis and cell proliferation and decreasing apoptosis. NF-κB is the transcription factor for COX2.

Several flavonoid compounds inhibit the expression of COX2, most likely through their inhibition of NF-κB activation. Additionally, certain flavonoid compounds inhibit the enzyme mPGES-1 that converts PGH into PGE_2; these include kaempferol, which is found in black beans, capers, cumin and cloves, and isorhamnetin, which is present in red and yellow onions and red wine.[522]

α-tocopherol increases the activity of phospholipase A2, and thus this form of vitamin E can increase the production of PGE_2 when there is a high ratio of n-6 to n-3 fats present in cell membranes.[523] The tocotrienol forms of vitamin E do not do this.

PGE$_2$ promotes cancer growth by activating β-catenin, VEGF, and epidermal growth factor receptor (EGFR) activation of ERK through a PI3K activated mechanism.[524]

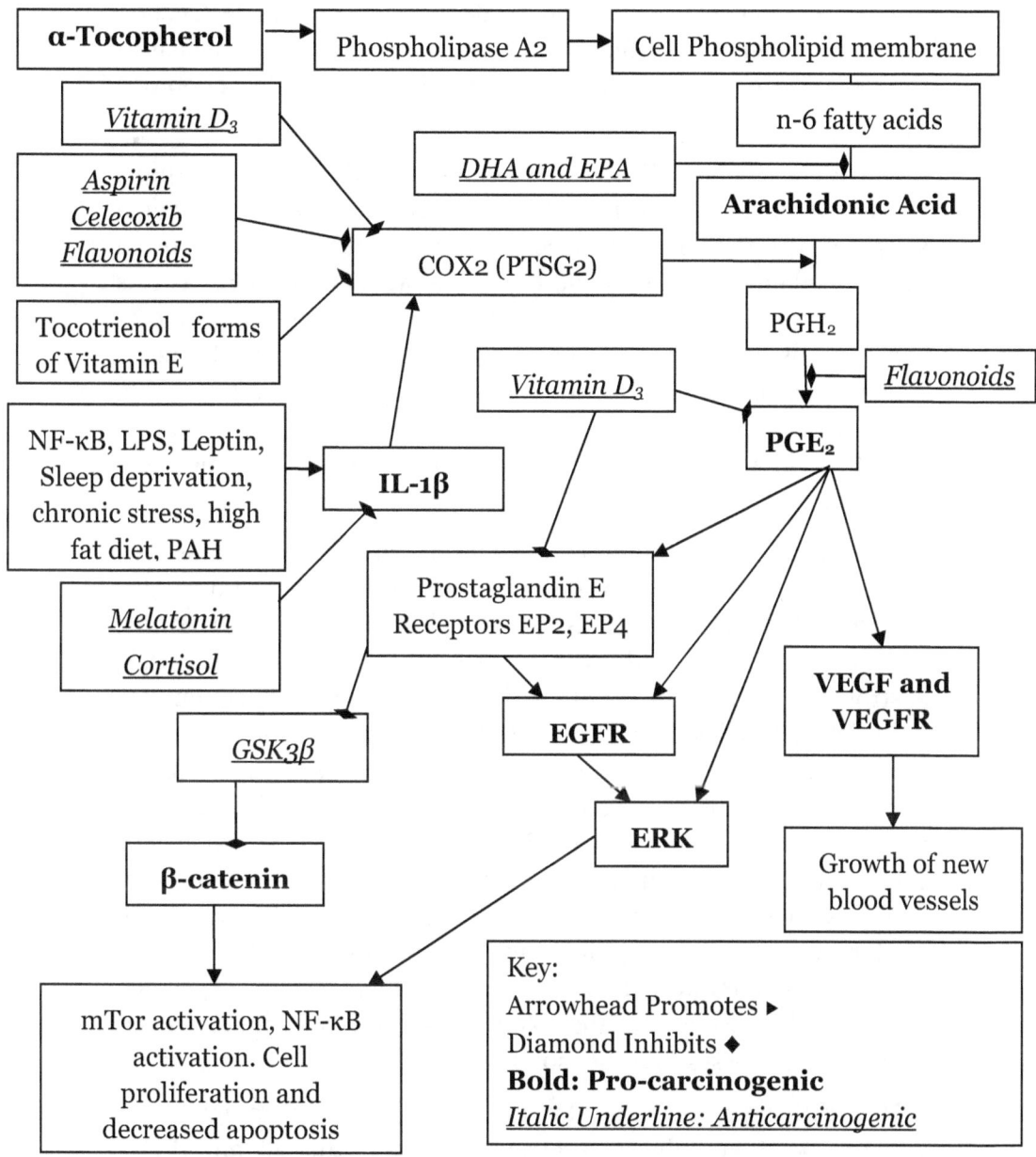

Figure 25-2: The Role of Inflammatory Prostaglandin E2 in Cell Proliferation and Angiogenesis. [525]

β-Catenin helps form a complex of proteins that constitute adherens junctions that bind cells to each other. These proteins maintain adhesion between cells and help regulate growth. β-catenin anchors the actin cytoskeleton. When β-catenin is not bound to the adherens junction, it acts as a signal indicating that the cell does not have a full complement of neighboring cells to adhere to and that growth of more cells is required. Free β-catenin thus can act as a signal for cell proliferation.[526]

PGE$_2$ activates Prostaglandin E receptors (EP$_2$ and EP$_4$), which phosphorylate glycogen synthase kinase 3 (GSK-3). GSK-3 prevents cell proliferation by acting in a protein complex that destroys free β-catenin. When GSK-3 is phosphorylated, it prevents its destruction of β-catenin, and thus, allows β-catenin to move into the nucleus of the cell where it promotes proliferation and impedes apoptotic signaling.[527]

The RTK receptor EGFR (endothelial growth factor receptor) stimulation by PGE$_2$ activates ERK. EGF also increases ERK through a separate, protein kinase-C dependent mechanism. ERK is involved in the regulation of mitosis and thus promotes cell division. PGE$_2$ is also a vasodilator and increases VEGF, and thus, it promotes angiogenesis and increases the blood supply to growing tissue.[528] Angiogenesis is needed to support a blood supply for tumor growth. These same signals are helpful for tissue repair after injury; nevertheless, they are not being beneficial when they promote unregulated growth or cancers.

Aspirin and COX2 inhibitors prevent the proliferation of cancer by preventing the formation of PGE$_2$ and its proliferative actions. This risk reduction, however, needs to be weighed against risks from side effects of these medications. In those with lower risk, gastrointestinal bleeding or other side effects of the medication may outweigh risks of cancer. Celecoxib, for example, increases risks of death from heart disease. Individuals with, or with high risk of, cancer may benefit from aspirin. Polyp formers or those diagnosed with colon cancer, those with Barrett's esophagus or esophageal cancer, and those with adenocarcinomas appear to benefit from lower risk of cancer proliferation and death by taking a baby aspirin (81 mg) a day.[529] Daily aspirin use decreases the risk of metastasis and death by 50% for adenocarcinomas, particularly pre-metastatic disease and for cancers of the colon and esophagus, with lower but significant decreases for other solid cancers.[530]

The PGE$_2$-associated risk for cancer can also be mitigated by vitamin D$_3$,[531] vitamin E tocotrienols,[532] and the vitamin E, γ-tocopherol[533] through the inhibition of COX2 enzyme activity.

If n-3 fatty acids are present in the lipid membrane, they compete for COX2 activity and produce anti-inflammatory eicosanoids in place of inflammatory ones. Additionally, the n-3 fatty acids eicosapentaenoic acid (EPA) and docosahexaenoic acid (DHA) inhibit the formation of arachidonic acid (AA). Oleic acid, found in olive oil, also inhibits the formation of AA.[534] In hepatocellular carcinoma cells, DHA and EPA inhibit cancer cell growth. DHA and EPA promote dephosphorylation and, thereby, activation of GSK-3β.

This causes degradation of β-catenin in these cancer cells, thus decreasing the cell's viability and ability to avoid apoptosis. Additionally, DHA down-regulates COX2 activity and increases the degradation of PGE_2 in these cells.[535]

In prostate cancer cells, vitamin D_3 was found not only to inhibit the expression of COX2, but it also up-regulated the expression of the enzyme, 15-prostaglandin dehydrogenase that inactivates prostaglandins. Vitamin D_3 also decreases the expression of the prostaglandin receptors EP and FP, which mediate prostaglandin signaling.[536]

Several vitamin E compounds downregulate the formation of PGE_2. The tocotrienols γ and δ have additional anti-carcinogenic effects. Both γ-tocotrienol and δ-tocotrienol have been found to inhibit the expression β-catenin protein in colon cancer cells,[537, 538] and cause apoptosis of these cells. γ-tocotrienol and δ-tocotrienol reduce the activation of ERK and MAP kinase activity in pancreatic cancer cells and induce apoptosis.[539] These tocotrienols have also been shown to arrest cell growth and cause apoptosis in human melanoma cells[540]. δ-tocotrienol suppresses angiogenesis induced by VEGF, while α-tocopherol, the form of vitamin E found in most supplements and food fortification, does not.[541] Rather than having an anti-carcinogenic effect, α-tocopherol inhibits the anti-carcinogenic effect of other forms of vitamin E by competing for their uptake into the tumor cells[542], and by increasing the activity of phospholipase A2, and thus, the formation of eicosanoids. Alpha-tocopherol supplements also outcompete other forms of vitamin E for intestinal absorption, causing other E vitamins to be eliminated from the body.

The n-6 fat, AA, induces leptin resistance and thus increases inflammatory signaling for growth, increasing both JAK2→STAT3 and PI3K→Akt signaling. Both STAT3 and Akt promote tumor growth and NF-κB activation.[543] Insulin stimulates Akt, and COX induces the formation of PGE2. PGE2, via the EP3 receptors, inhibits lipolysis, the utilization of fat for energy.[544] High n-6:n-3 diets are pro-inflammatory and promote obesity and tumor growth. They promote both leptin and insulin resistance and lower adipokinin production. High n-6:n-3 ratios in the cell membranes enhance PI3K activity and are associated with high levels of the inflammatory cytokines IL-1β, IL-6, and TNF-α. , that in concert, promote tumor growth. Thus, when an individual has cell membranes rich in n-6 fats, they are prone to inflammation and tumor growth.

In contrast, the n-3 fatty acids EPA and DHA block arachidonic acid formation that leads to inflammation. EPA and DHA promote insulin sensitivity by lowering Akt activation and increasing AMPK activation.[545] A dietary n-6:n-3 ratio of 5 to 1 or lower gives a more favorable, less-inflammatory cytokine level. The inflammatory propensity is even lower when the n-6:n-3 ratio is 1:1. In rats fed a diet that differed by n-6:n-3 ratio, those fed a 1:1 n-6:n-3 fat ratio diet had less visceral fat, lower inflammatory cytokines, lower c-reactive proteins, and less activation of TLR4 than those fed a 4:1 diet.[546] Muscle mass development was greatest with an n-6:n-3 ratio of 1:1 [547] Butter contains conjugated linoleic acids (CLA) that are converted by bacteria in the colon to n-3 α-linolenic acid. CLA inhibit the growth of breast cancer.[548]

The human diet in paleolithic times is estimated to have had an n-6:n-3 dietary fat ratio of about 0.8; thus containing more n-3 than n-6 fats. Prior to the 1960's the Mediterranean diet had an n-6:n-3 ratio of 2:1 or less and the Japanese diet currently has a ratio of 4:1. These diets are associated with the highest longevity. The American diet, in contrast, has an n6:n-3 fat ratio of about 17:1.[545] The ideal n-6 to n-3 polyunsaturated fat ratio is probably about one to one, with ratios above 4 to 1 being associated with increased visceral obesity, inflammation, and cancer risk.

Taking n-3 supplements, such as fish oil, generally fails to improve the situation as the supplement's impact on the n-6:n-3 fatty acids ratio in the diet is dwarfed by the vast consumption of n:6 fats. The quantity of n-6 fats and other (non-n-3) fats has to be reduced for most people to attain a favorable ratio. It takes months to change out the fats in the cell membranes, as these fatty acids are recycled in the membranes until converted to other compounds or broken down for energy. A low-fat diet or one very low in n-6 fats can aid in the speed of this turnover while a high-fat diet is likely to slow it.

Also, n-3 fat supplements easily oxidize; would you eat fish that sat out on the counter for a week? How long have those fish oil capsules sat, and how do they smell? Remember that lipid peroxides deplete glutathione and can form DNA adducts. It is best to get n-3 fats from eating fish, range-fed dairy products, and meat, and vegetables, although most vegetables are low in fat. Vegetable oils are not helpful, as most are too high in n-6 fats, and those rich in n-3 fats, such as flaxseed oil, oxidize and become rancid so fast that they would damage health. Cold pressed (expeller pressed) canola oil, with an n6:n-3 ratio of 2.2:1, has the lowest ratio of any of the available salad oils, but should not be used for frying as it breaks down easily to acrolein and other toxic compounds. Vegetable oils high in polyunsaturated fats are not health foods. Table 25-2 lists foods that have a low n6:n3 ratio. The goal should be to keep the ratio under two to one. The essential fatty acids, the polyunsaturated fatty acids, should come from food, not vegetable oil. If oils are needed, coconut and extra virgin olive oils contain low amounts of polyunsaturated fatty acids. Olive oil is high in the monounsaturated fat oleic acid that inhibits the conversion of linolenic acid to AA. Extra virgin olive oil has been found to reduce the risk of breast cancer.[1] Margarine should not be used. Butter is better.

Table 25-2: Foods with Favorable n-6 to n-3 (Omega-6 to Omega-3)[519]

Best: n-6 to n-3 Ratio less than 1:1	Good: n-6 to n-3 Ratio 1:1 to 2:1	O.K.: n-6 to n-3 Ratio 2:1 to 4:1
Seafoods; cold water and wild caught fish; shrimp, mollusks, and crustaceans Seaweed Winter squash, pumpkins Papaya, Mangos Beans: Mung, navy, pinto Turnips, Broccoli, Cauliflower Chia seeds	Free range chicken eggs Beans: white, kidney, black Milk, Butter, Natural cheeses (Not processed cheeses, avoid margarine)	Free range cattle Game: Deer and elk Cold pressed canola oil Lamb (grass fed) Free-range chickens Canola oil

Summary

Chapters 15 through 20 explained several ways that meat consumption can cause cancer, including the formation of DNA adducts with high cooking temperatures, and high levels of heme for individuals with a genetic propensity for iron overload. This chapter explains how the high amounts of n-6 fatty acids in meat and other foods can promote an inflammatory, pro-carcinogenic milieu in the body. Meat can raise cancer risk when the animal's feed is high in n-6 fats. This risk can be avoided by limiting meat consumption to range-fed animals and cold water fish. The content of n-3 fats in fish helps to explain why pescetarians, those who do not eat meat but do eat fish, have a longer life expectancy than vegetarians, vegans or meat-eaters.[4] Free-range chicken eggs also have low n-6:n3 ratios. Meat eaters should limit their consumption of meat to grass-fed and free-range animals to lower their n-6 to n-3 fat ratios. Since milk cows are usually grass fed, dairy products usually have a low n-6:n-3 ratio.

The meat of highest concern remains hamburger, especially less-expensive forms that have fat added during processing. Hamburger is composed of ground lean beef and fat, although connective tissue, blood vessels and "finely textured beef trimmings," also known as Pink slime, may be included. Since pink slime is acellular, the creatinine, amino acids, and glucose are free to form carcinogenic HCA when heated to high cooking temperatures.

Hamburger may be purchased ranging in fat content from lean meat with five percent fat, to that made with up to thirty percent added fat. At 30 percent fat, the hamburger provides 18 percent of its calories from protein, and 82 percent of its calories from fat.[295] The lower cost products, often used by the young and poor, have more fat. Recall that hamburger makes up the majority of meat consumed by adolescents.

Cows and chickens are not the only animals that n-6 fats increases the n-6:n-3 ratio in their muscles and other tissues. This is true not only of meat but with any dietart source of polyunsaturated fats. N-3 polyunsaturated fats are delicate and easily oxidized, and are thus unsuitable for vegetable oils. Furthermore, linoleic and linolenic acids promote phospholipase D activity, promoting cancer growth (Chapter 34).[549] Thus, vegetable oils high in polyunsaturated fats are unlikely to contribute to health, and should be avoided. That leaves extra virgin olive oil (EVOL) and coconut oil as the easily available ones for food preparation. Butter contains mostly short-chain saturated fats and is also a source of CLA that inhibits breast cancer growth. Thus, coconut oil, EVOL, and butter are the fats that are those recommended for dietary use.

Diets rich in foods from marine environments lower cancer risk and improve longevity. This includes fish, especially from cold waters, but also seaweed. Adding fish oil or other n-3 fat supplements has limited effect on health in a high n-6 fat diet. The ratio of n-6 to n-3 fats in the diet needs to be normalized to increase the incorporation of n-3 fats into the cell membranes. This usually requires a diet low in n-6 fats as well as a diet with sufficient n-3 fats from fish, dairy, and vegetables. Substitution of polyunsaturated fats by mono-unsaturated fats, such as those from olive oil, can also improve the n-6 to n-3 fat ratio. The low n-6:n-3 ratio oil, flax oil (linseed oil) goes rancid so quickly it is rarely used for food, and canola oil is not a good cooking oil. Dietary fatty acids affect the balance of eicosanoids that serve as pro- and anti-inflammatory signaling molecules. N-6 fatty acids, which are superabundant in the Western diet, increase the formation of PGE_2 while n-3 fatty acids decrease PGE_2 and favor the formation of non-inflammatory eicosanoids.

Vitamin D_3, certain forms of vitamin E, and the fatty acids EPA and DHA can help lower PGE_2 formation and mitigate inflammation. COX2 inhibitors can also be used to help slow the proliferation of some cancer cell lines. Preventing PGE_2-mediated chronic inflammation removes the support for maintenance of cell proliferation of some cancer cell lines.

26: Fruits and Vegetables

In a meta-analysis reviewing the entire medical literature, studies of bladder cancer and fruit and vegetable consumption were investigated. Nearly 7,000 published papers on the topic were reviewed, 166 were considered, but only 15 peer-reviewed studies met the inclusion criteria. When considering these, the overall effect of fruit consumption on bladder cancer risk was not significant. The massive European EPIC study, which studied the effect of diet on over half a million people for at least ten years, had the same outcome. However, there was a decreased risk among those consuming higher levels of citrus fruits (RR= 0.87; a 13 percent decrease in risk). Vegetable intake was associated with a decreased risk of bladder cancer with a 3% decrease in risk for each serving consumed daily. Much of the risk reduction from vegetables may have been from the consumption of cruciferous vegetables; this benefit for bladder cancer was most evident in non-smokers.[550]

Thus, while fruit consumption, in general, had no significant impact on bladder cancer, at least one specific class of fruits did. And while there was a small, significant benefit from vegetable consumption, most if not all the benefit came from a specific class of vegetables.

Folate

In the decades before 1990, about half of all Americans had folate levels (vitamin B9) low enough to increase the risk of heart disease and stroke, mostly as a result of elevated homocysteine (HCY) levels. We were not eating enough fruits and vegetables. Folate is needed to recycle HCY into methionine, which is needed for numerous metabolic processes. Low folate levels also cause neural tube defect in developing infants, as well as other devastating birth defects. Thus, the Institute of Medicine increased folate fortification of cereal products with folic acid in 1998. The incidence of neural tube defects fell by about one third after the increase in fortification started,[551] and was also associated with a decline in congenital heart disease,[552] and neuroblastoma in infants.[553] Consumption of fruit has been found to be associated with a decrease in risk of cervical, lung, stomach, and colorectal cancers. Much of this effect may be secondary to the high content of folate found in citrus fruit

Folate is the collective term for at least nine compounds that that body can use as or convert to vitamin B9. The most common folate in food is 6(S)-5-methyl tetrahydrofolic acid (5-MTHF), an active form of vitamin B9 that helps recycle HCY to methionine. Whole grains, fresh orange juice (OJ), broccoli, and carrots have most of their folates in the 5-MTHF form. Leafy vegetables and fermented foods predominately provide 5-formyl tetrahydrofolate (folinic acid). Other forms of folate in food include tetrahydrofolate (THF), 10-formyl folate, and folic acid (FA). FA is generally absent in fruits and vegetables but is found in naturally fermented yogurt.[554][555]

Whole wheat and brown rice contain 5-MTHF, but the vitamin is removed along with the bran when these grains are processed. Thus, fortification with FA is used to replace the folate that is lost. Like other B vitamins, folate is water-soluble vitamin. When foods are boiled, the folate is leached out, and often discarded with the water. Folate can also be destroyed by heat, so that boiling, and even more, frying temperatures partially degrade folate. With boiling and discarding the water, up to 85% of the folate can be lost; with frying a third can be destroyed.[556][557] Thus the diet is often low in folate. OJ is a good source as only about 2% is lost during pasteurization.[558]

Folic acid, folinic acid and 10-formyl folate are pre-vitamin folates, each requiring different enzymes for conversion to THF. THF is converted to 5,10-methylene THF before it can participate in the formation of nucleic acid synthesis or be further reduced by MTHFR to 5-MTHF to recycle HCY.

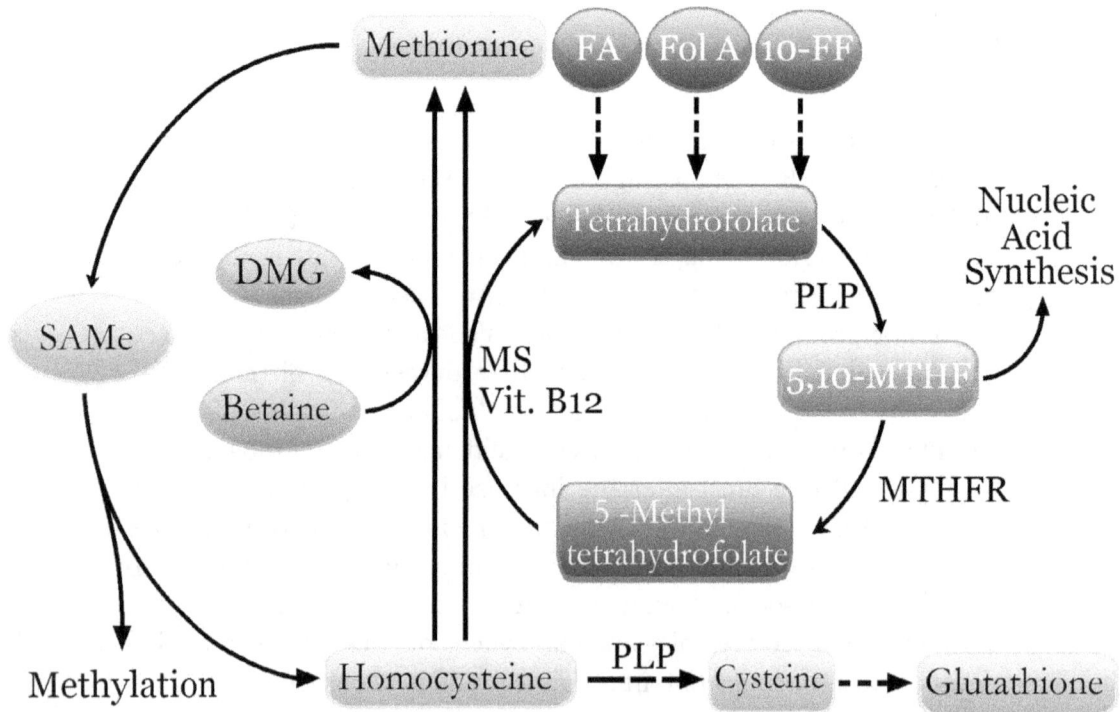

Figure 26-2: Folate-Methionine- SAMe Cycle. FA=folic acid, Fol A=folininc acid, 10-FF=10-formyl folate, 5,10-MTHF=5,10-methylene THF, MTHFR=methylenetetrahydrofolate reductase, MS=methionine synthase. PLP = pyridoxal-5-phosphate. Betaine gives up a methyl group and becomes dimethylglycine (DMG), also recycling homocysteine into methionine.

Before you go popping vitamin pills, know that since 1998 most cereal products (bread, pasta, breakfast cereals) in the United States are fortified with sufficient FA to provide an average 200 μg of folate a day, which when combined with dietary folate in food, gives most Americans adequate folate. It should also be understood that excess FA, the form of folate used in food fortification and most vitamin supplements, is associated with an increased risk of colon and other cancers, at least for those with pre-existing cancer cells.[559]

The body has limited capacity to absorb folate and has limited ability to process the rare folate, folic acid, into THF. Thus FA may prevent the absorption of other folates.[560] Consumption of more 200 μg of FA causes a build-up of unmetabolized folic acid (UMFA) in the bloodstream, especially for those with MTHFR allelic variants.[561] UMFA has no vitamin activity but may rather impede it, in part by increasing losses of active forms of folate into the urine and bile. In a study of lactating women, breast milk from mothers taking 400 μg of FA had UMFA levels 126% higher and 9% lower 5-MTHF levels,[562] putting them and their infants at risk of low folate activity. High FA intake reduces the number of NK cells in the bloodstream, the premier anti-cancer, antiviral WBC, and impairs NK cell function.[563] There is no evidence that other folates do have this effect, nor is there evidence that the 5-MTHF form folate supplement folate (Metafolin) increases cancer risk.

There are several common polymorphisms among the enzymes involved in folate metabolism, including methylation of the DNA, recycling of SAMe, and the formation of purines. I will discuss just a single example of these polymorphisms, as one is difficult enough to wrap my head around, without having to consider the possible interactions of multiple allelic differences.

Methylenetetrahydrofolate reductase (MTHFR) is the rate-limiting enzyme in the folate "one carbon cycle" in which homocysteine is recycled into methionine (Figure 26-2 above). The amino acid methionine is an essential "one-carbon" (methyl group) donor. The MTHFR enzyme usually has a cytosine in the 677 position (677C), but in some populations, cytosine is substituted with thymine. The 667T variant places the amino acid valine into the enzyme rather than the usual alanine coded into the 677C form. The 677T form of the enzyme works but is less stable.

Since we get one copy from each parent, individuals may have MTHFR 677CC, 677CT, or 677TT. Only one percent of African Americans have the 677TT form, about 10% of Caucasians do, and it is common among those of Hispanic and Italian descent; 20% of these individuals have the 677TT form of the MTHFR enzyme. Well over half of Mesoamerican Indians of southern Mexico have the unstable MTHFR 677TT form.[564] This correlates well with the high rate of neural tube birth defects among Hispanic, intermediate rate among Caucasian, and low rate seen among Black American infants.

Having adequate folate activity is important in the prevention of cancer; impaired folate metabolism associated with MTHFR 667TT is linked with breast,[565] colon,[566] head, and neck, lung,[567] pancreatic,[568] gastric,[569] and cervical[570] cancers, as well as some forms of leukemia.[571] If this were not bad enough, impaired folate metabolism increases the risk of a woman bearing a child with Down's syndrome,[572] severe neurologic birth defects, and autism.[573] I'm not done yet. Impaired folate function associated with MTHFR 667TT increases the vulnerability for Alzheimer's disease,[574] schizophrenia, bipolar disorder,[575] depression,[576] osteoporosis,[577] heart and vascular disease,[578] migraines,[579] and hearing loss.[580] Much of the disease caused by poor folate function may result from elevated HCY, a risk factor for many of the same diseases as low folate. HCY can cause DNA damage, ER stress and activation of acid sphingomyelinase, an enzyme that promotes inflammation.

People with the 677TT form of MTHFR bear a high disease risk from marginal folate levels. Alcohol also impairs the one-carbon cycle. Alcohol inhibits methionine synthase (MS), may inhibit several methyltransferases and methionine adenosyltransferase (MAT), and activates betaine-homocysteine methyltransferase (BHMT).[581] Additionally, alcohol may prevent the uptake of tetrahydrofolate from the small intestine. Thus, alcohol may act more potently as a carcinogen in individuals with MTHFR 667TT or who have other reasons for impaired folate metabolism.

Those with less active or poorly stable methylenetetrahydrofolate reductase (MTHFR) alleles need to maintain their levels in the upper half of the normal range to avoid a high risk of heart disease, strokes, cancers, and birth defects. This can be done with a diet high in foods naturally rich in folates, but folic acid supplements should be avoided. Metafolin, a 6(S)-5-MTHF supplement can be used, generally as a dose of 400 to 800 µg a day. As discussed in Chapter 11, alcohol reduces folate absorption and MTHFR activity, and thus should be avoided by those with compromised folate metabolism.

> Folate is a critical participant in the methylation of DNA. Methylation helps bind DNA to proteins called histones. Rather than a loose mess of thread that can get knotted and twisted, the DNA is neatly wound around histones that act like spools. There are large spools and small ones. These spools keep the DNA organized and protected.
>
> Take a string and wrap it around a cylinder two or three times, and tie it

with about two inches of extra string so that there is some slack in one loop, enough so that you can get your finger under it. You should have enough slack so that when you put your finger in the slack loop and flip your finger over, it tightens the string. That is how the DNA thread is when it is tied down by the small histone proteins. When your finger is removed, there is enough slack to lift any portion of the string from around the cylinder. This slack, created by the removal of the small histones, allows DNA segments that have been induced by transcription factors to be read and copied to mRNA but still allows the DNA to remain organized.

Folate participates in the methylation process helping protect the DNA by binding it to histones. A different process, upon induction of specific sets of genes, removes the methylation and frees the small histones, allowing groups of genes to be read and their proteins to be transcribed.

If there is insufficient folate, the DNA gets over-exposed and is more prone to breakage, putting it at risk of mutation. Excessive folate, however, may promote hypermethylation that keeps p53 from being expressed, and thus increases the risk for cancer.

Let's review: at least one in ten Americans has a polymorphism of a gene that impairs the folate function, and this increases the risk of cancer and many other diseases. MTHFR 667TT is just one of several polymorphisms that affect folate metabolism. Added to this, folate is one of the most common nutritional deficiencies worldwide, although now less common in the U.S.A., because of FA fortification in processed foods. Nevertheless, folate levels still remain marginal in many peeple. Alcohol additionally impairs folate absorption and function.

The fix for this would be simple, using easy to synthesize and inexpensive FA if it were not for the very real concern high amounts of FA decreases NK cell activity and may increase cancer and other disease risk. Part of this concern is that excess folate may cause hypermethylation that decreases the expression proteins such as p53 and BRCA1 that help eliminate aberrant cells that have DNA defects.

Taking a 200 – 400 μg supplement of folate a day was found to reduce the risk of aberrant p53-positive colon cancer; there was no additional benefit for those taking more. Seventy–five percent of colon cancers have p53 mutations. Nevertheless, an increase in normal-p53 colon tumors was demonstrated in patients with colonic polyps who consumed more than 400 μg of folic acid per day. This suggests that hypermethylation, which protects the gene from damage, also prevents its activation, increasing colon cancer risk.[582]

As with colon cancer, higher amounts of folate intake decreases breast cancer. However, the decrease in risk begins to reverse for those consuming over 400 μg of folic acid a day. The peak benefit is for those consuming 300 to 400 μg of folate daily. [583]

FA supplements for pregnant women have been found to decrease the risk of autism, several birth defects, and childhood cancers. Thus, there is benefit from low dose supplements, but excess FA increases the risk of disease. Consuming vitamins from food rather than tablets and avoiding mega or super-physiologic vitamin doses is recommended. Risk from natural dietary folates from any non-extreme diet is unlikely. The problem appears to be primarily from the folic acid vitaminer that the body has limited capacity to process, is present only in low quantities in natural foods, but is the form present in fortified foods and most vitamin supplements.

For those who are at high risk of folate impairment because of MTHFR 667TT or other impairment of the folate-methionine cycle, poor diet, pregnancy or alcohol abuse, Metafolin, a folate bioequivalent to the active form of folate 5-MTHF is an active vitamin, identical to the folate most common in food, and the form the body uses to recycle HCY. A physiological dose of 400 – 800 mcg per day is recommended. A trial of Metafolin is advised if testing reveals elevated homocysteine levels. And let me repeat here my call for universal genome-wide genetic testing for risk alleles will allow targeted treatment of 5-MTHF and other risk alleles.

> The following are easily available blood tests and their ideal levels. They are usually paid for by health insurance as long as a related diagnosis (even family history) is supplied:
>
> ϓ Serum Folate: 10 - 26 ng/ml (22.5 - 60 nmol/L) [584]
> ϓ Serum Vitamin B12: Over 540 pg/ml (400 pmol/L). [585]
> ϓ Vitamin D: 40 to 80 ng/ml (100 to 200 nmol/L) 25 OHD3
> ϓ HS-CRP: Less than 0.8 mg/L. [586]
> ϓ *Homocysteine: Action level - greater than 10 mg/L (74 μmol/L). Ideally less than 7.0 mg/L (52 μmol/L) (Some insurance companies no-longer cover this test)*
>
> A simple indirect screening blood test for adequate folate *function* is homocysteine (HCY) level. If the HCY level is high even when serum folate and vitamin B12 levels are in the normal range, it suggests poor folate-methionine cycling and indicates elevated disease risk. Ideally, HCY levels are less than 7.0 μmol/L. An HCY level of 10 μmol/L is associated with a 60 percent higher risk of vascular disease compared with having a level of 5.0 μmol.[587] It is not the use of folate and vitamin B12 supplements that reduces risk; it is normalizing function that does.

Lowered HCY levels are a demonstration of this normalization.

For most individuals with C677TT, folate (400µg/day) helps lower HCY. Riboflavin, another B vitamin, is also a cofactor for MTHFR. Some individuals may respond to supplementation with 25 mg of riboflavin.[588] Vtiamin B12 needs haptocorrin, a protein in the saliva for efficient absorption. Thus, oral B12 supplements should be dissolved in the mouth to mix with saliva, not just be swallowed.

FA needs to be absorbed twice to do any good. First, it is absorbed as a mix of folate compounds from the diet. It is then converted in intestinal mucosa and liver dihydrofolate (DHF), then to THF and finally to active coenzyme forms of folate, including 5-methyltetrahydrofolate (5-MTHF) used in the folate-methionine cycle. These active forms are then excreted in the bile into the small intestine where they can be absorbed by the small intestine mucosa cells and distributed by the bloodstream to the rest of the body for use. Conversion of pre-vitamin B9 folates to THF and then to 5-MTHF requires several enzymes, vitamins C, B6, and B3, and zinc as enzyme cofactors.[589]

HCY may be stubbornly elevated in individuals that have difficulty converting dietary folates into 5-MTHF, as may occur among those with liver or intestinal injury that precludes processing or absorption of the active forms of the coenzyme. Thus, supplementation with 5-MTHF is preferred, although finding and correcting the reason for folate dysfunction would be more helpful over the long run.

Pyridoxine (vitamin B6) is another vitamin cofactor that helps remove HCY from the folate-methionine cycle (Figure 2-26), converting HCY into cysteine. Adequate serum vitamin B6 (pyridoxal 5′ phosphate; PLP) levels and methionine intake are protective from breast cancer.[590]

If B6 levels are inadequate, a (25 mg) pyridoxine supplement may help. However; insufficient B6 activity is more often caused by inflammation rather than dietary deficiency. In this case, supplementation with the active form, pyridoxal-5'-phosphate, may help. Treating the inflammation is wise.

Betaine (trimethylglycine) is another B vitamin-like dietary compound that helps lower HCY levels.

Other blood tests: If low, it often takes 5000 i.u. of vitamin D3 supplements per day for adults to maintain these levels, as many people lose vitamin D3 during hepato-enteric circulation (Chapter 27). Hs-CRP is a heart disease and cancer risk marker (Chapter 36).

Choline

Choline is a critical nutrient and a semi-essential B vitamin. Our bodies can make it, well, at least most fertile women can, via a complex path (Figure 34-6), but this ability to make it is limited. Fertile women are able to convert phosphatidylethanolamine into choline using the enzyme PEMT (phosphatidylethanolamine n-methyltransferase). PEMT is induced by the estrogen response element. Thus, women who have sufficient levels of estrogen can go long periods with a diet low in choline without becoming choline-depleted. The same is not true for healthy men of the same ages. Choline is needed for brain growth and repair. The induction of PEMT in fertile women acts a safeguard to support fetal growth and development during thin times when sufficient quality foods are not available to support growth.[591]

There are also common genetic alleles of PEMT that do not work well. Fertile women with the misfortune of inheriting two impaired PEMT alleles are at high risk, those with one at medium risk, and those with two functioning PEMT alleles are at low risk of choline depletion on a low choline diet. Women with the impaired alleles are very susceptible to choline restrictions,[592] and if exposed to a choline-deficient diet during gestation, their offspring are more susceptible to neural tube defects and other birth defects. The rest of us are subject to choline depletion when we don't have it in our diet.

Choline deficiency can cause fatty liver, as it is needed for the export of lipoproteins from the liver. Choline deficiency can cause DNA damage. This deficiency has been noted to be the only nutritional deficiency that, on its own, can cause cancer.[593] At least in rats, choline deficiency causes hepatocarcinoma. Choline deficiency causes DNA damage so effectively in human lymphocytes that assessment of DNA damage in these cells has been suggested as a clinically useful measure of choline deficiency.[594] Choline acts as a methyl donor and helps stabilize the genome.[595] Choline deficiency may be particularly dangerous in those at high risk of cancer as DNA instability can lead to additional mutations that promote cancer.[596] For those with cancer, choline deficiency may add risk by increasing disease aggression and resistance to treatment.

Choline has several functions. It is a precursor of the neurotransmitter acetylcholine and a component of sphingomyelin, a component of the cell membrane and of the myelin sheath that surrounds and protects the axons of nerves. Choline can also be converted into betaine (trimethylglycine) that can donate a methyl group to recycle homocysteine into methionine. Choline deficiency can increase the risk of elevated homocysteine levels, a risk factor for ischemic heart disease, stroke, inflammation, and cancer. Choline is needed for the formation of phosphatidylcholine, a compound that acts as an energy auditing signal to let the cell know if there is sufficient energy available for cell growth.

Choline is critical for growth and development and for health. Americans usually get less than optimal amounts in their diets, as processed foods are usually low in choline. While there may be adequate amounts in wheat germ, there is very little to none in white wheat flour, white rice, white sugar, corn syrup, and fats. Shrimp, egg yolks, spinach, cauliflower, mushrooms, oysters, asparagus, fish, beef and chicken livers, and broccoli are just a few of the foods rich in choline.

Boron

Boron is a strange nutrient. We get it mostly from the consumption of fruits and nuts, but their content is dependent on the soil where they are grown. We know more about what it does than how. It helps strengthen bones and raises vitamin D and estrogen levels. Humans have no enzymes that use boron, however, our friendly gut bacteria do. Many of the effects of boron likely arise as a result of bacterial re-processing of vitamin D and estrogens that are excreted into the bile (as will be discussed in Chapter 27).

Men with higher intakes of dietary boron have about half the risk of prostate cancer risk as men with low boron intake. In mice, boric acid supplementation decreases PSA, IGF-1 and the growth of prostate tumors. Boron intake is inversely associated with risk of cervical cancer and associated with lower risk of lung cancer in female smokers.[597]

Boron inhibits HIF-1, and thus angiogenesis that supports tumor growth. Boron appears to get trapped in tumor cells dependent on glycolysis, and calcium fructoborate (CFB), a natural boron compound present in fruits and nuts, promotes apoptosis of breast cancer cells.[598, 599] Boron may also protect against genotoxicity and cytotoxicity during chemotherapy.[600]

A diet rich in boron during growth may decrease risk for breast cancer by increasing estrogen levels resulting in epigenetic down-regulation of estrogen receptors (ER). Boron supplements should be avoided in women with or at very high risk for ER+ cancers, other than in preparation for chemotherapy. Chelated boron supplements (6 mg/day) may be used to supplement boron, but the best source of boron is CFB from peanuts, tree nuts and fruit including grapes and stone fruit.

Phenolic Compounds

Folate is not the only compound in fruit that lowers cancer risk. It is likely the consumption of flavonoids, such as found in berries, some fruits, and tea that drives the associated between the consumption of these fruit with a decrease in risk of lung cancer.[601] In the EPIC study, the risk of lung cancer was reduced by fruit, but the reduction was limited to the consumption of berries; none of the other five categories of fruits were associated with lowered risk.[602]

Fruits high in phenolic compounds include berries and citrus fruits. A large portion of the flavonoid compounds in fruit are found in the fruit's skin. The phenolic compounds in the skin of the fruit inhibit bacterial and fungal growth; they act as a barrier helping to prevent the fruits from rotting. Phenolic compounds are also found in the skin of some root vegetables and some seeds; here too, they prevent rot. Many herbs are rich in phenolic compounds. The red to purple anthocyanidins pigments in fruits and vegetables are another group of phenolic compounds. This may be why berries are helpful in reducing risk; the skin is eaten.

The health benefits from red wine are derived mostly from the phenolic compounds in the grape skin. When fruits are eaten without their peel, they usually provide much lower amounts of flavonoids. Juicing may remove the skin and thus the phenolic compounds. Citrus fruits contain significant amounts of phenolic compounds, even though the skin is not eaten. Peeled apples, pears, and peaches, and bananas, melons, kiwi, and pineapples, for which the skin is not eaten, contain minimal amounts of phenolic compounds.

It is the berries and other small, thin-skinned fruit, and those with deep red or purple flesh that are highest in phenolic compounds. White and green grapes and wine made from them have much lower amounts of phenols than do purple and black grapes. Red onions have higher levels of phenols than do white or yellow ones.

Much of the phenolic compounds in unprocessed fruits and vegetables arrive in the form of complex polyphenolic compounds such as tannins and lignans. Polyphenolic compounds are a form of fiber. We lack the enzymes to digest these compounds, and they are very poorly absorbed. In the colon, some polyphenols are digested through bacterial fermentation, allowing the absorption of some of these compounds. In winemaking, the skin of the grape is fermented with the grape juice, allowing the release of small phenols into the wine, which increases their availability.

In a meta-analysis of other studies, both fruits and vegetable consumption was found to decrease lung cancer risk to a similar degree as that observed in the EPIC study. However, the risk reduction was limited to current smokers.[603] The modest risk reduction among smokers maxed-out with four servings a day. Nevertheless, the power of fruit and vegetable consumption in lowering the risk of lung cancer was much smaller than quitting smoking. Eating more fruits as a strategy to avoid lung cancer in smokers is absurd.

What is a fruit or a vegetable? I'm not questioning whether a tomato is a vegetable or a fruit. That question was settled by the court in California; it's a fruit. What I'm questioning is what people actually eat. The most abundantly consumed fruits are apples and bananas. The study measured consumption as quantity in grams; heavy fruits and vegetables counted most. Did anyone actually expect the most commonly consumed and massive vegetable, the potato, to prevent cancer? Should the serving of apple pie I had last night as a bedtime snack be counted as one or two servings of fruit?

In the EPIC study breast and ovarian cancers had near significant trends for *increased cancer risk with the consumption of fruit*. This could easily be noise. It is not unexpected to find a false positive relationship when 32 different cancer-food hypotheses are tested (as in this study) and where the significance boundary is set to one-in-twenty.

Still, could this effect be real? As discussed in previous chapters, fructose consumption may be a risk for cancer. Fruits high in fructose may present a risk. The most common of these would be apples, and its most noxious form would be apple juice.

When consumed as juice, large amounts of fructose can be quickly ingested and absorbed into the bloodstream. An eight-ounce glass of apple juice contains over 15 grams of fructose, more fructose than Pepsi or Coca-Cola that are sweetened with high-fructose corn syrup.[604] It takes three to six apples to make an eight-ounce glass of apple juice. That is a lot of apples to eat, but this much juice can be consumed easily. Two servings of fruit juice a day is enough to cause three to four-year-old children to become overweight. And my-my, my apple pie was not homemade. The apples were peeled, and the pie was sweetened with high-fructose corn syrup.

Apples, but not apple juice, contain pectin. Pectin is not digested by humans, but rather is fiber that is digested by our flocks of intestinal bacteria. Fiber consumption is associated with decreased risk of certain cancers. There are, however, several different classes of fiber, and these do not all provide the same benefits (Chapter 27).

In the EPIC study, women eating over 300 grams of vegetables a day, as compared to eating less than 100 grams of vegetables a day, had an eight percent lower risk of cancer, with much of this risk reduction for breast cancer. That is equivalent to three servings of vegetables a day. Both men and women eating over 200 grams of vegetables a day (about 7 to 8 ounces) had lower cancer risk than those eating less than 100 grams of vegetables a day. However, the anti-cancer effect was small, about a five percent reduction.

In men, but not women, eating fruit also was associated with lower cancer risk in the EPIC study. Men in the highest 20 percentile for fruit consumption, eating an average of 246 to 366 grams of fruit a day (about two apples, oranges or bananas a day) had a ten percent lower cancer risk than those in the lowest fifth of the population, who ate less than 90 grams of fruit a day. Women consuming this quantity of fruit had a non-statistically significant five percent decline in risk. If eating fruit is helpful in preventing cancer, European women are not eating enough fruit, or, at least, are not eating the right ones to prevent breast cancer.

> ### Grapefruit Caution
>
> The grapefruit is a hybrid of a pomelo and an orange. Both grapefruit and the less commonly consumed pomelo contain several compounds with unusual metabolic effects for food; they inhibit several cytochrome P450 enzymes in the intestinal mucosa and liver. Since these enzymes are responsible for the metabolism of several medications, consumption of grapefruit can affect the blood level and the activity of these drugs.
>
> When small amounts of grapefruit are consumed, only the enterocytes lining the intestine are affected. A ten ounce serving of grapefruit juice can impair enterocyte CYP3A activity for up to three days. Larger amounts can also affect P450 activity in the liver.[605]
>
> Consumption of grapefruit can inhibit the transformation of some medications into their active form, reducing their efficacy. For example, grapefruit can inhibit the activation of codeine, preventing it from providing analgesia. More commonly, however, the fruit may prevent metabolic elimination of a medication and create higher than anticipated levels or even dangerous toxicities. If you are taking medications and enjoy grapefruit, you should discuss potential interactions with your physician.
>
> Grapefruit inhibits CYP2D6, the enzyme that metabolizes tamoxifen into the much more active compound endoxifen. Women treated for breast cancer with tamoxifen who have a genetic polymorphism for

slow CYP2D6 have twice the mortality rate from breast cancer as those with the fast form.[606] Grapefruit impedes the activation of tamoxifen.

Consumption of grapefruit also alters the enterohepatic metabolism of estrogen in the gut, as it impairs CYP3A4, increasing estrone-3-sulfate and decreasing estradiol.[607] These changes in hormone may affect sex hormone-responsive cancers. Three different studies have evaluated the effect of grapefruit consumption on breast cancer risk. In one study, grapefruit consumption was associated with a 30 percent increase in breast cancer risk,[608] while no effect was found in two other studies.[609][610] Estrone-3-sulfate is associated aggressive prostate cancer.[611] Thus, grapefruit may increase the growth of prostate cancer.

Grapefruit also contains lycopene, lutein and other carotenoids, flavonoids, and other phenolic compounds that are associated with lower risk of cancer.[612] All told, the risks and benefits may cancel out. But to be safe, I recommend that those with a diagnosis of sex hormone-responsive cancer, those with BRCA gene alterations, and anyone treated with tamoxifen avoid grapefruit. The beneficial components of grapefruit can be found elsewhere. It should also be avoided for one week prior to chemotherapy.

Oranges and orange juice, likely prevent breast cancer without CYP p450 inhibition risk. In rats, orange juice inhibited breast cancer and the combination of orange flavonoids with tocotrienols (a form of vitamin E), or orange flavonoids with tamoxifen, inhibited breast cancer proliferation more than tamoxifen alone.[613] Tomatoes contain carotenoids such as lycopene and flavonoids that decrease the risk of developing prostate cancer [614] and decrease markers of prostate cancer growth in men with this cancer.[615]

Summary

Consumption of fruits and vegetables lowers cancer risks, but not dramatically. Anticarcinogenic effects are mediated in part by the folates and other B vitamins in the fruit and vegetables, and choline which is also found in meat and seafood. Additionally, phenolic compounds prevent cancer, but these may be lost when fruits and vegetables are peeling or processed. Fiber present in the fruits and vegetables may also lower cancer risk. Fruit juices that are high in fructose, and consumed in a form that is quickly absorbed, however, may increase cancer risk. Vegetables are high in minerals, some vitamins, and fiber. It appears to be, however, that most of the anti-carcinogenic benefits of vegetables are due to sulfur compounds found in cruciferous vegetables, garlic and onions. Cruciferous vegetables are discussed in detail in Chapter 24.

27: FIBER

In the EPIC study, the risk of liver, colorectal, breast, and prostate cancers were lower among those consuming diets high in fiber. The benefits from fruit and vegetable fiber are not limited to these cancers, but these highly prevalent cancers give us a platform for understanding the mechanisms by which dietary fiber lowers cancer risk.

Fiber is cool. Fiber is not one thing; it is many. Fiber is food matter that is not degraded by our digestive enzymes and thus, cannot be absorbed by the small intestine. This undigested biomass passes into the cecum and colon, where it is acted on by bacteria, and some of the fiber is digested, providing nutrients to the bacteria, and providing nutrients for the cells lining the colon.

To understand fiber, you need to understand that more than two-thirds of the cells in your body are alien life forms. In Chapter 4, it was explained that you have about 37 trillion cells in your body that were created according to data encoded in the DNA you inherited as a birthday gift from your parents. In addition to these, you also have another 50 trillion alien cells with non-human DNA that invaded your body soon after birth.

The word invaded is a bit strong, as *you invited them in*. As a newborn, you sabotaged your perfectly intact, healthy immune system by producing CD71$^+$ cells that intentionally weaken your immune defenses. This put you at risk for dangerous infections from *E. coli*, *Listeria*, and other gram-negative bacteria; and you did this just to let these aliens take root and colonize your innards.[616]

The average person hosts about 150 different species of microorganisms in their colon. We also have additional microbes living in our mouth, nasopharynx, and on our skin. With the exception of one common Archaea that can comprise up to ten percent of the microbial mass, these microbes are mostly bacteria. This population is comprised almost entirely of obligate anaerobes that only grow in low-oxygen environments.

Archaea are microbes about the size of bacteria but are genetically further away from bacteria than you are from a carrot. Archaea make of up about 20% of the Earth's biomass. They thrive in the mud of the arctic ocean floors, in volcanic vents, and under other extreme conditions. Although you may have just found out about them, they have been around for about three billion years. They are not known to cause disease or act as parasites. Archaea produce methane. When this light-weight gas is incorporated into the stool it can cause them to float and resist flushing.

There are about a thousand different species of bacteria that commonly colonize the human colon.[617] The 150 or so, which live in an individual's colon, depend on not only on which bacteria are swallowed, survive stomach acid and pancreatic enzymes, and gain entry to the colon, but just as importantly, on which species thrive in the colon's environment. Just as different plants are adapted to grow in different soils, terrain, and climates, and have to survive pests and competition with other plants; various bacteria thrive or disappear from the colon depending on its environment and the mix of other species present.

The microbial biome of the gut depends on the resources available to them, and what we feed them. The commensal, microbial biomes of various species of animals are linked to the animals' diets. Animals share similar microbial community clusters with other members of their species, depending on what they eat; carnivores, omnivores, and vegetarian have different clusters of bacterial species.[618] A change in diet can be accompanied, within a couple of weeks, by a bloom of new bacteria and a fall-off of other species of bacteria[619]. It is not the nutrients that are absorbed by our bodies, but rather, what is left over for the bacteria to ferment that affects which populations of bacteria thrive in the large intestine. A large portion of these leftovers is dietary fiber. What we eat, and more specifically, what doesn't get digested and absorbed, and thus enters the large intestine, affects the proliferation of the various species of microbes that comprise our enteric biome.

Dietary fiber, composed of plant materials resistant to our digestive enzymes, is not broken down into sugars or other absorbable compounds in the small intestine. These materials pass from the small intestine into the large intestine, the colon, where much of this material is fermented. Fiber that is easily fermentable by gut bacteria is called soluble fiber, and fiber, such as cellulose, that is only minimally fermented in the human colon is called insoluble fiber. Different species of microbes are capable of processing different compounds; those that find a favorable environment and nutrients, and are that are not out-competed by other organisms, feed, and multiply.

Not only do our microbes get the leftovers of digestion, but they also get old, sloughed-off cells from the intestine, IgA, dead bacteria, digestive enzymes, bile, and other residuals that make their way into the cecum and colon.

Several studies have shown that consumption of fiber is associated with decreased risk of colon cancer. However, not just any fiber will do. Whole grains, such as in whole-wheat bread, is associated with decreased risk of colon cancer.[620] This risk reduction is greatest for the distal colon and rectum, and when consuming two servings of whole grains a day.[621] Fiber from grain binds to bile and lowers the fecal bile acid concentration of the stool.[622] Eating more than one apple a day also decreases the risk of colon cancer, likely as a function of the pectin content in apples. The risk of esophageal cancer risk decreases with the consumption of dietary fiber, but only with soluble fiber from fruits and vegetables.[623] Other studies have shown that dietary fiber decreases the risk of breast and colon cancer, but here too, the type of fiber makes a difference.

Leftovers

Outside of malabsorption syndromes, only small amounts of digestible carbohydrates and very small quantities of fat enter the colon. The largest amounts of nutrients reaching the colon in health are resistant polysaccharides and resistant starches. These two classes comprise the most of the mass of fiber. Perhaps as much as 15 grams of protein enter the colon daily, but much of this comes not from food, but rather from the shedding of old intestinal cells, mucous, immunoglobulin, and digestive enzymes.[624]

Resistant polysaccharides, like other carbohydrates, are large molecules composed of sugars that are bound together by chemical bonds. These polysaccharides resist digestion because humans do not have the enzymes capable of cutting these bonds and disassembling the carbohydrates into simple sugars that can be absorbed. These resistant polysaccharides may also contain sugars our bodies can't use and don't absorb. These resistant polysaccharides are digested by bacteria that have enzymes that cut the non-digestible carbohydrate (NDC) into simple sugars and then use them for energy.

The bacteria in the colon have a far greater toolbox for metabolism and digestion than we do. The human genome contains about 20,000 protein-coding genes; the species living within the average individual's gut have an aggregate of about 536,000 different genes.[625] Many of these are genes for enzymes that can digest compounds that humans can't. A single common commensal colonic species, *Bacteroides thetaiotaomicron*, produces 172 different enzymes for the catabolism of various polysaccharides.[626]

Why are we so limited? The lowly ameba, *Amoeba dubia,* has a genome more than 200 times larger than ours. Why, as the most advanced creature in the solar system, do we have such a paucity of genetic breadth? It is because we are so darn smart!

Genes are susceptible to mutation, and damaged DNA can impair survival

> and cause disease. DNA damage in independent microbes that reproduce by the billions per cubic centimeter every few hours is not a critical problem for that species' survival. Some mutate, some may die, but plenty of others survive. The can rebuild their population in hours.
>
> Complex, slowly reproducing organisms, however, benefit from a safer and more efficient strategy; we hire out much of the metabolic work to the microbes that do the job best for us. And when we change our diet, we change our colonic bacteria as if we were changing our clothes for a change of venue.

Resistant starches are another form of NDC's that are not degraded in the small intestine. Although we have the required enzymes to cut the chains of sugars in resistant starches, the form of the starch prevents the enzymes from getting into the right position to do their jobs. This can occur because the starch is not fully gelatinized, as in the case of cooked rice that has been allowed to cool and crystallize. Some starch just has a shape that is resistant to enzymatic processing. About one-third of the starch in potatoes is resistant to digestion because of its structure. Different forms of resistant starches are fermented and support the growth of different sets of commensal bacteria.[627]

When we digest carbohydrates in our small intestine, we get about four Calories of energy per gram. Even though we don't digest NDC, we still get energy from them; typically between 1.25 and 2 Calories per gram. This energy comes from short-chain fatty acids (SCFA) released from the bacteria that digest the NDC. The rest of the energy from the NDC is used by the bacteria and archaea, spent in heat production, remains as non-processed biomass, or goes up in smoke: as gases, such as methane and hydrogen. Resistant starches, pectin from fruit such as apples, and soluble fiber such as oat bran are broken down into short-chain fatty acids, including butyric acid. Other types of fiber are also converted to butyrate, but less efficiently. Butyrate is also present in the diet from butter and cheese; particularly high butterfat aged cheeses such as Parmesan cheese. The short-chain fatty acids in dairy products are the result of ruminal fermentation of plant fiber in the animal.[628]

The cells lining the intestines get most of their nutrition snacking on the nutrients they absorb directly from the food we eat, rather than feeding on nutrients supplied from the bloodstream. Most of the nutrients from the diet are absorbed by the small intestine. Thus, there would be insufficient nutrients available for the mucosal cells lining the large intestine. An important source of energy for these colonocytes is the SCFA butyric acid (butyrate), which is formed by the bacterial fermentation of NDC fiber. Butyrate and other SCFA (acetate and propionate) formed from NDC by bacteria are absorbed into the bloodstream. Acetate is also used as fuel for the brain and propionate is taken up by the liver. The SCFAs provide energy and help decrease hunger between meals. Propionate also decreases cholesterol synthesis.

Butyrate helps colonocyte metabolic health and decreases risk of colon cancer.[629] Butyrate, (like sulforaphane and ITC) is a Class I HDAC (histone deacetylase) inhibitor.[630] HDAC1 enzymes repress the transcription several genes for large multi-protein complexes by promoting the transcription of co-repressors gene segments.[631] HDAC1 inhibitors enhance histone acetylation of the co-repressor, allow for greater transcription of these genes. Butyrate may prevent carcinogenesis by helping to reset epigenomic alterations that favor cancer and thereby increasing the production of p53, the pro-apoptosis protein that helps eliminate abnormal cells.[632]

> The human cecum has the capacity for a few ounces of fermenting biomass. Elephants, Earth's largest land animals, consume large amounts of poorly digestible leaves and tree bark for their nutrition. This requires a large volume for bacterial fermentation to supply the animal's nutritional requirements. The contents of an adult elephant's cecum comprise about 12 percent of the elephant's body weight. An adult elephant's cecum contains about 1200 pounds of fermenting vegetable matter.

Biofilms

Dietary fiber favors the growth of commensal bacteria over that of pathogenic species and discourages the formation of biofilms. A biofilm is a bacterial colony in which bacteria work together and become super bacteria. As a colony, bacteria produce a matrix gel that protects the colony from harm. The colony can produce enzymes and other compounds that the bacteria cannot produce as individuals. Almost all bacterial infections are the result of biofilm formation. Thus, although there may be many pathogenic species of bacteria living in a healthy person's gut, they are harmless..., until a biofilm forms.

The beneficial effects of *lactobacilli* and *bifidobacteria* largely result from their influence, modifying the intestinal environment, and hindering biofilm formation.[633] Different sources of fiber in the diet support different species of bacteria. Consuming fiber from a variety of plants promotes diversification of the bacterial species in the colon and lowers the propensity for "monoculture" or "oligoculture" where the biome is dominated by a small number of species that favor pathogenic biofilm growth. Use of broad-spectrum antibiotics that decimate many bacterial species in the colon also favors pathogenic biofilm production by selecting for the most resistant and spore-forming species that survive antibiotic treatment, thus favoring pathogenic bacterial overgrowth.

Ammonia and Toxins

Not all products of intestinal bacterial fermentation are benign. In normal adults with lactose intolerance, lactose from milk sugar is not digested or absorbed in the small intestine and instead passes into the colon where it ferments. The fermentation of lactose can produce toxic metabolites including alcohols, diols, ketones, acids, and aldehydes, such as methylglyoxal[634] that causes glycation and is atherogenic.[635] It also can cause bloating, foul winds, and diarrhea.

While carbohydrates are mostly fermented in the cecum and in the right side of the colon, protein fermentation occurs mainly on the left side of the colon. When proteins are broken down, the fermentation of amino acids can produce biogenic amines that are metabolically active and affect not only the gut but also the central and peripheral nervous system. Fermentation of amino acids can also produce ammonia and other toxic compounds.

While some protein normally passes into the colon, higher amounts can make their way to the colon if the pancreas does not produce sufficient protein-digesting enzymes, if there is malabsorption, or if the diet contains excessive amounts of proteins, particularly protein from meat. This may be more pronounced when meat is not cooked or if swallowed in large pieces.

Ammonia can be broken down by the liver in healthy adults, but infants and adults with liver disease accumulate toxic levels of ammonia. Ammonia produced in the colon is easily absorbed into the bloodstream and crosses the blood-brain barrier. In the brain, ammonia is toxic to astrocytes that serve as support cells for neurons. Ammonia can easily reach toxic levels and cause hepatic encephalopathy (HE) in those with liver cirrhosis. In HE, hyperammonemia causes irritability, memory loss, difficulty with concentration and tremor, and can result in death. In infants, even transient ammonia toxicity may be a cause of autism.[135]

Locally in the colon, ammonia is considered a marker for colon cancer risk. Ammonia may interfere with DNA synthesis and increase the risk of genetic damage in the colonic mucosal cells. Alternatively, it may be toxins other than ammonia, such p-cresol, indoxyl sulfate, or phenylacetic acid, which are associated with the fermentation of protein and amino acids that act as carcinogens.

Certain commensal colonic bacteria, such as some species of bifidobacteria, can utilize ammonia and convert it into amino acids for their own growth. Non-digestible carbohydrates support the growth of these bacteria and thus help decrease the exposure of the colonic mucosa to ammonia and its absorption into the circulation. NDCs also decrease the formation of p-cresol and other toxins associated with protein fermentation in the colon. This suggests that NDCs support the growth of bacteria that utilized amino acids from proteins that make their way into the colon.[636] The nitrogen from the amino acids is then passed in the feces, rather than being turned into ammonia.[637]

In a study using the non-digestible sugar, lactulose, production of nitrogenous compounds was halved.[638] This is why the NDC lactulose is used in the treatment of hepatic encephalopathy and may be the reason for lower rates of colon cancer in populations with diets high in resistant starches.[639] When resistant starches are added to the diet, fermentation of ileal effluent provides a higher production of butyrate and decreases the production of ammonia by two-thirds.[640]

In contrast, when amino acids are fermented without adequate NDC, other species of colonic bacteria produce ammonia and other amino acid-based toxins. Patients with liver cirrhosis and hepatic encephalopathy (HE) have very different populations of bacteria living in their colons than do those with liver cirrhosis but without HE.[641] Those with HE, have higher populations of amino acid fermenting, toxin-producing bacteria such as clostridia.

The Liver

In a healthy liver, the hepatocytes are laid out in nicely organized lobules; like well-planned neighborhoods. Blood flows, passing by each cell, and each cell is connected to the biliary "drainage" system. Blood from the intestine flows into the liver through the portal veins and the hepatocytes process the nutrients, proteins, and other compounds from the diet. The liver processes nutrients and makes new proteins, fats, and carbohydrates that are exported to the bloodstream. The liver also processes non-food compounds carried to it by the bloodstream.

Many toxic compounds are also processed by the hepatocytes. These processes include conjugation, where a compound is bound to another, making it easier to transport that compound. These conjugations often join a fat-soluble compound with a water-soluble one so that it can be eliminated by the kidneys, or make the compound more fat-soluble so that it is easier to cross cell membranes. Many compounds are processed and then dumped into the "dispose-all" drainage system, the bile ducts, which drain into the intestine. Here the intestine acts as a recycling center that sorts the trash from the recyclable goods. Compounds may be reprocessed or reabsorbed by the cells lining the intestine, processed by bacteria in the cecum and colon, or disposed into the feces. Bile contains bile acids that aid in the absorption of fat, including fat-soluble vitamins. Several vitamins and hormones rely on liver-bile-intestinal recycling. This recycling process is called enterohepatic circulation.

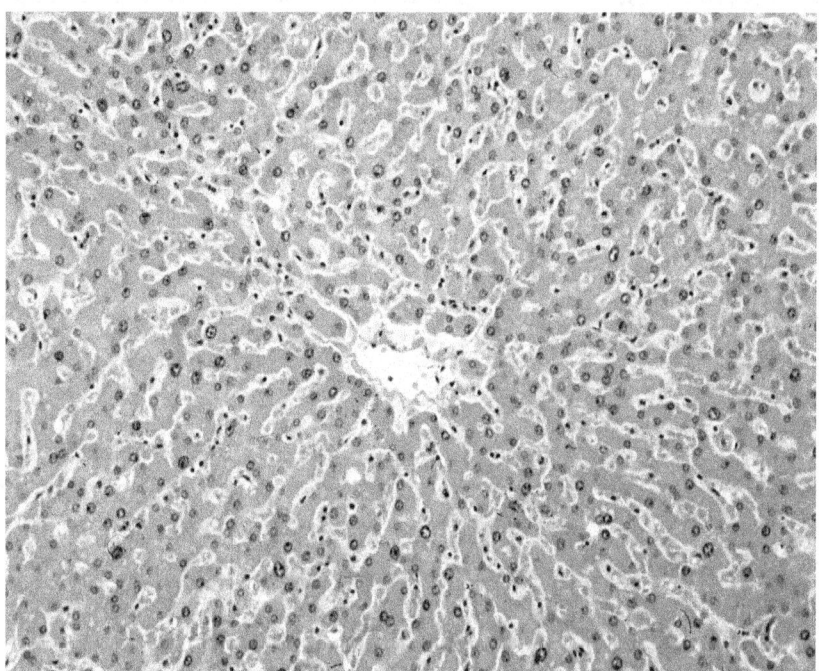

Figure 27-1: Liver cells organized around a central vein. Nutrients from the intestine flow in from the portal vein into the central veins.

Fiber and Estrogens

Most of the circulating sex hormones entering the liver are conjugated as glucuronide and sulfate conjugates. Conjugation inactivates these hormones. These conjugates may re-enter the circulation, but more than half of them are excreted into the bile. Although these conjugates may be taken up by other tissues and processed for reuse as active estrogens, glucuronide conjugates are highly water soluble and are quickly excreted into the urine. The sulfate conjugates are excreted more slowly, and thus more likely to be taken up by tissues where they have estrogenic effects.

More than half of the estrogen conjugates from the liver are excreted into the bile, some of these conjugates bind to dietary fiber. Once the conjugated estrogens reach the large intestine, these compounds can be de-conjugated by intestinal bacteria that produce the enzyme β-glucuronidase. This enzyme deconjugates those hormones, freeing them, and allowing them to be easily reabsorbed by colonic mucosa. This enzyme gives the sex hormones a divorce from their conjugates and puts them back into circulation in the dating scene. Conjugated hormones that are bound to insoluble, non-fermentable fiber are more likely to pass into the stool than those bound to soluble fiber.

Once reabsorbed into the colonocytes, the free estrogens are re-conjugated, allowing them to be absorbed into the bloodstream. Again, depending on the conjugate, some of these estrogens return to duty stimulating hormonal response, while others are eliminated in the urine.[642]

A high level of β-glucuronidase in the stool is a marker for pathogenic bacterial overgrowth in the colon, and it causes an elevated reabsorption of estrogens in women. Elevated levels of stool β-glucuronidase are associated with high-fat, low-fiber diets.[643] High-fat, low-fiber diets are linked to elevated risk of estrogen-sensitive cancers. The benefit from fiber is strongest for insoluble fiber that binds the hormone conjugates and carries them out of the body.

A high-fat diet, rich in phytoestrogens also increases the risk and growth of estrogen receptor-positive breast cancers. Phytoestrogens are present in plants as conjugates, and like endogenous estrogens, are conjugated by the liver and dispatched into the bile.[644] β-glucuronidase promotes their absorption. Phytoestrogens, such as genistein and daidzein, support ER+ cancer growth.[645][646]

> What!!!? Don't soy phytoestrogens decrease breast cancer risk?! They do when consumed during puberty and adolescence. (See Chapter 32) This protective effect may be even greater when consuming a high-fat diet during adolescence, as girls who are overweight during adolescence are also at lower risk of breast cancer later in life. The reason that soy phytoestrogens and being overweight during puberty decrease later breast cancer risk is that they raise estrogen levels during growth. The increase in estrogenic stimulus during breast growth and development is compensated for by an epigenetic down-regulation of estrogen receptor expression that persists for the woman's lifetime. Having fewer estrogen receptors on cells causes a decreased sensitivity for growth from estrogen and thus, less stimulus of growth of cancer cells bearing estrogen receptors. During adulthood, however, phytoestrogens and obesity add estrogenic effects. Boron, a mineral found in fruit, also increases estrogen and may act similarly.

The type of fiber consumed affects estrogen levels, and thus affects breast cancer risk differently for women at different times in their lives. Women that consume higher amounts of soluble, non-starch polysaccharide fiber had two-thirds higher levels of estrone (E1) and estradiol (E2) than those consuming low levels, and those consuming higher amounts of insoluble (non-fermentable) non-starch polysaccharides, had E1 and E2 levels that were about forty percent lower than those consuming lower levels.[647] Thus, consumption of soluble fiber, especially with a high-fat diet, increases estrogen levels, and consumption of insoluble fiber, such as those from whole grains, especially with a low-fat diet, decreases estrogen levels.

A diet high in (insoluble) fiber,[648] and faster intestinal transit times,[649] also helps lower circulating estrogen levels. These decreases in hormone levels may explain part of the beneficial role that fiber has on the risk of breast and prostate cancers. In contrast, soluble fiber, such as pectin, can more easily release the conjugates, and if there is an overgrowth of β-glucuronidase producing bacteria, these estrogens can be released and reabsorbed.

As explained in the box above, the age at which the diet is consumed plays a central role in the effect of diet on risk. For adult women, soluble fiber, especially when coupled with a high-fat diet, increases breast cancer risk and insoluble fiber decreases it. An inverse effect may occur during early adolescence when the breast is undergoing estrogenic-induced growth.

When bacterial overgrowth occurs in the colon, more steroid hormones are recycled. Overgrowth can be stimulated by a high-fat diet and unabsorbed proteins entering the colon. Thus, pathogenic bacteria overgrowth may increase the risk of hormone-sensitive cancers.

Vegetarian women consuming a diet with adequate fiber, with 30% of their caloric intake as fat were found to excrete three times more estrogen in the stool than do women who were omnivores and whose diet included 40% of their calories as fat. The vegetarian women also had 15 to 20 percent lower blood estrogen levels.[650]

Diets with higher fiber levels have been associated with a 13% reduction in breast cancer risk. The decreased risk was most clearly related to intake of soluble fiber from fruit[651] (pectin). Lignans, some of which are phytoestrogens, are associated with decreased risk of breast cancer.[652]

People who consume higher amounts of fiber and a higher diversity of fiber from different sources have lower amounts of β-glucuronidase from bacteria in their colons, and less β-glucuronidase to free conjugated estrogen and phytoestrogens.[653] Dietary fiber is thought to decrease cancer risk by improving insulin sensitivity, resulting in lower insulin levels,[654] and lower IGF-1 activity.[655] These hormones act along with estrogens to increase tumor growth.

Diets high in fiber are associated with a reduced risk of breast cancer.[656] Dietary fiber consumed during adolescence and early adulthood have the most pronounced effect on breast cancer. In a 20-year follow-up study of the dietary intake of over 90,000 young women, those in the highest 20% of fiber intake during adolescence or young adulthood had a 24% decrease in premenopausal breast cancer risk, compared to those with the lowest 20% of fiber intake. *Women in the highest quintile group for fiber intake group during both adolescence and young adulthood had their risk of premenopausal breast cancer incidence reduced by a third.*[657] The median fiber intake for the lowest quintile was 14.8 grams per day as compared to 25.3 grams per day in the highest fiber / lowest breast cancer risk group. Consuming over 20 grams of fiber a day significantly reduces the risk of breast cancer. *Even after the diagnosis of breast cancer*, women consuming higher levels of dietary fiber have a lower hazard of death from breast cancer as well as from other causes.[652] For reference, a medium apple has about 4 grams of fiber, and an orange has 3, and a slice of whole wheat bread has 2 grams of fiber. Both soluble and insoluble fiber decrease breast cancer risk. Thus, a diet rich in fiber from various sources is recommended.

Lignans, another type of fiber, supply polyphenols and phytoestrogens that may also decrease the risk of breast cancer. However, they likely only decrease risk when consumed during youth, before motherhood.

The bacteria living in the colon also stimulate our immune system, and over half of the immune cells in the body reside in the tissues lining the gastrointestinal tract. T-cells are an important part of the immune system response to melanoma and certain other tumor cells. T-cell activity, however, is held in check by a protein (CTLA4) that prevents T-cell over-activity and autoimmune disease. Several monoclonal antibody medications (such as ipilimumab) have been developed to stimulate the T-cells as anti-cancer medications. In a study of mice implanted with melanoma cells, only those mice with certain species of colonic commensal bacteria responded to these medications. Those without these bacteria failed to benefit from the medications.[658, 659] Since the various bacteria living in the gut depend on the nutrients (fibers) being supplied to them, the type and amount of fiber consumed greatly affects the presence of bacteria in the gut, and, thus, their effect on the immune system.

For colon cancer, as well, it appears that not all fiber is created equal. Of various sources of dietary fiber, consumption of whole grains is most highly associated with lower risk for colon cancer.[660] This risk reduction is greatest for cancers of the distal colon and rectum, and when consuming two to three servings of whole grain a day (1.25 servings per 1000 Calories of food intake).[661] Eating more than one apple a day is associated with a decreased risk of colon cancer,[662] as fruit fiber (pectin) decreases the risk of distal colon and rectal cancers.

Undigested proteins, such as meat fibers that reach the colon, have a different effect on bacterial growth in the lower intestine. In health, very little protein reaches the colon, as we have enzymes that break it down into amino acids that are readily absorbed. If an individual lacks digestive enzymes, has rapid small intestinal transit time that prevents adequate digestion, swallows large pieces of meat, or has other reasons that proteins are not digested, the proteins will be available for fermentation by colonic bacteria. When meat and other proteins ferment, it favors the growth of pathogenic bacterial biofilms in the distal colon. Similar to their action on sex hormones, enzymes from colonic biofilm-producing bacteria can also favor the deconjugation of carcinogenic heterocyclic amines that have been excreted into the bile, allowing these carcinogens to be "rescued" and absorbed into the mucosa, thus increasing cancer risk. Biofilm formation in the colon may explain some of the increased risk of cancer among those consuming larger quantities of red meat.

Individuals with malabsorption syndromes, irritable bowel syndrome with diarrhea, impaired digestion, or other conditions causing incomplete digestion of proteins should limit their meat intake as meat is harder than most proteins to digest. Individuals with pancreatic deficiencies can use enzyme supplements to aid digestion.

Bile Acids

Bile is formed from cholesterol, as are the steroid hormones, including sex hormones, cortisol, and vitamin D3.

Bile acids aid in the absorption of fat-soluble compounds such as triglycerides and fat-soluble vitamins. Bile acids are formed in the liver and excreted in the bile into the upper intestine when a meal contains fat. Bile helps break fat, in the form of triglycerides, into tiny particles that can be more easily processed by lipase enzymes into free fatty acids and a monoglyceride, which can then be absorbed by intestinal cells. After the fats have been absorbed, bile is reabsorbed from the distal small intestine and circulates back to the liver.

A small amount, normally less than five percent, of the bile acid pool, escapes reabsorption and passes into the colon. Here, the bile acids can be metabolized by bacteria and converted into the secondary bile acids lithocholic acid (LCA) and deoxycholic acid (DOC). DOC is easily absorbed from the colon; LCA is less soluble, and thus, a lower proportion of LCA is absorbed from the colon. Since bile recycles several times a day, the small portion of it that is converted to secondary bile acids tends to accumulate.

Bile release from the gallbladder is stimulated by fat in the diet; a high-fat diet increases the cycling of bile salts. This, in turn, increases the amount of bile salts entering the colon and metabolized by bacteria, and thus increases the proportion of secondary bile salts. As much as 35 percent of the bile pool may comprised secondary bile acids, predominantly DOC.

The problem is that LCA is cytotoxic and carcinogenic, acting through multiple mechanisms. Also, both secondary bile acids increase the generation of reactive oxygen and nitrogen species, cause the disruption of the cell membrane, damage the mitochondria, and induce DNA damage, resulting in mutations.[663] The secondary bile acids can damage enterocytes, the cells lining the intestines, and promote intestinal inflammation. DOC promotes the transcription of inflammatory proteins by stimulating MAPK, inhibits primary bile acid-induced apoptosis, and suppresses p53. DOC also prevents apoptosis and increases cell proliferation.[664]

Secondary bile acids increase the risk for cancer of the esophagus, stomach, small intestines, liver, pancreas, and biliary tract.

Dietary fiber has an important interaction with bile acids. Bile and other steroid hormones are absorbed by several types of dietary fiber in the small intestine. This prevents their reabsorption from the distal small intestine and carries them into the colon.

For many years, it was thought that bile bound to fiber was carried to a watery grave down the sewer pipes; however, the evidence does not bear this out. Although some bile is found in the stool, the amounts found neither correlates with the amount or type of fiber consumed nor with the degree of cholesterol lowering.[665]

Colonic fermentation of some types of dietary fiber lowers cholesterol by inducing transcription of the enzyme, cholesterol 7-alpha-hydroxylase, the first and rate-limiting enzyme in bile production.[666] Thus, fiber increases the conversion of cholesterol into bile, increasing the bile pools, diluting the secondary bile acids, and allowing more bile acids to pass into the colon. While the proportion of secondary bile acids falls with dietary fiber, the amount in the stool does not reliably change. This suggests that bile acids can disappear in the colon; they may be catabolized by bacteria.

The fermentation of primary bile acids that reach the colon may be affected by how easily fermentable the fiber the bile acid has adhered to is. If the fiber is more easily fermentable, the bile the bile acid may be freed. More important is which bacteria are doing the fermentation. When NDC fiber is present in sufficient supply, short chain fatty acids lower the pH of the colonic contents, and this inhibits the conversion of primary bile acids to secondary bile acids. Additionally, at least in vitro, *Lactobacillus* inhibits the conversion of primary bile acids into secondary bile acids, while *Bacteroides* increases it.[667]

This is the reason that some types of fiber can lower cholesterol level. The creation of new, primary bile acids by the liver depletes cholesterol from circulating lipoproteins. This also lowers the concentration of secondary bile acids in the bile pool, lowering the risk of cancers for the tissues that are most exposed to bile salts: the colon and liver.

Pectin, an NDC found in apples and other fruits and fiber from psyllium, a plant seed used for it high fiber content as a treatment of constipation, have been found to lower cholesterol levels.[668] While consuming an apple a day did not meet statistical significance, eating more than one apple a day was associated with a 47% decline in colon cancer incidence.[662] Fruit fiber (pectin) appears to decrease only the risk of distal colon and rectal cancers. The production of short-chain fatty acids (SCFA) by bacteria in the colon inhibits the production and absorption of secondary bile acids. This mechanism may help explain the anti-carcinogenic influences of SCFA in the colon.[669]

It is not a single form of fiber that lowers cholesterol or lowers the risk of cancer. It is a combination of different fibers that feed various populations of bacteria and the induction of cholesterol 7-alpha-hydroxylase and other proteins that creates an environment that inhibits the conversion of primary to secondary bile acids and favors the disappearance of bile acids.

The induction of cholesterol 7-alpha-hydroxylase (C7AH) by fiber is strengthened by the inclusion of pea and other legume protein in the diet.[670] Other researchers have found that dietary phytosterones, another form of plant fiber, also increase C7AH activity and increase the number of LDL cholesterol receptors in the liver. Phytosterones in vegetable matter may also lower the risk of cancer by decreasing the risk of metabolic syndrome, hyperglycemia, and hyper-insulinemia.[671]

Fiber from grain binds to bile and lowers the fecal bile acid concentration of the stool.[672] However, supplements with wheat bran fiber have failed to reduce the risk of recurrent adenomas in patients with high risk of colon cancer.[673] This data should not be used to suggest that other NDCs, such as resistant starch from grain, do not lower the risk of colon cancer. It may not be one or the other component, but the effect of the mix of fibers and other elements from whole foods that affect the microbial biome, rather than effects of a single fiber. Single fiber supplements may cause excessive dominance of certain types of bacteria at the expense of other species.

Malabsorption syndromes, where chyme (the mass of food and digestive juices) passes quickly into the colon before digestion can be completed, increase the conversion of primary to secondary bile acids. More protein is also moved into the intestine, where it can ferment into ammonia and other toxic and carcinogenic substances.

Meat and Potatoes

Bile is not the only carcinogen that binds to fiber in the gut. Various toxins also bind to fiber.

Mutagenic heterocyclic aromatic amines, created during the cooking of meats at high temperatures, adhere to both soluble and insoluble fiber. The more hydrophobic the HCA is, the more avid the binding. The binding is also highest for fiber that is more hydrophobic. Lignins (not to be confused with lignans,) are complex polyphenolic compounds found in the cell walls of plants. Lignins are a major component of wood, but also are found in the skin of potatoes and in wheat bran, as examples.[674] Waxy, hydrophobic substances in some lignins are especially effective in binding these HCA. These waxes help retain moisture in the leaves of some plants, in the skin of fruit, and in the seed coat of corn.

Yes, natural waxes in apple skin allowed them to be polished for a teacher in the 1840's, prior to the use of wax sprays now applied to preserve their freshness on the grocer's shelf.

Heterocyclic amines also bind to soluble fiber, such as the soluble fiber in oats and the non-digestible starches in potatoes.[675] This is great, as fiber may prevent the absorption of HCA from the diet by the small intestine. What is not great is that soluble fiber is degraded by colonic bacteria and this allows these carcinogens to be released into the colon. Here they can promote colorectal cancer or be absorbed and be transferred into the circulation.[676] Additionally, pH changes associated with fermentation can decrease the binding of HCA to fiber.[677] Formation of ammonia in the colon secondary to amino acid fermentation may also cause the release of the HCA from fiber.

Polycyclic biphenyl (PCB), dioxin, and similar carcinogens are also adsorbed to dietary lignin fiber.[678] Several vegetables, including cruciferous vegetables such as broccoli and cabbage, onions, spinach, kale, and perilla have also been found to increase fecal excretion of dioxins.[679] Notably, several of these are waxy vegetables. Even many years after exposure, consumption of these fibers increases the fecal excretion of dioxins in humans,[680] removing them from the enterohepatic circulation.

There are many different sources and types of fiber. Just as not all fruits and vegetables lower cancer risk, neither does all fiber. Consumption of the skin of fruits and vegetables may provide significant benefit as a result of their lignin content. Apple pie without the skins of the apple is not the same, nor is fruit juice.

Summary

The effects of fruits and vegetables on cancer risk may seem unimpressive. Most studies only show a few percentage points difference between those consuming higher or lower amounts of fruits and vegetables. Most likely, it is not the consumption of fruit and veggies that lower risk, but rather the consumption of adequate folate, phenolic and sulfur compounds, and fiber available from certain fruits and vegetables that lower cancer risk. Only some fruits and vegetables provide anti-carcinogenic benefits. Including these specific fruits and vegetables in the diet can not only decrease the risk of developing cancer but can also slow cancer growth.

Dietary fiber can help prevent some cancers. It does this by preventing the absorbing carcinogens, secondary bile acids, and hormones from the intestine. Bacteria in the intestine that rely on fiber for their nutrition and growth help stimulate the immune system and lower cancer risk.

Higher levels of dietary fiber intake have been associated with a 13% reduction in breast cancer risk. The decreased risk was most clearly related to the intake of soluble fiber from fruit (pectin for example).[656] Dietary lignans have been associated with increased survival after the diagnosis of breast cancer, specifically, in women with ER+/PR+. The lignan lariciresinol, which is found in the bran of cereal grains, flax seeds, and sesame seeds, is the lignin most clearly associated with decreased risk.[652] Lariciresinol, however, only decreases the risk of ER+/PR+ breast cancers.[681] Lariciresinol inhibits tumor growth and tumor angiogenesis and increased apoptosis.[682] Lignans are polyphenolic phytoestrogens that appear to act as competitive inhibitors of estrogen,[683] and may also promote NRF2 and the ARE.

Dietary consumption of the polyphenol, quercetin, has been associated with decreased risk of endometrial cancer,[684] as is the lignan secoisolariciresinol, which is found in high concentration in flaxseed.[685]

In studies of colon cancer it does not appear that just any fiber will do; rather, it is the consumption of whole grains that are associated with decreased colon cancer risk.[661, 686] Eating more than one apple a day also decreases the risk of colon cancer.[662] Fruit intake is associated with a decreased risk of gastric cancer that was stronger than the decrease in risk associated with consumption of cruciferous vegetables.[687] Raw vegetables, cruciferous vegetables, and citrus fruits were associated with decreased risk of esophageal cancer.[688] Dietary fiber can bind bile acids[689] that also can decrease the risk of esophageal and colorectal cancers.

Some risk reduction associated with diets higher in fruits and vegetables may be secondary to differences in dietary patterns; consumption of more fruits and vegetables may be inversely associated with a "meat and fried potato" pattern that carries a higher risk.[690] Most studies that have evaluated the association of food groups with cancer risk, however, have found that *low fruit and vegetable intake* to be a cancer risk factor.[691] Consumption of fewer than two servings of fruit a day, or of cruciferous vegetables less than once week, appears to be the relevant risk factor for cancer. This suggests that a deficiency of compounds contained in fruits and vegetables increases cancer risk. Thus, deficiencies of compounds present in fruits and vegetables increase the risk of cancer, much like how vitamin or trace minerals deficiencies cause disease; once there is an adequate supply of the nutrient, adding more provides little benefit.

Different fibers act through different mechanisms, with various fibers lowering risk for different types of cancer. A mix of trace minerals, phenolics, and other organic compounds from fruits, vegetables, herbs, and spices, supplies hundreds of different nutrients, both for our cells and for our internal microbial biome. A diet having a mix of fruits, vegetables, and whole grains is most likely to supply nutritional needs and lower risk of cancer and other diseases.

While dietary fiber has a smaller impact on cancer risk than some other dietary factors, it is important, as it is one of a few contemporaneous factors. Many cancer risk modifiers act during growth. Thus, by the time one has reached full adulthood, many dietary factors have already had their impact, and there is no going back to alter them. Dietary fiber may continue to act throughout life. While an industrial exposure that increases cancer risk by 1000% may seem more impressive than one that raises risk by 15%, the industrial exposure creates risk for very few individuals. Dietary fiber has an impact on the cancer risk of every person on the planet, and thus, low fruit and vegetable intake has a great impact on the number of cancers that occur in our population. Dietary fiber decreases the risk of cancer most significantly for colon, liver, breast, and prostate cancers.

The fermentation of certain types of dietary fiber by colonic bacteria provides energy for the cells of the colonic mucosa. The fiber also provides energy to bacteria that consume and others that decrease the production of ammonia and other toxins from the fermentation of protein in the colon. These toxins are carcinogens for the colon, and thus, their abatement lowers the risk of colon cancer. Bacteria in the colon may also free other phenolic compounds from polyphenols that reduce cancer risk. Many phenolic compounds found in vegetables have anti-inflammatory and anti-carcinogenic activities.

Bile acids are recycled, being reabsorbed and re-secreted by the liver. Certain types of dietary fiber bind to bile and other steroid compounds, causing their removal from the body, into the stool. Secondary bile acids are carcinogenic. Thus, eliminating secondary bile acids lowers the risk of both colon and liver cancer. When bile levels are low, they are replaced with new, primary bile acids that are not toxic. Since bile is made from cholesterol, this process helps deplete cholesterol and lowers blood cholesterol levels.

Binding of steroid compounds to fiber can also remove sex hormones from the body. This may decreases the growth of sex hormone-sensitive cancers. A more important role of fiber in the prevention of sex-hormone sensitive cancers and other cancers is the release of phytosterols (plant sterols) from another form of fiber, polyphenolic compounds. Some of these bind to sex hormone receptors and decrease the hormonal promotion of growth on tumor cells. The release of these compounds is dependent upon certain commensal bacteria and may require both the presence of the phytosterol and other nutritive substrates for these bacteria.

Consumption of foods containing dietary fiber lowers the risk of some forms of cancer. But do not forget that it is the consumption of foods that have been studied, and when isolated, processed fibers are added to the diet, cancer rates do not always fall. Caution should be used when interpreting the relationships of individual dietary components with disease risk. Dietary fiber may be associated with decreased cancer risk, but fruits, vegetables, and grains also contain numerous other compounds that may be affecting risk. Other compounds present in these foods may also contribute to lower risk of cancer, rather than fiber acting on its own.

Take Home Message

Consuming a variety of fruit, vegetable and grain fibers in the diet helps the body eliminate toxins and excess hormones that can promote cancer growth. Fiber supports a healthy commensal bacterial biome in the gut, and these bacteria can help metabolize and eliminate toxins that can cause cancer. A mix of various types of fiber throughout life can lower cancer risk.

Artificial Colorings

The US Department of Food and Agriculture (USDA) allows the use of artificial food coloring as they estimate that the amounts used are so small that they feel they do not pose a risk - but also because of industry pressure. Citrus Red No. 2 is a carcinogen used to dye oranges; dyed citrus fruit peel should not be consumed or used for making marmalade or zest.[135]

Designation	Name	E number	Cancer or Tumors in Rats or Mice	Color
FD&C Blue No. 1	Brilliant Blue FCF	E133	No	Dark Blue
FD&C Blue No. 2	Indigotine	E132	Brain	Blue
FD&C Green No. 3	Fast Green	E134	Bladder	Turquoise
FD&C Yellow No. 5	Tartrazine	E102	No	Yellow
FD&C Yellow No. 6	Sunset Yellow FCF	E110	Kidney Bladder	Orange
FD&C Red No. 3	Erythrosine	E127	Thyroid	Pink
FD&C Red No. 40	Allura Red AC	E129	No	Red
FD&C Citrus Red No. 2	(Used only to color citrus peel)	E121	Yes	Red
Caramel I and II	Caramelized sugar	E150A, B	No	Brown
Caramel color III and IV	Ammonia caramel: 4-methylimidazole	E150C, D	Yes	Brown

28: Liver Cancer

Among the most common causes of liver injury leading to cancer are viral hepatitis and toxins. In persons infected with viral hepatitis, immune cells fight the infection by targeting and killing liver cells that have gone viral. The immune cells produce free radicals used to help kill the cells, and the resultant pyroptotic cell death further increases inflammation and oxidative stress in the liver. Repetitive replacement of liver cells increases cancer risk.

The most consequential toxin in developed countries is excessive alcohol exposure and hepatitis C, but mycotoxins such as aflatoxin, other toxic substances, and other infections are also common causes of liver cell death. Liver cirrhosis from any cause can promote liver cancer. A common risk factor for liver cirrhosis is fatty liver disease.

Fatty Liver Disease

Fatty liver is a precursor to steatohepatitis (fat induced hepatitis). As in other causes of hepatitis, it leads to the death of hepatocytes and chronic inflammation that can lead to cirrhosis. Fatty liver is a risk factor for hepatocellular carcinoma (HCC) in patients with chronic viral hepatitis, as it promotes liver fibrosis. Fatty liver also impairs response to antiviral therapy.

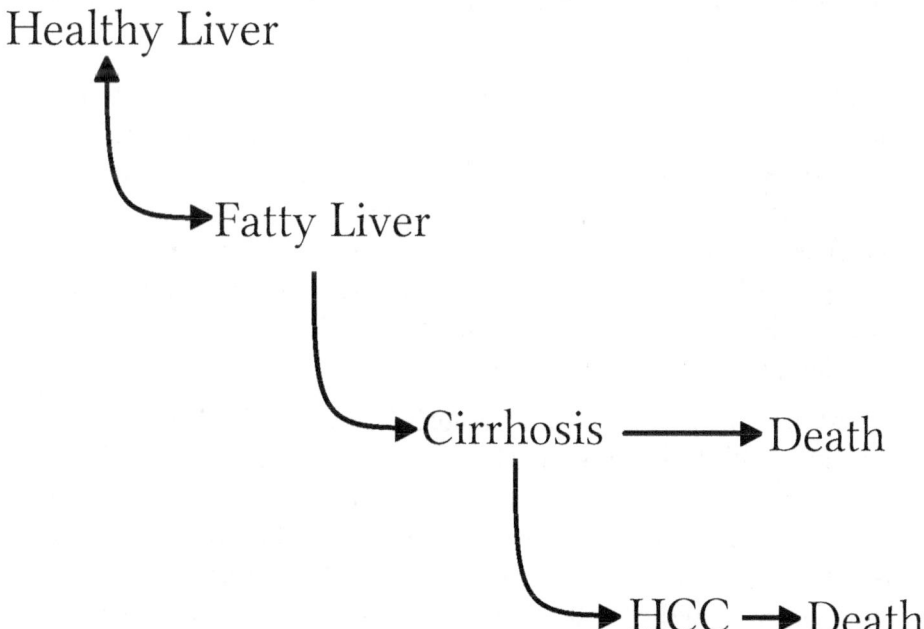

Figure 28-1: The path to Cirrhosis and Hepatocellular Carcinoma

The most common causes of fatty liver in the United States are alcohol abuse and obesity. Alcohol is a hepatotoxin that interferes with mitochondrial function in the liver. One effect of this is the accumulation of lipids, causing fatty liver and oxidative stress. Fatty liver is also common in metabolic syndrome, obesity, and diabetes. Although malaise, fatigue, and vague, right upper quadrant discomfort may occur, most patients with non-alcoholic fatty liver disease are asymptomatic and go undiagnosed.[692] Fatty liver by itself is reversible, so the diagram above shows a return arrow at this stage.

Fatty liver disease is associated with oxidative stress, insulin resistance, and production of the proinflammatory cytokines tumor necrosis factor-α (TNF-α) and interleukin-6 (IL-6). With time, this chronic inflammation, accelerated by common risk factors, easily progresses to steatohepatitis, a disease state in which the accumulation of fat and inflammation cause hepatic cell death and fibrosis.

The liver is damaged in non-alcoholic steatohepatitis (NASH) by inflammatory processes. This slowly turns a fatty liver into a cirrhotic one as healthy cells are replaced by fibrosis. NASH is a significant risk factor for cirrhosis, liver failure, and HCC. The added exposure to other risk factors - alcohol, mycotoxins, and viral hepatitis - greatly increases the risk of HCC in those with fatty liver or NASH. Twenty percent of obese persons have NASH, and it is common among those with type 2 diabetes, even when not obese. In 2010, 36% of American adults were classified as obese, having a BMI over 30.[693] This suggests that over seven percent of American adults have fatty liver disease and NASH.[692]

Repetitive liver damage, cell death, and replacement leads to liver fibrosis. Fibrosis occurs initially around the venules that drain the liver lobules. This may impede blood flow through the liver and cause portal hypertension. Repetitive or chronic liver injury also damages the bile canaliculi. They can become fibrotic and disorganized, causing stasis of bile in the liver. This irreversible fibrosis slowly fills the liver with scar tissue resulting in a hard, nodular, poorly functioning cirrhotic liver.

With fatty liver disease and cirrhosis, there is a decline in hepatic function. With this, there may be a loss of activation of dietary folic acid to the active form of folate. Other nutrients and hormones are also affected by hepatic recirculation, including the fat-soluble vitamins A, D, E, and K. Sex hormone metabolism and elimination may be impaired. With liver cirrhosis, there is an increased production of ammonia and decreased detoxification of endogenous and exogenous toxins, and secondary bile salts may accumulate in the liver. Thus, a poorly functioning liver raises the risk for cancer of the liver and of other organs.

Fructose and Fatty Liver Disease

Fructose is a natural sugar present in fruit. Just a few paragraphs ago, I stated that alcohol was the most common hepatotoxin causing liver injury in developed countries. I may have lied. That title might be earned by fructose, as dietary fructose is probably the most important cause of NASH. High fructose diets, especially in conjunction with a high-fat diet, are quite efficient for growing a plump, fatty, inflamed liver.

Fructose is sort of an invisible ninja. Fructose is not used by the brain, so the brain does not sense fructose in the blood, nor feel satiated by it. It tastes good, so we want to keep eating it, but the brain does not get satiated to tell us when we have had enough. Fructose is not seen by the pancreas either, so it does not stimulate insulin secretion.[694] The liver takes on the role of lowering fructose levels. It can use fructose for energy; however, if there are plenty of caloric nutrients around, the liver puts fructose into storage as energy for later use. The only thing it knows to do with excess fructose is to turn it into fat. Excessive fructose levels cause fatty liver. This effect is amplified on a high-fat diet when there is plenty of excess fat ready to be distributed throughout the body. If you happen to be a bear and want to put on a nice, warm layer of fat so that you can comfortably hibernate over a long subarctic winter, fructose is perfect.

PPARα is a transcription factor for enzymes that are needed for burning fatty acids for energy. Fructose decreases PPARα gene expression by 90% and causes a doubling in the expression of fatty acid synthase and alterations in the expression of several other genes that contribute to obesity and fatty liver disease. Fructose not only fills the liver with fat but promotes insulin resistance, inflammation, and fibrosis. A high-fructose, high-fat, diet can cause HCC without other risk factors.[695] A diet high in fructose is also a major risk factor for metabolic syndrome, leading to type 2 diabetes, gout, heart disease, and stroke.[696]

> Math note: a 90% increase in risk less than doubles the risk, while a 90% decrease in risk lowers risk by 10 times.

Immune-mediated oxidative stress from hepatitis increases the risk of DNA damage to hepatocytes. Insulin resistance raises the level of insulin and other cell growth promoters; together, they promote HCC and colorectal cancer.[697]

During the first half of the 20th century, Americans consumed about four to five percent of their caloric intake from fructose; this is about 20 grams of fructose and equivalent to 80 calories a day.

Twenty grams of fructose is the amount found in 40 grams or 3 tablespoons of table sugar. Before 1960, much of the fructose in the diet came from fruit that also supplied fiber, vitamins, phenolic compounds, and other nutrients that satisfy hunger.

By the year 2000, the *median* daily intake of fructose for an American adult had risen from 20 grams to over 65 grams a day; half of Americans consumed more. Much of this fructose was consumed as soda pop or other sweet beverages. Furthermore, this massive amount of fructose was consumed alongside a high-fat diet. Consider the iconic double juicy burger, large fries, and 20-ounce cola, as a common meal. The cola alone contains over 60 grams of fructose. That is similar to the amount of fructose in a dozen oranges.

Most people can consume as much as 10 percent of their caloric intake from fructose without it inducing disease risk, as long as it is not combined with a high-fat diet. Consuming 10 percent of daily calories as fructose is an enormous amount. It is like getting one-fifth of one's caloric intake from table sugar. Overweight and obese individuals and those with significant alcohol intake should keep fructose intake below five percent of their daily caloric intake.

Most of the injury from fructose may result when it is consumed in high amounts, that cannot be immediately used for energy or stored as glycogen in the muscles. In the muscles, and most cells, fructose is used much like glucose is. In the liver, fructose is not directly utilized as is glucose; it first must be metabolized into glyceraldehyde-3-phosphate, a process that depletes ATP and generates uric acid. Since fructose also depletes ATP in the hunger-satiation center of the brain, the hypothalamus, fructose increases appetite. Fructose is especially risky when consumed as a beverage, as this provides a quick release of nutrients for absorption into the bloodstream, and causes high blood fructose levels and places a higher load on the liver. Fructose consumed in the form whole fruits, especially those that are rich in phenolic compounds, eaten as a snack or as part of a meal when hungry, likely imparts little health risk. Fructose is more damaging when consumed along with fat, especially trans-fats and n-6 fats (linoleic acid for example), which are pro-inflammatory.

Betaine and Choline

Betaine (trimethylglycine) is a B vitamin-like compound present in some vegetables and available as a nutritional supplement. Betaine has been shown effective in treating nonalcoholic fatty liver disease in animal models. Betaine increases PPARα and normalizes most other changes in gene expression that are caused by fructose.

Betaine ameliorates fructose-induced hepatic lipid accumulation, gluconeogenesis, and inflammation in the liver and decreases damage.[698] Betaine has also been found to improve mitochondrial function and attenuate alcohol-induced fatty liver disease.[699] Betaine helps recycle the toxic and pro-inflammatory metabolite homocysteine back into SAMe, as illustrated in Figure 28-1.

Betaine is not a vitamin. Vitamins are compounds that the body cannot make, and thus are essential in the diet. Betaine can be made in the body from choline (Chapter 26). Deficiencies of the essential nutrient choline cause elevated liver enzyme levels and fatty liver. Betaine supplements thus spare or decrease the need for choline. Betaine is more of a co-vitamin.

According to the Institute of Medicine, the daily intake of choline needed to prevent a rise in the liver enzyme ALT is about 550 mg/day of choline for men and 425 mg/day for women.[700] I would submit for your consideration that the ideal intake of choline is likely higher than the amount needed to prevent liver damage. Nevertheless, the average choline intake is only 300 mg for American men and women, and the average betaine intake is about 100 and 120 mg in women and men respectively.[701] In a study of women in New Zealand, only 16% of women consumed the recommended amount of choline.[702] In the Nurses' Health Study, in the United States, less than 5% of women consumed the recommended amount of choline.[703]

The foods highest in choline concentration include shrimp, liver, eggs, cauliflower, broccoli, salmon, wheat germ, and soy. The foods with the highest concentration of betaine include dark green vegetables, such as spinach, wheat bran, wheat germ, beets, and quinoa.[704]

Citrulline

Citrulline is a nonessential amino acid. Like betaine, citrulline supplementation in animals has also been found to normalize the expression of genes altered by a high fructose diet.[705]

There is very little citrulline in the diet, but this does not mean that it is unimportant. Citrulline is synthesized almost exclusively by the cells lining the small intestine, mostly from dietary glutamine, during digestion. Citrulline is transported in the portal blood flow from the intestine to the liver. Citrulline sneaks past the liver and is carried into the bloodstream. About 80% of the citrulline is converted to arginine by the kidneys.

Citrulline takes part in the arginine-citrulline cycle for the formation of nitric oxide as well as the urea cycle, in which ammonia is converted to urea. By first creating citrulline and only later converting it to arginine, the body prevents first pass degradation of arginine into urea by the liver during absorption from the intestine. The liver is the only organ that can convert ammonia into urea. Ammonia can also be detoxified in the skeletal muscles by the amidation process for glutamine synthesis using branched-chain amino acids (BCAAs).[706] BCAA supplementation improves nutritional status, prognosis, and quality of life in patients with liver cirrhosis, in part, because of this.

> Citrulline levels in the blood reflect its production by small intestinal epithelial cells. As long as a person has normal kidney function, *the level of citrulline reflects the mass of small intestinal enterocytes.* (Renal dysfunction prevents citrulline → arginine thus raising citrulline levels.) The normal range for citrulline is 30 – 50 μmol/L. Citrulline less than 20 μmol/L indicates a severe compromise of small intestine enterocyte function. Low citrulline level indicates not only a loss of absorptive function and integrity, but also a loss of mucosa enzymatic activity, and increased colonic nutrient fermentation.
>
> Low plasma citrulline level is found and can be used in the diagnosis and management of diseases of the small intestine including celiac disease, Crohn's disease, short-bowel syndrome, and tropical sprue, and is useful for monitoring the efficacy of treatment of these conditions. Citrulline can also be used to assess damage to the intestine from radiation or chemotherapy during cancer treatment. Patients on parenteral nutrition can usually tolerate a return to an oral diet when citrulline levels rise above 20 μmol/L.[707]

Citrulline can be supplemented directly, or with a diet rich in, or supplemented with glutamine, as long as the intestinal mucosa is healthy.

Hepatitis C Virus and Homocysteine

Hyperhomocysteinemia and insulin resistance are risk factors for fatty liver.[708] Over 90 percent of HCV-infected patients have elevated blood levels of the toxic metabolite homocysteine (HCY). When patients are treated with antiviral therapy, those who respond to therapy, have a progressive and sustained drop in homocysteine levels.[709] Adequate levels of the B vitamins, folate, and cyanocobalamin (vitamin B12) are needed to prevent a rise in homocysteine level. Betaine can also help recycle HCY. The B vitamin pyridoxine helps convert homocysteine into cysteine, which can be used to make the antioxidant glutathione. (Chapter 26)

Coffee

Coffee provides anti-inflammatory, anti-fibrotic, and anti-oxidative benefits for the liver. Coffee lowers liver enzyme levels that are markers of liver disease. Coffee decreases progression to cirrhosis, lowers mortality rates in patients with cirrhosis, and has chemopreventive effects against hepatic cancer. In patients with chronic HCV infection, coffee consumption improves response to antiviral therapy.[710] Meta-analysis of multiple studies shows that drinking two cups of coffee a day decreases the risk of liver cancer by 31 percent among those without liver disease and by 44 percent in those with a history of liver disease.[711] These results have been replicated in Asia, South America, Europe, and America. Dark roasted coffees provide a better response than lighter roasts do. (Coffee is also discussed in Chapter 23.)

Trans Fats

High-fat diets, especially diets high in n-6 fats, are pro-inflammatory and contribute to fatty liver and NASH risk. Another type of fat, trans fats, are particularly dangerous. Consumption of trans fatty acids is associated with increased risks of several disease conditions, including heart disease, dementia, breast cancer, diabetes, and fatty liver. Studies cited by the U.S. FDA estimate that between 30,000 and 100,000 Americans die from heart disease in the U.S. each year, as a result of dietary trans fats.[712, 713] Trans fats also increase the risk of colon cancer[714] and infertility.[715]

Trans-fats (found in hydrogenated fats, which are used to increase shelf-life of processed foods), like fructose, not only cause obesity, they also cause non-alcoholic fatty liver disease and inflammatory cell death to hepatocytes.[716] Removing trans fats from the diet of animals allowed these fats to be dispersed from the liver (hopefully to areas of the body where they are less toxic) and resulted in the normalization of trans-fat associated fatty liver disease.[717]

Trans fatty acids occur in small amounts in nature, mostly as a result of rumination in cattle; however, almost all trans-fatty acids in the modern diet are created during the processing of long-chain unsaturated fats. Some trans-fat content is unintentional, as in the case of refining vegetable oil, but mostly, it is intentional. Vegetable fats are treated with hydrogen, a process not surprisingly called hydrogenation, to raise the melting temperature and improve shelf life. This makes for cheap (but toxic) butter (margarine) and easy to store lard (shortening) substitutes that offer processed foods a long shelf-life.

Shortening can contain from ten to over 30 percent trans-fats. In some human populations, a similar amount of the body fat is trans fats. When women breastfeed, trans fats they have eaten appear in their breast milk; in North America, 7% of the fat in mother's milk is trans fat.[718] Unfortunately, humans do not have enzymes for breaking down trans fats. Thus, these fats are not food, and we cannot use them for energy. Instead, they can be thought of as a slow poison, disguised as food, which accumulates in the body. Eating trans fats is something like checking into "Hotel California"; they are programmed to be received; you can check-out any time you like, but the trans fats will never leave.

Table 28-2: Typical Trans Fats Content of Processed Foods

Food	Serving size	Grams of Trans Fat[719]*
French fries	147 grams	8
Potato chips	Small bag 42 grams	2
Corn Chips	1 oz	1.5
Doughnut	1	5
Cookies (commercial)	3 (30 grams total)	2
Pound Cake (commercial)	1 slice, 80 grams	4.5
Candy Bar	40 grams (1.4 oz)	3
Shortening	1 Tbsp	4
Margarine (Tub)	1 Tbsp	0.5
Margarine (Stick)	1 Tbsp	3
Butter	1 Tbsp	0
Milk (whole)	1 cup	0
Mayonnaise	1 Tbsp	0

*Amounts vary significantly among food manufacturers.

U.S. law since 2006 has mandated labeling of the amount of trans-fats per serving. Many prepared foods now have "zero" trans fats. This is not your ordinary zero, but rather, a political zero. As long as a serving contains less than 0.5 grams of trans-fats, it can be rounded down to zero on the product label. Thus, 450 milligrams of trans fat per serving can be legally labeled as zero. One serving can be one cookie, a teaspoon of margarine, or a few potato chips. Each serving can be stated as having zero trans fats if it contains less than 0.5 grams, regardless of the number of servings or the total amount of trans fat likely to be consumed.

Thus, eating foods labeled as having zero grams trans fats per serving can still allow the consumption of several grams of trans fats per day. If this neither seems a significant quantity, nor provokes concern, then consider that the average American consumes only about 1.5 grams of the anti-inflammatory essential fatty acid, linolenic acid a day, and much of that may be burned for energy. The average American consumes only 0.07 grams of the n-3 fat DHA in their diet per day.[720] In June of 2015, the FDA finalized its ruling, determining that partially hydrogenated oils (PHOs), the major dietary source of trans fat in processed food, are not "generally recognized as safe." After June 2018, it will no longer be legal to *add* PHOs to food for sale in the United States.[721] Some manufacturers have already lowered the amount of trans fat in the foods they manufacture.

Summary

It is estimated that over 7 percent of the U.S. adult population has fatty liver disease, a precursor to liver cirrhosis and hepatocellular carcinoma. Fatty liver disease is common among the obese and diabetics, even those that are not obese. The most common causes of fatty liver disease in the U.S. are dietary: fructose, alcohol, and fats, especially trans fats.

Avoiding a high-fat diet, especially trans fats that are found in manufactured foods, margarine, and shortening, as well as fructose-laden sweet beverages and alcohol, can reverse fatty liver disease, and may slow the progression of liver fibrosis. Fructose should be limited to 10 percent of the caloric intake of non-obese individuals and to less than 5 percent of the caloric intake of obese individuals, as well as those with metabolic syndrome or fatty liver disease. Alcohol should also be avoided by those at high risk and limited to non-toxic levels in others. Alcohol is discussed in Chapter 11. As discussed in Chapter 9, effective medications are available for the cure of hepatitis C infection. Fungal liver toxins that increase the risk of hepatocellular carcinoma are discussed in Chapter 21.

Coffee, especially dark roasted coffee, betaine, and choline also prevent liver injury and disease progression.

29: OTHER ENVIRONMENTAL CAUSES

Much of the focus of this book has been the on things we put into our own bodies. Most of the risk factors for cancer described in this chapter are different; they are things we are exposed to in our work or home environments.

Air Pollution

Indoor air pollution from second-hand tobacco smoke is a cause of lung cancer. Even smokers are re-exposed to second-hand smoke, increasing risk of disease. Especially in less-developed areas, wood and coal are still used for heating and cooking. In many parts of the world, women still cook indoors over an open fire. Indoor air pollution from heating with coal, as is still done in China and some other regions, is associated with elevated risk of lung cancer. Bituminous coal produces more smoke than anthracite types and creates considerably higher risk than does the use of anthracite coal.[722] Long-term use of coal for heating or cooking more than doubles lung cancer risk. Use of wood for heating and cooking is not associated with the risk of lung cancer among individuals that don't smoke tobacco, but increases risk among those that do.[723]

In 2013, the World Health Organization officially recognized that *outdoor air pollution* (OAP) is a human carcinogen. Most studies have looked at the association of OAP and lung cancer. Long-term exposure to NO_2, NO, and SO_2 at a level of 2.5 parts per million are associated with an increased risk of lung cancer. Even so, most of the risk of lung cancer from OAP appears to be from exposure to smoke particulates.[724] The risk from air pollution is significantly elevated among those with occupational exposure to air pollution. Among professional drivers, lung cancer occurs 1.27 times more often than in the general population, from the exposure to vehicle exhaust.[725]

Lung cancer is not the only form of cancer caused by OAP. Oral, laryngeal, and pharyngeal cancers have also been associated with OAP.[726] Several studies have shown an increased risk of leukemia in children, in the United States and Europe, living near intersections or high traffic areas with high levels of OAP.[727] This risk has been attributed to benzene and NO_2 exposure from vehicle exhaust.[728]

Many of the studies on indoor and outdoor air pollution have been done in Asia and other areas that have poor pollution control. Thus, exposure levels and risk would be expected to be higher than in areas with better pollution control and lower exposure levels. Nevertheless, air pollution levels in the United States are linked to cancer rates. It is estimated that five percent of all cancer deaths in men and three percent of cancer deaths in American women between the years 1970 to 1994 were caused by air pollution.[729]

Plastic and Pesticide Endocrine Disruptors

A study of Canadian women to industrial exposures while working in different employment sectors found an increased risk of breast cancer among those working in five of 24 workplace settings: automotive manufacture if exposed to plastics; agricultural workers (growing crops); the food canning industry; working in bars and casinos; and metalworking. Women exposed to canning and to automotive plastics were over five times more likely to develop premenopausal breast cancer than were unexposed women.[730]

Table 29-1: Occupational Exposures Causing Breast Cancer

Industry	Likely Exposure	Breast Cancer Risks Ratio
Automotive (Plastics)	Plastics containing Endocrine Disrupting Compounds (EDC), solvents	5.1 (Premenopausal)
Agriculture	Organochlorine pesticides and chemicals that are EDC	3.1 to 7.3 for those working in fruit and vegetable farming
Canning (Foods)	Bisphenol A (BPA) and pesticide exposure; both of these are EDC	5.2 (Premenopausal)
Metalworking	PHA (heating of cutting oils), solvents, PCBs, that are EDC, heavy metals	1.7
Bars and Gambling	Shift work, sleep disruption. See Chapter 30.	2.2

For most sectors of agriculture, the risk of breast cancer was not found to be elevated. It was no different from the average background risk for women growing corn or working in the dairy industry. Women working in fruit and vegetable farming, however, were at high risk; especially if exposure occurred during puberty and adolescence.[730] DDT and other pesticides have chronic estrogen disrupting effects and can accumulate in the body.

Women working in the plastic and rubber industries, as well as those exposed to plastics in automobile manufacture, were also been found to have increased rates of breast cancer in several studies.

These women are exposed to endocrine-disrupting compounds (EDC) such as phthalates and polybrominated diphenyl ethers (PBDE). Occupational exposure to nylon fibers has been found to double the risk of breast cancer, and occupational exposure to acrylic fibers raises the risk 7.7 times. This sort of takes the pleasure out of that new car smell.

Endocrine disruptors (EDC) are chemical compounds that interfere with hormonal function. Exposure to them can cause birth defects, interfere with fertility, affect the nervous system and cause cancer. Some examples of EDC are phthalates, bisphenol-A (BPA), organochlorine compounds (such as vinyl chloride), many pesticides, polychlorinated biphenyls (PCBs), and dioxins. Many other chemicals used in plastic and rubber manufacture, such as BPA, butadiene, vinyl chloride, and several phthalates are known carcinogens.

PBDE are used as flame retardants. Phthalates are used as plasticizers to make plastic softer and more flexible. BPA is added to plastics to harden them and improve their clarity.

Phthalate exposure is associated with lower sperm counts and DNA damage in the sperm among men exposed to them. Children born to women with higher phthalate levels have smaller penises and testicles and have a smaller distance between the testes and anus, indicating an anti-androgen effect on the child. Girls exposed to phthalates were seven times more likely to have premature sexual development. Men with high phthalate levels are more likely to have abdominal obesity and insulin resistance.

BPA exposure is associated with an increased risk of breast and prostate cancers. It also affects neurological development in lab animals.

The elevated risk associated with food canning may be attributable to exposure to BPA that is used to line metal cans. When the cans are heated during the canning process, there may be a release of BPA into the air. The canning process reduces the level of pesticides present in foods, through washing, peeling, and cooking the produce. Women working in the canning industry may be exposed to pesticides from the fruits and vegetables they are preparing.

Metalworkers also have an elevated risk of cancer. It is not only women and not only breast cancer rates that are high in metalworkers; the risk is increased for cancers of the larynx, rectum, pancreas, skin, scrotum, bladder, and other organs.[731]

During metal machining, oils are used both as lubricants and coolants for the metals and metalworking tools as the metal is shaped or milled. During this process, the oils get hot, and some vaporize. Additionally, many processes cause a fine atomization of oil particles that get suspended into the air, causing exposure to the nasal cavity, lungs, and skin. A portion of these particles enters the oropharynx and are swallowed. Solvents used for cleaning metals also form volatiles and mists, causing airborne exposure.

When oils are heated, products of pyrolization, including carcinogenic polyaromatic hydrocarbons (PAH), are created and enter the air. Additionally, PCBs, organochlorines, and EDC, were previously used in metalworking. PCBs are oily liquids that conduct heat very well and have high flash point (ignition) temperatures. Thus, they were very useful in cutting fluids for machining.

PCB production was banned in the United States in 1979 and by the Stockholm Convention in 2001. PCBs, however, have a special property that causes them to be of continued interest. There are over 200 PCBs, and they have various metabolic effects. Also, like DDT, they are endocrine disruptors, persist in the environment for extended times, and bioaccumulate in the body, especially in fatty tissues. Since they last for such a long time, they are still with us and in us.

Most current exposure to PCBs is through the consumption of fish from contaminated waters and dairy and meat products from contaminated soils. Several PCBs are human carcinogens. And since cancer usually has a long latent period, it can take many years after exposure to manifest. Exposure to PCBs at levels currently present in the environment in many countries is associated with high risk of breast[732] and testicular[733] cancers. PCBs and other organochlorine compounds have been shown to interact with Epstein–Barr virus (HHV-4) in the causation of non-Hodgkin lymphoma.[734] PCB exposure is also a risk factor for myocardial infarctions and stroke. The risk for heart disease associated with this exposure may be lowered by consumption of foods rich in n-3 fatty acids.[735][736] Just make sure the fish rich in n-3 fats is low in PCBs, and not from a polluted lake or river.

Metal workers may also be exposed to toxic metals. Hexavalent chromium is a risk factor for nasal and lung cancers. It acts as an oxidizing agent that binds with glutathione, and this cogener forms DNA adducts.

The carcinogens that plastic workers and canners are exposed to are also found in our homes. When the general population is tested, over 90% of people have measurable BPA in their urine. Significant exposure to BPA can come from heating food in plastic containers as might be done in a microwave. Most plastics are not made for and are not safe to use in a microwave. Especially when heating acidic or oily foods in plastic containers, BPA, phthalates, and other toxins can leach from the plastic into the food. BPA is a major component in polycarbonate plastics, which have the recycling symbol with the number "7". Those marked "3" may contain phthalates.

Soft plastic containers, such as yogurt containers, are not microwave-safe to temperature; they can easily melt and may release toxins into the food being heated. Scratched, cracked, or multiple reused containers leach plasticizers such as phthalates more easily. Containers marked for single microwave use are not safe for reuse.

"Microwave-safe" plastic food containers are made without or with very much lower amounts of BPA and phthalates. Often, bisphenol-S (BPS) is used in these plastics as a substitute for BPA. BPS is a similar compound that is considered to be more resistant to leaching. BPS, however, has been shown to be a ten times more potent progesterone disrupter than BPA and to have similar androgenic and estrogenic effects as BPA.[737][738] Thus, microwave safe plastics are unlikely safe, but rather potentially less dangerous than other plastics. A much better choice is to avoid heating food in any plastic, and instead, use containers made from inorganic materials such as glass and ceramics for microwave heating. Natural fibers, such as cotton and paper may also be used to wrap or cover food in the microwave.

Although few readers are likely to try it, avoid hobo stove cooking, where food is cooked over a campfire in a BPA lined tin can.

Exposure to endocrine-disrupting compounds is especially filled with danger for the developing fetus, children, and during puberty and adolescence. Recall that it was women exposed to agricultural work during puberty and adolescence are at the higher risk for later development of breast cancer.

> The FDA banned BPA from baby bottles, but still, plastic baby bottles should not be heated in a microwave or heated in a bath of boiling water on the stove top to warm baby food. High temperatures can cause leaching of chemicals into the milk or baby formula. Additionally, the contents, especially when heated in a microwave, may have hot areas in the liquid that can scald the child's mouth.
>
> Infants do not need, and many do not prefer hot beverages. Most infants are happy with formula between room temperature and body temperature, while some enjoy their beverages cooler. The purpose of heating water for formula is to kill bacteria that might be present. When using a formula that needs to be added water,

> use water from the cold tap and let it run until the water is cool to lower the contents of contaminants such as lead and copper. Put the water into a clean pan and bring it to a boil to sterilize it; cover the pan to let the water cool to below body temperature. Then place the water and the formula into the bottle.
>
> Water from the hot water tap should not be above 49° C (120° F). This temperature is much less likely to leach compounds from baby bottles or from other containers than is a boiling temperature. A baby bottle can be warmed by letting it stand for a few minutes in a container with hot tap water and shaking it to distribute the heat before giving it to the child. Dishwashers can heat plastics to high temperatures that may cause the degradation of many plastics and thus, the release of EDCs.

Are non-agricultural workers exposed to dangerous levels of endocrine-disrupting pesticides? Those living in areas where there is aerial spraying of crops are exposed. Use of oregano pesticide bug spray in the home causes exposure. No joke - people will drown a roach in bug spray rather than step on one; when it would have taken a whiff of the poison to kill the bug, they use half a can. If a child is treated with lindane for head lice or scabies, they are exposed; this compound bioaccumulates and persists in the body. Any lindane you absorbed when you were treated for head lice when you were six years old is likely still with you. Insecticides and other organochlorine compounds are not just endocrine disruptors and carcinogens. Several are neurotoxins and associated with developmental disorders, Alzheimer's and Parkinson's diseases.[739]

The safest pesticides for domestic use are shoes, fly swatters, and magazines. Boric acid powder effectively kills roaches that scurry under the stove when you turn on the lights to get a glass of water at night. There are many non-genotoxic ways of preventing and eliminating insect infestations in your home, beginning with washing the dishes and cleaning countertops before retiring for the night.

Summary

Outside of occupational exposures, people may be exposed to carcinogenic organochlorine and endocrine disrupting compounds in their homes. Those of the most common sources of exposure are pesticides and plastics. Exposure to pesticides can be avoided, and safer methods of pest control are available. Heating or storing food in most plastic containers can allow carcinogens to leak into the food. Most plastics are not microwave or dishwasher safe, and may leak toxic and endocrine disrupting compounds after the container is heated or damaged with repeated use.

Table 29-1: Microwave Safe and Unsafe Containers

Microwave Safe	
Pyrex glass and most glass containers	Pyrex and most other glass containers as long as they do not heat when empty. To test, use another container with water in the microwave to prevent damaging the microwave from using it empty. Heat for 15 seconds to make sure that the empty container does not get hot.
Most ceramic containers	Ceramic containers (such as coffee mugs) as long as the container does not heat in the microwave when heated empty.
White paper plates, napkins, and towels	Avoid those with printed decorations.
Moistened cotton towel	Natural fibers do not contain EDC. Moistening the cloth decreases the risk of fire during heating.
Wax paper	Unbleached wax paper. Cooking parchment paper may also be used.
Not Microwave Safe	
Plastics	Most plastics are not microwave-safe, and even those marked as microwave safe may contain EDC that may leach into food with repeated use.
Brown Paper Bags	Contain recycled (unknown) materials including contaminants. Tiny fragments of metal in the recycled materials can start fires
Chinese cardboard and styrofoam take-out containers.	Metal wire handles can cause sparking and fire. Styrofoam is plastic.
Plastic wraps	Some plastic wraps are made to cover containers being used in the microwave; however, most are not. Those that are should not touch the food.
China with metallic trim	Metal heats and sparks in a microwave, and can damage both the china and the microwave.

30: SLEEP

The Need for Sleep

Sleep is essential to health. Lack of and poor quality sleep is a risk factor for cancer, including breast, prostate, colorectal, and brain cancers.

If lab rats are completely prevented from sleeping, they eat more but lose weight; their heart rates accelerate, they develop skin ulcers and die within a few weeks. Sleep is required for survival. Even tiny nematodes sleep. If sharks stop swimming, they suffocate. Thus, to keep swimming and keep water moving through their gills, sharks sleep half of their brain at a time. Porpoises need to come up to the surface to breathe; birds that migrate long distances across vast oceans also need to sleep but must stay awake to survive. Therefore, these animals also sleep half of their brain at a time. Although it may seem at times that some of us are only half awake, this trick does not work in humans; we need sufficient, quality, whole-brain sleep.

Humans sleep about one-third of their life away, or at least, we are healthiest and perform best when we do. When we have insufficient sleep, reaction times slow, attention lapses, the mood becomes labile, cognition foggy, and memory suffers. Decision-making can become faulty, and logic blurred.[740]

Excessive wake time impairs mood, judgment, and reaction time. Nineteen hours of sustained wakefulness is associated with a performance deficit equivalent to a blood alcohol level of 0.05%; the level at which it is illegal to operate a motor vehicle in most jurisdictions. After 24 hours of sustained wakefulness, the performance deficit is equivalent to a blood alcohol level of 0.1%,[741] a level sufficient to impair reaction times and gross motor control.

In addition to the need for sleep, our bodies have circadian cycles that tune the metabolism to daytime activity and nighttime quiescence. These cycles do much more than entrain the sleep cycle to help us wake and sleep coincident to dawn and nightfall. The circadian cycles are intimately tied to the release of at least a dozen hormones that control the body's energy use, activity, appetite, digestion, immune function, growth, and healing. Disrupting the circadian cycle can throw these hormonal cycles into disarray.

Sleep provides a quiet and undisturbed space for gleaning and interconnecting the relevant and salient information and processes encountered during the day. The various sleep stages make different contributions to learning. In the first part of the sleep cycle, SWS (short-wave sleep) helps to stabilize visual and declarative memory

("Just the facts, ma'am"). Stage 2 sleep helps reorganize the content that has been learned during the day and helps with learning motor sequencing and automaticity skills, such as playing a musical instrument or coordinated movements such as used in sports, dance or operating machinery. Throughout the night, REM (rapid eye movement) sleep enhances the memory, adds insights, explores interrelationships and helps reorganize information into associative networks.[742] These repetitive sleep cycles throughout the night allow for the iterative creation of memory and learning, and for winnowing the salient from the inconsequential. The brain is not relaxing during sleep – it is actively processing information.

Normally, the thyroid hormone T3 is released at night during sleep, and T4 form of the hormone is released in the morning. T3 is geared more for supporting growth and repair while T4 is more supportive of activity. T3 stimulates the wrapping of nerves with myelin by oligodendrocyte precursor cells,[743] and thus, is important for neurologic development, learning, and repair after injury. Sleep deprivation inhibits thyroid stimulating hormone release.

One reason that young people require more sleep is that they are more actively learning. Small children take frequent naps that help them learn motor and language skills more quickly. College students often try to learn more information in a sitting than they can organize and understand, much less integrate. Often, information learned during the day makes more sense the following morning. It may take two to three nights sleep to organize complex information into a gestalt. Adults that are actively engaged in learning have creative demands or require peak attention and reaction times need to dedicate eight hours per day to sleep.

Sleep Deprivation

Chronic sleep deprivation usually only causes a mild decline in subjective functioning. Nevertheless, it can cause a severe decline in attention and reaction times. When people are severely and chronically sleep deprived, however, they do not feel much worse than if they were only mildly sleep deprived. Regardless, their functioning can be seriously impaired. Maintenance of peak reaction times requires just over eight hours of sleep each night.

Many adults make do with much less sleep time without obvious problems. Even when sleep is restricted to only four hours a night, most adults will not complain of feeling fatigued or impaired, even after two weeks of curtailed sleep. It appears that there are different thresholds for feeling sleep-deprived for different individuals.[744] Nonetheless, those who feel well when sleep is limited are impaired by sleep deprivation; they just don't feel tired. They still suffer just as severe performance deficits as those who do feel tired.

Peak functioning, as measured by attention measurements, actually does not depend on sleep, but rather, on avoiding excessive wakefulness. Being awake too long diminishes focus. The effect of time awake is cumulative. Being awake an additional hour each day for 8 days in a row diminishes the level of focus and attention equivalent to missing one night's sleep; staying awake one extra hour daily for 16 days in a row will cause the difficulty in focus and attention that missing two night's sleep would. Performing at full attention and focus proscribes being awake for more than about 16 hours per day on average,[745] resulting in our need for about 8 hours of sleep.

Excitatory neurotransmitters, such as glutamate, associated with activity and alertness, are neurotoxic; when they accumulate, they can damage the brain. Sleep provides an opportunity for the brain to detoxify, replenish antioxidants, and repair itself. During sleep, the glymphatic system flushes wastes from the cerebral spinal fluid more quickly to help recover from the toxins and metabolites that accumulate during wakefulness.[746]

The CLOCK gene, which helps regulate circadian cycles, is involved in the growth and repair of muscles.[747] Sleep deprivation also impairs mitochondrial health. Deprivation of REM sleep can induce the loss of neuronal mitochondria through mitophagy,[748] a process in which the mitochondria, the energy production units of the cell, self-destruct. While an occasional sleep "fast" may help eliminate weak neuronal mitochondria, chronic sleep deprivation diminishes neuronal energy.

During sleep, an accounting of energy utilization and oxidative stress is made, and the results are used to plan and accommodate the next day's needs for energy and antioxidants. Energy use accommodation is provided through control of thyroid and other hormones to fine tune the metabolic rate and control the appetite. Sleep deprivation increases appetite.

Several of the genes involved in energy metabolism and for encoding antioxidant response element (ARE) proteins have increased transcription during sleep[749]. Melatonin, released from the pineal gland, not only helps induce and maintain sleep but also is an important antioxidant that helps protect neurons in the central and gastrointestinal nervous systems. Melatonin is a non-recyclable antioxidant for the nervous system; oxidized melatonin acts as a signaling molecule, through which the Nrf2→ARE pathway induces proteins that provide protection from endogenous and xenobiotic toxins and oxidative injury.[431]

Inflammation and Immunity

Sleep deprivation promotes inflammation. It causes increased levels of C-reactive protein, and of the proinflammatory cytokines IL-1β, IL-6, and IL-17. The changes in the appetite hormones leptin and ghrelin observed in sleep deprivation may result from increased levels of these cytokines. IL-6 is usually found to be elevated in fibromyalgia syndrome, a condition in which non-restorative sleep is common. The risk of heart disease is elevated in short-sleepers because of inflammation. C-reactive protein is a risk factor for heart disease and cancer. There is also an increased risk of dysrhythmias caused by increased adrenergic activity. IL-6 is an important cause of fatigue, and it causes a decrease in SWS.[750]

Sleep and circadian rhythms have a critical role in the development of immune function. The ROR (retinol-related orphan receptor) genes, which are subject to circadian influence, impact the differentiation of T helper cells into different lineages. Different types of T helper cells are used by the immune system to focus on specific targets, such as different types of infections or tumor cells. Sleep deprivation or disruption of the circadian cycle shifts T helper cell development towards T_H17 cell proliferation. T_H17 cells are involved in the chronic inflammatory and autoimmune diseases, including multiple sclerosis, rheumatoid arthritis, systemic lupus, inflammatory bowel disease, psoriasis, and asthma.[751] T_H17 activation promotes the development of food sensitivities. Thus, sleep deprivation may promote food sensitivities that cause migraine headaches, irritable bowel syndrome, depression, and other maladies. These are inflammatory disorders, and they act through the same inflammatory mechanisms that reduce apoptosis and promote tumor survival. Sleep deprivation is also associated with elevated B lymphocyte and lower NK-cell populations, thus affecting the body's immune response to infection and injury.

The immune system does not like to fight two battles on different fronts. When it is diverted and dedicating its resources to T_H17 immune cell functions, the immune defenses against cancer and other threats are compromised.

Inadequate sleep and disrupted circadian cycles promote inflammatory cytokines that impede apoptosis and promote the survival of cancer cells.

Table 30-1: Effects of Sleep Restriction on Hormones[752] and Cytokines[753]

Hormone	Effect of Sleep Deprivation	Effect on Health
Leptin (Satiation hormone)	Lower circadian peak leptin levels. Lower daily leptin production. Likely drives thyroid control (TRH).	Lower levels cause increased hunger, especially for high caloric, soft, palatable foods
(Acyl)-Ghrelin	Increased in short sleepers[754]	Stimulates hunger
Orexin (Hypocretin)	Increased with sleep deprivation.	Increases activity
TSH (Thyroid Stimulating Hormone)	Loss of circadian nighttime peak. Lower TSH and T3 output.	Fatigue and decreased energy use. Decreased myelination of nerves.
Cortisol	Decreases circadian cyclic variation (lower A.M. peak). Increases daytime and total cortisol output.	Increases inflammation. Increased abdominal obesity.
Sympathovagal balance	Increased sympathetic activity.	Increases resting heart rate, blood pressure, and risk for arrhythmia.
Insulin	Decreased glucose tolerance. Decreased insulin sensitivity.	Increased risk for Type 2 diabetes.
IGF-1[755]	Decreased production.	Decreased healing, increased mortality[756]
Interleukin-6[757] (IL-6)	Proinflammatory cytokine; increased in sleep deprivation. May decrease leptin output.	Chronic inflammation
Interleukin-1β (IL-1 β)	Proinflammatory cytokine	Chronic inflammation. Increased T_H17 immune function. Decreased T_H1.
Interleukin-17 (IL-17)	Proinflammatory cytokine; favors TH17 immune function.	Chronic inflammation, enteric immune system-mediated disease.
C-Reactive Protein	An inflammatory marker associated with risk of coronary artery disease.	Increased risk of coronary artery disease.
Melatonin	Decreased output. Melatonin is an antioxidant for the nervous system. It stimulates T4 and T8 lymphocyte production.[758] Helps with memory consolidation.	Decreased T-cell immune function. Impaired memory consolidation

When sleep and circadian cycles are normal, there is a surge of glucocorticoid hormones each morning that helps down-regulate inflammation. This is particularly relevant for individuals with a BRCA1 mutation, as these individuals have a decreased expression of glucocorticoid receptors,[759] and thus are less responsive to the diurnal anti-inflammatory signal.

Energy Balance

Individuals sleeping fewer hours are more likely to become obese. Children who sleep less than ten hours a day are 89% percent more likely to be obese than children who get more sleep, and adults who get less than six hours sleep are about 55% more likely to be obese than adults who get more than six hours of sleep.[176] The association between short sleep time and obesity has been found in more than 30 studies performed on six continents; this effect is not limited to the North American or Western lifestyle.

Obesity is also associated with longer sleep time because obesity greatly increases the propensity for snoring. When snoring becomes severe, it can disturb sleep and is often associated with sleep apnea. In obstructive sleep apnea, the person's breathing becomes obstructed momentarily, and sleep is disturbed. Heavy snorers with sleep apnea may experience dozens of semi-awakenings throughout the night but have no recollection of them. These frequent arousals result in poor quality, non-restorative sleep as the sleeper spends little time in deep, restorative, Stage 2, SWS and REM sleep. Thus, although patients with sleep apnea may spend more time in bed and more time sleeping, they can still have large sleep deficits and feel sleepy and fatigued during the day. In a vicious cycle, the sleep deficits from sleep apnea promote inflammatory cytokines that increase appetite and thus obesity that worsens snoring and sleep apnea.

Obviously, a lack of sleep leads to fatigue. It is not only the lack of sleep, especially short wave sleep, but disruption of the diurnal cycle of thyroid hormones, growth hormone, and cortisol, and the increase in inflammatory cytokines that cause fatigue. The fatigue, lack of energy, and decrease in muscle function act to dissuade many short sleepers from exercise; this leads to another vicious cycle of obesity and poor health.

Sleep Deprivation and Cancer

Obesity, lack of exercise, oxidative injury, inflammation, and a decline T-cell function – the immune cells most closely linked to targeting cancer cells: all of these are risk factors for cancer.

In a study sampling two million people enrolled in the Taiwanese national health insurance program, sleep disorders were associated with a seventy percent increased risk of cancer. Individuals with obstructive sleep apnea (OSA) had a greater than doubling in the hazard for breast, kidney, bladder, and thyroid cancer. Suffering from OSA was associated with 3.69 times higher hazard of prostate cancer. The risk of prostatic hypertrophy is also elevated among men with sleep apnea.[760] Colorectal cancers were increased by 55 percent in persons with OSA. Cancer risk was similarly elevated among those with chronic insomnia or parasomnias.[761]

> Parasomnias are abnormal movements, behaviors, emotions, perceptions, and dreams that occur while falling asleep or during sleep. They usually involve a state of partial arousal. They include sleepwalking, teeth grinding, night terrors, and restless leg syndrome.

Another study found that OSA was associated with a doubling of breast cancer incidence among women aged 30 to 59 and a tripling of incidence among women over sixty.[762] The risk of primary brain cancers has been found to be raised by seventy percent among persons with sleep apnea.[763]

Shift Workers

Shift work has been found to be associated with increased risk of cancer. A review of 25 studies found a nine to 48 percent increased risk of breast cancer among women who do night/shift work, especially among women doing night shift work for more than 20 years.[764] Doing three or more nights of shift work a month was sufficient in increase breast cancer risk among nurses.[765] Night shift work raises the risk of breast cancer by about *three percent for every five years* of exposure.[766] The risk is potent enough that *women who have been diagnosed with breast cancer are advised not to do night shift work*.[767] The increased risk of prostate cancer from night shift work is similar to that for breast cancer: *2.8 percent increase in risk for every five years* of exposure.[768]

Night shift work has also been found to be associated with an increased risk of colorectal cancer; here the risk is considerably higher, with an 11 percent increase in risk for every five years of shift work.[769] The risk of colorectal cancers may be especially elevated in night shift workers because of its disruptive influence on the circadian cycle of the intestines.

The motility of the gastrointestinal system is mediated by CLOCK genes expressed in intestinal epithelial cells and in neurons in the enteric nervous system, which help control circadian rhythms.[770]

Yes, the gastrointestinal system has its own brain that controls the GI tract. Gastric emptying times are longer for solid foods in the evening than in the morning. The propagation of contractions in the small intestine is slower at night; moving only about 2.9 cm/minute, as compared to 6.4 cm/minute during the day.[771] Colonic motility is low at night but increases in the morning, aiding in defecation. Melatonin, released from enterochromaffin cells in the gut, increases blood flow and acts as an antioxidant[772] that protects the enteric nervous system. The enteric nervous system produces more melatonin than does the pineal gland in the brain. Disruption of the circadian cycle by alterations in sleep time and meal times can cause intestinal dysmotility. This is why shift work or time zone traveling can lead cause gastrointestinal bloating, abdominal pain, diarrhea, or constipation.[770]

Irritable bowel syndrome and gastrointestinal reflux are associated with sleep disorders and common among shift workers. Nurses on rotating shifts are twice as likely to have a functional bowel disorder as those working day shifts[773]. Missing meals during the day or feeding at night may also disrupt gastrointestinal circadian cycles.[774, 775]

Glucose, insulin, ghrelin, leptin, and GLP-1 (glucagon-like peptide-1) levels follow meal patterns.[776] Nighttime eating can offset the intestinal circadian rhythm, and nighttime meals result in increased blood sugar and triglyceride levels, compared to the same meal consumed during the day.[777] Disruption of the circadian cycle causes changes in appetite that increase risk for obesity.[778] Shift work also results in elevated triglyceride levels; increased BMI, waist circumference and obesity; and blunted response to insulin.[779] Indeed, in addition to the risk of cancer, circadian disruption in shift workers increases the risk of depression, metabolic syndrome, diabetes, cardiovascular disease, cognitive impairment, and premature aging. [780, 781, 782]

In the previous chapter, data was presented that showed that women working in bars had an increased risk of breast cancer. Male waiters have also been found to be at increased risk of cancer. The availability of alcohol and exposure to secondhand cigarette smoke may partially explain this risk. Shift workers, especially younger men doing shift work, are more likely to binge drink than their non-shift-working peers, perhaps in an attempt to help induce sleep.[783] Night workers also tend to smoke more[784] and eat more foods associated with inflammation.

I recommend that women with breast cancer or at high risk for breast cancer avoid night shift work. Those at high risk include women with high-risk BRCA alleles, with a strong family history of breast cancer, or with a personal history of breast cancer. Since night shift work is also a strong risk factor for colorectal cancer, those with a family history of colorectal cancer should also avoid night shift work.

Light and Melatonin

Melatonin is a multifunctional substance produced in the body from the neurotransmitter serotonin. Melatonin is a hormone that helps with sleep but is also an important antioxidant for the central, autonomic and enteric nervous systems. The pineal gland, located deep within the brain, releases melatonin when the level of light reaching the retina of the eye is low. Exposure to light at night disrupts melatonin production. Women living in areas with high levels of outdoor light at night are at increased risk of breast cancer.[785] Nightime light exposure and melatonin disruption are designated by the World Health Organization as probable human carcinogens.

Melatonin inhibits human breast cancer cells that are stimulated by estrogen, decreasing estrogen-induced gene transcription.[786] Melatonin also prevents the uptake of linoleic acid (LA) by breast cancer cells. LA is a n-6 fatty acid that supports tumor growth. LA is converted to 13-HODE, which amplifies the activity of the EGF → MAPK pathway that leads to cell proliferation.[787] This is especially relevant for the 70 percent of breast cancers that are estrogen receptor alpha (ERα) positive. Light at night induces disruptions in the circadian rhythm and output of melatonin. This, at least in part, explains the increased risk of breast cancer in shift workers.[788]

Over 30 percent of women with ERα-positive (ERα+) breast cancer are intrinsically resistant to tamoxifen and similar anti-estrogenic medications used in the treatment of breast cancer. Eventually, most breast cancer patients develop resistance to these medications. In animals implanted with ERα+ human breast cancer cells, light-induced melatonin disruption increased tumor growth and conferred resistance to tamoxifen treatment. Animals exposed to dim light at night and given melatonin did not become resistant to tamoxifen. Melatonin supplementation was able to re-establish the sensitivity of ERα+ breast tumors to tamoxifen and promoted tumor regression.[789] In another quite ingenious experiment, human ERα+ breast tumors implanted into rats were perfused with blood from healthy women. When this blood was drawn from women during the daytime or at night after exposure to fluorescent lighting, it increased tumor metabolism. Blood drawn at night from women during darkness decreased tumor energy use, lowering cAMP by

86%, and decreased tumor DNA content by about 70 percent. However, blocking melatonin allowed the tumor activity that had been inhibited by the blood drawn from women during a dark-night.[790]

Women with ERα+ breast cancer should avoid shift work as there is substantial evidence that it promotes tumor growth and promotes resistance to anti-estrogen therapy. Additionally, these women should carefully avoid light during their sleep cycle.

The circadian drive is most sensitive to blue light with peak sensitivity to light at wavelengths about 480 nm. Low levels of light in this region of the spectrum help calm us and get us in the mood to sleep. Melatonin suppression appears to result from non-image-forming retinal cells containing the pigment melanopsin.[791] Melanopsin has its peak sensitivity to light with a wavelength around 480 nm. Melanopsin has little sensitivity to red light, above 600 nm. Blue light around 480 nm helps entrain the circadian cycle. The amount of light required to suppress melatonin output is much higher than the amount of light needed to alter circadian cycles.

Melatonin and melanopsin are separate, but complementary pathways. In a natural environment, melatonin is released shortly after sunset as a result of dimming light. It prepares us to wind down from the activities of the day and promotes the onset of sleep about three hours later. Similar to melanopsin, melatonin is most sensitive to blue light. Exclusion of exposure to light waves shorter than 530 nm prevents melatonin suppression. This is light between yellow-green and violet.

Women who do shift work can use melatonin around three hours before bedtime. This may mitigate cancer risk caused by the circadian disruption. The use of low dose melatonin is considered to be essentially risk-free,[792] other than it may interfere with blood thinners. Women with ERα+ breast cancer should discuss the use of melatonin with their physician, especially if using tamoxifen or similar medications, or if the woman has failed to respond to it.

Melatonin also suppresses prostate cancer growth. Sleeping in the dark suppresses prostate cancer proliferation, at least in lab rats. Exposure to bright light during the day, especially light in the blue range, increases nighttime, dark-cycle output of melatonin several fold. Exposure to bright daylight, associated with increases nighttime melatonin output, delays the development of human prostate cancer xenografts in rats and slows the cancer metabolism and growth.[793] Underexposure to sunlight during the day, and overexposure to light in the evening and during sleep at night promotes cancer growth.

Getting exposure to midday sunshine also creates vitamin D3 in the skin. There are ROR and RZR receptors in the pineal gland that help mediate melatonin production as well as other proteins that are involved with sleep.[794] Vitamin D is a ligand for the ROR and RZR receptors,[795] and thus, vitamin D made in the skin during the day by sunlight may help with the production of melatonin and with other aspects of the circadian cycle. Vitamin D's effect on the pineal gland may partly explain why sunshine makes us feel good.

Vitamin D may be helpful in the primary and secondary prevention of circadian and other sleep disorders. If vitamin D supplements are taken, midday is likely the most advantageous time.

Vitamin B_{12} amplifies the response of light in resetting the circadian clock,[796] and is helpful for some individuals with circadian rhythm disorders.[797] Vitamin B_{12} levels should be checked when investigating sleep disturbances and in patients with cancer.

I'm Only Sleeping

Whether studying Americans, Europeans or Asians, the lowest mortality rates, when assessed by daily sleep duration, are between six and eight hours per night.[798, 799, 800, 801, 802] Sleeping less than six hours is associated with a slight increase in mortality, and more than nine hours of sleep at night is associated with an even higher risk. More sleep is probably associated with higher risk of mortality among adults for the same reasons that they require more time to sleep; their sleep is low quality or fractured. Retired persons tend to sleep more, perhaps because of less demanding schedules, but this may also be due to poorer health. Even after adjusting for multiple risk factors, five hours of sleep in men and six hours for women appears to be sufficient to prevent an increased risk of mortality as compared to seven or eight hours. Less than four hours of sleep is a risk factor for higher mortality, similar in magnitude to the risk of nine hours sleep.

The optimal sleep time for adults appears to be about 7 hours and 45 minutes. This is about the length of time that adults will sleep if they have no impediments to sleep, a quiet, dark place, no appointments or scheduling imperatives or night-time disturbances. Most people take another 15 minutes to fall asleep and spend 15 minutes lying awake in the morning before arising. This is reflected in the 7.7 hours average sleep time, and 8.3 hours average time in bed observed in studies of healthy Americans.

Restoring Circadian Rhythm

Keeping regular meal times helps maintain the gastrointestinal circadian rhythm and helps with regular sleep. This is especially important in small children. Avoid large meals within 3 hours of bedtime. A small protein/carbohydrate/calcium snack, ice-cream for example, an hour before bedtime can induce production of serotonin and melatonin, and help with sleep onset.

Adhering to a regular wake and rise time is fundamental to improving nocturnal sleep efficiency and daytime alertness

Low dose melatonin (0.3 to 0.5 mg) given several hours prior to sleep has been found helpful to restore circadian rhythms. Low-dose melatonin has also been found to be helpful in preventing "sundowning" delirium in the elderly.[803] Larger doses of slow-release melatonin (3 mg to 6 mg) may be helpful for maintaining sleep in patients with early morning waking. The underlying cause of sleep disturbances should be investigated and treated. Lower doses of melatonin, below 1.5 mg) may be more effective than larger doses to assist sleep. Between 0.3 and 1.0 mg of rapidly absorbed, sublingual melatonin at bedtime is a reasonable dose to promote the onset of sleep. Up to 6 mg, usually in slow release form, may be used to maintain sleep, although 1.5 mg is sufficient for most people.

As a natural product, present in animals and some plants, melatonin is sold as a food supplement. Endogenous production of melatonin requires serotonin and the B_6 vitamin, pyridoxine-5-phosphate. Most people have adequate B_6 vitamin levels, but low levels are associated with increased risk of colon cancer.[804]

Melatonin is useful in the treatment of many enteroimmune and inflammatory diseases including fibromyalgia, IBS,[805] metabolic syndrome,[806] GERD,[807] migraine,[808] and cluster headaches,[809] and protects against Alzheimer's disease and depression.[810]

Having adequate vitamin B_{12} levels is important for a full circadian response to light. Vegan diets do not contain vitamin B_{12}. People with dry mouths and those with poor dentition that do not chew meat well enough to mix it with saliva can have low B_{12} absorption. Haptocorrin, a protein present in saliva, protects vitamin B_{12} in the diet from destruction by stomach acid. For those needing an oral supplement, sucking on a B_{12} tablet to mix it with saliva increases the amount that can be absorbed by over 100 times. Individuals with sleep disturbances and those with cancer should be tested to make sure vitamin B_{12} levels are adequate. Supplementation should be used to maintain vitamin B_{12} levels between 540 and 1200 pg/ml.

Vitamin D_3 level should also be tested in individuals with sleep disturbances and in cancer patients. Vitamin D_3 levels optimal for cancer prevention are over 100 nmol/L (40 ng/ml) of $25OHD_3$, and perhaps as high as 120 nmol/L (48 ng/ml). Low vitamin D levels may also cause the parasomnia, Restless Leg Syndrome (RLS). Normalization of vitamin D levels has been found to improve symptoms in RLS patients that have low vitamin D levels.[811] A dose of 2000 I.U. of vitamin D_3 daily is sufficient to raise $25OHD_3$ above this 90 nmol/L in many adults,[812] although a dose of 5000 I.U. is commonly required in patients with asymptomatic malabsorption syndromes. Boron supplementation can increase intestinal absorption of vitamin D_3.[597]

Vitamin D2, from mushrooms and synthetic vitamins, does not prevent cancer.[813] Note: The strongest effect of vitamin D on cancer mortality has been seen in studies with follow-up greater than 5 years.[813] In some studies, vitamin D3 levels were not associated with a change in cancer incidence but were associated with a decrease in cancer and overall mortality. This suggests that vitamin D may slow cancer growth.[814]

Iron deficiency is commonly associated with sleep and cognitive problems in children.[815] Sleep disturbances in children with autism may improve after correction of the iron deficiency[816]. Iron deficiency also affects sleep in adults. In a study of patients with anemia, heart failure, and sleep disturbances, treatment for anemia including iron not only improved heart function but also caused improvements in sleep deprivation and improved both central and obstructive sleep apnea.[817] Iron deficiency is associated with RLS, difficulty falling asleep, and daytime fatigue.[818] Iron deficiency not severe enough to manifest as anemia can still be severe enough to cause delays in neurodevelopmental milestones,[819] thus sleep disturbances in infants and young children should be investigated with blood tests for ferritin. Testing for anemia is not adequately sensitive to rule out iron deficiency severe enough to cause sleep disturbances. Serum ferritin levels should be over 50 ng/mL. Iron overload, a cancer risk factor is discussed in Chapter 20.

Caution: Most studies of vitamin supplementation in adults show an increased risk of cancer for adults taking them. High levels of some B vitamins can increase the risk of DNA errors and many vitamins and mineral supplements increase cancer risk. The supplements mentioned in this chapter should be only used to raise vitamin levels to correct deficiencies and bring levels to their optimal level for metabolic function. While vitamin D levels between 100 and 200 nmol/L are probably not associated with increased risk, vitamin B_6, folate, and B_{12}, have U-shaped curves for risk, with increased risk at both low and high levels.[820] The best source of vitamin B_6 is a healthy diet. Most American adults do not get enough sunlight to form sufficient vitamin D. Vitamin B_{12} inadequacy is common in vegans and in the elderly. The elderly often have difficulty in absorbing vitamin B_{12}.

Getting Better Sleep

Fatigue is no fun. Sleep disturbances, such as sleep apnea, are medical conditions that require treatment. Most sleeping medications, however, do not restore normal sleep cycles and should be avoided. If an adult dedicates eight hours to their pillow and still does not get sufficient quality sleep to wake feeling refreshed, there is a problem that should be addressed.

Waking in the wee hours of the night with worries and ruminations is a common sign of depression. These symptoms recover with treatment. Snoring and OSA should be treated early to prevent fibrosis of the muscles of the throat that worsen this condition.

ADHD (Attention Deficit Hyperactivity Disorder) should be assumed to be a sleep disorder or secondary to sleep deprivation until proven otherwise. At least 50% of children with ADHD have sleep disorders; it is safe to assume that sleep deprivation causes a similar effect on college students and adults. For children, just adhering to a calm evening and bedtime routine, lowering of the lights, avoiding electronic screen exposure in the evening, and having a set bedtime with a routine of tooth brushing, a warm bath, a story, hugs and kisses, and lights out, improves the symptoms of ADHD.

Exercise: Getting sufficient physical activity during the day helps with sleep. Part of this may be the brief rise and subsequent lowering of IL-6 levels that occur with exercise. Exercise helps improve sleep efficiency and decreases sleep fragmentation in the elderly.[781] Vigorous or strenuous exercise, however, should be completed several hours before regular sleep time, preferably before 2 P.M., as it stimulates wakefulness.

Obesity: Sleep deprivation is an important cause of obesity. Obesity increases the risk of snoring and sleep apnea and thus, can worsen the sleep disorder. Treatment of other contributing factors of obesity can also help break the circuit of obesity and sleep deprivation.

Avoid Stimulants: Coffee is a healthy food for most people that, among other things, stimulates the production of antioxidant enzymes and lowers cancer risk. Studies of moderate coffee intake show that coffee drinkers are less depressed, more active, and live longer. Moderate amounts of caffeine (200 to 400 mg per day) are associated with longevity and health (about 2 to 5 cups of coffee a day). Caffeine is the world's favorite stimulant; it is used to ward off sleep.

Our bodies have two sleep drivers, the homeostatic drive that makes us sleepy after we have been awake too many hours, and the circadian drive that responds to daylight. Adenosine is a metabolite that makes us feel tired, and an important part of the homeostatic sleep drive. Adenosine builds up during wakefulness and is eliminated during sleep. Caffeine blocks the adenosine receptors in the brain, and thus, enhances wakefulness. Caffeine does not work against the circadian sleep drive. When taken in the morning or early enough in the day, caffeine can be used to enhance the homeostatic diurnal drive by helping to time activities to the desired alert-awake/drowsy-sleep cycle. Caffeine is a major cause of insomnia when used later in the day. Caffeine in the evening is more likely to cause stomach upset. The irritability, fatigue, depression, and heart arrhythmias that may be associated with caffeine use appear to be the effect of disturbed sleep rather than being directly caused by caffeine itself.

Caffeine consumed in the morning is rarely a problem for night sleepers. But it should not be used less than about eight hours before bedtime to prevent it from disturbing sleep. For the average person, the half-life of caffeine in the body is about 6 hours. If two cups of coffee are consumed after supper at 7:00 PM, 63% of the caffeine will still be present in the bloodstream at 11:00 PM. Persons that metabolize caffeine more slowly than average take longer to eliminate caffeine, and may even have trouble sleeping if coffee is consumed in the late afternoon.

Caffeine causes habituation that can be associated with rebound headaches if a dose is late or missed. To alter a coffee habit, wean the dose slowly over several days.

Chocolate contains some caffeine, but much less than coffee. Chocolate also contains the alkaloid theobromine, a molecule very similar to caffeine, but it contains several times more theobromine than caffeine. Like caffeine, theobromine binds to adenosine receptors, promotes wakefulness, and can cause insomnia. Caffeine is, in part, metabolized into theobromine. Theobromine has a seven-hour half-life for most individuals. Although less active, theobromine also blocks the homeostatic sleep drive. Chocolate can cause insomnia when large amounts are consumed late in the day.

Avoid Nicotine: Banish tobacco. Not only is tobacco highly addictive and carcinogenic, but it is also a stimulant that can disturb sleep. Nicotine can reset the circadian clock to the wrong time.

Avoid Alcohol: Although alcohol is often used to self-medicate to help initiate sleep, it is not an effective agent for treating insomnia. Alcohol use impedes deep, restorative sleep stages and causes fragmentation of rapid eye movement (REM) sleep. Alcohol consumption desynchronizes circadian rhythms, thus making regular sleep more difficult.[821] Alcohol also prevents light from resetting the circadian clock.[822] This adds to the risk of breast cancer caused by alcohol.

When the alcohol begins to wear off, glutamine levels in the brain rebound and act as a stimulant, causing shallow, non-restorative sleep or wakefulness. Alcohol also blocks vasopressin production in the pituitary, leading to increased urine output, promoting nocturia (nighttime urination), sweating, dehydration, and dry mouth. Alcohol depletes glycogen stores in the liver, briefly raising blood sugar, followed by a fall in blood sugar that causes fatigue. Once habituated to alcohol, stopping its consumption can temporarily induce insomnia and nightmares, deterring efforts to avoid it. Alcohol should be avoided for at least 3 hours before expected sleep time.

Stress Relief: Stress can disrupt hormonal circadian rhythms, and the disruption may continue long after the original stressor is no longer present.[823] Disturbances in the circadian cycle can cause sleep deprivation and poor response to stress. Stressors should be identified and eliminated, or accommodated.

Don't fret: Wanting to fall asleep not only makes it harder to fall asleep but also increases the chances of awakening during sleep and increases sleep fragmentation.[824] If unable to sleep, just relaxing in a dark, comfortable environment provides benefit. Meditate on things that make you happy. Clocks should not be visible from the sleeping position, as clock watching keeps sleep fretters awake. Most people overestimate the amount of time they are awake at night; even if you think you are lying awake for hours in the dark of the night, if you are not drowsy or fatigued during the day, you may actually be getting plenty of sleep.

Create a Restful Sleep Environment: The purchase of a well-made, new car, with proper maintenance, care and luck should provide about 4000 hours of service; 4000 hours at an average of 50 MPH gives 200,000 miles, costing about $25 per hour, accounting for typical expenses. A good mattress provides about 30,000 hours of comfortable service at a cost of about six cents an hour. A comfortable bed is an inexpensive luxury and investment in health and productivity.

Make sure your bed is comfortable and service it frequently (turn the mattress according to the manufacturer's instructions, twice a year). Get comfortable sheets and pillows and replace them when they are worn out. Pilled sheets are irritating, and old pillows are uncomfortable and downright nasty, as they accumulate saliva, skin, and dust mite feces. Doctor's orders: replace them. Polyester pillows should be washed every three months and replaced after six to nine months. Memory foam pillows can last from 18 months to three years.

To promote sleep, the temperature of the bedroom should be pleasant and several degrees cooler than the daytime room temperature. The body temperature needs to fall about 3° F (1.7° C) to help initiate sleep and a bedtime room temperature cooler than the environment in which the person spent their day is conducive to this. The room should be dark, and quiet, without distractions. There should not be a TV or computer in the bedroom; reserve those distractions for a different location.

Darkness and Light: Exposure to bright light in the evening and night disrupts the circadian clock through its effect on the circadian sleep driver.

Fluorescent and LED lights have more energy in the blue end of the spectrum than do incandescent lights, and it is this blue light that most potently disrupts the circadian rhythm and melatonin release. Fluorescent light is used in most workplaces, and now they are used in the home. In the workplace, these lights decrease fatigue and increase productivity. In the home, they are used to save energy. Thus, in recent years, household lighting has a greater negative impact on the circadian drive in the hours before bedtime than in the past when incandescent lights were the norm. Use of computer monitors, tablets, phones and televisions adds to the exposure of blue light on the retina in the evening hours.

The image below shows the spectral output of sunlight, as well as white LED, incandescent, and fluorescent lights used in the home. Commercial fluorescent tubes have an even larger peak in the blue spectrum than do compact fluorescent lights (CFL).

Notice in the image that the sunlight has a large fall-off at the violet end of the spectrum; this is UV light, which the human eye cannot see, but which causes the formation of vitamin D3 in the skin, as well as sunburn and skin cancer with excessive exposure. The image also cuts off the infrared spectrum above where we can see it. Note the large amount of invisible infrared light from sunlight and incandescent lights. Some infrared light is felt as heat. For the incandescent light, 90 percent of the energy is wasted as infrared light and heat, and thus, these lights have poor energy efficiency.

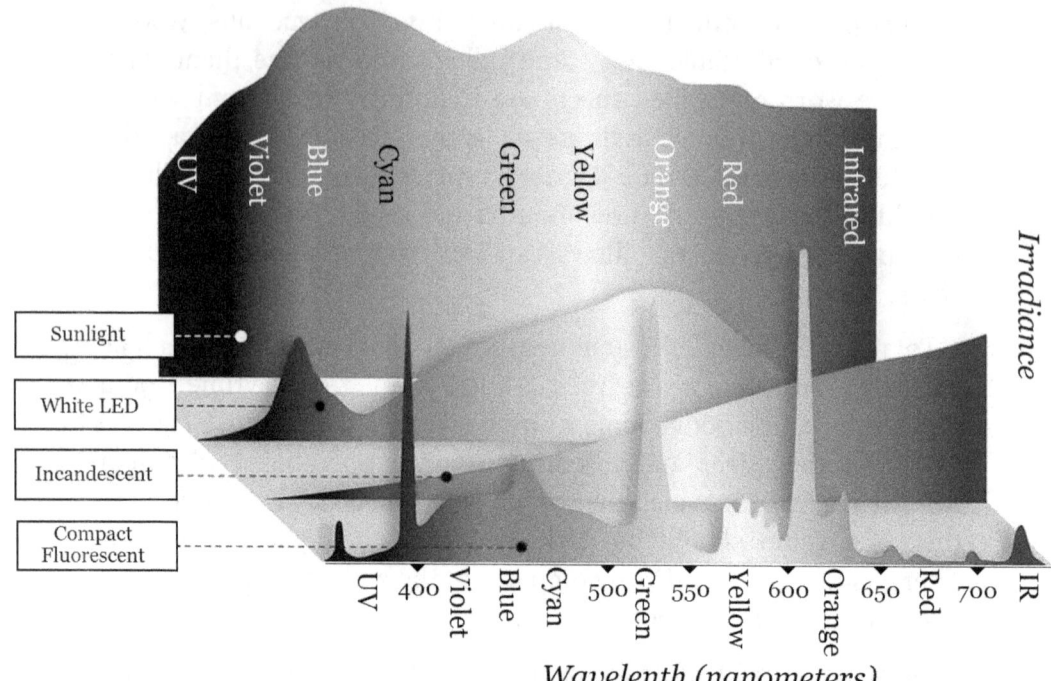

Figure 30-1: Spectral Output of Various Light Sources

Standard white LED and fluorescent lights are made by having a blue or UV light excite phosphors that glow in the green to red area of the spectrum, so that when combined, they give a white light. Depending on the mix of phosphors, the light can be daylight (bluish), or have warmer colors that have more light from the red end of the spectrum. Alternatively, LEDs can create white light by mixing colored LEDs, typically blue, green and red LEDs.

A problem with most white LED lights and all fluorescent lights is that the peak of light in the blue spectrum keeps us awake. Incandescent lights are being phased out in the U.S. to improve energy efficiency. As can be seen in the illustration, incandescent lights have much less light in the blue area of the spectrum and have much less effect on delaying sleep. When children are exposed to the fluorescent and standard white LED lights in the evening, it is much more difficult to get them to settle down and go to sleep. LEDs can be made with dimmable blue content or with much lower amounts of blue light, and controllable ones are available.

The problem with blue light in our homes in the evening is not limited to light fixtures. Televisions, computers, and smartphones also have high levels of light that impede the onset of sleep. Even electronic-paper readers project a great deal more blue light into the eye than is encountered reading a paper book with room light. Do you like to read a few pages of a book before falling asleep? Reading an ebook around bedtime reduces sleepiness, increases sleep delay time, decreases melatonin output, and reduces next-morning alertness compared to reading a printed book.[825] Computer monitors are problematic because of their close viewing and televisions are increasing in size. This should be expected to raise the incidence of sleep and circadian disturbance and their associated disorders, which include mood disorders, ADHD, bipolar syndrome, premenstrual dysphoric disorder, and cancer.

Light Remedies

Yellow or amber-tinted glasses worn in the evenings or night help prevent disturbing the circadian cycle and diminish the decline in melatonin output.[826] They are known as blue-blocking glasses. Yellow (not dark amber) glasses are also helpful for reducing glare when driving at night.

Computer apps are available that automatically change the screen to a "bedtime mode" by diminishing blue light from the monitor at a set time in the evening.[827] These can help decrease the effect that computers and phones have on delaying sleep. LED lights can be made to diminish the blue content in the evening hours or made with less blue light content.

Lighting in a "smart home" could shift lighting to lessen the sleep delay caused by blue light. Lighting at around 200 lux with attenuated blue light that still appears white was found to only lower melatonin 6% more than 3 lux light. This lighting would not be appropriate for most work settings, as there was a decrease in alertness,[827] but it would be appropriate for home use in the evening, and help get the kids calmed down for bed.

Bright light in the mornings and the use of "natural sunrise" can help entrain the circadian clock. "Alarm clocks" are available that gently increase light in the room, simulating a natural sunrise.

For sleep, the bedroom should be very dark to permit adequate melatonin production. If the bedroom windows let in excessive light from streetlights or other light pollution at night, blackout or other light impervious blinds are recommended. Aluminum blinds do a good job of blocking light well, whereas plastic blinds do not. There should be no more light in the bedroom at night than what is required to see large shapes after the eyes are adjusted to the dark.

To avoid blocking nighttime melatonin production, the bathroom should be equipped with a light, for use when getting up at night, that when illuminated allows safe use of the toilet and sink. A dim orange or red LED light, bright enough to use the facilities but that limits light to wavelengths over 550 nm should not impact melatonin output. A dim red LED in a smoke detector should not be a problem in the bedroom.

Napping: Snatching a siesta can help one catch up from a sleep deficit. Napping has anti-inflammatory effects, helping to decrease the level of inflammatory IL-6.[828] Napping is a healthy activity for adults and can be used to increase performance and learning. Naps are an effective sleep supplement that increases vigor and alertness, decreases information overload, and boosts mental performance and memory.

A "power nap" lasting from six to 30 minutes provides mainly Stage 2 sleep; it is refreshing and improves motor skills and declarative memory.[829, 830] These short naps, of less than 30 minutes, avoid sleep SWS and thus, avoid the sleep inertia and grogginess upon awakening that can last 30 minutes. Nevertheless, longer naps that include SWS provide more sustained cognitive performance than do short naps.[831] Napping for 60 to 90 minutes can provide an entire sleep cycle, thus allowing the napper to awaken from Stage 1/REM, refreshed without sleep inertia. A supine position is better than a seated position for napping,[832] as sleeping supine increases the glymphatic flow and clearing of toxins from the brain. Falling asleep in a recliner at night should also be avoided for this reason. It is best to avoid napping after four P.M. or within six hours of bedtime to avoid disrupting the nighttime sleep cycle.

Summary

Night shift workers are at increased risk for cancer, likely because of disruption of circadian rhythms and loss of melatonin output. This in part may be due to meal times that disrupt the circadian rhythm of the GI tracts.

Women with breast cancer, or at high risk of breast cancer from a BRCA variant gene, should avoid night-shift work, and try to maintain a regular day-awake, night-sleep cycle. In the evening and at night, exposure to bright light or light in the blue end of the spectrum can prevent melatonin release and delay sleep onset. Melatonin is a non-recyclable antioxidant that stimulates the NRF-2 Antioxidant Response Element (Chapter 23) and helps prevent cancer. Not only is a loss of melatonin output a risk factor for cancer, but it may also even prevent the efficacy of tamoxifen in preventing breast cancer growth.

Sleep is essential for health. This chapter reviewed strategies for getting better sleep.

Table 30-2: Nap Guide

6 to 30 Minutes Stage 2 Sleep	Quick refresher. Avoids SWS and waking groggy. Use an alarm to prevent oversleeping. A cup of coffee taken just before the nap can enhance awakening with energy as it takes about 30 to 40 minutes for the caffeine to be absorbed.
30 to 60 Minutes SWS Sleep	Generally, *avoid naps of this duration*; they result in waking during SWS sleep and grogginess which can last for 30 minutes.
60 to 90 Minutes Full sleep cycle	Allows a full sleep cycle and waking refreshed during stage1/REM sleep. Use an alarm set for 90 minutes, or use a smartphone app or another device that monitors motion and wakes the sleeper during the light, stage-1, sleep. Phone apps such as "Sleepbot," "Sleep Cycle," or "Sleep" may be used to monitor sleep at night. Some apps can even alert the user that they may have sleep disorders.

31: Breast And Colorectal Cancer Screening

Ductal Carcinoma in Situ

DCIS (Ductal Carcinoma in Situ) is a very early stage of breast cancer. Here, the cancer is still localized to the milk ducts of the breast. DCIS is also known as stage zero cancer. This is the best time to eliminate it. Since it is detectable by mammography followed by breast biopsy, doctors now can detect and treat it when the cancers are tiny. In 2009, 62,000 American women were diagnosed with DCIS. The downside of this high detection rate, early diagnosis, and treatment is that about fifteen percent of these women did not actually have breast cancer, but underwent the trauma of a cancer diagnosis, mastectomy, and treatments for a condition that was not a problem.

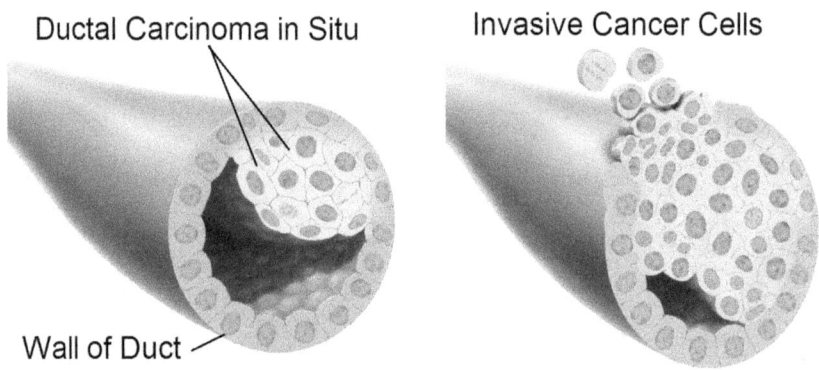

Figure 31-1: The Development of Ductal Carcinoma of the Breast

Cancer Over-Diagnosis

In Korea, the rate of thyroid cancer is considerably higher than it is in North America or Europe. In response, the Korean government began paying for ultrasound screening for thyroid cancer. Between 1980 and 2011 the rate of thyroid cancers diagnosed and treated increased by 15 times. There was an epidemic of thyroid cancer! Nevertheless, thyroid cancer mortality rates were unchanged.[833] Thyroid cancer is a rather slow-growing cancer, and less metastatic than many other cancers. Examining the lack of change in cancer death rates, it can be estimated that around 93% of the thyroid cancers diagnosed through this program would not have progressed and would have never become disease. In recent years, more caution is being used in the screening and diagnosis of thyroid cancer in Korea. As a result, and the number of thyroid cancer surgeries have fallen by 35% in just a few years.[834]

Before mammography was common, finding breast cancer was based mostly on changes in the breast, such as retraction of the nipple, dimpling of the skin, or other changes (See Figure 31-3). Now, 80% of the cases are found by mammography. A difficulty with mammography is that screening determination for breast cancer can be based on small, calcified lesions that look like a few grains of salt. A biopsy follows, and the diagnosis is made from the appearance of a small sample of cells. Sometimes the cells clearly have the characteristics of cancer, and other times, clearly not. Sometimes, it is a toss-up. If you are a pathologist responsible for calling the diagnosis, and the biopsy is neither normal nor clearly cancer, on which side of the fence do you err? A false-negative determination can allow the cancer to progress. This could be a death sentence for the woman and a lawsuit for the pathologist. A false-positive report, however, can inflict significant harm from additional testing, surgical procedures, chemo, and psychological distress.

About 20 to 30% of DCIS that are left untreated progress, becoming invasive breast cancer. This may take decades to occur. Or the DCIS may progress more quickly. Thus, DCIS has a wide range of disease risk.

Mammography screening that allows for early diagnosis of DCIS has increased the breast cancer rates, as some lesions that would not have progressed into an invasive cancer are diagnosed as cancer. Stage zero breast cancer now accounts for a significant proportion of breast cancer diagnoses. This is good, as the cancer is being detected and eliminated at an early stage before it becomes invasive. It is also bad because some stage zero breast cancers are not cancer at all. The incidence of DCIS increased 800% in the U.S. in the two decades between 1980 and 2000.[835] And since it is rather easy to treat a lesion that would not have caused invasive cancer, and call it a cure, breast cancer treatment has become "more effective." Computer-aided mammography is even more sensitive for the detection of DCIS.

While the diagnosis of breast cancer has become more common, the rate of invasive breast cancer has remained the same.[836] Some estimates suggest that 70,000 women each year are over-diagnosed with breast cancer. Forget for a moment the anguish, terror, disfigurement, and financial burden from unnecessary breast cancer treatment; the treatment itself, with radiation and chemotherapy, increases the risk of subsequent cancer and impairs the immune system.[837] Breast cancer is more invasive and deadly than thyroid cancer and screening can save lives, but over-diagnosis of breast cancer causes needless suffering.

During the interval from 1978 through 2006, the incidence of metastatic breast cancer declined eight percent in the United States. However, much of this decrease may have been due to actual improvements in the treatment of stage I and stage II cancers, rather than the result of screening. There is serious debate among epidemiologist as to the value that screening has had on the incidence of invasive breast cancer and its outcome.[838, 839] It is estimated that 31% of the cases of breast cancer diagnosed in the United States in 2008 were "over-diagnoses": tumors detected on screening mammograms that would never have led to clinical disease.[840] More intelligent screening for breast cancer can lead to a lower frequency of over-diagnosis while still protecting women's health.

Understanding Mammography

Mammography is the central tool for early diagnosis and prevention of progression of breast cancer. When cancer is diagnosed early, before it has spread, it can be treated, and usually cured. When breast cancer is diagnosed as a localized (Stage 1) lesion, it has a 98.6 percent five-year survival rate. However, if breast cancer is discovered after it has metastasized to areas beyond the lymph nodes for the breast, the 5-year survival rate is only one-in-four.

The mammogram is an X-ray that looks for features typical of breast cancer. Calcium is radiodense, meaning calcium is less transparent to X-rays than other tissues, and thus, calcium deposits appear as white areas on X-rays. On X-rays, the shadow areas appear white; when the X-rays pass through tissue, it exposes the film, turning the area dark. The bones are high in calcium and this is why X-rays show bones as white areas, while the soft tissues that allow X-rays to pass more easily are dark. The X-ray is thus a negative image of radiodensity.

When cancers grow in the breast, small blood vessels are needed to supply growth; the rapid turnover and replacement often leaves calcium deposits when these cells die. Especially early on, these deposits may appear as tiny specks, like scattered grains of salt. Later, they accumulate and show larger densities, often with typical patterns suggestive of breast cancer. Other injuries, infections, and diseases of the breast can also leave calcium deposits, some of which are similar and others that are dissimilar to the appearance of breast cancer. It is the job of the radiologist to recognize different patterns and identify those that cast a shadow suggestive of cancer.

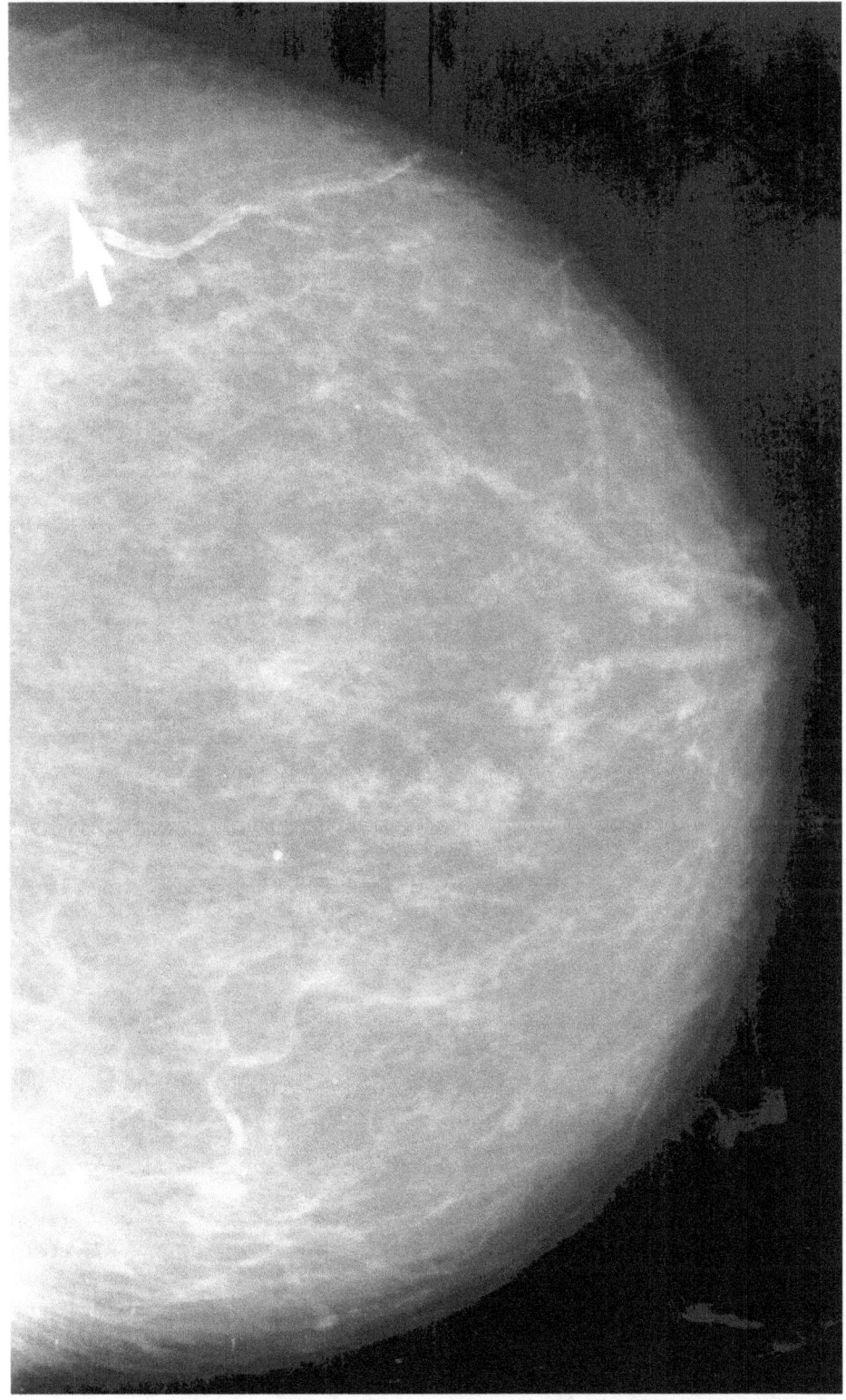

Figure 31-2: Mammogram showing breast cancer lesion

Mammograms are graded into 9 categories that indicate the likelihood for breast cancer. They are also scored into four breast density classes:

Table 31-1 BI-RADS Mammograms Breast Density Scoring

BI-RADS Density Score	Description
A or 1	The breasts are mostly fatty tissue of low density.
B or 2	There is scattered fibro-glandular breast tissue.
C or 3	There is mixed breast density, which may obscure small masses.
D or 4	The breast is extremely dense or has very dense areas. These make it difficult to see small calcifications and thus lower the ability to find cancerous lesions on the mammogram.

Table 31-2: Mammography Category Scoring

Mammogram Category	Interpretation
Category 0: Incomplete	Needs additional information or imaging
Category 1: Negative	Virtually zero likelihood of cancer
Category 2: Benign	Nearly zero likelihood of cancer
Category 3: Probably Benign	Less than 2% chance of cancer
Category 4a: Low Suspicion for malignancy	Between 2 and 10 percent likelihood of breast cancer
Category 4b: Moderate suspicion for malignancy	Between 10 and 50 percent likelihood of breast cancer
Category 4c: High suspicion for malignancy	Between 50 and 95 percent likelihood of breast cancer
Category 5: Highly suggestive of Malignancy	Over 95 percent likelihood of breast cancer
Category 6: Biopsy proven Malignancy	Previously confirmed diagnosis; use for follow-up after surgery

The denser the breast tissue is, the harder it is to see suspicious lesions on a mammogram, and thus, the less sensitive the mammogram is for detecting disease. The four density classes are not evenly distributed. About 12% of women have class A, low-density breast tissue, 45% class B, 35% class C and about 8% class D. Younger women have denser breasts, making mammograms less sensitive to cancer detection in women below the age of 50 by obscuring small lesions. Class A through D density scores are also referred to as Class 1 through 4 density scores (Table 31-2).

Moreover, breast density is related to the amount of connective and glandular tissue (fibro-glandular tissue) present in the breast, in contrast to less-dense fatty tissue. The amount of fibro-glandular tissue in the breast is directly correlated with the risk of breast cancer. More cells, more cell reproduction, more chance for mistakes to be made during cell cycling. Women with the highest breast density have breast cancer risk about four times higher than those with low-density breasts.

Breast density tends to be similar among women in the same family, and it is thought that about two-thirds of the variation in breast density is familial. Breast density is also mediated by obesity; although counterintuitive, breast density rises when weight is put on and declines with weight loss. Additionally, combined estrogen/progestin therapy is associated with increased breast density and cancer risk, while estrogen therapy alone is not. Tamoxifen, an anti-estrogen, lowers breast density and lowers breast cancer risk.[841] Breast density also falls with age after menopause. Breast density is a major risk factor for breast cancer, and as such, screening protocols should take density into account to make screening more effective.

The American Cancer Society recommends annual screening mammography for women age 40 and older, for as long as they are in good health. This view is not supported by most researchers. For many women, annual screening creates unnecessary risk from over-diagnosis and radiation exposure, added expenses, and discomfort.

A protocol for mammography breast cancer screening developed by researchers at the University of California, San Francisco, and the University of Minnesota that takes breast density into account is shown in Table 31-3.[842]

This model is for women who do not carry an altered BRCA gene. Note that this is for asymptotic screening for breast cancer, and does not suggest that any physical signs of breast disease should be ignored.

Under this screening protocol, a baseline mammogram is done at age 40 that acts as a reference point and determines breast density. The two additional risk factors considered in this screening protocol model are:

1) Family history of breast cancer, and
2) Personal history of breast biopsy.

Table 31-3: Protocol for Screening Mammography[842]

Normal mammography at age 40

Density 1	Next screening mammogram at age 50
Density 2, 0 or 1 risk factors	
Density 3 or 4, 0 risk factors	
Density 2 and 2 risk factors	Screening mammogram every 2 years, reassess at age 50
Density 3 or 4, 1 or 2 risk factors	

Mammography at age 50

Density 1, 0 risk factors	Next screening mammogram at age 60
Density 1, 1 or 2 risk factors	Screening mammogram every 3 to 4 years, reassess at age 60
Density 2, 0 risk factors	
Density 2, 1 or 2 risk factors	Screening mammogram every 2 years, reassess at age 60
Density 3 or 4	

Mammography at age 60 and older

Density 1, 0 or 1 risk factors	Screening mammogram every 3 to 4 years. Reassess risk at age 70 and 80. Stop screening when life expectancy falls below 10 years.
Density 2, 0 risk factors	
Density 1, 2 risk factors	Screening mammogram every 2 years. Reassess risk at age 70 and 80. Stop screening when life expectancy falls below 10 years.
Density 2, 1 or 2 risk factors	
Density 3 or 4	

The US Preventive Services Task Force 2015 recommendation for mammography screening states that there is insufficient current evidence to assess the balance of benefits and harms of screening mammography for women aged 75 or older. The utility of breast cancer screening, in terms of years of life gained, begins to diminish after the age of 74 and provides no benefit after the age of 90, as the risks and side effects of overdiagnosis and treatment outweigh any benefit gained.[843] Overdiagnosis increases with age, as there is a higher proportion of slower growing lesions. The risks incurred from the treatment for breast cancer also increase with age. As people age, they have slower healing, more cognitive decline, toxicity, fatigue, ischemic heart disease, and increased mortality as a result of breast cancer treatment. Also, mortality risk from breast cancer falls in relation to other causes of death. Thus, it has been recommended that screening for breast cancer should stop when a woman's life expectancy falls below 10 years.[844] To be clear; this is not a recommendation not to treat breast cancer, but rather a recommendation not to screen for preclinical disease among patients with short life expectancies.

The lower the risk a person carries, the more likely that any positive diagnosis will be an over-diagnosis or false positive diagnosis. Over twenty percent of all breast cancer diagnosed through screening mammography are over-diagnoses. It is estimated that 1.3 million American women have been over-diagnosed with breast cancer over the last 30 years.[840] An over-diagnosis can be devastating, subjecting the women to disfiguring surgery, radiation therapy, and chemotherapy; severe emotional distress, financial hardship, and possible divorce; and increased risk of disease, cancer, and of death; all for a radiographic finding that would have never caused disease. Targeted screening provides more benefit at lower risk. Risk factors can be used to determine who is at risk or how high a person's risk for a disease is. Thus, risk factors can be used to determine screening protocols. Some risk factors can also be used to target lifestyle-associated risks that can be modified.

> Do the Math: Screening can do more harm than good. Screening for disease runs the risk of false-positive results and overdiagnosis. In false positives, the screening diagnoses disease when it is not present; in overdiagnosis, a lesion is present but does not represent a clinical threat that would harm the patient.
>
> Let's assume that two cases in 1000 are false-positives or over-diagnoses in a very *high-risk* population, while 60 cases are true positives. Here, 60 persons benefit from an early diagnosis, but two people are harmed. This gives a 30:1 benefit to harm ratio.
>
> Now let's assume that 1000 women are screened in a *low-risk* population, and two false positive or overdiagnosed cases are diagnosed, but since it is a low-risk population only two women are correctly diagnosed with breast cancer. Here, half the women that have been diagnosed would be treated for cancer unnecessarily.
>
> Cancer and other disease screening should target high-risk individuals and

> be much more cautious with low-risk individuals. Screening can cause harm (such as radiation exposure in the case of mammography, or injury in the case of colonoscopy) and a false diagnosis and treatment of something that would have never caused harm can cause serious injury or even death.

Screening mammography is different from diagnostic mammography, in which case, there are clinical signs suggestive of breast cancer. It is the same test but used to visualize and assess a clinical lesion, such as a breast lump, change in the skin, nipple retraction, or peau d'orange skin. Here, cancer is suspected; the mammography is diagnostic, and the risk of a false positive or over-diagnosis is very much lower.

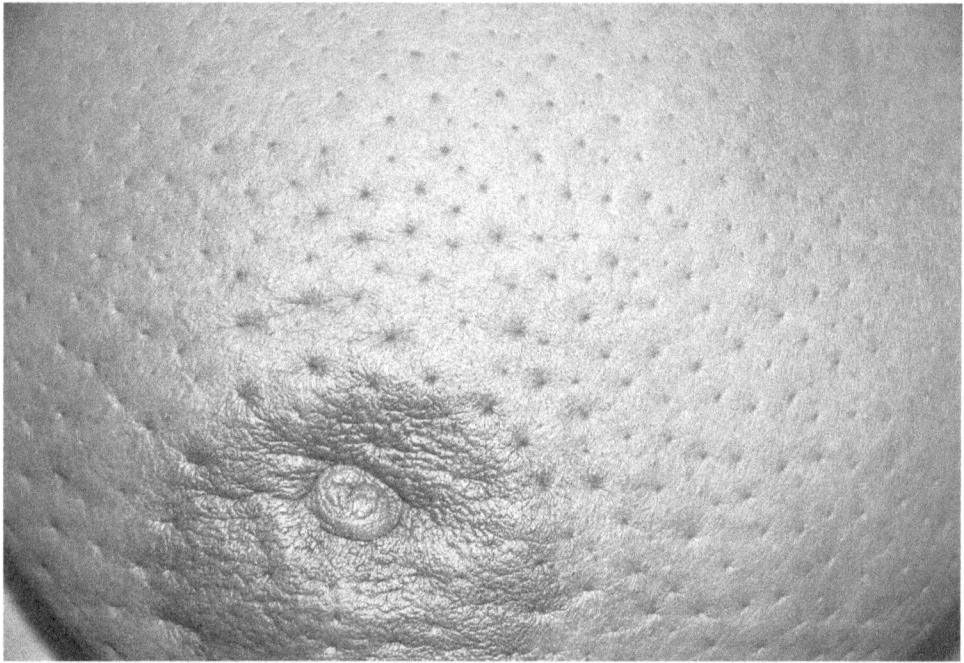

Figure 31-3: Image of breast showing nipple retraction and peau d'orange skin in a woman with breast cancer.[845] Peau d'orange is French for orange peel; the pores appear dimpled in the skin of the breast from swelling due to lymphatic obstruction. This pattern can also occur in cellulitis caused by soft tissue infection.

Colorectal Cancer Screening

In Figure 4-1, it can be seen that colorectal cancer (CRC) mortality in the US has fallen by nearly half since 1978. This decline may be attributed to higher survival rates due to earlier and more efficacious treatment, screening and removal of precancerous lesions, and by a reduction in the incidence of cancer as a result of secular trends.[24]

CRC screening allows detection of early colon cancers, but more importantly, it finds and permits the removal of adenomas, small abnormal growths that have the potential to develop into cancer. Since they sometimes bleed, they often may be detected by stool tests for occult blood (FIT testing). Annual FIT testing and follow-up decreases CRC mortality by 14%. Screening sigmoidoscopy, which is almost as efficient as colonoscopy, reduces CRC mortality by about 28%.[24] However, even now, only half of adults over the age of 50 are screened. Screening and removal of early dysplastic lesions only explain a small portion of the decline in CRC mortality.

> Endoscopy is only as good as the physician performing it. Doctors giving careful colon exams during colonoscopy (CS) and flexible sigmoidoscopy (FS) are more likely to find and remove adenomas. The patients of doctors that have an *Adenoma Detection Rate* (ADR) of over 33.5% for CS (meaning that they find at least one adenoma for every three patients they scope) have a 62% lower CRC death rate than do persons whose doctors had an ADR of less than 23.9%.[846] Patients of doctors with an ADR of over 14.4% on FS had 65% fewer CRCs.[847] How effective is your doctor in finding adenomas? Ask for the doctor's Adenoma Detection Rate before you schedule your appointment to find the most persnickety, meticulous doctor you can for this test. Look for a physician with an ADR over 28% for CS and 14% for FS.
>
> Additionally, schedule the colonoscopy for early in the morning. The ADR falls continuously throughout the day as the doctors become fatigued and begin to rush as they get backed on their schedules. ADRs in women are about twice as high at 7:00 A.M. as they are at 4:00 PM, while the decline in men is about half as pronounced.[848] This is likely true for most medical procedures.

The U.S. Preventive Services Task Force recommends that individuals of average risk, (those without strong family history or other significant CRC risk factors) between the ages of 50 and 75, have annual FIT testing and FS once every ten years. Persons who form adenomas (polyps) tend to develop many and will be placed on a tighter schedule for colonoscopy, while FS, a simpler, easier, and less costly exam suffices for those at low to normal risk. Those who have not formed polyps by the age of 75 are unlikely to develop them. A newer stool test, gFOBT (Cologuard), detects occult blood and DNA markers of colon cancer. It has a higher sensitivity (92% for cancer detection) than does FIT (with 74% sensitivity) and has largely replaced the use of FIT testing. Annual Cologuard testing is paid for for those on Medicare. A downside of improved sensitivity is that Cologuard is that it comes with a higher false positive rate. Thirteen percent (one in 8) positive tests are false positives, leading to more colonoscopies, which carry a low but real risk of colonic perforations and splenic injuries. [849]

Colonoscopy is much more effective at finding polyps, which is essential for those at high risk. CS detects 95% of large polyps, Cologuard 42%, and FIT oly 24%.

Treatment for colorectal cancer has become more effective. The 5-year survival rate for CRC has increased from 51.2% to 65.1% since 1980.[850] This is due in part to earlier detection and more efficacious treatment. Earlier detection and treatment, however, can only explain a fraction of the decline in mortality from CRC. Most of the decline in CRC deaths in the U.S. since 1980, however, are due to a fall in the incidence of CRC as a result of lower exposure to CRC risk factors. Among these risk exposures, is the consumption of beef, which has fallen about 40% over the last 35 years.[26]

32: Breast and Ovarian Cancer Risks

Risk factors for breast cancer begin at a young age. Even fetal exposures to carcinogens can increase risk of breast cancer as an adult. Exposure to breast cancer risk factors should be vigilantly avoided at the times that they impart high risk. To protect women from breast cancer, lifestyle risk-factor management should be implemented by the age of eight. The breast is most susceptible to cancer-causing mutations during growth and cellular turnover in the breast. This can be divided into five periods (Table 32-1).

Table 32-1: Age and Breast Cancer Development Risk

Age	Risk Events
Fetal	Breast tissue develops and may be responsive to maternal hormones. High susceptibility to mutagens and carcinogens.
Childhood	There is very little breast tissue growth and very little risk of promoting breast cancer during this period; however, this period of growth gives high risk for the development of mutations that can cause cancer in other organs.
Puberty: Thelarche to Menarche	This period begins at the onset of puberty and onset of breast development (thelarche) at the beginning of puberty until the onset of menstruation (menarche).
Adolescence: Menarche to first completed pregnancy	During this time, the mammary glands continue their development. Maturation of the breast tissue is completed by hormonal activity that occurs during the first half of a woman's first pregnancy. The risk of breast cancer is related to the number of menstrual cycles that occur during this period, as there is cell proliferation with each cycle. If there is no pregnancy, risk increases until the woman is in her early thirties. Thus, pregnancy at an early age decreases the number of at-risk cycles and of breast cancer risk.
Adult (Premenopause)	The risk of new stem cell mutations is much lower, but do occur. Cancers can develop and grow. About a quarter of all breast cancer is diagnosed during this period.
Postmenopausal Adult	With a decline in female hormone production, risk for new mutations is even lower. However, DNA repair mechanisms and immune function may not be working as well. The accumulation of errors over time increases the risk of cancer development. Hormones, obesity, and inflammation act as growth promoters for cancer cells.

Breast Cancer Risks During Puberty

Puberty is a period of growth associated with the development of secondary sexual characteristics. In girls, the onset is marked first by the development of the breast buds, disk-shaped nodules below one or both nipples. Adrenarche, the development of axillary and pubic hair, usually follows soon after. Puberty in girls usually begins around the age of 11, with thelarche as the first indication. Puberty lasts for 2 - 3 years. Estrogen drives this process.

The age of puberty has changed significantly over the last century. The typical onset of menstruation (menarche) was 15 in 1900. From this comes the traditional quinceañera (15th birthday) celebration in Latin America that marked the transition from childhood to womanhood. The average age of menarche in the U.S is now 12 years 5 months. Menarche occurs at an earlier age in girls that are obese or who exercise little. It also occurs at a younger age in girls raised in a stressful situation, those exposed to cigarette smoke, and in girls who were not breastfed as infants.[851] Obesity causes an increase in estrogen production by fat cells. The epidemic of childhood obesity has caused an alarming rise in early breast development in girls in the U.S. Ten percent of Caucasian girls, and nearly a quarter of African American girls begin breast development by age 7![852] Early puberty puts these girls at higher risk of teenage pregnancy and higher lifetime risk for breast cancer.

Since it can take longer than a scientist's career for cancer to develop, and also because lifestyle history, such as what a person had for lunch 40 years before cancer presented, can be unreliable, indirect markers for risk are sometimes helpful for the study of disease causation. It is known that benign breast disease, which develops in late adolescence, is a risk factor for the later development of breast cancer. It is much easier to study the lifestyle of girls and the association of benign breast disease over the following five to ten years than wait for 30 to 60 years to see if breast cancer develops. Thus, there have been several studies examining the association of the lifestyle of pubertal and adolescent girls with benign breast disease (BBD).

BBD comes in three flavors: non-proliferative BBD, which is not associated with future breast cancer risk; proliferative BBD without atypia, which is associated with a 1.3 to 1.9 times increased breast cancer risk; and proliferative BBD with atypia, which is associated with a 4.1 to 5.3 times risk of breast cancer.[853] The frequency of BBD increases with age until midlife and then falls.

The risk of developing future cancer from exposure to carcinogens during puberty is high. This is a time of rapid growth of the breast's ductal tissues, and exposure to carcinogens imparts risk, especially for ductal carcinomas.

Usually, being tall is a sign of health, and a good thing and obesity is a sign of poor health and not such a good thing. However, short and heavy are associated with decreased pubertal risk of BBD. Both bone and breast ductal tissues respond to estrogen and insulin-like growth factor (IGF-1) for growth. It appears, however, that variation in the expression of estrogen receptors in the breast and bone tissue, rather than circulating estrogen levels, imparts the greatest impact on the growth on these tissues. The rapid long bone growth and early epiphyseal closure of these bones, which stops girls from continuing to grow taller, is correlated with future risk of ductal carcinoma.

The hormonal changes associated with an early age of menarche confer cancer risk. Rapid growth in height during puberty is associated with increased risk of BBD when comparing those with the most rapid growth in height to those with the slowest growth. It is also associated with increased risk of breast cancer. Women who attain their complete adult height by the age of 12 have a 40 percent higher risk of breast cancer than do those who complete their growth after their 17th birthday.[854] We stop growing taller when the bone plates close, and this is triggered by estrogen in both males and females. Although not completely understood, it appears that estrogen interacts with growth hormone and IGF for both the growth of the breast ducts and bones.

Breast cancer risk associated with high peak pubertal growth rate and early epiphyseal closure is probably mediated by the same mechanism as the rapid growth of ductal tissue in the breast. The form of breast cancer most associated with this risk is ductal carcinoma, and it is more highly associated with estrogen receptor-negative tumors.

Consumption of soy products is associated with lower risk of breast cancer. The strongest protection imparted by soy products occurs before menarche. In girls under the age of 12, consuming soy products more than 6 times a month (compared to less than 3 times monthly) decreases the future breast cancer risk by 60 percent. Consuming soy products, such as tofu, just once a week lowered risk nearly this much. Soy consumption during adolescence or adulthood, however, while still beneficial, only lowered risk by about 20 percent and then only when consuming at least eight servings a month.[855] This and other studies suggest that the soy isoflavones have little, if any, beneficial effect on breast cancer when consumed as an adult. Most, if not all, of the benefits from soy consumption, occur from pubertal soy consumption.

There are several different soy isoflavones; several are phytoestrogens, plant-based compounds that can bind to estrogen receptors. Although they bind to the receptors and may mimic the effect of estrogens, they may block or diminish estrogenic activity in some tissues, by getting in the way of more active estrogens. Thus, they may have both estrogenic and anti-estrogenic effects at the same time. It is likely that the estrogenic effect of soy during puberty and growth causes a life-long down-regulation of the estrogen receptor (ER) population of the cells developing ERs. The effect of soy on the breast is most relevant during the thelarche phase of breast development.

Additionally, isoflavones in soy affect the expression and activity of several p450 enzymes that metabolize estrogens into multiple products, altering the estrogenic activity of hormone-sensitive tissues.[856] This activity may increase the conjugation of estrogens, helping to move estrogens into bile, and then out of the body. Thus, phytoestrogens may modify endogenous estrogen levels.

Care should be taken to limit exposure to all mutagens and carcinogens during the pubertal period of rapid ductal growth. It takes both cell growth (division) and errors (which can be caused by mutagens and oxidative stress), as well as impaired DNA repair and cell culling to develop cancer.

There is no evidence that the decrease in risk from consumption of soy isoflavones during early puberty does not apply to women who carry altered BRCA1 and BRCA2 genes. We should assume that soy products provide even greater protection for girls that carry the altered BRCA genes.

There is great variation in the amount of isoflavones present in soy-based foods, depending on their preparation, but also on the maturity of the bean used. Alcohol-extracted soy protein has about one-eighth the amount of soy isoflavones as that processed by water extraction. Mature soybeans have about five times the concentration of isoflavones as do immature (edamame) beans.

It takes about 3 servings of soy milk to get the same amount of isoflavone content (about 8 mg) as one 100 gram serving of soft tofu (about 24 mg). A soy burger has about half as much as tofu.[857]

Breast Cancer Risk Factors for Adolescents

Adolescence is the period between puberty and adulthood. More specifically, herein it refers to the developmental period beginning at the full development of the breast, which roughly coincides with menarche, and the completion of breast maturity that occurs during a woman's first pregnancy.

Pregnancy (to midterm) promotes the completion of mammary gland development. It decreases the number of hormone-sensitive luminal cells and down-regulates the *Wnt*-signaling pathway in basal stem cells and progenitor cells, making breast tissue much less susceptible to carcinogens. The span of time from thelarche to the first completed pregnancy is one of high risk for the breast, as this is the time of rapid growth and cell cycling. The thelarche to menarche pubertal time span is limited to two to three years, while the duration of the adolescence, menarche to pregnancy, can be significantly longer.

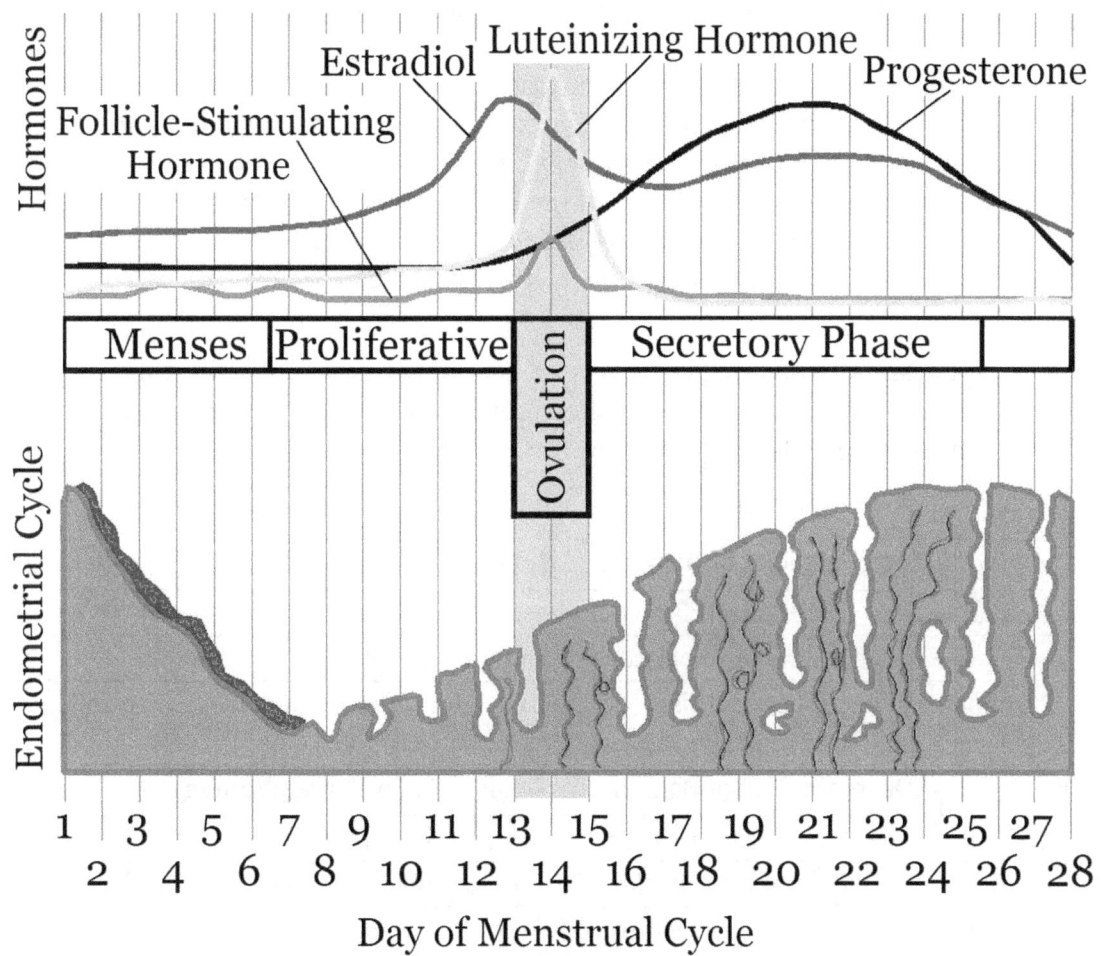

Figure 32-1: Hormonal Fertility Cycle

The breast has a cyclic, monthly variation in female hormone exposure, and this is illustrated in Figure 32-1. Estradiol levels rise during the mid-cycle (days 10 through 15) of a 28-day cycle beginning on the first day of menses. Estrogen increases the growth of ductal cells in the breast. Progesterone and hydroxyprogesterone levels are elevated during the second half of the menstrual cycle (days 14 to 25) and increase the growth of the milk-producing glands of the breast, as well as increasing growth of endometrial glands and blood vessels in the uterus. It is progesterone that causes swelling of benign fibrocystic lumps and tenderness in some women's breasts the week before her period. With each cycle, there is growth, and with this cellular proliferation, comes risk for mutations. The risk to the breast from exposure is greatest during the secretory phase of the menstrual cycle. Thus, exposure to X-ray radiation, intoxication with alcohol, and exposure to HCA in foods are more likely to cause mutations in the breast during these proliferative days: days 12 to 25 from the first day of menses.

Exposures that result in mutations in ductal cells are most likely to occur when estrogen levels are elevated (days 10 to 16). Lobular cells (the milk-producing glands) are most susceptible to mutations during days 14 to 26 of the menstrual/breast cycle. The duration of the adolescent phase of breast development correlates with risk for lobular carcinomas and hormonally responsive cancers, such as ER+ tumors. Estrogen stimulation of the breast ducts has fewer risk days each month than does progesterone activity and its promotion of glandular (lobular) tissue, which last almost 2 weeks out of each cycle.

Several dietary factors have been associated with BBD, and thus are probable risk factors for later breast cancer when consumed as an adolescent. They are given in Table 32-2.

Table 32-2: Dietary Benign Breast Disease Risk Factors for Adolescents

Increase Risk of Benign Breast Diseases in Young Women	
Animal Fat	Increased risk for highest quartile intake (33% Increase)[858]
Meat	Three or more servings a day (50% increase)[859]
Alcohol	Increased risk: 35% increase for 3 drinks per week or more for women aged 18 to 22[860]
Decrease Risk of Benign Breast Diseases in Young Women	
Vitamin D	Decreases risk for highest quartile intake (21% decrease)[861]
Fiber	Decreases risk for highest quartile intake (25% decrease)
Peanut butter and other nuts	Decreases risk for one serving every three days compared to none (44% decreased risk)[862]
Sweet Corn	Decreases risk for one serving every three days compared to none (37% decreased risk)
Vegetable Fat	Decreases risk for highest quartile intake (27% decrease)

Although animal fat appears to be a risk factor for BBD, the studies did not separate the risk from the animal fat from risk from the consumption of meat, and the two are obviously closely linked. Dairy product consumption does not appear to impact the risk of benign breast disease.[863]

Note that while a diet high in vegetable fat, presumably high in n-6 fatty acids, is associated with a lower risk of BBD, this association is no longer significant after accounting for peanuts, nuts, corn, and other vegetables in the diet.

Corn (sweet corn) refers to the vegetable rather than field corn which is used as a grain and for oil manufacture.[862] In two studies, carotenoids were found to be inversely associated with risk of proliferative BBD, but this benefit disappeared after adjusting for vitamin D, nut, and fiber intake.[864]

Breast Cancer Risk Factors for Adult Women

The most important risk factors for adult women are those factors that promote the growth of tumor cells and those that impair the body's ability to eliminate those aberrant cells. After the completion of breast growth and the decline in stem and progenitor cells in the breast, the risk of mutations falls. During adulthood, the major risk factors are those that promote and sustain growth. These include IGF-1 and female hormones for hormone-sensitive tumors. Once cancer has developed and is growing, however, mutagens increase the risk of the cancer becoming more aggressive.

Major risk factors for breast cancer during adulthood are obesity and lack of exercise. As explained in Chapters 12 and 13, these are, in many ways, the same risk factor. They are also part of the same risk factor as chronic inflammation and metabolic syndrome. It is not obesity per se that causes cancer risk, but rather the gaining of weight, elevated IGF-1 and leptin, and the associated inflammatory processes, and increases in circulating estrogen associated with a high-fat, low-fiber diet. A healthy weight-loss, from overweight at the end of adolescence to normal weight as an adult, lowers breast cancer risk.

Inflammatory signaling and inflammatory cytokines, mediated through NF-κB,[865] induces mTOR signaling and promotes cancer growth, invasion, and metastasis. A diet and lifestyle that promote weight gain and inflammation promote breast cancer in adult women. This will be further discussed in Chapter 34.

The US 1870 Census detailed the causes of 492,263 deaths; a rate of 1,276.7 per 100,000 persons. Most deaths were caused by infectious diseases. Cancer was uncommon, with only 6,224 deaths, a rate of 16.1 per 100,000 persons. Breast cancer was listed as the cause of 630 deaths that year, a rate of 1.6 per 100,000 persons. Falling objects killed 712 persons that year, and lightning killed 202.[866]

Table 33-3: Modifiable Breast Cancer Risk Factors for Adult Women

Increase Cancer Risk	Chapter
➢ High Fructose Diet	28
➢ High Fat Diet, especially high n-6 fats and trans fats	25
➢ Sleep Deprivation,	30
➢ Shift work	30
➢ Low amounts of high demand physical activity	13
➢ Low fiber diet	27
➢ High Homocysteine (HCY) levels	26 and 28
Lower Cancer Risk	**Chapter**
❖ Vigorous exercise and hot baths	13
❖ Nrf2 inducers (garlic, phenolic compounds, cruciferous vegetables, coffee, olives*	23, 24, and 35
❖ Extra virgin olive oil, tree nuts*	Herein*
❖ Uric Acid (xanthine oxidase) inhibitors (Flavonoids)	23
❖ A nutritionally balanced diet, with adequate n-3 fats, folate, B12, betaine, and choline, to maintain a low HCY level.	26 and 28
❖ Fasting	37

*In a trial among mostly postmenopausal, overweight, Spanish women that were considered to be at high risk of heart disease, those provided and consuming two tablespoons (about 240 Cal) of extra virgin olive oil (EVOL) daily had a 68% reduction in breast cancer compared to women not given the olive oil. Another group of women consuming 30 grams (about one ounce) per day of walnuts, hazelnuts, and almonds had a 49% reduction in breast cancer cases as compared to the control group.[1] For those who would prefer not to consume that quantity of EVOL every day, four or five green Spanish olives contains a similar polyphenol content as does two tablespoons of EVOL. However, the oleic acid in olive oil may also contribute to its anti-carcinogenic effects (Chapters 25 and 34). EVOL and nuts likely act by different mechanisms; adding both to the diet may lower breast cancer risk even further.

Breast Cancer Risk Factors for Older Women:

Many risk factors for breast cancer, such as the age of menarche, the age at first pregnancy, breastfeeding, and breast density have less impact on breast cancer development among women over the age of 65. Obesity, bone density, and lack of physical activity remain as risk factors for breast cancer. The risk from combined estrogen/progestin hormone-replacement-therapy associated falls within two years of discontinuing these medications. Family history remains a risk factor, which may increase in relevance as a woman's relatives age and risk is revealed. Late menopause also increases the risk of breast cancer by about 6% per year.[867]

> Math note: This does not add a 6% risk of breast cancer per year, but rather multiplies the woman's risk. Thus, for a woman with a lifetime risk of one in 10 of developing breast cancer, a 5-year delay in menopause raises a woman's risk by 3 percent, from 10 to 13%.
>
> $1/10 \times (6\% \times 5 \text{ years}) = 10\% \times 30\% = 3\%$

The modifiable risk factors for postmenopausal breast cancer are similar to those given in Table 27-3. Heavy alcohol use appears to be a risk factor in older women more than during middle age. This may reflect inflammatory, anti-immune, and anti-nutritive effects from alcohol intake.

BRCA1 and BRCA2 Genetics

BRCA1 and BRCA2 germline alterations strongly increase the risk of breast cancer. The risk for BRCA1 alterations is so severe that few women who carry a dysfunctional copy of this gene live to the age of seventy without developing cancer. Fortunately, inheriting a dysfunctional copy of this gene is fairly rare. Among Ashkenazi Jews, a population that has particularly high prevalence, about one in one hundred persons is a carrier of a high-risk BRCA1 allele. A similar percentage of the population carries a high-risk BRCA2 alteration. The prevalence in the general population is much lower, closer to one in a thousand for each of these gene alterations. Very rarely, an individual may have the misfortune of carrying a high-risk mutation in both the BRCA1 and BRCA2 gene.

BRCA1 and BRCA2 gene alterations are not only risk factors for cancer, but they are also risk multipliers. Fifty-eight percent of women with BRCA1 will develop breast cancer by the age of 70, and 34% will develop ovarian cancer. Fifty-one percent of women with BRCA2 will develop breast cancer by the age of 70 and eleven percent will develop ovarian cancer. The risk is not limited to women. BRCA2 alterations increase the risk of breast cancer in men by 80 times. Table 27-4 shows the risk ratio for carriers compared to those without the altered genes. For the most part, the risk factors for hormonally sensitive tissues are similar for women with or without BRCA alterations; these gene alterations just amplify the risk. Thus, alcohol, HCA, shift work and weight gain increase cancer risk in BRCA carriers, but the effect is multiplied.

Table 33-4: Cancer Risk Ratios for BRCA1 and BRCA2[868]

Cancer Risk Ratios	BRCA1	BRCA2
Female Breast	9.1	7.8
Ovarian	31	10
Male Breast	8.0	80
Prostate <65 years	1.82	7.33
Prostate ≥65 years	.84	3.39
Pancreas <65 years	3.1	5.54
Pancreas ≥65 years	1.54	1.61

Ovarian Cancer Risk

Ovarian cancer risk is also highly associated with certain germline genetic alterations. In addition to BRCA1 and BRCA2, there are other heritable germline mutations that increase the risk of ovarian cancer. RAD51 is a protein that helps in the DNA repair process. These are a relatively rare mutation; however, women carrying an inactive RAD51C or RAD51D allele have a 5.2-fold and 12.0-fold risk for ovarian cancer, respectively. The inactive RAD51D allele also increases the risk of breast cancer by 30 percent.[869]

As would be expected, ovarian cancer is associated with fertility, but there is more to the feedback loop than just the monthly hormonal cycle. Surprisingly, to me at least, just having a tubal ligation lowers the risk of ovarian cancer slightly, as if the procedure was telling the ovary to relax, you don't have to work so hard pumping out those eggs each month. Tubal ligation decreases risks of ovarian cancer in women with BRCA1 alterations by over 60 percent, but it is not clear if the risk reduction occurs with BRCA2 alterations.[870]

Childbearing lowers ovarian cancer risk slightly, but there are easier ways to lower risk more effectively. Breastfeeding for a year or more also lowers risk modestly, likely because it temporarily puts ovulation on hold. Early menarche and late menopause are risk factors for ovarian cancer; more ovulatory cycles impart more risk.

The most effective method for ovarian cancer risk reduction is to remove the ovaries (oophorectomy) along with the tubes (salpingectomy). During the process, a woman can also remove the risk of endometrial and cervical cancer by having a complete hysterectomy (removal of the uterus and associated tissues). This is not recommended for most women as means of controlling cancer risk; however, it can be recommended for women with the BRCA1 gene after they have completed their family or around the age of 35 if they have chosen not to, or have been unable to have children. In women with the BRCA1 gene, oophorectomy also decreases the risk of breast cancer by about 50%. Oophorectomy, however, causes the immediate onset of menopause. Estrogen replacement does not appear to increase breast cancer risk in women with BRCA1, nor does current alcohol use. Sufficient data on the risk effect of estrogen replacement is not yet available for BRCA2 carriers.[871]

Oral Contraceptives

Oral contraceptive (OC) use also lowers the risk for ovarian cancer. A meta-analysis of over 20 studies showed that the risk of ovarian cancer falls by 10 to 12 percent for each year oral contraceptives are used, for up to 5 years, yielding as much as a 50% reduction in ovarian cancer risk. The pills with higher progestin levels are apparently more effective in cutting this risk than are low progestin pills. Progestins with less androgenic (testosterone) effect were equally effective as those with higher androgen effect. This reduction in risk also protects women with BRCA1 variants, and likely protects women with the BRCA2 variants.[872]

Oral contraceptives also greatly lower the risk of endometrial cancer, and this risk reduction continues for many years after cessation of use of the pills. Several studies have shown an 80 to 90 percent decline in uterine cancer with long-term use of OC. In one of the most recent studies, which reflect the use of more current OC formulations, use of OCs for over 8 years decreased the risk of uterine cancer by 90%. IUDs (intrauterine devices) also lower the risk of endometrial cancer.[873]

OC use lowers the risk of colon cancer by about 14 percent. On the other hand, oral contraceptive use is associated with a slight increase in the risk of cervical cancer among women infected with HPV.[874] This may be because of an enhanced environment for HPV viral replication.

On the flip side, OC use can increase the risk of breast cancer, depending on the formulation. Birth control pill formulations have evolved with time, and they are not all the same. OC formulations that were used in the 1960's had high doses and provoked high risk for blood clots and thromboembolic events, such as stroke and pulmonary embolism. They also raised the risk of breast cancer. The average ethinylestradiol dose now used in OC's is less than half of what it was in 1972, and some pills use different artificial forms of hormones. These changes in formulations make the study of long-term outcome difficult; the goal here is to make recommendations for women today to lower future risk, rather than to place blame on past formulations.

Some formulations of OC's have the same estrogen and progestin dose in each hormone pill; these are called monophasic. Triphasic OC's contain three estrogen and progestin dose combinations that are used in phases during the menstrual cycle. In the Nurses' Health Study II, OC use and breast cancer were studied among over 100,000 women from 1989 through 2001. In this study the greatest risk was among women using triphasic oral contraceptives containing the progestin levonorgestrel; this formulation tripled the risk of breast cancer![875] In a more recent study examining recent and current OC use, triphasic OC with levonorgestrel raised breast cancer risk by 90% and triphasic OC's with higher doses of norethindrone raised breast cancer risk by 3.1 times (310%). Overall, triphasic OC's increase breast cancer risk about 20 percent more than monophasic OC's do. Overall, OC's raised the risk of breast cancer in recent and current users by about 50 percent.

Low dose estrogen formulations (less than 30 mcg ethinylestradiol (EE)) have not been found to be associated with increased breast cancer risk. Meanwhile, moderate dose EE formulations, on average, raise risk by 80% and high dose estrogen formulations (over 50 mcg EE) raise risk several times. Moderate EE dose OC's with low norethindrone doses were also not associated with breast cancer risk. The following table contains some OC formulations with OC doses that were not associated with increased breast cancer risk in the Group Health Cooperative study of recent OC users.[876] Unfortunately, data on third-generation progestins was not included, and little data are available on their impact on breast cancer risk. Some women may experience breakthrough bleeding on these lower dose regimens.

Table: 33-5: Monophasic Oral Contraceptives with Doses That Are Not Associated with Increased Breast Cancer Risk.

Trade Name	Mcg EE	Progestin	Mg	Maker
Alesse	20	Norethindrone acetate	1.0	American Home Products
Loestrin 1/20	20	Norethindrone acetate	1.0	Parke-Davis
Ovcon 35-21	35	Norethindrone	0.4	Bristol-Myers Squibb
Modicon	35	Norethindrone	0.5	Ortho
Brevicon 21 day	35	Norethindrone	0.5	Searle
Nelova 0.5/35	35	Norethindrone	0.5	Warner Chilcott

These low-dose OCs have been found to be more effective in lowering ovarian cancer risk than high-dose oral contraceptives.[877]

When assessing OC-related health risks, health benefits provided by these medications should also be taken into consideration. These include reproductive planning and avoidance of the many risks associated with pregnancy. OC's are useful for the regulation of menses and decrease dysmenorrhea and the risks of benign breast conditions. Most of the breast cancer risk from OC's is from current or recent use, and for most young women, this risk is low. Some oral contraceptives increase the risk of breast cancer, but this risk diminishes with time, and risk among previous users is similar to never users after 10 years. Since OC's are principally used to prevent fertility, the risk of breast cancer is mostly among younger fertile women, and not postmenopausal women. Nevertheless, OC's are sometimes used in the management of menopause.

For most young women, 5 years of use of *low dose* OC's to delay fertility would be expected to reduce ovarian cancer risk by 50% without increasing the risk of breast cancer. When a woman is done having her children, women may use an IUD for many years of contraception without the need for hormonal contraception. If a woman does choose to use OC's during the years between 30 and 50, low dose OC's should be selected to avoid any increase in breast cancer risk. In women with very high risk of breast or ovarian cancer, oophorectomy may be appropriate after the woman is done having children.

Breast cancer risk increases with the exposure time between menarche and the first pregnancy completed to at least mid-term. During each menstrual/breast cycle during this time span, there is a proliferation of breast cells, and with it, the risk of mutations. Extended-cycle oral contraceptives, such as *Seasonale,* that limit menstrual cycles to only four cycles per year may decrease the risk of developing breast cancer in the future among young women who wish to delay their fertility by limiting the number of ovulatory and proliferative breast cycles. No published clinical study, however, gives guidance on this.

Summary

Breast and ovarian cancers are under hormonal influence, and the age at exposure influences risk factors for these cancers. This chapter describes how women of different ages can lower their risk by avoiding those risk factors most relevant to their age and hormone status.

Women using OC's should be first tried using those forms of OC's that are not associated with increased breast cancer risks. OC's that impart higher risk should be reserved for situations where lower risk medications are ineffective.

33: Bladder Cancer

Bladder cancer gets its own chapter, mostly because it has its own special carcinogens: azo dyes. Azo dye exposure is highly associated with transitional cell carcinoma of the urinary bladder.

Hairdressers have been shown in the past to have an increased risk of bladder cancer. The black hair dyes that were identified as carcinogens were removed from the market many years ago, and the risk of the associated bladder cancer among hairdressers has fallen since that time. Rates remain high in hairdressers, but this may be a residual effect as this cancer has a long latency period. In metal workers exposed to azo dyes, the latency period from initial exposure to the diagnosis of bladder cancer averaged 29 years, with a range of 17 to 45 years. Cancers that were diagnosed in the year 2010 may have been caused by exposure to chemicals banned and removed from use in the 1970's. More than a quarter of the workers that had been employed at a German benzidine production facility that was shut down in the 1960's, presented with bladder cancer in the 1990's.[878]

Hairdressers also have an increased risk of lung cancer, but this has been attributed to higher smoking rates within this population.[879] Although many azo dyes have been removed from the market because of their carcinogenicity and general toxicity, at least some of the azo dyes that are still in current use as temporary hair dyes have been found to be genotoxic.[880, 881] Hairdressers performing hair-wave treatments more than once a week have been found to have shorter telomeres, suggestive of genotoxic exposure.[882] These workers may still be exposed to significant levels of carcinogens. Home use with temporary hair dyes has not been shown to increase cancer risk.

Some metal workers exposed to azo dyes, used to detect cracks in metal products, were found to have increased bladder cancer risk. Dye is used to help see very fine defects in metals. Some azo dyes are made, or in the past were made, with now-banned, carcinogenic, aromatic amine solvents.[883] Benzidine, a chemical used in the manufacture of azo dyes, is associated with risk of bladder and pancreatic cancers. It was banned from production in England in 2002, and the European Union banned 48 benzidine-based dyes from use in 2006. The U.S. Environmental Protection Agency is much more cautious when it comes to banning substances where there is the potential for harm to commerce. The agency pointed out in 2010 that *some* of those 48 benzidine-based dyes are not likely to degrade into carcinogenic amines.[884] Thanks, Dad.

The azo dyes are used in the production of textiles, such as carpets and clothing; leather; paints; printed materials including paper; inks for marking pens; ink-jet dyes; and pharmaceuticals. They are most potent when inhaled or when the skin is exposed. While they may not be directly absorbed through the skin, they can be metabolized by skin bacteria into forms that are absorbed.[884] House painters, leather workers, and workers involved in dyeing textiles and leather are at increased risk of bladder cancer.

The exposure age of highest concern is for infants and children who are at highest risk for cancer development. One concern is that babies who suck on the corner of their blanket to comfort themselves may absorb some of the dye.[884] Marking pens contain azo dyes and solvents that are not intended to be used on the skin, and should not be used by children to decorate themselves. Unless you wear Italian shoes made after 2006, wear socks that can be washed over those sweaty feet. I have seen feet blackened from the dye from shoes.

As noted above, not all azo dyes are thought to be carcinogenic. Those that decompose into benzidine are. The risk of bladder cancer is particularly high from benzidine, but benzidine is also a risk factor for cancers of the skin and liver.[885] Use of hair dye is also associated with higher risk of non-Hodgkin lymphoma.

Non-permanent hair dye use is unlikely to be a cancer risk factor for adults having their hair colored. There is more risk for hairdressers who work with it multiple times a day. Nevertheless, hair dye should not be used during pregnancy or during lactation. This is especially true for women who work as hairdressers. "Progressive" hair dyes that gradually darken the hair contain lead acetate. They are labeled "not to be used" on the mustaches or eyebrows. Some hair dyes contain p-phenylenediamine (PPD) that is activated with hydrogen peroxide. PPD is a sensitizer that can cause severe, even life-threatening, allergic reactions or blindness. For these reasons, PPD is being replaced by 2,5-diaminotoluene. Diaminotoluene is listed by the CDC as an animal carcinogen and a potential occupational carcinogen.[886]

Several companies advertise non-PPD, natural hair color products that are based on plants. These are usually not permanent and may fade more quickly than chemical based dyes.

Tobacco smoke is the most important risk factor for bladder cancer in the general population. Tobacco smoke contains aromatic amines, including β-naphthylamine, 4-aminobiphenyl, and o-toluidine which are carcinogenic. Polycyclic aromatic hydrocarbons (PAH) present in tobacco smoke also increase the risk of bladder cancer. Truck and bus drivers, rubber workers, mechanics, and other workers exposed to petrochemical combustion products, such as diesel fumes and pyrolyzed oil, are also at increased risk for bladder cancer.[887] Early hair dyes were coal dyes that contained PAH.

Another very potent carcinogen for the bladder is cyclophosphamide. This is a chemotherapy drug used in the treatment of lymphomas and some forms of leukemia and brain cancer. It is also sometimes used in the treatment of life-threatening autoimmune disease. Cyclophosphamide causes alkyl adducts in the DNA that interfere with DNA replication by causing DNA cross-linking. Cyclophosphamide increases the risk of lymphomas, leukemia, skin cancers, bladder, and other cancers. The latency period for acute myelogenous leukemia after cyclophosphamide treatment is 3 to 9 years, and it is 4.5 years for bladder cancer.[878]

Bladder cancer risk is lower in men who drink six cups of water a day. This is likely because the water dilutes the carcinogenic compounds and encourages voiding the bladder more quickly, causing lower exposure to the carcinogens.

This may not apply to chlorinated water; drinking chlorinated water for 40 years increases the risk of bladder cancer by 20 percent.[888] This risk is likely due to organic materials (humus) present in some municipal water sources that form Mutagen X, (yes, that's its real name), and halo-acetic acids when exposed to chlorine. Water filtration can effectively remove these compounds.[889]

Read labels and follow directions if using hair colorants. The FDA recommends:
- Follow the directions in the package. Pay attention to all "Caution" and "Warning" statements.
- Do a 24-hour patch test for allergic reactions before putting the dye in your hair *before every use*. A person may become allergic at any time and reactions can suddenly become more severe with repeated use. Not having a reaction does not guarantee that a person will not have an allergic reaction the next time they use the dye.
- Wear gloves when applying hair dye.
- Don't leave the hair dye on the head longer than the directions state.
- Rinse the scalp thoroughly with water after use.
- Never mix different hair dye products. This can hurt your hair and scalp.
- Never use hair dye to dye your eyebrows or eyelashes. This can harm the eyes. It may cause blindness. The FDA *does not* permit the use of hair dyes on eyelashes and eyebrows.

34: MTOR

Work on this book was progressing fairly easily until it came time to explain mTOR. There was not a nice path for avoiding mTOR, a protein central to understanding cancer. It had come to the point where it needed to be discussed, but I avoided it for weeks. Instead, I studied the parasites of parasites, read about lipid production in the organelles of toxoplasmosis, and studied the effects of domestic quantitative easing on international inflation. I raked my yard. I went to hear the Brooklyn Riders in a midday concert and listened to a steel drum orchestra. Then, there was an Ansel Adams photography exhibit just across the state line I did not want to miss. I wrote letters and called friends I had not spoken to in 20 years. I took macro photos of thistle flowers. I went zip-lining 60 feet over a alligator-filled lake. I found energy and motivation to do all sorts of activities to avoid this Chinese puzzle with its variety of interlocking parts. Did I mention that mTOR is both central and complex?

This is my attempt to make it simple.

The enzyme mTOR acts within two different enzyme complexes: mTOR Complexes 1 and 2. The enzyme complex mTORC1 is a central mediator of protein synthesis and cell reproduction, autophagy, and programmed cell death. It is the great decider between expansion, contraction, and dissolution. When the enzyme complex mTORC1 is activated, it increases the translation of DNA into messenger RNA (mRNA), thereby increasing protein and lipid synthesis. Additionally, it decreases autophagy (the turn-over of older proteins in the cell), blocks apoptosis and decreases insulin sensitivity so that more glucose is available to fuel the cell's growth and for forming proteins and lipids. MTORC1 helps move the cell through the cell growth cycle.

You might want to read that paragraph again. Did you notice the part about decreased insulin sensitivity and increased glucose availability? It sounds a lot like Metabolic Syndrome. MTORC1 hyperactivity occurs in insulin resistance, obesity, and type 2 diabetes. MTORC1 decreases insulin sensitivity, increases lipid (fat) production and increases the reproduction cells, including fat cells. It is involved in the aging process as it impedes the elimination of old proteins and organelles from the cell and the elimination of old worn-out cells.

MTORC1's normal role is to promote growth and repair; but, if things go amiss, it can also do a swell job of promoting cancer proliferation, as well as obesity, diabetes, and other metabolic syndrome diseases. The same system that helps us grow helps promote the diseases of aging.

The mTOR complexes are present in normal cells; however, their activity is kept at a very low level except when stimulated by growth factors. Some of the signals that inhibit mTORC1 and its activities include low energy availability, lack of certain amino acids, hypoxia (low oxygen state), or damaged DNA.

One might imagine that proteins used to promote cell division would only be produced by the cell when by growth factors, hormones signal for growth. But these are multipurpose proteins and protein renewal in the cell is constantly and rapidly occurring. Thus, like many cell regulators, mTOR protein is always available but is inhibited. Its function is turned off, like a car in the driveway, ready to take you to work. You just need a key to turn it on.

The key to turning mTOR on requires a cascade of events that may include growth factors, hormones, and enzymes that keep the process in balance (at least when everything is behaving). Thus, many of the proteins are ready to go, but their activity is blocked; similar to how the little plastic safety caps inserted into electrical sockets keep toddlers from sticking paper clips into them. You need to pry out the safety cap before you can plug in the vacuum cleaner. Having multiple inhibiting proteins allows multiple factors to act as checks and balances in mTORC1 activity.

If the cell decides to undergo mitosis and split into new cells, it first needs to make sure that everything is ready. One would not want to begin building a house and then find out, half-way into the building project, that there were blunders in the blueprints, a scarcity of copper wire for wiring, a paucity of pipes for the plumbing, a shortage of shingles or sheetrock, or a deficit of doors. What good is a half-built house that cannot be occupied except by roaches and raccoons? MTORC1 acts like a general contractor, making sure that everything is ready before protein production starts and before the cell moves from the resting G1 phase of the cell cycle into the reproduction phase (described in Chapter 5).

The inhibitors of mTORC1 prevent its activation until there are cellular signals indicating that there are no gross errors in the DNA and that there are adequate protein and energy supplies to support growth. MTOR also signals for the growth of new blood vessels to support growing tissues. Thus, mTORC1 integrates several signals and coordinates the decision for the cell to hold-off or commit to reproduction.

> MTOR is named after a chemotherapy agent; it stands for mammalian "Target of Rapamycin". Rapamycin is an antibiotic that was derived from a soil bacterium that causes protein binding with mTOR in a way that prevents mTOR's activation.

We want to be able to grow, repair injured tissue, and replace worn-out cells. We don't want unregulated or cancerous cell growth. Thus, the multiple factors and proteins involved in regulating mTOR are essential to control abnormal growth and development.

Upstream of mTOR activation are the various hormones, enzymes, proteins, and other compounds that activate or inhibit mTOR activity. Downstream from mTOR are the proteins mTOR activates, and these proteins promote cell growth.

TIME OUT!!!

If you are not interested in molecular biology, or just want to wait for another day when you have more time to savor the delicious details, feel free to skip ahead to the next chapter. A summary is given, followed by how the information may be used to prevent cancer and slow its growth.

The mTORC1 complex is composed of several proteins. First and foremost is mTOR. The other proteins include raptor (regulatory-associated protein of mTOR, aka RPTOR or raptor), MLST8 (mammalian lethal with SEC13 protein 8), PRAS40, and DEPTOR.

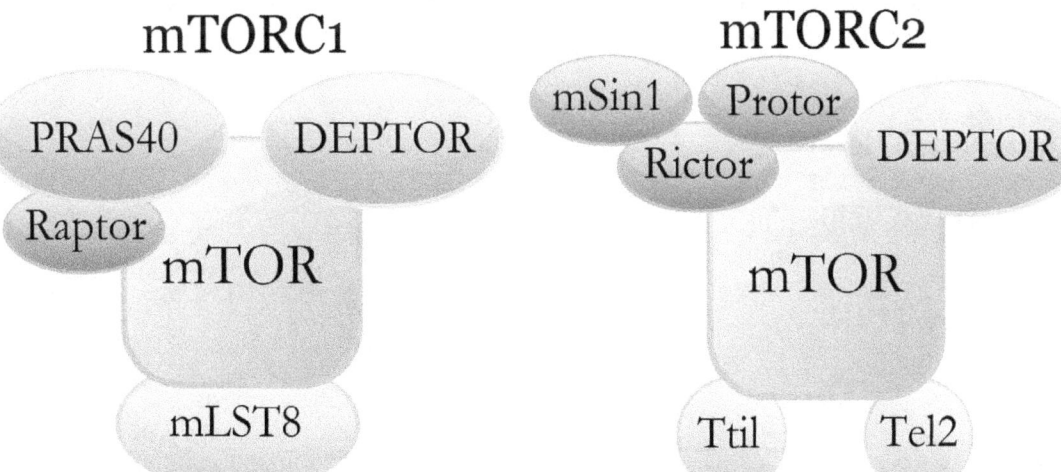

Figure 34-1: MTOR Complexes 1 and 2. (Blue indicates that the protein in its inactive state inhibits activity, red promotes.

PRAS40 and DEPTOR are inhibitors of mTOR for mTORC1. Raptor acts as a sensor for nutrients and mitochondrial uncoupling, mLST8 promotes cell growth, by phosphorylating 4E-BP1, blocking its hold on EIF4e, and thus increasing mRNA transcription.[890][891]

MTORC2 is less well understood but also participates in cell growth regulation. It shares some overlap in its activation but has different downstream activities. MTORC2 likely helps in the regulation of insulin response and glucose uptake by cells, promotes cell survival, and participates in cell cytoskeletal organization.

The mTORC2 complex may control cell structure and polarity. It is likely not insignificant that most human cancers occur in polar cells – cells that require proper orientation to function correctly, such as those lining the mucosa and glands. Installing these cells upside-down would be like installing a toilet upside; it doesn't work. But cancer cells don't build working organs; they are unregulated growth. In many cancers, mTORC1 is overactive but mTORC2 appears underactive. Normally, activation of S6K by mTORC1 inhibits DEPTOR and thus activates mTORC2. CaMKKβ activation may promote mTORC2 activity over that of mTORC1. The TTI1 and TEL2 proteins components of mTORC2 help repair and may elongate the telomeres of the DNA, allowing a greater number of cell reproductions. Our discussion will focus on mTORC1.

What mTOR Does

First, let's start with the downstream effects of mTOR. Two proteins activated by mTORC1, the proteins eIF4E and S6K1 are of particular interest as they increase mRNA translation, the biogenesis of ribosomes for the manufacture of proteins, initiate protein production, and promotes cell replication, all of these things are needed for growth.

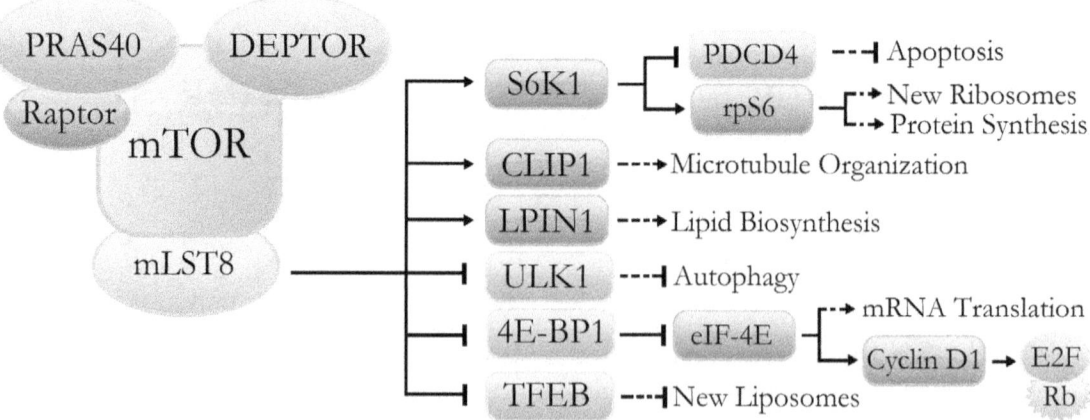

Figure 34-2: MTORC1 Downstream Activities.[892] See also Table 34-1.

Table 34-1: MTORC1 Downstream Activity

mTOR Complex 1	Inhibits 4E-BP1 and TFEB, and promotes S6K1, CLIP, and LPIN1. Together, these factors promote new protein and lipid production and prepare the cell for replication. It inhibits autophagy and apoptosis, promotes energy use and the growth of new blood vessels.
S6K1	Promotes the formation of ribosomes and mRNA reading by the ribosome via rpS6 activation. Causes the degeneration of PDCD4, thus preventing apoptosis. Blocks RBX1, thereby inhibiting ubiquitination and protein recycling.
PDCD4	Programmed cell death protein-4 promotes apoptosis
CLIP	Promotes microtubule assembly for mitosis
LPIN1	Lipin1 Promotes the generation of new lipids for cell membranes
ULK1	In its inactive form, ULK1 prevents autophagy, recycling of intracellular proteins and organelles. During G1, the cell can build up enough proteins for two cells.
4E-BP1	A protein that is normally present in the cell that inhibits eIF4E activation.
eIF4E	Removes a hairpin segment from newly transcribed mRNA allowing it to enter the ribosome and begin protein translation. Promotes Cyclin D1 activation that frees Rb from E2F. Rb then allows the cell to move into the S phase.
E2F	Binds to Rb, preventing the cell from moving into the S phase. Once activated, it also induces Cyclin A and E that help move the cell through G2 and mitosis.
Rb	A protein that acts as an energy auditor and prevents cell growth until there is evidence of sufficient energy and protein supplies.
TFEB	A transcription factor for the creation of lysosomes. Lysosomes recycle unwanted cell parts. Suppressed for cell reproduction.

A key protein activated by mTORC1 is S6K1. S6K1 increases the formation of ribosomes for protein manufacture, and together with eIF4E, activates ribosomal reading of the mRNA. Thus, S6K1 and eIF4E together provide a double check, impeding protein production, until both are activated. S6K1 also has other potent activities. It causes degeneration of the protein PDCD4 (programmed cell death protein 4). Eliminating PDCD4 prevents the cell from undergoing apoptosis. Additionally, it blocks the activity of RBX1, a protein involved in the ubiquitination of proteins in the cell; thus, S6K1 activation prevents ubiquitination and the removal of older proteins from the cell, as the cell is now trying to accumulate enough proteins for two cells.

S6K1 activation signals for a decrease in the number of insulin receptors in some cells and blocks the activity of glycogen synthase, preventing storage of glucose as glycogen. Both these actions cause elevation of the blood sugar and liberate more energy for cell growth.

S6K1 activation is part of the mechanism by which insulin resistance increases the risk of cancer. Excess dietary protein, branched chain amino acids BCAA in particular, may support obesity, insulin resistance, and cancer promotion. The BCAA include leucine, isoleucine, and valine.

The branched-chain amino acids make up about 40 percent of the essential amino acid mass; about 35 percent of the mass of muscle protein is composed of BCAA. Thus, a paucity of the branched chain amino acids would be an accurate indicator to the cell that there is an insufficient supply of amino acids to embark on a protein-building project. The presence of insulin indicates that sufficient glucose is available to serve energy needs for the building of proteins and creation of lipids required for cell new membranes; both of these are energy intensive processes. Glucose is the primary energy source for this.

Certain amino acids increase mTORC1 activity. Specifically, leucine increases mTORC1 activity by about 60%. Leucine causes a non-enzymatic interaction of inositol polyphosphate multikinase (IPMK). IPMK is an mTOR cofactor involved in maintaining the binding of mTOR with raptor; leucine-mediated signaling stimulates mTOR activation by stabilizing mTOR:raptor binding in the mTORC1 complex [893] The amino acid leucine is required for S6K1 activation.

Leucine helps with protein production, muscle function and repair, and cognitive function.[894] Branched chain amino acid supplements are used in very ill patients to help them recover as they help with cell growth and rebuilding muscle mass.

The enzyme 4E-BP1 is inhibited by mTORC1 activation. Inhibition of 4E-BP1 (the safety cap), allows activation of eIF4E (eukaryotic translation initiation factor 4E), an enzyme that clips a hairpin-shaped loop off the end of messenger RNA (mRNA) that has been transcribed from the DNA. This hairpin loop (microRNA) prevents the mRNA from being threaded into the ribosome, and thus prevents translation of the mRNA into protein. Activation of eIF4E not only requires mTOR but also requires the presence of insulin plus a BCAA. However, mTORC1 and leucine can activate eIF4E activity without insulin.

EIF4E also promotes the export of cyclin D mRNA out of the nucleus into the cytosol, so that it can be transcribed into protein. Cyclin D protein, returning to the nucleus, promotes the hyperphosphorylation of Rb, causing it to be released from the Dimer Rb:E2F Multiplex (a.k.a. the DREAM complex), that has kept the cell sleeping in the G1 phase. The release of E2F allows Rb to move the cell past the G1 checkpoint that audits for DNA damage, and into the S phase of DNA replication. E2F also promotes the activation of Cyclin E and Cyclin A that help move the cell through cell division.

Another protein, TFEB, is inactivated by mTORC1 activation. TFEB is a transcription factor for the creation of lysosomes, the recycling centers for cells. Activation of TFEB increases the number of lysosomes and thus, increases autophagy of older and worn-out proteins and organelles in the cell. During growth, the cell is trying to make enough proteins for two cells, not eliminate redundant ones.

MTORC1 activation increases the transcription of the hypoxia-inducible factor 1A (HIF1A). S6K1 inhibition of RBX1 helps activate HiF1A. Hypoxia usually keeps cells from growing and differentiating. In most situations, one does not want to waste energy or risk having a bunch of starving cells that can't get enough blood or oxygen to survive. HIF1A, however, allows some cells, such as those in the growth plate of bones, to survive in low oxygen conditions.

Under normal oxygenation, HIF1A is inactivated and degraded through ubiquitination. When stabilized by mTORC1 activity, HIF1A stimulates glycolysis (via FOXO1 activation). Glycolysis, while inefficient, allows ATP production independent of oxygen level. NF-κB, a transcription factor for inflammatory proteins, can stabilize HIF1A even when oxygen levels are below normal. This allows inflammatory white blood cells to do their work, even if the oxygen supply in the area is lower than normal. Unfortunately, the mTOR → HIF1A→ Glycolysis cascade also allows cancerous tumors to survive in lower oxygen conditions.

HIF1A also induces the formation of VEGF (vascular endothelial growth factor) that promotes angiogenesis. The formation of new blood vessels is essential for the development of the vasculature in embryos, and VEGF is essential for the growth of new tissues and healing after injuries. VEGF also allows for delivery of a new blood supply to support tumor growth and invasiveness. Without VEGF, tumors don't usually get larger than the size of a pea. They just can't grow very large without having their own blood supply.

> Phenethyl isothiocyanate (PEITC), a naturally occurring isothiocyanate product of gluconasturtiin, is present in some cruciferous vegetables. (PEITC) inhibits HIF1A, perhaps through suppression of NF-κB.[895] This is one of the ways that cruciferous vegetables prevent and help limit the growth of cancers.

In summary, mTOR activation supports cell reproduction. It is central to cancer cell proliferation. mTOR activation slows the recycling of old proteins, prevents apoptosis, and promotes the growth of new blood vessels. Activation of mTOR increases the availability of glucose and promotes protein and lipid production. The downstream activity of mTOR depends on an adequate supply of branched-chain amino acids, and most critically of leucine and glucose supply.

Upstream Activation of mTORC1

Now that we have an idea of what mTORC1 does, let's see what motivates it. mTOR activation is modulated by several proteins.

MTOR is encased in several proteins that together form the mTOR complex 1 (mTORC1). Some of these proteins keep mTOR from being activated and modulate where and when mTOR is active. mTOR activation requires the simultaneous disinhibition of these proteins. This process allows rapid activation, but also provides redundant protection from activation.

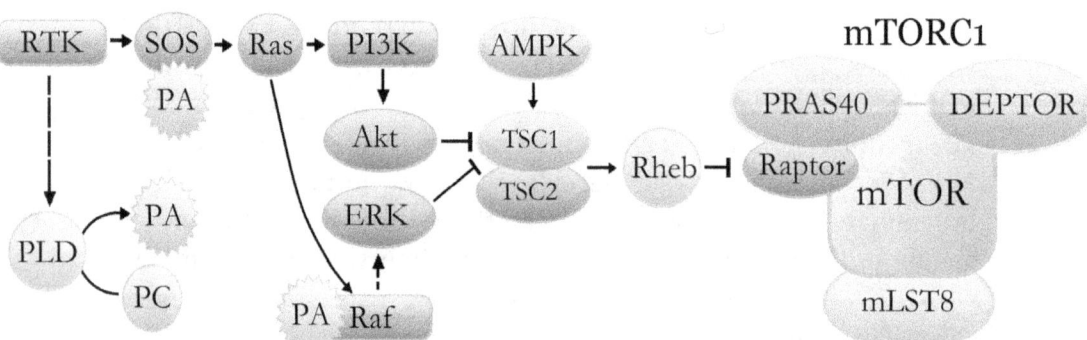

Figure 34-3: Upstream Activation of mTORC1.
Arrows promote, T's inhibit, and dashes indicate intermediate steps.

The protein complex, TSC1:TSC2, prevents mTOR activation. When TSC1 is bound to TSC2 it keeps the enzyme TSC2 from converting active Rheb-GTP to inactive Rheb-GDP; Rheb-GTP stops mTOR activity, so inactivation of Rheb-GTP by TSC2 activates mTOR. Separating TSC1 from TCS2 starts the mTOR activation cascade. It's all so very simple! Once TSC2 is free from the restraints of TSC1, it inactivates Rheb, and this activates mTORC1.

The central factor controlling <u>deactivation</u> of mTORC1 is AMPK. Intracellular stress, such as hypoxia, low glucose levels, and several other factors inactivates mTORC1 via AMPK.

AMPK, when activated, strengthens the bond between TSC1 and TSC2, thus preventing the dissolution of the TSC1:TSC2 complex, and mTOR activation, illustrated in Figure 34-4. AMPK activation also causes the mTORC1 to disassociate from the lysosome membrane where it exerts its effect, thus incapacitating it further.

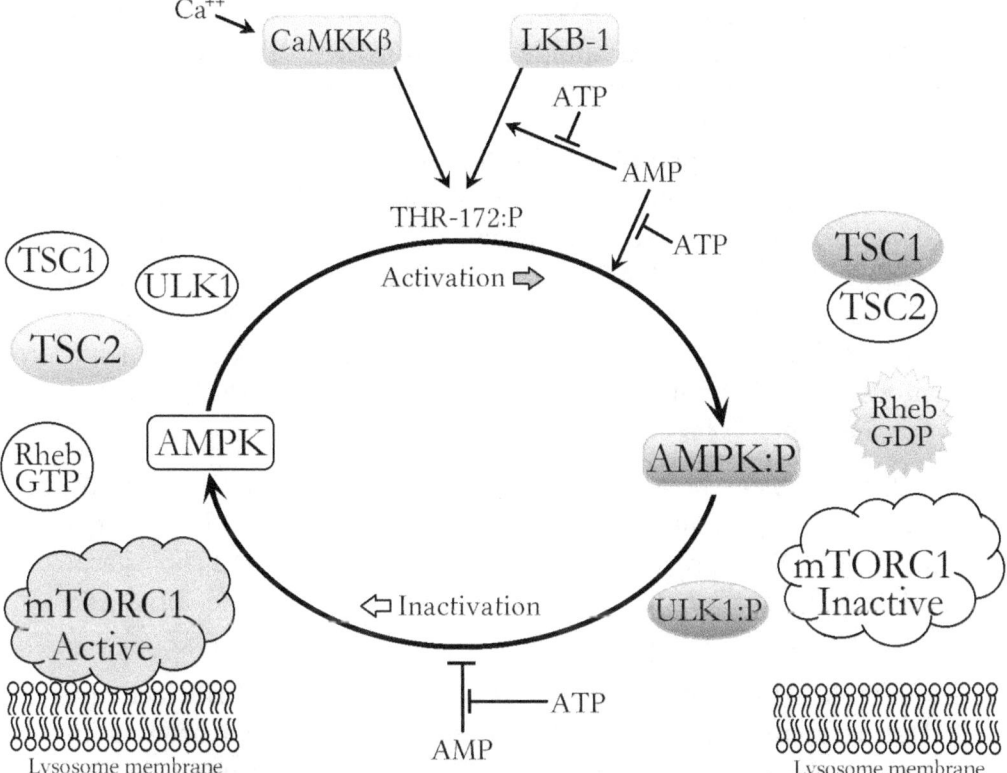

Figure 34-4: AMPK activation by the addition of a phosphate group.
White indicates inactive, and tinted active, states. Activated AMPK strengthens the bond of TSC1 to TSC2, thus preventing the activation of mTORC1. When mTORC1 is active, it sits on the lysosome membrane, inactivating the recycling of proteins and lipids. Activation of AMPK also activates ULK1 that promotes autophagy.

AMPK, in turn, is activated and inactivated by other proteins and processes. *If we can hack the activation of AMPK, we can control a central factor in cancer growth.*

AMPK acts as a metabolic master switch that regulates several aspects of energy supply to the cell. When energy levels in the cell are low, AMPK switches on catabolic processes that generate ATP and turns off ATP-consuming pathways such as protein synthesis and cell proliferation. AMPK helps regulate cellular uptake of glucose, the burning of fatty acids for energy, and the energy-producing activity of the mitochondria.

> Numerous enzymes are either activated or inactivated by the addition of a phosphate group at specific locations on the protein molecule, and this activation or inactivation may be reversed by removal of the phosphate group.
>
> Kinases are enzymes that transfer a high-energy phosphate group from a donor molecule, such as ATP, to another molecule, a process termed phosphorylation. Phosphatases are enzymes that do the inverse; they remove a phosphate group from their substrate.

AMPK senses the energy status of the cell through the ratio of adenosine mono-phosphate (AMP) to adenosine tri-phosphate (ATP). When a high-energy phosphate bond in ATP has been depleted, it is converted to adenosine di-phosphate (ADP) and then further depleted to AMP. AMPK (AMP-activated protein kinase) senses this low energy status by the AMP:ATP ratio, and when the ratio is high, activates cellular processes for energy conservation and production. It stimulates the catabolic processes of breaking down fats and proteins for energy.

AMPK also prevents energy consumption by inhibiting unnecessary protein building by constraining mTOR when energy levels are low. It prevents the synthesis of fatty acids and cholesterol which are needed for the creation of the cell and organelle membranes.

Muscle activity is one of the main stimulators of AMPK activity. During exercise, ATP is converted to ADP. ADP is not used as an energy source directly, but instead, one phosphate group from ADP can be transferred to ATP, resulting in one ATP molecule and one AMP molecule. The newly formed ATP can then be used for energy.

$$ADP + ADP \rightarrow ATP + AMP \quad (A2P + A2P \rightarrow A3P + A1P)$$

The effect of exercise may only occur, however, when ATP availability to the muscle is sufficiently depleted that it raises the AMP:ATP ratio to the point that AMPK is stimulated. When an individual is adapted to a moderate exercise routine, this depletion may not occur at moderate exercise workloads. Thus, a variation in exercise routine on different days or vigorous exercise helps maintain the efficacy of exercise in depleting ATP and raising AMP levels.

AMPK is activated about 100-fold by the tumor suppressor protein LKB1 and CaMKKβ in the presence of sufficient AMP. ADP increases AMPK activity by about 10 times, and AMP increases it by 100 times.

AMP can also bind at a second site on the AMPK protein complex, giving a greater than 1000-fold increase in activity of AMPK. ATP inhibits AMPK activity. The concurrent stimulus of LKB1 and CaMKKβ gives additive AMPK activation.

AMPK Activators

There are various ways that compounds can activate AMPK:

1. Mitochondrial inhibitors: These inhibit mitochondrial production of ATP, providing the cell less ATP and more AMP and ADP. These inhibitors may act at different steps in ATP production. Resveratrol and quercetin inhibit mitochondrial ATP synthase. The anti-diabetic medication metformin inhibits mitochondrial electron chain Complex 1 activity, also decreasing ATP production.

2. AMP analogs: These compounds are converted in the cell to monophosphate compounds that attach to at least one of the AMP sites on AMPK, and thus mimic its activity.

3. Direct AMPK activators: These compounds directly activate AMPK. Two agents that have been reported to have this activity are salicylic acid and gallic acid. Aspirin, which has some anticarcinogenic activity against adenocarcinomas, is rapidly converted into salicylate in the body. Gallic acid is found in fruits, black tea, and other plants and vegetables. Gallic and salicylic acid are hydroxybenzoic acids, a class of phenolic compounds. At least 27 hydroxybenzoic acids have been identified in various foods, and some of these may also activate AMPK.

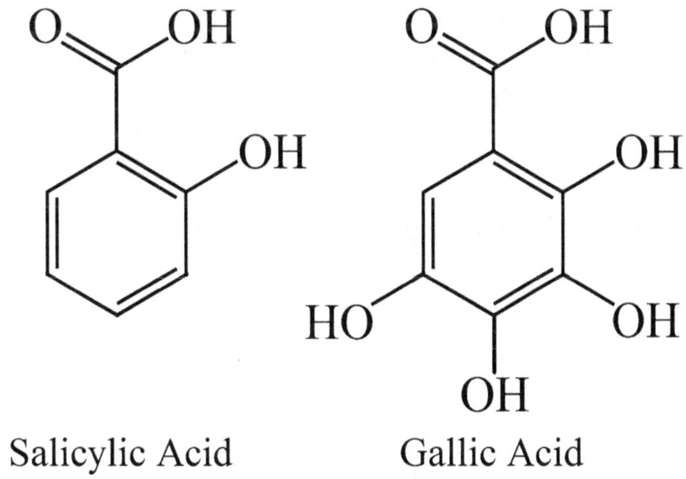

Figure 34-5: Two hydroxybenzoic acids that activate AMPK

> **Hacking and Stacking:** When metformin and salicylate, which activate AMPK by different mechanisms are used together they synergistically activate AMPK.[896, 897] This means that a greater AMPK activation occurs than would be expected as an additive effect of the two agents. Thus, combining low doses of agents that stimulate AMPK activity at different points in its activation may allow a stronger effect with less risk of toxicity.

4. Fat cell hormones: Leptin, the satiety hormone is produced by fat cells when they have had plenty to eat. They signal the brain to let it know they feel stuffed, and it's time to stop eating. Ghrelin is a hunger hormone that does the opposite; it is produced by the stomach when it is empty and tells the brain that the stomach can handle another meal. Ghrelin does not encourage us to eat more, just more frequently. Although ghrelin does not directly regulate hunger, it increases food intake.

Leptin impedes AMPK activity in most tissues. It may do this by stimulating fatty acid oxidation as an energy source for the cell, thus increasing the supply of ATP.[898]

Adiponectin, like leptin, is secreted by the fat cells. Adiponectin, however, is secreted by the adipocytes when they get hungry, as occurs during caloric restriction. Adiponectin activates AMPK. Adiponectin decreases the utilization of amino acids and favors the use of lipids for energy. It also increases the uptake of triglycerides and glucose into the cell. Adiponectin also has an anti-inflammatory effect, as it suppresses AKT and ERK → NF-κB signaling.[899] Adiponectin has been found to suppress cancer cell growth or induce apoptosis in several cancer cell lines. Adiponectin appears to inhibit cancer growth for many forms of cancer.[900] Adiponectin appears to be activated by thiazolidinedione medications, used in the treatment of diabetes.

5. THR-127 Phosphorylation by LKB1 or CaMKKβ: Phosphorylation of the threonine at the 127th amino acid (THR-127) in the AMPK molecule may be activated by either LKB1 or CaMKKβ.

LKB1 is known as a tumor suppressor protein, as it participates in the activation of AMPK, and thus slows the growth of tumors. LKB1 (aka STK11) activates AMPK by adding a phosphate group to the "THR-127" segment of AMPK, thus activating it. Metformin's inhibition of ATP production activates LKB1, and thus slows cancer growth, but only when LKB1 activity is intact. Several cancers have been found with mutations in the LKB1 gene, causing this protein to be dysfunctional.

LKB1 suppresses cell growth and proliferation when nutrient and energy resources are scarce. LKB1 production is inhibited by androgens, so androgens such as testosterone act as growth promoters.

The CaMKKβ protein is a separate, AMP:ATP-independent AMPK activation pathway that, like LKB1, adds a phosphate group to the "THR-127" segment of AMPK, thus also activating it. CaMKKβ is activated by elevation in intracellular calcium. Typically, this occurs as the result of influx through calcium channels. Different cell types have different calcium channel membrane proteins and thus, can respond according to the needs of the cell and its functions. The activation of CaMKKβ requires the protein calmodulin and magnesium.

> Munchies: CB2 receptor (cannabinoid receptor type 2) activation, through calcium influx, activates CaMKKβ. In the hypothalamus, CaMKKβ mediated AMPK activation stimulates the production of the appetite-stimulating hormone neuropeptide Y, thus explaining the effect of CB2 agonists on appetite.

Several compounds have been demonstrated to activate AMPK via CaMKKβ. These include baicalin (a Chinese herbal medication), the flavone luteolin,[901] lipoic acid,[902] S-allyl cysteine (from garlic),[903] and the thyroid hormone T3 (triiodothyronine).[904] Calcium is required for, and magnesium assists in, CaMKKβ enzymatic activity. CB2 agonists also stimulate CaMKKβ. Certain cannabinoids have been shown to have anticarcinogenic properties and likely act through this mechanism.[905] CB2 agonists do not cause psychotropic highs.

When amino acid levels in the cytosol of the cell fall, it triggers an elevation of intracellular calcium and CaMKKβ activation of AMPK. This activation causes the phosphorylation of ULK1 that initiates autophagy.[906] In this way, the cell acts to increase the availability of amino acids to maintain production of essential proteins required for cell survival.

CaMKKβ can activate AMPK even in the presence of ATP levels that inhibit LBK-1 activation. Either a lack of energy in the form of ATP or lack of the amino acids building materials for proteins, perhaps specifically methionine, can activate AMPK and shut down the cell growth cycle.

Choline and Cell Growth

Phosphatidylethanolamine (PE) and phosphatidylserine (PS) activate, but phosphatidylinositol (PI) and phosphatidic acid (PA) strongly inhibit CaMKKβ.[907] This effect likely occurs as PS and PE activate calmodulin. In contrast, phosphatidylcholine (PC) does not activate calmodulin.[908] [909] CaMKKβ signals the presence of low amino acid levels and promotes autophagy via AMPK and ULK1. Since CaMKKβ, but not LBK-1, activation of AMPK signals autophagy, its signal also acts in the phosphorylation and activation of ULK1, an enzyme that promotes autophagy.

PS, bound to the inner lipid membrane, under enzymatic control flips to the outer side of the cell membrane during apoptosis, and here, acts as a "come and get it" signal for macrophages to engulf the dying cell. The enzymatic shift occurs with Fas-triggered apoptosis when ATP is depleted or when 2-deoxy-D-glucose (2-DG) accumulates in the cell.[910]

> Although 2-DG looks like glucose, most cells can't use it for energy. It tends to accumulate in cancer cells, as they have a high uptake of glucose and 2-DG gets absorbed along with the glucose. 2-DG, however, decreases the production of ATP and lactate by the cell, thereby promoting apoptosis.[911] 2-DG used as an oral medication prior to radiation therapy makes the cancer cells more sensitive to radiation and promotes survival in lab animals with cancer.[912]

When sufficient specific amino acids are present in the cell, PS is converted to PC by SAMe. Generation of SAMe requires the amino acid methionine. Thus, in the presence of sufficient methionine, the addition of three SAMe molecules can methylate PS, converting it into PC. PC can then be cleaved into PA and choline by the enzyme Phospholipase D. As stated above, PA strongly inhibits the activation of calmodulin and thus prevents CaMKKβ activation. PA is an important precursor for creating lipids for the cell membranes, as is needed for growing and dividing cells.

If there is insufficient methionine or choline in the cell, PS and PE dominate, thereby increasing AMPK activation via CaMKKβ. When there is plentiful methionine, SAMe, or choline for PC and PLD formation and activity, AMPK is inhibited, and autophagy is down-regulated and lipid construction is active. The amino acid serine is used in the conversion of PA into PS.

Phospholipase D (PLD) transcription is stimulated by various growth factors via both the NF-κB and Wnt-β-catenin/TCF pathways. The product of PLD, PA, is a signaling factor for normal growth, as well as for inflammation and invasive tumor growth. PA has been found to be essential for the growth of colon cancer cells. PA promotes the (Raf→ERK and β-catenin/TCF) induction of protein transcription, including for that of PLD.[913] Thus, it can create a positive feedback loop if left unregulated.

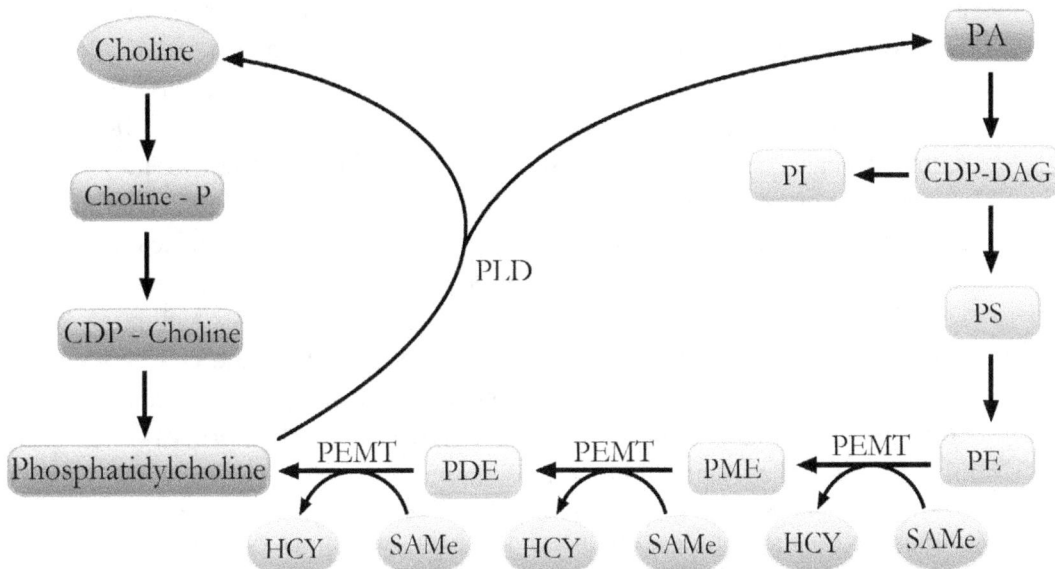

Figure 34-6: Choline – Phosphatidylcholine Recycling

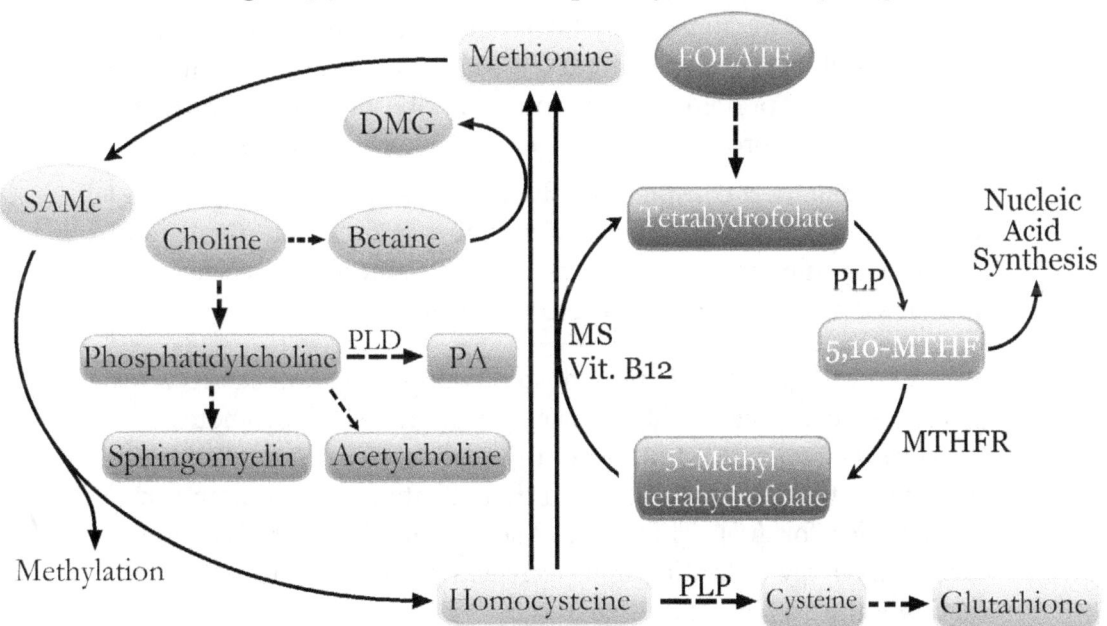

Figure 34-7: Methionine –SAMe – Homocysteine Recycling

Vitamin D3 inhibits the Wnt/β-catenin pathway in colon cancer,[914] and the dietary phenolic compounds, quercetin, and caffeic acid downregulate the transcriptional activity of β-catenin/TCF in human colon cancer cells, causing the arrest of the cell cycle and promotion of apoptosis.[915][916] Resveratrol directly inhibits PLD activity by preventing its movement from the cytosol to the inner cell membrane, its site of action.[917] Other phenolics may act in this same way.

Longevity of lab rats can be greatly increased by dietary restrictions. In early experiments, it was found that a 40% caloric restriction increases longevity. Later, it was found that it was only dietary protein that needed to be restricted by 40% to get the life extension effect. Follow-up experiments determined that nearly the same increase in longevity could be accomplished through dietary restriction of a single amino acid, methionine. Among its other activities, methionine acts as a signal that the cell has a sufficient pool of amino acids to build proteins. A depletion of methionine signals the need to recycle redundant and worn-out intracellular proteins to increase the supply of amino acids so that the cell can make critical survival proteins. This spring-cleaning gives the cell a tune-up and gets it functioning more efficiently. This process of autophagy is likely signaled through ULK1.

> One of the most potent poisons is abrin, which is present in a tropical pea. A tenth of a milligram, about the amount of a single grain of table salt, if injected or inhaled is enough to kill a full-grown man. It would probably take a dose the size of two or three grains of salt if ingested. Abrin and the similar toxin ricin act in the cell by blocking protein production by the ribosome. When protein production can't proceed, the cells begin to die within a few hours.
>
> The cells require a constant supply of amino acids to produce the proteins they need to survive. Methionine and choline depletion signal that supplies are low and triggers autophagy to harvest proteins that are not non-critical for survival.

Lipoic acid promotes the phosphorylation of AMPK. It also promotes the expression of the protein PCG-1α, which promotes the biogenesis of mitochondria, likely through the activation of AMPK. In animals, this increases the utilization of both fat and protein from the muscles for fuel. Thus, lipoic acid-induced AMPK activation increases energy utilization and decreases protein synthesis. It may do this at the expense of muscle mass.[918]

Table 34-5: AMPK Actions

- Inhibits mTORC1, and thus, synthesis of proteins and lipids.
- Activates ULK1, a protein that initiates autophagy.
- Stabilizes p53 and cyclin-dependent kinase inhibitors p21 and p27; thus, it arrests the cell cycle at G1 and prevents proliferation.
- Down-regulates HIF-1α and prevents cell growth during hypoxia.
- Impairs glycolysis in most tumor cells and promotes the energy efficient oxidative respiration in mitochondria that is used by most non-proliferating cells.
- AMPK activation makes life hard for tumor cells.

TSC1:TSC2 Destabilization

AMPK is the principal agent that stabilizes the TSC1:TSC2 complex that prevents mTORC1 activity. But what factors destabilize the TSC1:TSC2 complex? The kinase enzymes, Akt and ERK, deactivate TSC1 and destabilize the TSC1:TSC2 complex. TSC2 is then free to inactivate Rheb, allowing for the activation of mTORC1.

Activation of Akt and ERK begins with RTK signaling. Recall that insulin and IGF-1, and many other growth factors, act via receptor of tyrosine kinase (RTK) membrane receptors that activate tyrosine kinase. The tyrosine kinase enzyme sits on the inner surface of the cell and can trigger a cascade of intracellular events.

One of the common RTKs that trigger Akt activation in cancer is the IGF-1 receptor; however, many RTKs stimulate SOS, which activates PI3K. PI3K causes the formation of the phospholipid, PIP3, which helps activate Akt. Akt activation causes the destabilization of TSC1 from TSC2; Akt also blocks another mTORC1 inhibitor PRAS40. Additionally, Akt activates IKK that activates NF-κB; inhibits caspase 9, Bad, and p53, evading apoptosis; and blocks p27 and p21, thus, promoting proliferation. See Figures 34-3 and 36-1.

ERK can also inhibit and destabilize TSC1. It too is activated via SOS, but down a separate pathway branch only indirectly involves PI3K. Ras activates Raf → MAPK → ERK. ERK not only blocks TSC1, but it also activates c-Fos and c-Jun that form a proliferative form of AP1. The c-Fos:c-Jun form of AP1 increases the transcription of survival and proliferation proteins. ERK moves into the nucleus and activates transcription factors for VEGF and IL-8 that promote angiogenesis, CyclinD1 that promotes the cell cycle from G1 to the S phase, and for phospholipase A2 that releases arachidonic acid from the cell membrane for the formation of PGE2.

At this point, let me mention that I have greatly simplified these pathways and their branches and ramifications. Many other pathways are in play in cancer. Consider these data as the highlights of how ERK and AKT work to activate mTOR and promote cell proliferation.

The RTK pathway for growth promotion includes phospholipids that help in signaling. Raf, in the ERK pathway, is activated by phosphatidic acid (PA). PIP3, as mentioned, helps activate Akt, but this also requires PA. The formation of PIP3 appears to require enzyme activation by PA. MTORC1 may also require PA directly for its activation.[9,19] Thus, PA appears essential for growth and cellular proliferation. PA is made available by its release from phosphatidylcholine (PC) by the enzyme PLD. Lysophosphatidic acid, made from lysophosphatidylcholine by the enzyme "autotoxin," appears to play a very similar role in other pathways. PA strongly inhibits CaMKKβ, thus inhibiting AMPK, and thereby inhibits the binding of TSC1 to TSC2.

PA is formed when PC is hydrolyzed into PA and choline by the enzyme PLD. Its activity is enhanced by ATP and GTP, the presence of its substrates, linoleic and linolenic acids, and sphingosine. PLD is inhibited in humans by ceramide, curcumin, oleic acid, resveratrol, and alcohol.[920]

When PC is in short supply, AMPK is activated, and Akt and Raf are inactive, promoting DSC1 binding with DSC2; preventing mTORC1 activation. Thus, without PC, the cells cannot grow. PC can thus act as a central indicator of cellular resource availability for growth. PC is formed from a phospholipid plus choline or a phospholipid plus SAMe. The formation of phospholipids requires high energy phosphate groups from ATP. Thus, it occurs when the cell has energy resources. Choline either comes from the diet or can be made, especially in fertile women, when sufficient SAMe is present.

Inflammation

Avoiding growth factors can help avoid mTOR activation. Inflammation also increases the activation of ERK and Akt. Inflammation has overlapping mechanisms with cell proliferation and activates many of the same signaling molecules. Thus, inflammation increases the risk of cancer and impairs the chances of recovery.

Normally, the inflammatory process helps us. We want our white blood cells to be healthy, to go forth, and multiply enough to continue their work of killing pathogens and eliminating parasites. Then, we are pleased to have them switch gears into clean-up mode and take out the trash, removing dead pathogens and dead cells. And finally, like any nice house guests, the inflammatory cells politely go away. They should only be active as long as the intruder is about, or during the clean-up, and then they should volunteer for apoptosis and be recycled. While they are needed, inflammatory signals keep the WBCs going. These signals prevent apoptosis, not only for the immune cells fighting a localized infection but also impede apoptosis of immune cells elsewhere in the body so that may ready if needed.

Inflammatory signals inhibit apoptosis – not only for inflammatory cells but for any cell that has cytokine receptors for the inflammatory ligands. This inhibition of apoptosis by interleukins, TNF-α, prostaglandins, and growth factors occurs in all cells other than red blood cells and platelets.

If a person has just a few mutated cells ready to give up the ghost, but inflammatory signals come along and say, "Wait! Don't go," they may stick around. If there is already a tumor, inflammation can deter apoptosis and help spread cancer.

In addition to RTKs, Toll-like receptors (TLRs) and other inflammatory receptors induce protein transcription through the ERK and Akt pathways. Although these do not cause metastatic growth in normal cells, they prevent apoptosis and promote proliferation.

Bacterial cell wall antigens stimulate PLD1 through TLR4 and signal the production of the tumor necrosis factor-α (TNF-α).[921] Many opioid medications activate the TLR4 receptor, inducing the inflammatory pathway, and the mu-opioid receptor stimulates phospholipase D2.[922] Bacterial overgrowth in the colon increases the production of the compound lipopolysaccharide (LPS) that activate TLR4. *Helicobacter pylori* produce LPS that activates TLR4. TLR2 is activated by cell wall components from gram-positive bacteria, and other compounds from parasites, viruses, and infectious fungi. Several of the infections discussed in Chapter 9, including *Schistosomiasis, Chlamydophila pneumoniae*, HBV, HCV, tuberculosis, malaria, and herpes virus activate TLR2. TLR2 receptors are found in epithelial cells of the lung, kidney, bladder, and skin. Thus, chronic infection can promote proliferation and impede apoptosis of these epithelial tissue cells. TLR activation by chronic infection helps promote the proliferation and survival of cells and including the survival and growth of cancer cells with these receptors.

Several phenolic compounds inhibit the NF-κB pathway through inhibition of TBK1-kinase. TBK1-kinase, similar to IKK, can phosphorylate IκBα. This allows NF-κB to migrate into the nucleus where it acts as a transcription factor for inflammatory cytokines, some of which participate in cancer growth by impeding apoptosis. IKK can also stimulate mTORC1 activation. By inhibiting TBK1-kinase, certain phenolic compounds prevent the release of IKK from NF-κB and thus allow for its ubiquitination and destruction.[923] Some phenolic compounds also inhibit the proliferative cascade by inhibiting the enzyme PLD. Other phenolic compounds appear to prevent the cell surface assembly of the TLR4 receptor. [924,925,926] Melatonin inhibits TLR4 inflammation at the MyD88 level.[927] Vitamin D and betaine have a similar effect by inhibiting TLR-4 signal induction.

Summary

Growth factors acting on receptors can initiate a cascade of events that support growth, whether it is a good idea or not. For infants and children growth is great. I want my wounds to heal, my hair to grow; I want new cells lining my intestines and replacing my skin. I want to replace old cells with new. I don't want tumors or unregulated growth.

Cell growth is regulated by the activation or inhibition of the mTORC1 protein complex. Activation of mTOR promotes cell growth by increasing the formation of ribosomes, the transcription of proteins, prevention of apoptosis, and by allowing the cell to move past the G1 checkpoint.

Insulin-like Growth Factor-1 (IGF-1) and other growth factors promote growth, including tumor growth. IGF-1 promotes cell proliferation and survival by inhibition of apoptosis via RTK activation of Ras → PI3K → Akt activation, as well as through Ras → Raf → MAPK → ERK activation. ERK and Akt both inhibit the TSC1/TCS2 complex, allowing for activation of mTORC1.

During the RTK activation, phosphatidylcholine (PC) is converted to phosphatidic acid (PA) by the enzyme phospholipase D (PLD). PA is an essential cofactor in the activation of Akt and ERK, and thus for mTOR activation. PA also strongly inhibits CaMKKβ-induced activation of AMPK that would inhibit mTOR activation.

A sufficient supply of PC thus acts as an auditor making sure that there are sufficient energy and nutrient resources for building two cells from one. It takes energy to synthesize PC, but also the vitamin choline from the diet. Some PC can also be made from SAMe if sufficient methionine, especially in fertile women, or betaine are present in the diet.

Activation of the downstream mediators of mTOR also requires specific amino acids, notably leucine and the other branched-chain amino acids, isoleucine, and valine.

35: Hacking mTOR and AMPK

For those that made their way through the previous chapter, I give my cheers and condolences. If you skipped up to this point, welcome back.

We can prevent and slow the growth of cancer cells by activating the energy auditors AMPK and mTOR. For a recap:

Growth depends on having an adequate supply of ATP for energy, amino acids for building new proteins, and lipids for building membranes. New tissues need glucose for energy to help survive low oxygen while developing new blood vessels. They can do this by glycolysis of glucose, an inefficient but strategic use of energy.

AMPK and mTORC1 act as auditors to make sure there are sufficient materials and energy to build new cells both in health and in cancer. Upstream of mTORC1, AMPK determines whether there is a sufficient cellular supply of ATP, lipids, and proteins for current operations and for growth. If supplies are insufficient, AMPK prevents growth by inhibiting mTOR activation and promotes autophagy. Autophagy recycles proteins and organelles within the cells to maintain critical operations. AMPK activation also has the cell recycle lipids from organelle membranes and burn them as fuel. It is like having a garage sale to help pay for rent, utilities, and groceries during hard times.

The mTOR1 complex also determines the external support for the growth of the cell through signaling from growth factors and the systemic availability of glucose through sensing of insulin and sensing the availability of amino acids needed for protein construction.

Inflammation creates intracellular signals that overlap with those triggered by external growth factors, and thus supports cell survival and impedes apoptosis. Inflammation can thus promote cancer cell growth.

Hacking AMPK

Now that we have a grip on how AMPK and mTOR function, let's see how to hack them. To prevent cancer, we can boost AMPK activity. This will promote autophagy and mitophagy, and inhibit mTOR promoted growth. Mitophagy is the selective elimination of old, feeble, and poorly functioning mitochondria. Old geezers tend to make and leak free radicals, ROS and RNS, which damage intracellular proteins and lipids, and that can cause DNA damage. Mitophagy allows the culling of weak mitochondria and the reproduction of strong, healthy ones.

There are several ways to boost AMPK activity.

Several phenolic compounds have been demonstrated to activate AMPK. These mostly act indirectly, and often through multiple mechanisms. Some of these agents activate AMPK through the formation of ROS by inhibiting mitochondrial function[928]. This may also induce mitophagy. These compounds also inhibit the activation of NF-κB, Akt, and ERK. Some of those documented to activate AMPK are listed in Table 35.3.

One group of phenolic compounds, the hydroxybenzoic acids (HBA), appear to act directly or through activation of LBK1. Aspirin is rapidly metabolized to salicylate, an HBA that has this effect. Epigallocatechin gallate from green tea activates LKB1, thereby activating AMPK. This compound breaks down into gallic acid and Epigallocatechin. Gallic acid is another HBA that activates AMPK.[929] Salicylate, from willow bark, activates AMPK [930] after it is metabolized into 4-hydroxybenzoic acid.

Several compounds have been demonstrated to activate AMPK via CaMKKβ. Lipoic acid is a nutritional supplement. Only the R-isomer is naturally present in nature; the L-isomer appears to block the activity of lipoic acid. Thus, only R-lipoic acid (sodium stabilized) is recommended. A dose of 50 to 100 mg appears to be as effective as 600 mg of alpha-lipoic acid. Lipoic acid is an antioxidant, however, and may impede the activity of oxidative stress-inducing drugs used in chemotherapy. Thus, it should be avoided during chemo. S-allyl cysteine (present in garlic) and T3 (triiodothyronine) also activate CaMKKβ. T3 output may be impeded by sleep deprivation.

The medication metformin activates AMPK and has been found to slow the growth of cancer. Most cancer patients with, or at risk of adult-onset diabetes should be taking metformin. In a study of non-diabetic women recently diagnosed with breast cancer, those placed on metformin had a decreased risk of developing metastatic tumors.[931, 932] Metformin should be avoided during chemo.

Leptin, the satiety hormone released from fat cells when the cells are full, tells the brain they have had plenty to eat. It also blocks AMPK activation in most cells. Leptin resistance, a condition associated with obesity, causes high leptin levels, and supports cancer growth, while ghrelin, a hormone that stimulates the feeling of hunger, activates

AMPK.[933] Adiponectin, a hormone secreted by fat cells when they get hungry, also activates AMPK. Factors that increase or decrease the production of leptin and adiponectin are given in Table 35-1.

Many of the flavonoids and other substances found in the diet that activate AMPK also raise the level of adiponectin. Flavonoids act at multiple steps in the cellular processes that control growth and inflammation.

Table 35-1: Modifiable AMPK Activity Factors

	Promote AMPK Activity	Impede AMPK Activity
Leptin	Decrease Leptin Levels: ❖ Fasting (24-72 hours) ❖ Exercise training[934]	Increase Leptin Levels: ➢ Sleep Deprivation, Sleep apnea ➢ Obesity and Insulin ➢ High-fructose, high-fat diet ➢ Psychological stress[935] ➢ Estrogen
Adiponectin	Increase Adiponectin Levels ❖ Exercise training ❖ N-3 fatty acids: EPA and DHA ❖ Berberine, Curcumin, ❖ Capsaicin, Gingerol, ❖ Catechins	Decrease Adiponectin Levels ➢ The combination of obesity with sleep apnea or sleep hypoxia.[936] ➢ Uric acid (when elevated, such as with high-fructose diets)

Sleep deprivation is a risk factor for cancer as discussed in Chapter 30. Reduction in sleep time, and especially limitations of deep sleep (slow-wave sleep, SWS) time, increase insulin resistance and risk of diabetes. Lack of SWS may occur during sleep apnea, patients in pain, or those who are stressed and have frequent nighttime arousals.

One reason that sleep deprivation promotes cancer is its effect on appetite hormones. Sleep restriction decreases leptin and increases ghrelin levels, both of which increase feeding. Sleep deprivation may also favor the selection of high-caloric, palatable foods.[937]

Patients with sleep apnea have been found to have leptin levels twice as high as control subjects.[938] The combination of sleep deficits and obesity causes low adiponectin levels. Successful treatment of sleep apnea helps normalize both adiponectin and leptin levels. Exercise training, especially vigorous exercise, lowers leptin levels, decreases insulin resistance, and increases adiponectin levels. This effect is especially pronounced in overweight and obese persons and those with high levels of markers for inflammation.[934, 939]

Melatonin can decrease leptin levels[940] or increase it. Normally, melatonin lowers appetite during the night and lowers leptin levels. Light exposure in the evening or during the night that disrupts melatonin production increases leptin. Circadian disruption likely increases leptin levels. In contrast, however, if insulin levels are elevated, melatonin increases insulin's effect on leptin resistance and raises leptin levels. This effect is amplified by high levels of corticosteroids.[941] Most of the body's melatonin is made in the gut, where it slows digestion during sleep.

Since insulin raises leptin levels at night, it would be advisable for cancer patients and anyone with insulin resistance to avoid late evening meals, sweet desserts, or bedtime snacks that raise blood sugar and maintain high insulin output during the sleep period. Excessive fructose (more than required for current energy needs) increases leptin production, most likely through its promotion of obesity and insulin resistance.[942]

Individuals that have higher leptin levels are more likely to skip breakfast.[943] Thus, if you do not wake up hungry, or are often able to go until lunchtime without feeling hungry, you may be eating too much too late in the day, causing increased nighttime leptin and decreased adiponectin, and raising cancer risk. If this is the case, try shifting daily food consumption to earlier in the day, eating a lighter dinner, and if hungry in the evening, try a small, high protein/fat snack, such as nuts or a piece of cheese.

A high-fat, high-fructose diet can cause leptin resistance within a few weeks. It can also be reversed within a few weeks by a diet containing a healthful fat content and limited fructose content. Fructose is not inherently evil. If one consumes a moderate amount of whole fruit when hungry and when blood sugar is low, the fructose will be slowly absorbed and utilized as energy and will not promote disease. Eating an apple as a snack is not the problem. Fructose consumed in whole fruit, when eaten when feeling hungry, is much more likely to be utilized for energy.

The problem arises after a meal; the body is flooded with nutrients and the blood sugar (glucose) levels rise. Insulin is released to direct traffic and sends glucose into various cells for use and storage. Fructose is not metabolized as easily, and can only be stored as fat. This process creates uric acid as a side effect. Fructose in liquid forms, such as fruit juice or soda pop, is the most dangerous as it is quickly absorbed. It is especially problematic when the drink is used to wash down a meal that causes the blood sugar to be elevated. It is even worse when added to a high-fat meal.

AMPK Hacks:

- Avoid midnight snacks and evening desserts if one is overweight.

- Increase the amounts of phenolic compounds shown in Table 35-3 into the diet. Keep in mind that many phenolic compounds act through hormesis as low-dose toxins or pseudo-toxins. There is no evidence that doses above those found in a healthy diet provide benefit, and they may create risks. One-quarter of a 3.5 ounce 65% chocolate solids dark chocolate bar every other day likely provides the dose with the maximum health benefits, not more.944

- Optimize CaMKKβ activity by making sure the diet has sufficient calcium and magnesium. Check the vitamin D3 blood level (25-OHD3) to help assure that calcium is being absorbed from the diet. Garlic also stimulates CaMKKβ. R-lipoic acid supplements may help. Garlic in the diet helps.

- Avoid things that raise leptin levels or decrease adiponectin levels. (Things that cause weight gain, sleep deprivation, and/or high blood sugar at night).

- Get plenty of sleep. Most SWS occurs during the first 4 hours of sleep at night. You want this sleep to be deep, and not polluted with a high blood sugar, or with light. Chapter 30 explains how light in the evening can decrease melatonin production. T3 is also released at night.

- If you have sleep apnea, get and use treatment. If you snore heavily, get tested for sleep apnea. If you have insomnia – get instructions (not medications) from a sleep specialist.

- If you have cancer, avoid night shift work.(Chapter 30)

- Avoid high-fat, high-fructose diets.

- Get rid of chronic inflammation. If you have a chronic infection, get it treated. If you have intestinal bacterial overgrowth, a low-fat diet, high in fiber from a mix of sources should help.

- Wake up with an appetite for breakfast. Don't overeat in the evenings. Get vigorous exercise. See Chapter 13 for more explanation. If exercise is not making you short of breath, it is unlikely to lower cancer risk. If you are unable to do vigorous exercise, or just enjoy them, hot baths may provide many of the benefits of exercise.

- If you are at high risk for diabetes or cancer, or have have type 2 diabetes or cancer, ask your doctor about being placed on metformin. If you have type 2 diabetes and cancer, a thiazolidinedione medication may be appropriate.

- ☞ Fast. Modified fasting to impede mTOR activation will be discussed in the next chapter.

- ☞ One way you may be able to tell if these hacks are working is if they are helping with weight loss in an overweight person or helping with blood sugar control in a diabetic.

- ☞ Chill. Perhaps the most seemingly useless advice is to avoid stress. But stress can be avoided. Appendix C provides useful advice on lowering stress

For best results, do all of these "hacks" that apply to you. The more mTOR activation is slowed, the more likely you are to stop the progression of tumor cells before they grow.

Table 35-2: Compounds that Activate CaMKKβ

CaMKKβ Activators	Foods Containing High Levels of CaMKKβ Activators
Luteolin	Globe artichokes, oregano, thyme, sage, black olives
S-allyl cysteine	Garlic
R-lipoic acid	Small amounts are present in many foods. Therapeutic doses are most easily available from supplements. Avoid the more easily found, racemic, alpha-lipoic acid. Use R-lipoic sodium acid supplements. Typical therapeutic doses range from 50 – 100 mg for adults.
Minerals	Calcium and magnesium are required for CaMKKβ activation.[945] Make sure the diet has enough. The typical American diet has plenty of calcium but is low in magnesium. Many people benefit from a 200 mg daily dose of magnesium citrate, which is better absorbed than other forms of magnesium. Calcium is one of few supplements that have been found to be associated with a decreased incidence of cancer. Boron supports magnesium and calcium absorption.

Table 35-3: Phenolic compounds shown to Activate AMPK

Phenolic Compound[946]	Food Sources
Epigallocatechin gallate[947]	Green tea, oolong tea, pecans, hazelnuts
Quercetin	Chocolate, capers, elderberries, orange juice, cloves, oregano, shallots, red onions,
Genistein	Soy products (tofu, tempeh, etc.)
Resveratrol	Muscadine grape wine, other red wine, cranberries, red currants, loganberries, strawberries
Punicalagin	Pomegranates. This is another hydroxybenzoic acid. [948]
Hispidulin	Oregano, sage, thyme, rosemary
Curcumin	Turmeric (found in curry powder)
Theaflavins	Tea (black, green)
4-hydroxybenzoic acid	Loquat, green olives, red wine, coconut, green tea. It may also be formed during the metabolism of catechins
Gallic Acid	Very high levels: Chestnuts, chicory, walnuts, cloves, blackberries High levels: Oregano, black tea, red wine, sage, chicory,
Catechin	Chocolate, red wine, drupes (peaches, plums, prunes, apricots, cherries), black grapes, strawberries, broad beans, red beans, pecans.
Capsaicin	Chili peppers
Gingerol	Raw ginger root. Dried ginger.
Nootkatone[949]	Nootkatone found in grapefruit; activates AMPK.
Berberine	A yellow pigment found in several plants including goldenseal. Berberine-rich plants are used in traditional Chinese medicine. It is present in barberry but otherwise uncommon in foods. It is allergenic.

> Caution: The phenolic compounds commonly found in food are generally safe; however, note that many of them have bitter tastes and are avoided by children. There may be a good reason for children not to like the taste of these foods; they may impede growth.
>
> While encouraging a diverse, nutritious diet that includes foods containing phenolic substances, it should be kept in mind that they may

impede growth in children or fetal development in pregnant women. I advise against the use of refined or concentrated phenolic substances in children and pregnant women.

These substances may be toxic in high doses. High doses may provide no advantages over the amounts encountered in foods, and may even be less effective or detrimental. Unless clinical trials have shown both safety and efficacy, I recommend avoiding the use of refined or concentrated phenolic extracts.

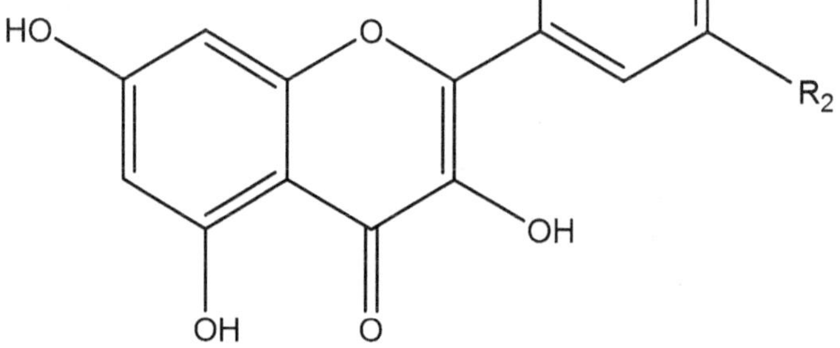

Flavonol	R_1	R_2
Isorhamnetin	OCH	H
Kaempferol	H	H
Myricetin	OH	OH
Quercetin	OH	H

Figure 35-5: Example of Polyphenol Structures:

The structure of a flavonol polyphenol. Each phenyl ring with at least one OH group represents a phenol group. The substitutions in R groups make for different compounds.

36: CHEMOTHERAPY

The behavior and growth of the cell types from which cancer clones develop greatly influence which hormones, cytokines, and other mediators will affect that cancer's growth. Cancers arising from different cell types respond to different treatments. Table 31-1 lists examples of common chemotherapy regimens used for various cancers.

Table 36-1: Examples of Common Chemotherapy Regimens

Cancer Type	Chemotherapeutic Combination	Acronym
Bladder cancer	Methotrexate, vincristine, doxorubicin, cisplatin	MVAC
Breast cancer	Cyclophosphamide, methotrexate, 5-fluorouracil	CMF
Breast cancer	Doxorubicin, cyclophosphamide	AC
Colorectal cancer	Folinic acid, 5-fluorouracil, oxaliplatin	FOLFOX
Lung cancer	Cyclophosphamide, doxorubicin, vincristine	CAV
Hodgkin's disease	Mustine, vincristine, procarbazine, prednisolone	MOPP
Hodgkin's disease	Doxorubicin, bleomycin, vinblastine, dacarbazine	ABVD

How easy it would be if it were only that simple.

In addition to developing from a wide variety of cell types, let me repeat that several hundred mutations in genes underlie and drive cancer development and that on average, an adult-onset cancer cell has alterations in six to ten of these "cancer-driving genes. Certain mutations, or cluster of mutations, are common in some cancer types. However, this does not mean that there are no additional cancer-driving mutations in most cancers. These mutations can affect how the cancer behaves and how it responds to treatment. As cancer progresses, additional mutations make this even more complex.

One of the great difficulties in treating cancer is that no two cancers, even when of identical cell origin and cancer type, are guaranteed to respond to the same treatment. Think about it. You may respond to a medication differently than your cousin, because you metabolize the drug differently, even though you are closely related. Cancer cells have altered genes, and they may be as different from those of the host, as are the genes of a different species of animals.

While we can share many of our foods and medicines with our pets, others will kill them. It only takes a couple of sugar-free Tic Tacs or sugar-free chewing gum sweetened with xylitol to kill a large dog.[950] Cats cannot metabolize aspirin, making it easily toxic for them. Avocados are deadly to birds. In dogs, grapes and raisins can cause renal failure, and consumption of garlic and onions causes rupture of their red blood cells.[951] Different species and different cancers may metabolize and respond differently to various compounds.

Most cancers have growth factors and mutations characteristic of their cell type of origin. This does allow selection of chemo agents that the cancer type generally responds to. However, there are no guarantees. Additionally, by the time cancer has been diagnosed, the cancer is usually no longer composed of identical clones, but has undergone further mutations, and may have mutated into several different "species", some of which may be more resistant to a specific treatment. Chemotherapy can also drive the selection process to increase mutations that cause treatment resistance.

Describing cancer as different species is actually misleading. As cancers accumulate mutations, they progressively lose genetic stability, increasing the number of mutations present among the now numerous cell lines. Most mutations do not assist survival, and many mutations kill the aberrant cells. Some mutations, however, aid in the cancer's survival and progression. As mutations accumulate, the surviving cancer cells progressively de-evolve from specialized cell type and function, into more primitive, primordial cells that more readily adapt to changes in their environment. The more adaptive these cells are, the more likely Darwinian selection is to favor the growth of cell lines adapted to rapid cell cycling, metastasis, and to develop treatment resistance.[952]

For these reasons, treating cancer early in its development, when the mass is small, and there are few cancer cell lines, greatly improves cure rates. Also, some cancers are easily cured by surgical removal when they are caught early on.

The goal in chemotherapy is not to kill cancer cells but rather to irreparably damage them so that they cannot reproduce; this damage impels those cells to undergo apoptosis. The difficult part is damaging cancer cells without harming normal cells.

We are currently in our third generation of chemotherapy agents used in the treatment of cancer.[953] The first generation of chemotherapy targeted quickly growing cells. These drugs were often selected on the basis of their side effects, with little understanding of their mechanisms of action. When Dr. Sydney Farber began inducing remission of acute lymphoblastic leukemia in children in the 1940's, protein was thought to be self-replicating, and DNA was, at most, believed to act as a support structure for protein. In the early days, the search for chemotherapeutic agents often began with the selection of compounds that would selectively damage quickly growing cells while sparing other tissues. The chemotherapeutic agent vinblastine was originally tested as a potential anti-diabetic drug but caused fatal infections in rabbits. When it was discovered that the cause was a decline in white blood cells, it was then tested as an anti-cancer drug. The most effective chemotherapeutics, still used today, were discovered by a search for agents that killed quickly growing cells.

Most first-generation chemo drugs are alkylating agents which have two sites that form covalent bonds with DNA strands. Since they bind two strands, they cause cross-linking between or within DNA strands. This prevents DNA replication or causes the strands to break during DNA repair. Since these damaged cells cannot replicate, they undergo apoptosis. Alkylating agents also damage proteins and RNA. They damage cells during G1 as well as during cell division. These agents are among the most highly genotoxic of chemotherapeutic agents; they can cause new cancers.

> The first alkylating agents were derived from the blistering chemical warfare agent mustard gas. The name of this gas comes from the garlic – mustard odor of the gas, not from the seed or the plant with the name. Most well known for its use by the Germans in World War I, mustard gas causes severe, painful blistering of the skin, eyes and respiratory tract, which does not occur until several hours after exposure. It was also observed to suppress the production of blood cells, which suggested its use for the treatment of lymphoma. Those surviving gas attacks during the war were found to be at increased risk of cancer years and even decades later. These agents continue to be illegally used in warfare and terrorism.

Anti-metabolic chemo drugs impede the synthesis of DNA and RNA. Several of these chemicals are structurally similar enough to DNA synthesis building enzymes or coenzymes, that they block the enzymes function, or are incorporated into the DNA or mRNA. When incorporated into the DNA, they block DNA replication and thus promote apoptosis.

Some of the anti-metabolites are antifolate drugs that prevent the cell from forming a precursor for purines needed for forming DNA (adenine and guanine). Even before DNA was understood, it was known that methotrexate blocked folate metabolism. However, it was not understood at the time that folate was needed for DNA synthesis. 5-Fluorouracil blocks thymidine synthesis, required for replicating DNA. Cisplatin causes cross-linking of the DNA, interfering with mitosis. Thus, the antimetabolic agents act and are only effective during the S phase of cell reproduction.

Anti-microtubule medications prevent the assembly or function of the microtubules that separate the two sets of chromosomes into the opposite ends of the cell during mitosis. Microtubules during this process are continually being formed on one end of the microtubule and being disassembled at the other end. The vinca alkaloids prevent microtubule formation. They bind to tubulin molecules during the S-phase and prevent M-phase cell progress, thereby causing cell cycle arrest during mitosis, which induces apoptosis. These drugs may additionally inhibit topoisomerase. In contrast, the taxanes prevent microtubule disassembly but similarly induce apoptosis.

Topoisomerase inhibitors prevent DNA de-twisting that results in DNA breaks, leading to apoptosis. If you coil a cable or cord, and then unwind it, you may have noticed that the process creates twisting in the line. The same occurs when DNA is wrapped around histones and then unwound. The enzymes topoisomerase I and topoisomerase II cut and re-attach the DNA strand to remove these kinks. When drugs block these enzymes, it causes the DNA strand to break during DNA replication.

Table 36-2: Examples of First Generation Chemotherapeutic Agents

Chemo Class	Representative First Generation Chemo Agents
Alkylating agents	Nitrogen Mustards: cyclophosphamide, melphalan, chlorambucil, ifosfamide and busulfan. Nitrosoureas: carmustine (BCNU), and lomustine (CCNU) Cisplatins: cisplatin, carboplatin, and oxaliplatin
Antimetabolites	Antifolates: methotrexate and pemetrexed Fluoropyrimidines: 5-fluorouracil and capecitabine Deoxynucleoside analogs: cytarabine and gemcitabine Thiopurines: thioguanine and mercaptopurine
Anti-microtubule	Vinca alkaloids: vincristine and vinblastine Taxanes: paclitaxel and docetaxel,
Cytotoxic antibiotics	Anthracyclines: doxorubicin, daunorubicin, and epirubicin Bleomycin, and Mitomycin
Topoisomerase inhibitors	Topoisomerase I: irinotecan and topotecan Topoisomerase II: etoposide and doxorubicin

Cytotoxic antibiotics also interrupt cell division but kill cells through additional mechanisms. Anthracycline drugs, such as doxorubicin, prevent DNA transcription and replication and inhibit RNA synthesis by binding to and crosslinking to DNA and RNA, similar to alkylating agents. They also generate free oxygen radicals that cause cellular stress and DNA damage.

The cells lining the intestine, hematopoietic cells of the bone marrow that produce the red and white blood cells and platelets, and the mucosa and skin cells are quickly growing. These are the cells most susceptible to injury by traditional chemotherapy agents. Damage to these cells by chemo drugs causes hair loss, sores in the mouth, itching, nausea, vomiting, and diarrhea. The loss of white blood cells and other quickly responding immune cells puts patients treated with chemo at high risk of infection.

These chemotherapeutics are genotoxic to dividing cells; they promote DNA damage, as well as other injuries during the synthesis and mitotic phases of the cell cycle. Cells that are in the S and M phases at the moment that chemo is applied are much more susceptible to injury, mutation and death than are cells in other phases of the cell cycle. However, alkylating agents can also damage proteins, mRNA, and DNA in cells in the G1 phase.

While some cancers, especially those derived from very quickly dividing cells such as testicular cancer, choriocarcinomas and several forms of leukemia, respond very well to chemo and are usually cured. Most other cancers have a varied prognosis after chemo. Most solid cancers are not as quickly growing as white blood cells or intestinal mucosal cells, and most cancer cells are not actively dividing at any one time. More slowly growing cancers have a significant population of cells that are not actively dividing, and thus, are less susceptible to chemo.

Genotoxic chemotherapeutic agents preferentially kill cancer cells because cancer cells have more difficulty in repairing DNA damage than do normal cells. That is often, in part, how they got to be cancer cells in the first place. Normal cells are considerably more likely to identify DNA errors, stop growth at checkpoints, and undergo apoptosis than are cancer cells. Chemo causes new, often lethal, mutations. Cancer cells that survive chemo are also more likely to have additional mutations.

Chemotherapy, almost by design, kills growing cells. Thus, the most visible adverse effects of chemo are for tissues with quickly or constantly growing cells. First generation chemo agents remain the most used and most successful chemo agents, despite their considerable side effects and drawbacks.

The second generation of chemotherapy is known as targeted therapy. These drugs target specific components of growth and survival pathways. An example of these is poly ADP-ribose polymerase (PARP) inhibitors that inhibit DNA repair and replication. Most second-generation chemo drugs are genotoxic. An advance within second generation chemotherapy is the targeting of two pathways simultaneously, as cancer cells are much less likely to have the ability to get around both critical pathways. Second generation chemotherapy agents often use a combination with agents that suppress growth.

The third generation of chemo agents targets cell function rather than DNA replication. Many of these pathways were discussed in the mTOR chapter (Chapter 34). Many of these agents stress the cancer cells and interfere with their metabolic processes.[954] These include cell membrane RTK inhibitors EGFR (cetuximab; Erbitux), HER2/neu (trastuzumab; Herceptin), and VEGF (bevacizumab; Avastin) cell receptors. Proteasome inhibitors block the breakdown of proteins in the cell which promotes paraptosis. The proteasome inhibitor bortezomib is used in the treatment of multiple myelomas. The monoclonal antibody rituximab specifically targets a protein on the surface of B lymphocytes and likely acts by inhibiting their maturation, thus inducing apoptosis. It is used in the treatment of lymphoma and leukemias.

Hormone therapies might be included in the philosophy of the third generation agents; however, they have long been used in cancer treatment.

Additionally, many drugs modulate the production of ceramide, an inducer of programmed cell death. Several first generation chemo drugs increase ceramide production, but so do many drugs that are not genotoxic chemotherapeutic agents. The corticosteroid, dexamethasone, is used in cancer treatment as it inhibits cell growth; in part by increasing the formation of ceramide and sphingosine that activate caspase-8 and promote apoptosis.[955] Appendix B discusses medications and supplements that modulate the ceramide pathway, and its conversion to S1P, which increases proliferation. Many other medications affect the ceramide pathway, including THC, but are not yet utilized in chemotherapy.

Some forms of cancers respond very well to chemotherapy and have high cure rates with chemo. Other cancers will go into partial remission with treatment, and still others are difficult to treat. The treatment for cancer depends on the type of cancer as well as on many other factors, such as the patient's underlying health and age.

Sadly, chemotherapy often only provides a partial response, knocking cancer into temporary remission, but not completely eliminating it. Cancers that are more resistant to chemotherapy or treated later, when the cancer has grown larger, are less amenable to treatment. Brain cancers are difficult to treat with chemo; the blood-brain barrier keeps many chemo drugs out. Second and third generation medications are neither necessarily more successful nor more benign in their side effects than the older drugs.

The more bacteria present in an infection, the more likely it is that one or more bacterium will be resistant to an antibiotic, just based on probabilities. Additionally, the lower the dose of antibiotic given, the more likely that clones of bacteria that are partially resistant to the antibiotic will survive. Those survivors may further mutate to develop even greater antibiotic resistance. This is also true for cancer cells and chemo. The larger the cancer cell population, the higher the likelihood of multiple lineages, and that one or more lineages will be resistant to a given chemotherapy. The bacteria, or cancer cells, that are most susceptible to the treatment are killed leaving the resistant ones to survive and multiply. Just as antibiotics can help select resistant bacteria, chemotherapy can help select resistant cancer clones.

Chemo even goes further, as it contributes to the genetic instability of the cancer cells and those cells that survive chemo often have mutations that make them resistant to the medication. The average remission time for a metastatic cancer is 9 to 14 months. While a patient may respond to the second round of chemo or to an alternative chemotherapy agent, few cases have a vigorous response to the third round of chemotherapy. By this stage, the cancers have often become very diversified, aggressive and resistant. Especially when the diagnosis has been late, the outcome is often devastating. Thus, it is essential to minimize mutations and to optimize killing of the cancer cells with the first round of treatment.[956]

The second round of treatment may give another extension, but a third round of the same drugs would be futile. Use of an alternative chemo regimen, using alternate drugs, may help, but often adds little to survival time, as the multiple cancer lineages present at this stage have numerous resistance mechanisms.

Chemo is dangerous. Although modern chemo has become less toxic, it is still fraught with problems. Chemo is not only toxic to quickly growing cells. Some agents cause oxidative stress damage to the "immortal" cells of the heart and brain. Many chemo agents, both old and new, cause neurotoxicity.[957, 958] Peripheral neuropathy is a common side effect but may improve with time. Chemotherapy often causes neutropenia, lymphopenia, and immune suppression. It can take 6 months or longer for neutrophils counts to return to normal. Some survivors have a permanent degradation in immune function. The decline in immune function not only places the patient at increased risk of infection, but it also decreases immune function that might help eliminate cancer cells.

Anthracyclines can kill stem cells in the heart. This can lead to cardiomyopathy and heart failure several years after treatment.[959] Trastuzumab (Herceptin) can also damage the heart. Although there are medications that can prevent toxicities from chemo,[960] some of these treatments, such as the use of antioxidants, may also spare cancer cells, rendering the treatment less effective. Chemo can be toxic to the liver and kidneys, as these organs concentrate and metabolize these agents as they try to clear them from the body.

Chemo can be quite expensive. Newer chemo medications cost between $200,000 and $300,000 per quality life year attained through treatment.[961] I guess that's why one of my med-school classmates was doctoring the chemo, watering it down, and pocketing the change. Her justification was that the medication wasn't going to change the outcome. She was mean in med-school, and I doubt her life in the federal penitentiary has changed her.

As stated above, chemo becomes less effective with cancer progression and with treatment. Treatment selects more aggressive cancer cell clones. Chemo causes mutations in normal cells that can cause the development of new cancers. The success rate of chemo for most stage three and four cancers is poor and especially poor for those with recurrent cancers (that have returned) or *reoccurrent* cancers that have newly developed after the initiation of cancer treatment.

Apoptosis

Before moving on to how to make cancer treatment safer and more effective, we should revisit apoptosis. In Chapter 4, apoptosis was described as ranging from being intrinsic and initiated in the nucleus of the cell, to being extrinsic and being initiated in the cytosol and/or external to the cell, or being a blend of both.

Let me remind you that intrinsic apoptosis allows cells in a tissue to retire gracefully when they are no longer needed by the tissue or when they have aged out. This is how the mucosal cells lining the intestine are replaced every several days; they shrivel up and take a great leap into the dark lumen of the intestine. In other tissues, there is no place to shed to, and these cells methodically break themselves down into tiny fragments that can be absorbed by surrounding tissues or washed away without triggering immune processes.

Table 36-3: Adverse Effects of Chemotherapy

Organ	Adverse Effects	Prevention/Treatment
Bone Marrow		
Red Blood Cells	Anemia, Fatigue	Transfusion, erythropoietin
Platelets	Bruising and bleeding	Platelet transfusion
Neutropenia	Immune suppression and infections	Granulocyte-colony-stimulating factor (F-CSF)
Pancytopenia	Myelosuppression (Loss of blood cell production)	Bone marrow transplant
Gastrointestinal Tract		
Gastroenteritis	Nausea, vomiting, diarrhea, cramping, constipation. May lead to dehydration.	*Sanafast*™ diet. Avoid dehydration.
Stomatitis	Dry mouth, mouth sores	The *Sanafast* diet
Neutropenic enterocolitis	A life-threatening infection of the cecum caused by immune suppression, and overgrowth of gram-positive bacteria usually associated with antibiotic use. More deadly than most cancers. The food emulsifiers carboxymethylcellulose and polysorbate can disrupt the mucous layer that protects the colon from bacteria.	The *Sanafast* diet. Avoid artificial emulsifiers. Prebiotics (foods with mixes of fiber) Probiotics for those on antibiotics or antibiotic chemo.
Skin – mucosa		
Hair loss	Usually temporary hair loss, but may be permanent. Hair re-growing usually begins several weeks following the end of treatment. Severity depends on the treatment regimen.	2% topical minoxidil and scalp cooling may decrease the severity of hair loss and speed recovery.[962]
Pruritus	Itchy skin	The *Sanafast*™ diet
Neurologic		
Chemo Brain	Post-chemotherapy cognitive impairment (PCCI), "brain fog". Mild cognitive impairment occurs in 10 to 40 percent of women treated for breast cancer and often lasts four years or longer. It typically affects visual systems, word memory, attention, concentration, and coordination.[963]	Chemo Preconditioning (below, in this Chapter). The *Sanafast* diet (Chapter 37), including curcumin, and flavonoid compounds,[964] Chapter 35. Accurate dosing using blood-level testing.
Peripheral Neuropathy	Chemotherapy-induced peripheral neuropathy (CIPN) Numbness and tingling, usually sensory nerves, but may also involve motor nerves causing weakness.	
Ototoxicity	Injury to the cochlea of the inner ear can cause dizziness and vertigo	

Other Organs	Adverse Effects	Prevention/Treatment
Tumor lysis syndrome	When chemotherapy kills large numbers of tumor cells, as may occur in leukemia and lymphoma, high levels of uric acid, potassium and phosphate may be released and may cause toxicity and cardiac arrhythmias and renal damage.	Adequate hydration, monitoring in hospital
Cardiotoxicity	Anthracyclines kill stem cells in the heart. This can result in cardiomyopathy years later as heart cells normally slowly replace themselves from these cells.	Chemo preconditioning, the *Sanafast*™ diet
Liver Toxicity	The liver metabolizes most of the chemotherapy agents, and may be injured by them.	Preconditioning diet high in choline and Nrf2 stimulants.
Kidney Damage	May be direct, especially by drugs metabolized or cleared by the kidney, or secondary to tumor lysis syndrome and the accumulation of toxic metabolites.	Maintain hydration
Infertility	Some chemo drugs are highly toxic to ovaries but others much less so. If the patient wants to preserve their fertility, this needs to be discussed with the oncologist before treatment.	Drug selection, GnRH analog induced suppression, egg cryopreservation
Teratogenicity	Chemotherapy can cause severe birth defects during the first trimester of pregnancy, and can induce genetic mutations in the child. Abortion is generally recommended if a first-semester pregnancy is compromised by chemotherapy	Birth control initiated in fertile women at the time cancer is diagnosed in them or when their mate starts chemo.
Secondary Cancers	Genotoxic agents cause cancer. For older adults, the risk is mostly limited to acute myeloid leukemia, as they usually do not survive long enough (20 to 30 years) to develop secondary solid tumors. Childhood cancer survivors have a greater than 10 time the normal risk of developing cancer during adulthood.	Avoidance of genotoxic chemotherapeutics when possible, Preconditioning, the *Sanafast*™ diet, boron, vitamin B12.

Nuclear-initiated apoptosis allows pollywogs to lose their tails and us to have fingers without webs and eyelids that open, as the cells that are no longer needed voluntarily do themselves in, without leaving a trace.

Extrinsic apoptosis is not a voluntary retirement for cells that are no longer useful; it is rather more like martyrdom. These cells self-destruct, not because they are senile or no longer needed, but because they have become a danger to their community. Rather than becoming a vector of destruction, they detach themselves from their neighbors and turn evidence to the immune system.

For example, the presence of DNA in the cytosol outside of mitosis, generally from intracellular bacteria or viruses, is sensed by a cluster of proteins, the inflammasome, as a dangerous abnormality. Inflammasomes also react to bacterial cell wall components that have no business inside a healthy cell and thus indicate an intracellular infection. Activation of the inflammasome enzymatically promotes procaspase-1 to caspase-1, which initiates an inflammatory cascade that moves the cell towards apoptosis. The inflammasome also induces the cell to make and activate inflammatory cytokines, including interferon-γ (INF-γ), IL-1β, and IL-18. The release of these cytokines sounds an alarm for neighboring cells and encourages them to undergo extrinsic apoptosis if things are amiss within. The cytokines also summon killer T-immune cells to the area.[965] [966] These immune cells insert the protein perforin into the cell wall of the target cell creating a pore through which the immune cell injects granzyme B, which cleaves several proteins that maintain cellular integrity.

Caspase-1 cleaves and inactivates several enzymes for glycolysis that reside in the cytosol blocking energy production from glucose.[967] Caspase-1 then triggers the relocation phosphatidylserine (PS) from the inner wall of the cell membrane to the outer wall; this is a dinner-bell for phagocytic immune cells to come and consume the cell. This allows lymphocytes to process the cellular components, including the intracellular viruses and bacteria for immune recognition. Thus, the extrinsic apoptotic mechanism is part of the innate immune system that is geared to cause infected cells to self-destruct in a way that brings the immune system running and that alerts its neighbors to be on the lookout for invaders.

Inflammasomes are activated by recognition of pathogen-associated molecular patterns (PAMPs), but can also be activated by recognition of other danger-associated molecular patterns (DAMPs). Cathepsin-B, a proteolytic enzyme that is usually restricted to phagolysosomes in the cells, can act as a DAMP if released from the lysosome. This can occur when the lysosome gets damaged by proteins or other substances it is unable to digest. Amyloid-β protein may cause this as part of the process of neuronal loss in Alzheimer's disease, and α-synuclein may do the same in Parkinson's disease.[968] Misfolded proteins and proteins damaged by ROS can also activate the inflammasome, either directly as DAMPs or secondary to the damage they may cause to lysosomes.

Towards the end, whether initiated in the nucleus or cytosol, there is a common pathway that mediates the cell's death, involving several proteins that act as representatives in coming to a consensus whether to push the self-destruct button or not. There are several apoptosis-regulating proteins. Bax and Bak prevent apoptosis until activated by Bid. P53 is a transcription factor for these proteins. Bid causes Bax and Bak to join with each other or with similar proteins that form a pore in the outer membrane of a mitochondrion, which allows the release of cytochrome C that activates caspase self-destruct enzymes. Release ROS, mitochondrial DNA, and cardiolipin from the mitochondria also contribute to activation of the inflammasome.

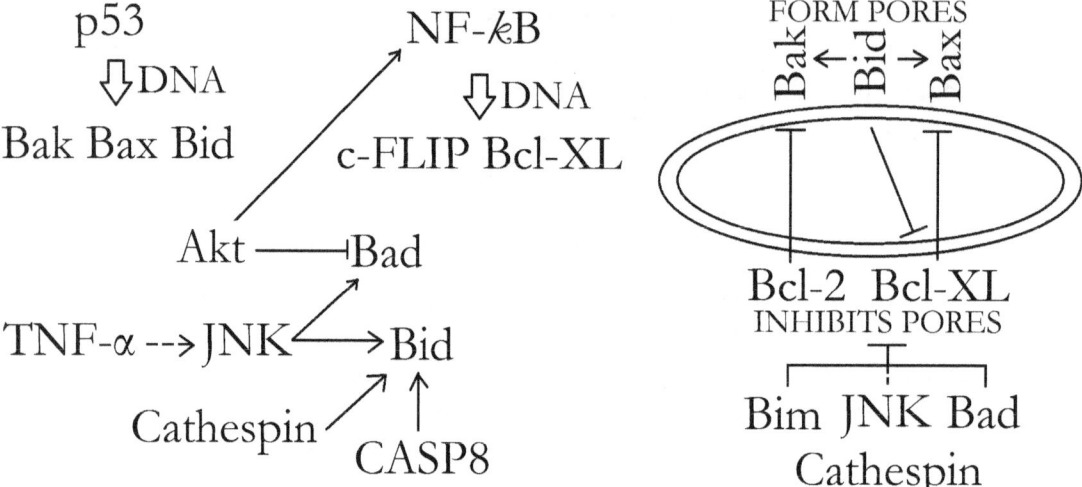

Figure 36-1: Bak and Bax form pores in the mitochondrial membrane.

Bcl-XL and Bcl-2 are proteins that inhibit the formation of pores in the mitochondrial membrane, and thus, inhibit apoptosis. The proteins BAD, Bim, JNK, and cathepsin can deactivate Bcl-Xl and Bcl-2, allowing apoptosis to move forward. JNK, cathepsin, and CASP-8 also activate Bid, and thus, pore formation. Akt inhibits apoptosis both by deactivating Bad and by inducing the pro-survival proteins c-FLIP and Bcl-XL via NF-κB. Various cell types have other mitochondrial pore-regulating proteins. One example is Bim that acts in the cytosol and is activated by stress.

The process of programmed cell death is complex and democratic. It is not cell suicide on a whim with a quick bullet to the brain. It takes the interaction of many cell regulators, involves the orderly production of inflammatory proteins, and allows for a range of outcomes.

The RTK ligands, such as IGF-1, VEGF, and EGF, activate the PI3K → Akt and Fos → Erk pathways that promote the activation of mTOR and cell growth. The RTK ligands not only stimulate growth, but they also prevent apoptosis through the nuclear, intrinsic pathway. The pro-apoptotic protein BAD is inhibited by Akt, and thus, Akt also inhibits extrinsic pathway programmed cell death. (Note: Fos should not be confused with Fas ligands that activate receptors on the cell surface, discussed below)

Toll-like receptors on the outer cell membrane activate NF-κB, which promotes inflammation and survival through suppression of nuclear apoptosis. Other cell membrane receptors, such as cytokine and Fas ligand receptors for TNF-α, IL-1β, and INF-γ, can promote either inflammation and replication, or apoptosis primarily via the promotion of the extrinsic apoptotic pathway. The choice depends on the strength of inflammatory signaling and stimuli for growth.

Preconditioning for Chemo

Now let's get back to cancer and chemotherapy. The same DNA errors that chemo is promoting to trigger genotoxic self-destruction also create mutations that can make cancer more dangerous and aggressive. It can also cause mutations among healthy cells, turning them into pre-cancer cells. Additionally, it kills the very immune cells that we need to fight infections and cancer. In spite of its problems, chemo remains the treatment choice for most patients with invasive cancer.

This does not mean that a person undergoing chemo has to just lie down and accept the side-effects of chemo. Efforts can and should be made to both protect the patient as much as possible from the harms associated with these treatments, and to increase the efficacy of chemo against cancer.

Which sounds like a better apoptotic strategy for killing cancer cells: the nuclear option where the cell self-destructs without a trace or cytosolic self-detonation that alerts the immune system?

For single, mutant cells, nuclear self-annihilation is the best option. It gets rid of the problem before it becomes one. It avoids autoimmunity. The bad cell is gone, and we never knew it was even present. For cancer treatment, however, the nuclear option is not ideal.

Treatment that triggers extrinsic apoptosis not only convinces the cell to commit suicide, it also preps neighboring cancer cells to do the same and recruits the immune system to recognize cancer cells as foreign and dangerous. Some traditional chemotherapeutic agents, while genotoxic, also induce apoptosis through the induction of cellular stress. A non-genotoxic approach would be best for slowly growing solid cancers, especially those with less risk of progression during the patient's lifetime.

In general, genotoxic agents act through intrinsic, nuclear-based apoptosis, and non-genotoxic anti-cancer agents act by inducing extrinsic, cytosolic-induced apoptosis. There is considerable overlap for many agents, however.

Making Chemotherapy More Effective

Effective Dosing: Dosing of these highly toxic medications has usually been based on a calculation of the patient's body surface area (BSA) using a patient's weight and height. In obese patients, that can lead to such high doses that some doctors limit the dose in an attempt to avoid toxicity. The available evidence, however, strongly argues for using the full dose based on a patient's actual BSA. While lower doses may lower toxicity, they are less effective and have poorer survival outcomes. Since different patients process and clear medications at different rates, when possible, blood level testing of the chemo medications should be done to find the most accurate dosing of the medication for the patient.[969] Blood level testing is available for carboplatin, busulfan, methotrexate, 5-FU, docetaxel and paclitaxel.

- ❖ Personalizing chemo dosing by blood level monitoring has been demonstrated to decrease toxicity and side effects. For example, using the FOLFOX regimen in colorectal cancer when compared with BSA dosing, individualized dosing greatly reduced diarrhea, mucositis, and neutropenia,[970] increased disease-free survival,[971] and was cost effective.[972]

- ❖ When possible, target only the cell type or organ that the cancer originated in.

- ❖ Treat early when the cancer cell mass is smaller, hence having a lower probability of mutations.

- ❖ Enhance susceptibility of the cancer cells to apoptosis while protecting normal tissues by differential preparation.

- ❖ Precondition the patient to decrease side-effects of the treatments.

- ❖ Slowly growing cancers with low-risk of progression should be treated with agents that have low genotoxicity, lower risk of inducing mutations, and that are more likely to promote cancer death through stress-induced extrinsic apoptosis.

- ❖ If the target cancer is not derived from immune cells, medications that are less toxic to immune function should be selected.

- ❖ Cancers that are highly susceptible to genotoxic chemotherapy should be treated hard and fast.

An example of targeting the organ or origin and cell type is thyroid cancer. Here the treatment usually begins with surgical removal of the cancer or of the entire thyroid gland, depending on the mutations present in that cancer and the age of the patient. Radioactive iodine, when used, is specifically taken up by the thyroid gland, thus targeting thyroid tissue, and avoiding damage to other tissues. The thyroid can also be specifically targeted by hormones that suppress thyroid activity and growth. Testing of DNA abnormalities in thyroid cancer has further allowed targeted therapy of the genetic defects underlying the cancer. For example, medullary thyroid cancers often have a defect in RET receptor for tyrosine kinase (RTK) that can be treated with vandetanib, an inhibitor of vascular endothelial growth factor receptor (VEGFR) and epidermal growth factor receptor (EGFR).

Chemo Preconditioning

Most solid, difficult-to-treat cancers are still relatively slow growing at the time that they are detected. A several-week delay in treatment of these cancers usually has little impact on the cancer growth or on patient survival. The weeks leading up to treatment can be used to prepare the patient and make the treatment less damaging and more effective. Even if several weeks are not available, there are several things that can be done to protect the patient and improve outcomes.

Cardiovascular exercise training in the weeks leading up to chemo adapt the body to oxidative stress and protect the heart from damage associated with doxorubicin,[973] without lowering antitumor efficacy.[974] Exercise preconditioning appears to decrease damage to skeletal muscles, the brain,[975] immune system,[976] and other organs associated with doxorubicin treatment.[977] Exercise preconditioning can protect normal cells from injury from chemotherapeutic agents that act through the induction of oxidative stress. Exercise improves insulin sensitivity associated with visceral obesity, and lowers insulin and IGF-1 levels and also increases IGF-binding protein-1, decreasing the cancer growth-promoting effects of IGF-1. Patients who are unable to exercise may get some of the benefits of exercise through the use of hot baths as described in Chapters 13 and 38.

Most of the strategies for enhancing AMPK activity discussed in the preceding and following chapters will help protect normal cells from injury during chemo treatment. An exception is the use of metformin.

Metformin prevents gluconeogenesis by the liver, helping to lower blood sugars. It also acts on the mitochondria, inhibiting Complex I activity in oxidative phosphorylation, and reducing ATP production and energy availability for normal and cancer cells. This decreases the ATP:AMP ratio, and helps activate AMPK. Combining short-term starvation with metformin enhances the down-regulated glucose consumption and increases oxidative stress in cancer cells. This effect may, however, be short-term as the cancer cells start to adapt.[978]

While metformin *may be used prior to or after chemo* to slow cancer growth, stopping metformin a couple of days prior to chemotherapy treatment may specifically put the cancer cells at higher risk of toxicity and genome damage, making chemotherapy more effective..., at least in theory. This has not been tested in clinical trials. Metformin during chemo also may increase the risk of lactic acidosis. Metformin should be avoided with the use of trastuzumab (Herceptin) and other agents that decrease cardiac output.

Phytochemicals that enhance the antioxidant response element (ARE) may also help precondition the patients to protect normal cells from oxidative damage from chemotherapy.[979] Many phenolic compounds are anti-carcinogenic on their own. Gallic acid, (present in black tea, cloves, chicory, and other plant sources) activates AMPK, thus slows growth, protecting normal cells during chemotherapy. Gallic acid inhibits HIF-1α and VEGF expression in human ovarian cancer cells.[980] Gallic acid has also been found to induce apoptosis and enhance the cancer-killing effect of the chemo agent cisplatin in small-cell lung cancer.[981] Another phenolic compound, curcumin from turmeric, has been shown to be synergistic with several chemotherapeutic agents in decreasing proliferation and inducing apoptosis in retinoblastoma cells.[982] Thus, these compounds may protect normal cells through preconditioning and increase the sensitivity of cancer cells to chemotherapy. Many flavonoid compounds inhibit activation of NF-κB, and thus, reduce NF-κB's anti-apoptotic, pro-survival influence. Foods rich in these substances can be used during Chemo Precondition™ and as a part of the *Sanafast*™ diet used just prior to and during chemo.

Phytochemicals found in cruciferous vegetables, garlic and onions have also been found to potentiate chemotherapeutic medications. Sulforaphane, found in broccoli, has been shown to protect the brain and retina from reperfusion injury after ischemia,[983] and to protect the stem cells of the heart from chemotherapeutic drugs. Consumption of cruciferous vegetables during preconditioning should help protect these tissues from oxidative stress.

Choline protects the brain and nerves from the oxidative stress injury.[984] In the weeks before chemo, the diet should contain a minimum of 550 mg per day for men and 425 mg per day of choline for women.[985] Broccoli and cauliflower, by the way, are excellent sources of choline.

Allium and cruciferous vegetables, such as garlic[506] and broccoli;[483] boron;[600] and adequate vitamin B12 levels;[986] protect the body from chemotherapy-induced cytotoxicity and genotoxicity and enhance chemo efficacy. Vitamin B12 level should be checked to assure that it is replete (over 540 ng/ml) prior to chemo. Boron supplements (6 mg/day) can be used leading up to chemo, but calcium fructoborate from fruits and nuts is far better. Garlic and cruciferous vegetables should be part of chemo prep, and as directed, as a part of the *Sanafast*™ diet, explained in Chapter 37.

Enhance Cancer Killing

Elevated insulin, IGF-1, and leptin levels are found in insulin and leptin resistance. These hormones support cell growth and survival and inhibit apoptosis, while adiponectin, which is inversely associated with leptin levels, inhibits mTOR-mediated survival. Insulin and leptin resistance may decrease the efficacy of chemotherapy agents that promote stress-induced cell death. As discussed in previous chapters, insulin and leptin resistance can be reversed in six weeks by a low-fat, low-fructose diet and with adequate quality sleep. If there is not sufficient time or compliance, patients with metabolic syndrome or isolated high uric acid levels may benefit from treatment with allopurinol. This medication prevents the decline in adiponectin caused by fructose and helps prevent the associated insulin resistance.

As discussed in previous chapters, the goal is not to lose weight during preconditioning and cancer treatment, but rather to normalize metabolic function. Cancer patients should get counseling and encouragement to follow a diet that helps reverse insulin and leptin resistance.

Sleep also makes a great contribution to normal leptin and adiponectin levels. The patient should be encouraged to get to bed early enough to get eight hours of quality sleep and feel refreshed in the morning. If the patient is suspected of having sleep apnea, they should be treated prior to initiating chemotherapy, in order to lower leptin and raise adiponectin levels. Chapters 12, 13 and 35 provide more details on leptin and adiponectin. Shift workers should be switched to daytime work at the time of a cancer diagnosis, and certainly before chemotherapy is initiated. Inadequate sleep and a disrupted circadian cycle promote inflammation that increases the level of inflammatory cytokines. These inflammatory cytokines impede apoptosis of cancer cells.

If the patient has a hormone-sensitive tumor, such as breast or prostate cancer, hormone therapy should be initiated prior to chemo or radiotherapy to decrease the survival enhancement provided by these hormones and to increase the susceptibility of the tumor cells to stress-induced cell death. In young women being treated for non-hormone-sensitive cancer, such as leukemia, gonadotropin-releasing hormone (GnRH) may be given and then withdrawn prior to chemo to down-regulate ovarian activity, and help decrease damage to the ovaries from chemo.

Phytochemicals may also be useful to enhance the cancer-killing potential of chemo. DIM (3,3'-diindolylmethane), a product formed from I3C (indole-3-carbinol) found in cruciferous vegetables, has been shown to potentiate the anti-tumor effect of paclitaxel on gastric cancer cells.[987] DIM activates growth arrest and DNA-damage-inducible protein (GADD45), a signaling factor for cell stress, that "votes" for apoptosis. IC3 in combination with genistein (from soy), has been shown in some lines of breast cancer cells to decrease the expression of estrogen receptors and trigger apoptosis.[988] Sulforaphane (SFN) has been shown to potentiate the effect of the stress-inducing chemotherapy in cancers without increasing the agent's toxicity to normal cells.[989] In mice, feeding SFN 24-hours prior to ischemia reduced injury. These can be included in the diet in preparation for chemo, but only certain ones can be used in the *Sanafast*™ diet because of choline restrictions.

Phytochemicals that reduce NF-κB activity should increase the efficacy of chemo in promoting apoptosis of cancer cells. The flavonoid compounds, quercetin, luteolin, kaempferol, and resveratrol have been found to promote autophagy.[990] These include highly available forms of phenolic compounds such as those in green olives, capers, cloves, and currants.

Although the in vitro studies combining phenolic compounds from a variety of plants; and sulfur compounds from cruciferous vegetables, garlic, and onion; with chemotherapy are encouraging and support this as a direction for research, to date, no human studies have been published. This is an area that merits research, but that cannot be relied on as a treatment option until more is known.

The following chapters will detail the use of fasting, diet, and hyperthermia to protect normal cells differentially while increasing the sensitivity of cancer to chemotherapy.

Enhance Immune Killing

Sub-toxic doses of chemotherapeutic agents that kill the most susceptible cancer cells may stimulate an immune response against cancer.[991] Efforts to protect immune function should be made so that the immune cells can help eliminate tumor cells. This may be done by selecting chemo agents that are less genotoxic, especially to the bone marrow, and using agents that rely on stressing the cell to promote extrinsic apoptosis.

Timing and Cycling

In the day of tall sailing ships, the ships would leave port in the morning to time their departure with the outgoing tide and offshore breezes. It is much easier to sail downwind and to swim with the tide than against it. In targeting cancer, advantage can be gained by aligning treatment with natural cycles.

Cancers that respond to female sex hormones can be targeted in premenopausal women by treating in sync with the fertility cycle. Genotoxic agents would be more effective when estrogen-responsive tumors are under the growth-promoting influence of the hormone at their peak levels. See Figure 31-2. For other cancers, it is best to treat during the menses when hormone levels are low. For cell stress-inducing agents that promote extrinsic apoptosis, the nadir of hormonal influence would put the cancer at highest risk of apoptosis. This timing can be used for various forms of cancer treatment, including chemotherapy, radiation, and hyperthermia.

There is a natural immune cycle that lasts six to seven days, depending on the person. The immune system has a peak of activity followed three to three and a half days later with a low in immune activity. This cycle can be determined by drawing hs-CRP values every several days of the week for two to three weeks. C-reactive protein (CRP) is an inflammatory mediator that not only indicates cancer risk but also promotes cancer growth. In cancer patients, a high CRP level is associated with a worse prognosis.[992] Hs-CRP is a routine, easily available and relatively inexpensive blood test covered by insurance. There is also a daily immune activity cycle with a peak at about 3 P.M.[993] The nadir of immune activity is around 8:00 AM when cortisol levels peak in individuals with a normal circadian cycle.

The inflammatory cycle can be used to time cancer treatment. Apoptosis is most likely to occur in a low inflammatory milieu, as apoptosis is inhibited NF-κB. Treatment can be timed to be done at the nadir of the 7-day immune cycle, and in the morning when natural cortisol is at its peak and inflammation is at its lowest. This is true for both genotoxic and non-genotoxic chemotherapy, as dosing at the immune nadir may prevent injury to the immune cells and enhance the antitumor activity of the agent.

An even more robust combination or convenient alternative is to use the corticosteroid medication dexamethasone. Dexamethasone, which is often given to decrease toxicity during chemo, has been found to enhance chemo's efficacy for several types of cancer.[994] [995] [996] This effect may be mediated via the increase in ceramide as well by the downregulation of the NF-κB-mediated inflammation.

Patients with BRCA1 mutations or with cancers with de-novo BRCA1 mutations have decreased expression of glucocorticoid receptors. Functional BRCA1 is essential to develop an efficient glucocorticoid signaling, and thus, this signaling is impaired by BRCA1 mutations.[997] These tumors may have little or no pro-apoptotic response to dexamethasone. In these patients, alternative treatments that down-regulate NF-κB and increase ceramide can be applied. Curcumin, flavonoids, and similar compounds may help down-regulate NF-κB. Ceramide-affecting agents are discussed in Appendix B.

Timing should also be used for drug delivery. For example, RTK antibodies and Fas ligands administration should be timed so that peak activity occurs simultaneously with other treatments. If hyperthermia is used as a treatment, medications should be administered so that its peak level occurs in coordination to hyperthermia. One study found that hyperthermia should be initiated 38 minutes after administration of bortezomib to maximize efficacy,[1063] to coordinate their maximal effects.

General Measures

Bed rest, opiates, or beta blockers may protect the heart from chemotherapeutic drugs while the agent is present in the body, by lowering the heart's metabolic activity.[998] Maintaining hydration during chemotherapy can prevent concentration of some chemotherapy toxins in the kidney. Avoiding nausea, vomiting, and diarrhea associated with chemo can help, as they promote dehydration. Gastrointestinal side-effects of chemo can be prevented by fasting or modified-fasting as discussed in the following chapter. IV fluids may be needed to maintain adequate hydration in some patients. Most of the risk factors for cancer growth discussed in previous chapters will worsen outcome for chemo; most of the preventive factors will prevent damage and aid in chemo's success.

Throughout this book, genetic testing has been advocated to help prevent cancer. Cancer cells can also have their genome tested.

Genome testing can determine which cancer-driving genes are in play for the cancer growing in a patient. Even if new mutations occur, it is very unlikely that those present early on will revert to normal. As we learn, more cancers will have their treatment guided by knowledge of which mutations are driving the cancer's growth and survival.

Knowing which gene alterations are present in a cancer can help guide the selection of treatments, allowing more specific and successful targeting of therapy. Knowing which RTKs are misbehaving allows for specific targeting of them. Knowing which enzymes or regulators are up- or down-regulated in a cancer that promotes growth and survival can allow them to be specifically targeted with medications. Cancer may evade toxicity from chemo by up- or down-regulation of certain genes. If we know the mutation, we can target therapy, increasing the specificity of the chemo and avoiding unneeded side-effects and risk of new mutations.

A round of second or third generation chemotherapy can easily cost $300,000 per year of life gained, while genome testing of a cancer should only cost a couple of thousand dollars. Surely, cancer genome testing should be a routine component of treatment, until we move on and find better methods.

37: Modified Fasting

Notice: The information presented in this chapter is based on emerging data in 2016. It is based almost entirely on animal data with only a few human cancer trials. As with any emerging area of science, which we are just beginning to evaluate and understand, may not develop as expected. Consult with your physician before using this information as part of and cancer treatment.

Although I'm confident that you were enraptured by the chapter on mTOR, it wasn't just for fun. In normal cells, growth is promoted by pro-growth effects of Akt and ERK, and inhibited by the effect of AMPK on mTOR. AMPK restricts growth to times of sufficient building materials for new cells, but most cancer cells don't follow these rules. Many cancer cells ignore p53, BRCA, and other checkpoint stop signs telling the cell not to enter into S phase of growth with DNA replication and not to undergo mitosis; situations where the cell is extremely susceptible to DNA and chromosomal errors.

What if we could convince normal, healthy cells, such as the intestinal cells, to take a vacation during chemotherapy so that they avoided being poisoned by chemo? This could protect the intestine and prevent the patient from getting sick from chemotherapy. It would also decrease the risk of healthy cells being damaged by chemo, and lower the risk of chemo causing mutations in healthy cells that could later cause a new cancer. If we can persuade normal cells to take a vacation and stay in the G0 or G1 phases during chemotherapy, we can avoid injury to those cells from genotoxic chemotherapy or radiation treatment, and reduce the risk of treatment-induced cancer.

It turns out that we may be able to go one step better than this. We may be able to construct a diet that selectively baits cancer cells during chemo, increasing the damage to them. We can use diet to differentially stress cancer cells exposed to chemotherapy, pushing them towards apoptosis.

The extracellular growth factor IGF-1 stimulates RTK and cell growth. In lab animals, dietary restriction lowers IGF-1 levels, slows cancer growth, and greatly increases apoptosis of cancer cells. IGF-1 inhibits apoptosis and supports mTOR activation.[999] Injections of this hormone, sufficient to restore the normal fed-levels of IGF-1 in calorie-restricted animals with cancer, restore cancer growth.[1000] Caloric restrictions not only lower the production and circulating levels of IGF-1, but also lower the level of another RTK hormone,

VEGF (vascular endothelial growth factor), a hormone that supports the development of new blood vessels for cancer and its metastatic tumors.[1001]

A difficulty with this diet is that slowing of cancer growth requires restricting caloric intake to less than 60% of the animals' normal dietary intake. This diet starves the cancer of its growth factors. It is easy to restrict the diet of an animal in a cage. People are not that easy, and starvation comes with its own problems, especially since this would require long-term calorie restriction. Additionally, the 40 to 80% caloric restriction needed to lower IGF-1 levels can take months to become effective.[1002] Even if a person were to reduce their dietary intake severely, it could easily be a wasted effort. Severe caloric restrictions do not lower IGF-1 levels in humans without causing malnutrition. Cancer patients would be hungry, weak, and irritable; they would become depressed, aggressive, have significant weight loss, loss of muscle and bone mass, and have slower healing and high susceptibility to infectious diseases. And even though these severe caloric restrictions slow tumor growth, they do not stop the disease.

An alternate-day fast-and-feast diet can allow an individual to consume a healthful diet in amounts according to hunger and satiety. In this diet, on a fast day, the diet is restricted to 20% of the estimated daily caloric requirements, and the next day, food is consumed freely to satisfy hunger and make up for energy deficits. The fast-and-feast diet allows the individual to consume a healthful diet in amounts according to hunger and satiety, without malnutrition. Alternate-day fasting can raise adiponectin levels,[1003] and lower IGF-1 levels.[1004] Alternative daily fasting has been demonstrated to lower markers of oxidative stress and inflammation in humans with asthma.[1005]

Alternate-day fasting has been demonstrated to be as effective as long-term caloric restriction in reducing cell proliferation but with many fewer detrimental side effects.[1006] Data from various experiments suggest that alternate-day fasting is sufficient to provide protection from chemotherapy toxicity and improve outcomes, and it has been recommended that such a diet be used for a few weeks prior to chemo to provide its benefits.[1007]

Another alternative that has better results than long-term calorie restriction is short-term starvation. Short-term starvation (fasting) lowers IGF-1 and raises the level of IGF-binding protein-1 (IGFBP1) in the bloodstream. Raising IGFBP-1 decreases the accessibility of IGF-1 to cells. The decrease in IGF-1 stimulation differentially protects normal cells from several chemotherapeutic agents, while not protecting cancer cells.[1008] Short-term starvation (fasting) is considerably easier than long-term caloric restrictions and does not cause chronic, prisoner of war, death-camp type weight loss. It has also been shown to be more effective in the treatment of (animal implanted with human) cancers. *Cycles of short-term starvation (STS) are as effective as chemotherapy in slowing cancer progression in these animals.*

An even better treatment is the combination of STS with chemotherapy; it has provided long-term cancer-free survival in animals that had been implanted with fast-growing human cancers.[1009] In cancer treatment, fasting not only protects normal cells from damage from chemotherapeutic agents but also makes the cancer cells more susceptible to the toxin. Five days of fasting can provide this benefit.[1010] Fasting is not only helpful for the traditional, highly toxic chemo agents, but also for the tyrosine kinase inhibitors, such as imatinib. For these agents, fasting for more than two days (48 to 60 hours) with only water has been found to increase the drug's efficacy and reduce toxicity to non-cancer cells.[1011] This is great, but a several-day, water-only fast does not qualify as easy and is likely to be accompanied by hunger, irritability, poor decision making, and weakness.

STS during chemotherapy also allows animals to survive higher and more effective doses of chemotherapy that kill animals in the fed state. In animals, short-term starvation prevents damage to the stem cells of the small intestine, providing faster recovery of intestinal function after chemotherapy.[1012]

In human trials of fasting with chemotherapy, a total fast (water only) has been used for 48 to 72 hours prior to treatment and continues for 24 more hours after chemo. The continued fast after chemo is important, as feeding would spur the growth of normal cells while the chemotherapy agent was still in the body. This could cause toxicity to normal cells and raise the risk of DNA damage that might cause resistant or new cancers. The duration of fasting after chemotherapy depends on the half-life of the drug and how long it takes to be cleared from the body.[1009] Thus, the duration of the fast after treatment depends on the medication used and the patient's health and ability to clear the medication from the body. If fasting is used to prevent injury from radiation, eating can resume as soon as the radiotherapy dose has been given, as the exposure is over.

Published reports of STS with chemotherapy are very limited, but their results are encouraging. STS during chemotherapy decreased the intensity of many of the side effects of chemotherapy. It decreased fatigue, weakness, mouth dryness, and mouth sores by more than half. It greatly reduced nausea and abdominal cramping and eliminated post-chemo vomiting and diarrhea. The data suggests that STS during chemo can reduce post-chemotherapy cognitive impairment (PCCI, aka chemo brain); patients who fasted had fewer headaches, and less severe short-term memory impairment, numbness, and altered sensation.[1013]

The short-term trials that have been published only provide data on the immediate toxicity from chemo, and they have not yet provided information on whether STS during chemo in humans provides a cancer survival advantage.

Among the classes of nutrients, including carbohydrates, fats, and proteins, only protein restriction lowers the production of IGF-1.[1014]

When you take a look at steaming, warm, roast beast-steak, it is easy to think about the protein in the meat as a stable structure. And there are proteins such as collagen, which are fairly stable structural proteins. Our muscles seem to be relatively stable from day to day. Most proteins, especially regulatory proteins, however, are quite dynamic and ephemeral. When you consider that the lifespan of some white blood cells can be less than 12 hours, you can appreciate that all the proteins required for the cell to function have to be produced quickly, and are just as quickly disassembled into their parts.

The cell cycle of bread yeast involves over 3,700 proteins. The half-life of proteins in yeast ranges from two minutes to more than twenty hours, with an average of five and a half hours.[1015][1016] But yeasts are just barely animals and have no muscles or bones. Surely, our proteins must be longer lived. Not so much. On a survey of one hundred human proteins, the half-lives ranged from 45 minutes to 22.5 hours.[1017]

Chapter 3 explained protein production, and how tRNA delivers amino acids to the ribosome for protein building. What happens when a required amino acid is missing? The protein production line stops, and the cell can be in deep trouble. This usually does not happen, as the cell senses low amino acid levels; AMPK is activated, puts the brakes on growth-oriented protein production and starts an autophagy recycling program that frees up amino acids to make essential services proteins needed to keep the cell alive. Restricting carbohydrates and triglycerides does not provide protection to healthy cells from chemotherapy; this requires protein restriction.

Restricting protein intake to 0.95 grams per kilogram a day (from 1.67 g per kg) lowers IGF-1 levels by nearly 25 percent,[1018] a difference that would be expected to slow cell growth. A separate study demonstrated a decline in IGF-1 when comparing 1.0 g per kg of protein a day to 0.66 g per kg.[1019]

While IGF-1 measurement is convenient, as it can be measured in the blood of animals and humans, the effect of protein restriction is not limited to circulating levels of growth factors. Short-term starvation also differentially increases the oxidative stress caused by chemotherapy and promotes apoptosis in cancer cells. The reasons for this become apparent when considering the information presented in previous chapters; when normal cells lack resources, AMPK becomes activated, and mTOR gets shut down. This slows the production of new proteins for cell growth and promotes apoptosis.

Before we get into the details of fasting for chemotherapy, there is another reason for fasting; to prevent cancer and prevent aging.

Fasting can cause cells to do spring cleaning by promoting autophagy. In autophagy, the cell tags older proteins and organelles for recycling; the amino acids and lipids are used as fuel and for building new proteins and organelles. The cell components may be slimmed down for a less active but more efficient cell during times of famine. Why carry a load of twice as many mitochondria, or twice the useful capacity for protein production during lean times? Autophagy allows the cell to get rid of old, worn-out parts. Production can be increased with new parts when richer supplies of fuel and construction materials are available. This gives the cells a tune-up. The internal and external cellular membranes, proteins and organelles can all be replaced. Even the mitochondria get refreshed, and the old weak ones get culled and replaced by healthier ones. Even though it is the same cell, if it has all new parts, it is almost like a new cell.

Almost but not quite; it is more like a new car, with the same old driver and his luggage. The DNA, although it may be repaired, does not get replaced with a new DNA. Old errors will still be there, but healthier cells make fewer *new* DNA errors. And then there is the luggage. As cells age, they tend to accumulate lipofuscin.

Lipofuscin is a mix of waxy substances that are composed of oxidized lipids the cell does not know what to do with. Much of this oxidative damage comes from poorly functioning mitochondria leaking ROS. The cell does not have enzymes that can process lipofuscin, so it just accumulates in the cell as long as the cell lives. This is as long as we live for most of our neurons, retinal cells, and heart cells.

Lipofuscin is sort of like linseed oil-soaked rags sitting in a corner. They can catch fire and burn the house down. Accumulation of lipofuscin eventually kills cells, likely by damaging liposomes and causing the release of cathepsin-B that, along with a strong oxidative stress, promotes the activation of the inflammasome. Thus, a strong oxidative insult in old cells that have accumulated too much lipofuscin can trigger cell death. This can happen in elderly persons who suffer a severe febrile illness. It can occur in the non-renewable cells of the heart, retina, and brain with chemotherapy. Thus, preconditioning for oxidative stress prior to chemotherapy or hyperthermia can prevent the death of these cells.

Periodic fasting can be used to prevent cancer as well as treating it, as it promotes autophagy and mitophagy, making cells healthier. It also promotes apoptosis of unhealthy and DNA-compromised cells, helping to rid the body of pre-cancerous cells.

Thus, fasting, exercise, hot baths, phenolic compounds in food, and other agents that stimulate an AMPK response can stimulate the urban renewal that prevents lipofuscin accumulation and aging of the cell. This should be done throughout the lifetime to keep cells healthy and vigorous. Frequent housecleaning through autophagy throughout a person's lifetime can prevent poorly functioning mitochondria from leaking free radicals that cause lipofuscin formation and DNA damage.

At the beginning of the book, I promised to make things easy, but fasting is hard and inconvenient, and hunger is unpleasant. Most of us have busy lives with demands from jobs and family and going hungry while at work or caring for your family is not prudent. It makes people more aggressive. In the flight or fight response, the evolutionary imperatives side with going toe-to-toe and fighting over that hambone when we are hungry, rather than backing off or fleeing; a hungry person is more likely to act aggressively.

What if you could have the benefits of fasting without having to go hungry?

Now that we know that carbohydrate and fat restrictions do not lower IGF-1, and only protein restriction does, it may occur to you that only protein fasting is required for STS to be effective in lowering IGF-1. This would allow a fast that permits starches and fats. Oh yum! But fortunately, we can tweak the diet a bit further.

We understand that protein availability affects cell proliferation and is key for growth. Furthermore, it is not protein per se, but rather certain amino acids present in proteins.

An adequate supply of methionine appears to be needed upstream of mTORC1 for its activation. Methionine participates in the uncoupling of Tsc1 and Tsc2.[1020] AMPK prevents the separation of Dsc1 from Dsc2, and thus, mTOR activation. CaMKKβ is stimulated when methionine levels are low, activating AMPK. On the flip side, the ERK or Akt pathways activate the dissociation of Dsc1 from Dsc2 and activation of mTOR. Critical to the activation of ERK and Akt is an adequate supply of phosphatidic acid (PA). The availability of PA is limited by the supply of phosphatidylcholine. Phosphatidylethanolamine (PE) can be recycled into PC but three molecules of methionine are required to supply S-adenosyl-methionine (SAMe) needed as methyl donors.

Additionally, when there is a deficit of methionine, the cell looks for amino acids by triggering autophagy, which breaks down older or redundant proteins and organelles. The key to autophagy, the intracellular recycling mechanism, is activated by a short supply of three nutrients; the essential amino acid methionine, betaine, and dietary choline, which can be converted into phosphatidylcholine.

Phosphatidylcholine (PC) is of great interest here, as it is part of the signaling transduction for cell growth. RTK tyrosine kinase activity stimulates PLD enzymatic conversion of PC to PA that activates Akt and ERK and impedes AMPK activation. PA thus activates mTORC1 and the production of proteins; promotes the formation of lipids for the formation of new cell membranes from glucose, and impedes apoptosis.

Choline deficiency can promote apoptosis. It promotes the generation of ROS and oxidative stress.[1021] Through activation of Akt, PA prevents BCL-2 signaling for mitochondrial pore formation and the leaking of cytochrome C and apoptosis.[1022] The enzyme choline kinase-α is involved in the synthesis of phospholipids and in the development of some cancers. Choline kinase-α inhibiting drugs are being developed as potential chemotherapeutic agents and have been shown to induce apoptosis in cellular and animal models.[1023]

Choline is also used in the production of sphingomyelin and can be metabolized into betaine. Betaine (trimethylglycine) can provide a methyl group to recycle SAMe, just as methionine can. Phosphatidylinositol (PI) plus three molecules of SAMe can be used to form PC, or it can be made of one molecule of PI plus one of choline. Betaine also protects cells from osmotic stress that can promote apoptosis. Thus, choline is a rich alternative to methionine, and may be the salient signal of adequate energy and vigor for cell growth. Remember that when SAMe gets used and donates its methyl group, it becomes homocysteine that can be recycled into SAMe if sufficient methyl providers (methionine, betaine or choline) are present.

Homocysteine promotes inflammation in large part by activating an enzyme, aSMase (acid sphingomyelinase). ASMase causes the release of ceramide from the sphingomyelin that is stored in cell membranes. The release of ceramide can promote cell growth and proliferation or promote apoptosis. When there is sufficient energy, ceramide is converted into S1P or C1P that promote multiple growth pathways.

Especially when energy levels are low, ceramide promotes apoptosis via the activation of cathepsin and ASK1 and inhibition of Akt. Ceramide can be converted to sphingosine, which promotes apoptosis by activation of caspase 8.[1024] Additionally, the enzyme PAP can hydrolyze S1P into sphingosine, C1P into ceramide, and PA into diacylglycerol, plus a phosphate in each reaction. PAP is stimulated by fasting and inhibited by ATP.[1025]

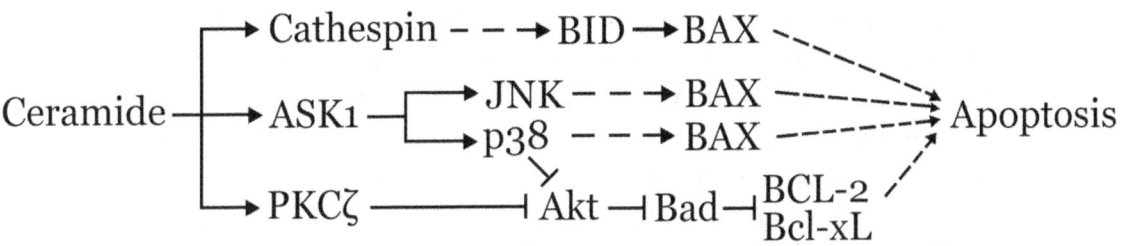

Figure 37-1: Ceramide pathways and apoptosis.[1026]

Thus, ceramide helps to promote the growth of well-nourished energetic cells and promotes the death of weak, feeble and senescent ones. Curcumin, a flavonoid-like compound, increases ceramide synthase activity and promotes apoptosis.[1027] TNF-α also promotes aSMase and ASK1) activity but also promotes sphingosine kinase that converts ceramide into the pro-proliferative compound S1P.[1028]

Since choline is a component of cell membrane phospholipids, well-nourished cells have a store of choline at their disposal. At least in men, however, blood choline levels fall within a few days on a choline-depleted diet. This depletion can injure hepatic cells sufficiently to raise liver enzyme levels within a couple of weeks.[1029] Thus, in growing cells, where new cell membranes are needed, choline deficiency can rapidly occur. In one cell culture study, choline deprivation increased apoptosis by 16 times during a 48-hour incubation.[596]

Thus, choline restriction during a modified fast may increase cell stress in rapidly growing cells, such as cancer cells, and induce apoptosis. Quiescent cells are less prone to damage from short-term choline depletion. Nevertheless, choline restriction may be less effective for fertile women undergoing chemotherapy. Estrogen stimulation gives these women the capacity to form choline from other phospholipids. This process requires SAMe; thus, methionine and betaine restriction should limit this ability. An estrogen inhibitor used as part of chemotherapy for estrogen-sensitive cancers may limit this. Thus, a methionine, choline, and betaine fast can promote a choline deficit that impedes growth and promotes apoptosis, via the limitation of PA and the induction of ceramide.

MTORC1 provides signaling for protein synthesis, cell cycling, and inhibition of programmed cell death. Dietary restriction can also affect the downstream signaling of mTORC1. While a deficit of any amino acid can stop the translation of mRNA in the ribosome to protein, the cell uses certain amino acids as signaling agents to determine if there is an adequate supply of amino acids. This helps keep the cell from embarking on futile cell building projects.

In the presence of insulin, a higher concentration of amino acids increases S6K1 activity. Downstream of mTOR activation S6K1 and eIF4E require the presence of specific amino acids for their activity. The amino acids leucine and arginine are both required for normal activation of S6K1, and a deficit of either one impairs S6K1 activity even when all other amino acids are present in adequate supply. Even if other AA are sufficiently present, a leucine deficit reduces S6K1 activity by nearly 90%, and lack of arginine reduces its activity by about 70%.[1030] Impeding S6K1 activity impairs mRNA translation for proteins and promotes apoptosis via PDCD4 (programmed cell death protein 4).

4E-BP1 phosphorylation activates eIF4E. EIF4E prepares the mRNA so that it can enter the ribosome for protein transcription. 4E-BP1 phosphorylation depends on certain amino acids; the branched-chain AAs (BRAA): leucine, isoleucine, and valine. BRAA are the only amino acids whose levels rise in the peripheral bloodstream in proportion to their content in the diet after a meal. Thus, BRAA signal the presence of protein availability. Other AAs are mostly retained in the liver and gut and released as needed. The BRAA are also among the amino acids with the highest concentrations in the muscles. BRAA give a good indication of the availability of AA's available for growth.[1031]

There is one more AA worth mentioning here. The amino acid glutamine also plays a unique role in mTOR activity. Glutamine is a rate-limiting AA for mTOR activation in normal cells since it is the exchange AA for leucine and other branched-chain amino acid. The sodium-dependent carrier protein LAT1 transports glutamine out of the cell in exchange for importing leucine and other BCAA and aromatic amino acids into the cell.[1032] Glutamine is a non-essential AA except during times of high demand such as physiological stress. Glutamine is plentiful in the diet and can be formed from glutamate and certain other amino acids and other compounds. Since this is an energy-dependent process, glutamine serves as yet another indicator of the abundance of energy available to the cell.

LAT1 is a dimeric protein composed of SLC1A5 and SLC3A2. SLC1A5 is expressed on many tumor cells and required for their survival.[1033] Glutamine deficiency can induce apoptosis.[1034] Glutamine synthesis and transport blocking agents are being studied as possible targets for cancer treatment for melanoma, leukemia, lung, prostate and other cancers.[1035] [1036] Glutamine synthetase inhibitors,[1037] along with dietary restriction of glutamine, may have potential in the treatment of cancer; however, adequate dietary restrictions of glutamine alone would be ineffective. Furthermore, glutamine synthase inhibition may greatly increase the risk of neurotoxicity during cancer treatment.[1038] [1039] Glutamine synthase production is induced by glucocorticoids such as cortisol and dexamethasone, growth hormone, triiodothyronine (T3), and insulin. Glutamine synthase production is inhibited by interleukin 1β and tumor necrosis factor-α.[1040] Although glutamine restricts the cells access to BRAA, since it is easily made by the cell, dietary restrictions of this AA do not appear to be a favorable target. Activation of AMPK, however, should limit the formation of glutamine in the cell.

Thus, there are two choke points for cell growth that can be manipulated by dietary restriction of two amino acids and one-and-a-half vitamins. A methionine – choline – betaine restriction will promote autophagy and slow growth. This diet could be used as a fast to promote health and prevent cancer on its own. A 40% methionine-restricted diet decreases mitochondrial ROS production and free radical leak from mitochondria measured in the brain and kidneys of laboratory animals,[1041] and increases the lifespan lab animals almost as much as does a 40% restriction of total calories.[1042] For a double whammy on cancer, a methionine – choline, branched-chain AA diet would greatly decrease growth. Leucine is the most critical of the branched chain AAs, as it helps activate S6K1 and thus inhibits PDCD4.

Restricting leucine while permitting isoleucine and valine, which allow eIF4E activation may promote unbalanced and futile promotion of DNA replication in the nucleus of cancer cells, and begin the futile threading of mRNA into the ribosome. These activities would put these cells at further risk of damage from cell stress and may promote apoptosis, at least in theory. It likely makes little practical difference as most low-leucine foods are also low in other branched chain AAs.

Thus, as promised, here is the *Sanafast*™ diet, an almost easy, possibly palatable, hunger-avoiding, anti-cancer "modified fast" that can be used to enhance cancer treatment. One more restriction will also be added to enhance the methionine - choline - leucine restriction; choline can be converted in the body into betaine (trimethylglycine), which can donate a methyl group to recycle homocysteine into methionine, as shown in Figure 26-2). The nutrient betaine spares choline, and recycles methionine, and thus, should also be restricted.

NOTE: The *Sanafast*™ diet is a modified-fast is designed to impede growth. This diet is not recommended for pregnant and lactating women or growing children except under the advice and care of their personal physician for the treatment of disease. Furthermore, the dietary requirements for protein are higher in children and pregnant and lactating women. While the World Health Organization (WHO) estimates a daily intake of 0.45 grams of protein per kilogram (0.204 grams per pound) of ideal body weight as the minimum daily protein intake required for maintaining nitrogen balance, it estimates a requirement more than three times higher for pregnant adolescents.[1043] This modified fast is not intended as a regular diet but as a short-term therapeutic fast for intermittent use.

Calculations for the Diet

Ideal Body Mass (for Dietary Requirements)

Men: 106 lbs. + (6 lbs per inch over 60" in height)

48 kg + (1 kg per cm over 150 cm in height)

Women: 100 lbs. + (5 lbs per inch over 60" in height)

45 kg + (0.85 kg per cm over 150 cm in height)

Several studies indicate that a forty percent long-term protein restriction is sufficient to effect the metabolic changes that increase lifespan through the induction of autophagy. The standard in these diets is about equivalent to the dietary *recommendation* for 0.8 grams of protein per kilogram, and thus, a 40% restriction would be 0.48 mg/Kg, almost identical to the WHO estimate for protein *requirement*; below this level, adults begin losing muscle mass. Protein needs vary among individuals, but a diet with 0.3 mg/Kg protein creates a protein deficit pretty universally.

However, we are concerned with only certain amino acids, the branched-chain amino acids, particularly leucine, and methionine. Thus, we will want to restrict the amino acid content of the fast to a level that assures a deficit in order to promote autophagy and facilitate apoptosis.

37-2: Dietary requirements for amino acid balance

Nitrogen Balance[1043]	Per Kilogram Ideal Body Mass	Per Pound Ideal Body Mass
Protein: Balanced	0.45 grams	0.204 grams
Methionine Balance	10.4 mg	4.7 mg
Leucine balance	26 mg	11.8 mg
Isoleucine balance	26	11.8
Valine balance	14	6.4
Methionine 2/3 of balance	6.93 mg	3.15 mg
Leucine 2/3 of balance	17.3 mg	7.88 mg

A 5'8" tall man would have an ideal body weight of 154 pounds (70 kg) and would have a (0.45 × 70 =) 31.5-gram daily protein requirement to maintain muscle mass. Individuals who are building muscle or growing may need three times this much protein in their diets. He would need 728 mg of methionine and 1,820 mg of leucine. We are also going to assume a 2200 kcal intake for this individual.

A two-thirds restriction has been selected to push this diet into a protein deficit. The 0.45 g/Kg requirement for protein balance is thus limited to 0.3 mg of protein per Kg per day.

A methionine deficit diet that supplies two-thirds of the methionine needs for a 70 Kg ideal body weight man would limit methionine intake to 485 mg a day. A leucine deficit diet that supplies two-thirds of the leucine needs for that person would limit leucine intake to 1211 mg a day.

The 485 mg of methionine supply two Calories, and the 1121 mg of leucine supply five, in a diet of 2200 kcal. A restricted diet would limit foods to those with less than 22 mg of methionine and less than 51 mg of leucine per 100 kcal. These may seem odd metrics, but they come in handy for planning meals.

Other amino acids are much less important, and may even allow for further depletion of methionine and leucine, as these amino acids may be incorporated into proteins, helping to deplete methionine and leucine. When specific amino acid data is not available, food total protein may be used to gage foods use in the *Sanafast*™ diet.

Foods with less than 1.0 gram of protein per 100 kcal are acceptable; however, caution must be used for rounding, as 1.45 grams a protein may be displayed as 1 gram on a label.

The effects a low-methionine diet has on autophagy, impairing cell growth, and apoptosis likely depends largely on methionine being used to recycle homocysteine into SAMe, and SAMe helping to form phosphatidylcholine. Thus, choline and betaine need to be restricted in the *Sanafast*™ diet. In this diet, choline should be restricted to less than 5 mg/Kg per day and betaine to less than 2.5 mg/Kg, to maintain a deficit of these nutrients.[1044]

Appendix A lists several food ingredients that meet the criteria for this diet: These foods have a leucine and methionine contents less than 51 and 22 mg/ 100 Calories, respectively. Choline + (Betaine/3.375) content of the food should be no more than 15 mg per 100 Cal, and preferably less than two-thirds this amount. The *Sanafast*™ diet also includes foods that promote autophagy and apoptosis, such as garlic, broccoli sprouts, and certain foods high in phenolic compounds. Nutrition data for specific foods can be found online at http://nutritiondata.self.com/tools/nutrient-search.

Prevention of Cancer and Aging

The *Sanafast*™ diet can also be used to prevent cancer and aging. It promotes autophagy and mitophagy. Mitochondria have a turnover time of about seven days, a renewal cycle of about once a week. This methionine, choline, betaine, and leucine, (MCBL) restricted fast, one (long) day a week, along with vigorous exercise, or a hot bath if you are feeling feeble, should be enough to cull the weakest and most polluting mitochondria and other worn out organelles. If the *Sanafast* diet is started with an MCBL-restricted supper, through the following day and until breakfast the next morning, it would give a one day's fast, plus two nights; thus, a 40 hour (long) one day fast.

Such a fast once a week or every two weeks should keep the cells fit. A seasonal, two-day, three-night deeper cleaning may be used for turnover of more organelles to help slow aging and prevent cancer.

After a *Sanafast*™, a diet with a very low n6:n3 fat ratio should be implemented. The *Sanafast* diet depletes polyunsaturated fats from the cell membranes. Breaking this fast gives an excellent opportunity to replenish the cell membranes with anti-inflammatory n-3 fats from fish and other sources (Table25-2).

Preconditioning for Chemotherapy

The *Sanafast*™ diet is designed for *preconditioning for chemotherapy*. The goal is to prevent oxidative stress of "immortal" cells in the heart, brain, retina, and cochlear cells of the ear to avert damage from oxidative stress due to chemotherapy. Older patients and those with a history of exposure to oxidative injury, such as smokers and those with a history of high alcohol consumption, are at especially high risk. These individuals often have higher loads of lipofuscin that can trigger programmed cell death when exposed to a strong oxidative stress. Preconditioning for chemo can be done by using the MCBL-restricted *Sanafast* one or two days a week for several weeks prior to starting chemo. Try to get in five 40-hour fasts, at least three days apart, before chemo.

The *Sanafast*™ for Cancer Treatment

The goals for this diet are to restrict normal cell growth and activity to protect them from injury from chemotherapy, to promote apoptosis in cancer cells, and to decrease gastrointestinal and other side-effects of chemo. It is recommended that the *Sanafast* begin with supper, three to four days preceding cancer treatment with radiation, chemotherapy, or hyperthermia. The diet should continue for the day of treatment, and the day after treatment for chemotherapy so that the medication can be cleared from the body before returning to normal cell activity. Return to a normal diet can begin immediately after radiation therapy.

> Note: Not all cancers behave the same. Some cancers have mutations that allow them to grow in spite of low IGF-1 levels or have other mutations that may circumvent the effects of fasting. Additionally, fasting does not protect normal cells from all chemotherapy agents.
>
> Most cancer cells depend on glycolysis for the generation of ATP. In the liver, glucagon released from the pancreas during a fasting state inhibits the glycolysis enzyme pyruvate kinase. Thus, fasting may have a different effect on liver cancer cells than on cancer cells from other organs.

Avoid Artificial Emulsifiers

The food additives polysorbate (PSB) and carboxymethyl cellulose (CMC) are not degraded during digestion and cause a detergent action the disrupts the mucous layer that protects the cells of the colon,[1045, 1046] increasing the risk of neutropenic enterocolitis. PS (Tween, PEG) and CMC may be found in ice cream. PS may be found in whipped crèmes, barbecue sauces, pickles and cottage cheese.

CMC is used in some baked goods, chewing gums, peanut butter, margarine, toothpaste. Read the labels of all manufactured foods before eating them. These agents should be completely avoided in the days before and after chemo, and most other days of our lives.

The natural emulsifier lecithin should during a *Sanafast* because of its high choline content.

Ceramide and aSMase

The enzyme aSMase induces the release of ceramide from sphingomyelin. Ceramide can induce apoptosis and inhibit Akt and activation of mTORC1. Curcumin, found in turmeric, promotes aSMase activity and is thought to have anticarcinogenic potential, at least in part, through the induction of apoptosis. It can be included in an anti-cancer diet. The inclusion of curcumin and other phenolic compounds enhance the MCBL restrictions of the *Sanafast*™ diet.

There are a few natural plant compounds that inhibit aSMase; one of interest here is tomatidine, found in tomatoes. Tomato-based foods should be avoided for the 24 hours before and after chemo to prevent reduction of its efficacy. Also of concern during cancer treatment are about 100 medications that effectively inhibit aSMase. These include medications commonly used among cancer patients, including Zoloft, Claritin, tamoxifen, and promethazine. Avoiding these agents when possible by using alternative medications during cancer treatment may help promote cancer cell death. Ceramide metabolism and medications affecting it are further discussed in Appendix B.

Vitamin D, the B vitamin pyridoxine-5-phosphate (P5P), and magnesium are cofactors in the metabolism of ceramide into other compounds. P5P and magnesium are cofactors for many enzymes, and on balance lower the production of S1P and C1P, thus decreasing inflammation and cancer cell promotion.

The B vitamins, folate, B12, betaine, and choline promote recycling of homocysteine by SAMe and thus decrease the activation of aSMase and ceramide production. Lipoic acid also prevents activation of aSMase by homocysteine. These nutritional compounds may inhibit the efficacy of cell stress induced by chemotherapy from inducing programmed cell death. They should be avoided in the days leading up to and during chemo to increase cancer killing.

Vitamins and minerals should come from food in a balanced, nutritious diet. Vitamin supplements should only be used to correct nutritional deficiencies, after testing the blood.

38: Hyperthermia

In Chapter 10 on exercise, the use of hot baths to mimic some of the cancer preventive effects of exercise was briefly discussed. It was mentioned that hot baths can help with the control of diabetes.

What do you do when you get the flu and have a fever? Most of us take an antipyretic such as Tylenol, Motrin or aspirin. Fever is the body's reaction to infection, and it is not without purpose. The use of an antipyretic in patients with viral influenza is associated with a 5% increase in mortality,[1047] and in critically ill, septic patients, the use of an antipyretic may also decrease survival.[1048] Fever helps fight infections by activating immune cells and increasing WBC population growth, survival, and migration to the site of infection. An elevated environmental temperature even helps cold-blooded lizards fight infections more efficiently.[1049] Fever increases the susceptibility of infected cells by bacteria and viruses to pyroptosis. On the other hand, fevers cause high metabolic demands and may worsen ischemia to stressed organs, such as the heart and brain. During myocardial ischemia, stroke, or other brain injuries, fever should be treated.

In the pre-antibiotic era, fever was sometimes used to treat certain chronic infections. Along with other agents used for syphilis treatment, sterilized skim milk was injected to cause a fever increasing treatment efficacy.[1050] In the pre-chemotherapy era, fever was used to treat cancer, and *this therapy was as effective as modern chemotherapy is today.* Yes, this sounds like one of those internet conspiracy stories claiming that the government is withholding a secret technology that allows a car to get 300 miles per gallon, or that the FDA banned an effective cure for cancer. (It kinda did.)

William Coley was a young doctor at New York Memorial Hospital in the 1890's. Very early in his career, he had an 18-year-old woman only a few years younger than himself as a patient. She presented with a minor injury to her right hand that was not healing. It turned out to be a sarcoma. There was no evidence of metastasis, so the arm was amputated in an attempt to save her life. She spent the next three months in hospital.

In his words, Coley watched "a disease that starting from an insignificant injury, attack(s) a person in perfect health, in the full vigor of early maturity, and in some insidious, mysterious way, within a few months, destroy(s) life." He watched this young woman develop numerous painful metastases and die during the months she spent in the hospital under his care.

Dedicating himself to research sarcoma treatment, he learned of another patient that had been treated by a senior colleague at the hospital, who had assisted in the young woman's care. This previous patient had a large sarcoma tumor on the face that was surgically removed; however, the cancer returned, and the tissue and surrounding surgical excision became infected with erysipelas, a soft tissue infection caused by *Streptococcus pyogenes*. In the late 1800's, without antibiotics, there was little to do to treat the infection. The patient had had two bouts of high fever from erysipelas, followed by a rapid regression of the tumor and healing of the wound. After hearing about the patient, Coley spent weeks searching for the man on New York's Lower East Side. He found him in good health seven years after his hospitalization, but with a large scar on his face,

With further research, Coley found reports of several other cancer cases in which patients apparently healed after erysipelas infection. In 1893, Coley published a few case studies of cancer patients intentionally inoculated with the pathogen.[1051] With some success and some deaths from infection, Coley realized that he could achieve better results with lower risk by injecting killed bacteria into the patients.

Coley was not the first to treat cancer with infections. In Europe in the 1700's, patients with ulcerating cancers were sometimes treated with bandages from patients with infections. (Yuck!) By killing the bacteria first, Coley avoided having the infection kill the patient.

Coley's treatment involved daily or every-other-day injections of two species of killed bacteria that, in most patients, caused high fevers, fatigue, and weakness. The in-hospital treatments continued until the tumors resolved, sometimes requiring several weeks. The five-year survival rate was about 60% for those responding with a fever of 38.5° to 40° C, but only 28% for those who did not attain temperatures above 38.5° C.[1052]

The "vaccine" caused high fevers, but if it failed to cause fever, it failed to kill the cancer. Remarkably, cancer-associated pain abated sufficiently after the first fever that narcotics could usually be stopped.

Over his career, Coley treated more sarcoma patients, perhaps, than any other physician of his time. Before 1930, the five-year survival rate for inoperable sarcomas and carcinomas treated by Coley's vaccine was similar to current survival rates with the use of modern chemotherapy.[1053] Although it was an accepted method of treatment for sarcoma until 1963, Coley's treatment was not widely used, as radiation therapy was easier, less expensive, seemed more modern, and was less uncomfortable for the patient. Never mind that radiation was rarely effective. And yes, the FDA did put the kibosh on the vaccine. The newly implemented FDA rules in 1963 required a new drug application, but without a patent and a deep-pocketed champion to benefit financially, it never happened.

Now that medicine has a better knowledge of the underpinnings of biomolecular science, do we understand how Coley's vaccine worked, and can we use that knowledge to cure cancer? We are getting there. Coley's vaccine contained pyrogens that caused fever, bacterial toxins, and immunogens. Our current understanding is that bacterial toxins in the vaccine provided no treatment benefit.

Additionally, Coley's vaccine promoted an immune response. Immunogens from the cell wall components of the killed bacteria activate the TLR4 receptors on the cell walls of white blood cells. Toll-like receptors recognize specific microbial compounds. This increases the immune activity, growth, and survival of immune cells that help eliminate cancer cells.[1054] TLR4 receptors are also present on some solid cancer cells, including breast cancer, so the cell wall components may impede apoptosis for these tumors. Certain small segments of bacterial single-stranded DNA are recognized by TLR9. Since TLR-9 is only expressed on B-cell lymphocytes, the bacterial DNA only stimulates B-cell activity and development of antibodies that may help in the immune response to a tumor. TLR-9 stimulus, however, may promote the growth and development of lymphomas.

As we knew from Coley's experiments, the fever was critical. Heat exploits inherent weaknesses of cancer cells; the genes that are permissive of mutations because they fail to stop mutations from reproducing also allow for critical errors. Heat stress induces changes in the expression of thousands of proteins in the cell. In a comparison between normal and cancerous breast cells, there were hundreds of proteins that were differentially expressed in cancer cells after heat exposure. Heat treatment of breast cancer cells in culture found that most of the cell deaths occurred in cells during the G2/M phase of cell growth. This appears to be the phase at which cells are most susceptible to heat-induced damage.[1055] Cell death during the G2/M phase, however, is unlikely to explain the resolution of solid cancers, as most cells are not actively growing at any one time in these cancers.

At 45° C (113° F), cells die a necrotic death. They die from a lethal systemic collapse of functions. This is not a programmed death, and it kills all cells, not just cancer cells. Between 42° C (107.6° F) and

43° C (109.4° F) cells die orderly, programmed cell deaths.[1056] Exposure to mild hyperthermia, 40° C (104° F), levels that usually do not cause injury, creates stress that that actually induces thermotolerance and protects the cell from endoplasmic reticulum (ER) stress-induced apoptosis.[1057] These low, fever level temperatures appear to spare normal cells from damage. Fever, by design, promotes apoptosis of cells containing aberrant proteins, RNA, and DNA from viruses and bacteria, while sparing normal cells.

Fever also activates the immune system. White blood cells are more active and efficient at fever temperatures, even in animals that do not mount fevers in response to infection. A desert iguana was found to have a 75% decrease in survival from infection if prevented from raising its core temperature 2° Celsius through muscular activity. The poliovirus replication rate in cells is 200 times lower with a fever of 40 to 41° C than at normal body temperature. White blood cells have increased activity at fever temperatures of 39.5° C.[1058]

While cancer cells may have less than a dozen "cancer-driving mutations" they may have ten times as many other mutations. These mutations may cause protein misfolding. Fever can exploit this difference. Maintaining a fever or heating the tumor area with a short pulse of moderate hyperthermia at 42° C increases apoptosis of tumor cells. Heating tumor cells induces the release of misfolded proteins from the ER. This release can activate the inflammasome and act as chemokines, drawing white blood cells to the tumor.

Fever increases the metabolic demand of the body. For every 1°C increase in temperature, the cells increase their metabolism by 10 to 12%.[1058] This means the cells need ten percent more oxygen and fuel, and this may disproportionately affect cancer cells that often have a tenuous oxygen supply. Cancer cells may also be less capable of adaptation to heat and less able to develop thermotolerance to protect themselves from stress-induced injury. Coley's success, using sequentially increasing doses of bacteria during hyperthermia therapy over many days, would suggest that development of thermotolerance by the patient does not impede successful treatment of cancer, however, it is not clear that cancer does not become thermo-tolerant with repeated exposure to mild hyperthermia or other non-lethal stress.

Most of the attention to heat-induced killing of cancer cells has centered on Heat Shock Proteins (HSP). The name "heat-shock proteins" was given, as subjecting cells to heat, akin to high fever temperatures, induces the production of numerous proteins in the cells, many having to do with stress reactions. Heat shock proteins (HSP) are induced by heat, and also by some other cell stressors. There are many HSP; some are associated with further advanced and more invasive cancers, while others are not.[1059][1060] The job of most HSP is to protect the cell from stress; the increase in HSP corresponds to an increase in the level of these proteins when the cell is stressed, and heat is one of the stressors HSP respond to. Heat shock proteins protect cells, both normal and cancer cells. Treatment of cells with quercetin, an inhibitor of HSP-70, sensitizes cancer cells to hyperthermia-induced apoptosis without increasing the risk to normal cells.[1061]

One heat sensitive system is the Heat Shock Factor:Heat Shock Protein complex; when paired, this complex resides in the cytosol and is inactive. When this complex senses misfolded proteins (MFPs) in the cell, it dissociates releasing the HSP. The HSP helps refold MFPs back into their correct and functional form. Misfolding of proteins can be caused by several cell stressors, such as pH change, reactive oxygen species (ROS), or excessive heat. If many MFPs are detected in the cell, and many HSF:HSP complexes are activated, there will be a sufficient quantity of newly freed HSF molecules to bump into each other and form triplets. These triads can migrate into the nucleus, where they act as a transcription factor for stress proteins, including more HSF. The newly minted HSF will bind to HSP and when in balance, they return to their inactive state.

Since heat can cause proteins to denature, temporarily disrupting hydrogen bonds that then randomly reform, often aberrantly, heat can cause a massive wave of MFP and a massive activation of HSP triads of Heat Shock Element protein transcription.

The optimal temperature for formation and binding of the heat shock element (HSF:HSF:HSF) to the DNA is 42° C, at about 15 minutes after the start of heat exposure. Few MFPs are created at 41°C, and at temperatures of 43° C or higher, DNA translation becomes impaired.[1062] The peak of MFPs occurs after about 25 minutes of hyperthermia. It does not take this much time to misfold the proteins, but rather, 25 minutes of hyperthermia provides sufficient time to exhaust the supply of HSP for protein repair. The peak for new HSP and HSF protein production occurs about 110 minutes after initiation of heating, although the heat does not need to be applied this length of time. It may be possible to avoid thermo-tolerance by using short pulses of heating.[1063] Thus, 42° C appears to be the Goldilocks spot to cause MFPs.

Some cancers are sensitive to lower temperatures, and may have decreased survival at 40° C; however, others are more resistant.[1064]

Many proteins in the cell are rendered dysfunctional by oxidative or heat stress. Some HSPs help protect or restore proteins that are bent out of shape by oxidative or heat stresses.

Heat Shock Proteins, such as the HSP70 and HSP90, act as protein chaperones in the cell. They help shape proteins, aid in reshaping misfolded ones and mark damaged proteins that cannot be repaired for disposal. HSP also protects the cell from apoptosis.

Another heat-sensitive protein, HSPA5, acts as a chaperone in the endoplasmic reticulum, preventing premature protein folding, and thus, protein misfolding, in the endoplasmic reticulum. During protein production in the cell, mRNA is translated into a primary protein strand, a simple chain of amino acids, by the ribosome. The ribosomes are attached to the endoplasmic reticulum and feed the nascent protein strands directly into the ER. In the ER, HSPA5 prevents premature and incorrect folding of various sections of the protein, so that they can be folded in the proper sequence for the folding proteins into their secondary forms and helps join proteins to form mature tertiary or quaternary protein structures that give the proteins their function. Protein folding is a bit like origami; the same piece of paper might be folded into a butterfly or a cat if folded in a different order, but if the order is wrong, it just ends up as trash. After proper folding, the proteins are then ready for release from the ER into the cytosol.

The HSPs surround specific areas of the proteins, preventing certain sections of the strand from interacting with other areas, and thus from being folded prematurely. The term "chaperone" is a nice analogy, as it guards the immature protein against premature liaisons. HSP also helps repair proteins that have become misfolded after exposure to stressors that dislodge the protein's hydrogen bonds and allow for random refolding.

Another HSP, mortalin, protects the mitochondria. Although mitochondria have their own DNA, most of the proteins in mitochondria are made outside of it. Mortalin helps fold and import proteins. Dysfunctional mortalin causes dysfunctional mitochondria. Oxidative damage to mortalin likely contributes to the development of diseases involving immortal cells, such as Alzheimer's, and Parkinson's, and aging.

BiP and Mortalin also protect cancer cells from apoptosis. Overexpression or phosphorylation-inducing activation of HSP is often found in cancer cells, which use this adaptation to enhance survival. Disruption of the HSP is a target of cancer treatment. Since most HSP are responsive to heat, heat can be used to target these proteins.

When released from damaged cells, HSP70 can act as a distress signal. It induces tumor cells to produce chemokines that attract immune cells to them and activate TRL4 receptors on the immune cells. Thus, it helps mount immune activity against the tumor.

A study of HSPs found that heat-shock induces changes in the expression of about 1500 genes, and a number of these changes coincided with effects of TNF-α activity. Many of these genes involved the cytokine-mediated functions of NF-κB. NF-κB activation promotes the induction of gene transcription for proteins that enhance cell survival. The NF-κB pathway is frequently up-regulated in cancer cells, and contributes to their resistance to anticancer treatment.

NF-κB is present in normal cells in an inactive form, as it is bound to IκBα. Various signals in the cell, including PI3K, Fos, and TLR pathways, can activate the enzyme IKK that causes IκBα to disassociate from NF-κB, releasing it and allowing NF-κB to pass into the nucleus where it promotes the transcription of pro-survival proteins.

Heat shock proteins are also present in the cytosol of normal cells in inactive clusters. Heat and other intracellular stressors can break up the cluster, allowing the HSP to perform their stress-induced functions and for HSF1 to migrate to the nucleus where it induces the transcription of various genes, including those for chemokines that attract immune cells to the area. One of these functions is to prevent activation of IKK and the freeing of IκBα from NF-κB, thus preventing its activities. Nevertheless, even when HSP prevents IKK's activity, NF-κB can be freed by an alternative activation route involving the TNF-α pathway.[1065]

TNF-α receptor activation is not a simple, one-way reaction; it activates NF-κB and MAPK8 pathway via the protein TRAF, which under most circumstances promotes survival and proliferation, but which can also activate intrinsic apoptosis, depending on other cellular influences. TNF-α receptor activation also activates caspase 8 via FADD, and this activates caspase 3 and BID. Both of these are strong pro-apoptotic influences. Thus, TNF-receptor activation can stimulate apoptosis under certain conditions or promote proliferation and inhibit apoptosis, under other conditions. TNF-α and the protein p53 additively promote apoptosis while NF-κB, which can be activated by TNF-α, promotes resistance to apoptosis.

IKKα-mediated phosphorylation of CREB binding protein (CBP) changes the CBP binding preference from p53 to NF-κB. This increases NF-κB-mediated gene expression and decreases p53-mediated gene expressions, and thus, leads to the promotion of cell proliferation and tumor growth. CBP phosphorylation is inhibited by IL-1β and LPS. LPS activates TLR-4, which stimulates IKKα activity. Both IL-1β and LPS activate NF-κB, and thus, promote cell proliferation in the presence of TNF-α.[1066]

IκBα is bound to NF-κB in the cytosol of the cell, inactivating it. The enzyme IKKα can phosphorylate IκBα, freeing NF-κB, which can then be translocated into the nucleus where gene transcription occurs.

Several dietary compounds have been found to inhibit NF-κB activity, including dark-roasted coffee,[1067] thyme, oregano,[1068] and cloves.[1069] Anthocyanins, (blue, red or purple plant pigments), curcumin, resveratrol, and other plant phenolic compounds have been found to prevent phosphorylation of IκBα, and thus, these compound inhibit the translocation of NF-κB from cytosol to the nucleus.[1070,1071,1072] This explains part of the anti-inflammatory and anticarcinogenic effects of phenolic compounds. At least some of these phytochemicals inhibit TNF-α activity by a mechanism that appears to be downstream of TRAF, and thus, may inhibit the survival influences of TNF receptor activation while sustaining the pro-apoptotic caspase-8 activity. The bioflavonoid quercetin inhibits phosphorylation and transcriptional activity of the heat shock transcription factor HSF1, thus reducing HSP expression.

It's taken several paragraphs of gobbledygook to get here; there is a point. Hyperthermia activation of HSP proteins can be synergistically enhanced with the co-administration of certain phytochemicals, including some phenolic compounds, such as quercetin.[1054]

A limitation to the successful use of oral administration of phytochemicals is their absorption into the bloodstream. Although an agent may have low toxicity and high efficacy in a culture dish, a potent agent that is poorly absorbed may have less efficacy than a less potent agent that is well absorbed. Three times as much quercetin 3-O-beta-glucoside is absorbed from an oral dose as quercetin, while two other forms of quercetin have little to no absorption.[1073] When used for therapy, flavonoid compounds should be selected that have high bioavailability.

TNF-Related Apoptosis-Inducing (Fas) ligand (TRAIL) is a member of the TNF receptor family that promotes apoptotic cell death, primarily in tumor cells. TRAIL binds to and causes three Fas and TRAIL ligand proteins in the outer cell membrane to come together, forming a "death-inducing signaling complex" (DISC) composed of three death domains (DD). In humans, eight of the 30 Fas receptors contain DD's. Others can act as signals for inflammation; thus, one signaling molecule can have different effects in different cells.

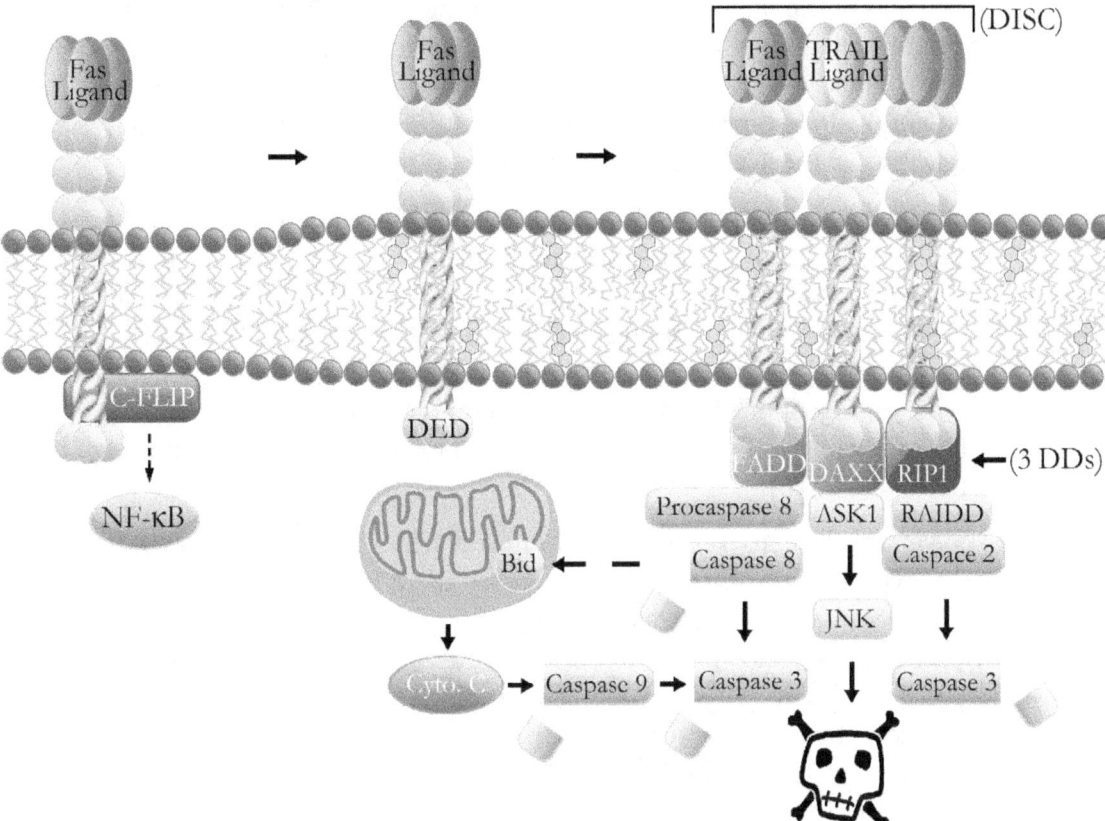

Figure 38-1: Lipid Rafts and Death Domains

The formation of DISC, with the DD FADD, activates the conversion of procaspase 8 to caspase 8, promoting extrinsic apoptosis, as illustrated in Figure 38-1. Several non-genotoxic anticancer agents have been developed that activate the Fas ligands, but they have little efficacy.[1074] The cell has means of protecting itself from Fas-ligands and being indiscriminately goaded into extrinsic signaling for apoptosis.

C-FLIP (aka CLFAR) is a protein that binds to the DED (death effector domain) of the Fas-Death domain (FADD), thus blocking the access of DED-procaspase 8 to FADD, and preventing the activation of caspase 8. C-FLIP tethers Fas receptors to areas of the cell membrane that are thinner, rather than to the thicker "lipid raft" areas of the membrane that contain more sphingolipids and cholesterol. Receptors located in lipid rafts are protected from certain membrane enzymes, and thus often behave differently. The impoundment of Fas receptors to the non-lipid raft areas by c-FLIP alters the action of these receptors and blocks the assembly of the DISK complex. When activated within a lipid raft, DISC the activation of caspase 8 activates both caspase 3 and Bid, which activates pores in the mitochondria, causing the release of cytochrome C. In contrast, when tethered by C-FLIP to non-lipid-raft areas of the membrane, activation of the TRAIL ligand by TRAIL or the Fas ligands by Fas promotes cell survival via activation of NF-κB.[1075] Thus, c-FLIP makes Fas activation by TRAIL or Fas ligand pro-survival and pro-inflammatory. C-FLIP acts similarly on the activation of the TNF-α receptor, TNF-R1.

Many cancers evade the Fas-induced apoptosis because of c-FLIP. This protein is highly expressed in many tumors, at least in part, because its transcription is induced by NF-κB via Akt. PKC, which activates Akt, also induces the phosphorylation of c-FLIP, preventing its ubiquitination and destruction. Thus, many cancers resist endogenous TRAIL-induced apoptosis because of c-FLIP. Hyperthermia inhibits c-FLIP activity and restores the pro-apoptotic effects of TRAIL.[1076]

Over the last 30 years, several clinical trials have demonstrated that hyperthermia increases the efficacy of radiotherapy treatment of cancer and improves patient survival. However, use of hyperthermia has been limited because of challenges in its application during radiation treatment. Hyperthermia during radiation therapy increases apoptosis by down-regulating Akt signaling.[1077] This is likely via a c-FLIP inhibitory mechanism.

The inhibition of cFLIP occurs at moderate (fever-like) hyperthermia of 40° C (104° F), a level that is safe in the short term, and likely of physiologic significance. Inhibition of c-FLIP may be part of the adaptive reason the body uses fever to fight infections by inducing apoptosis of intracellular infections. Hyperthermia frees c-FLIP from FADD, and it then undergoes ubiquitination and is eliminated.

The most effective temperature for c-FLIP inhibition appears to be 42° C (107.6° F). Thirty minutes exposure to hyperthermia at 42° C decreases c-FLIP by about 50% and greatly increases tumor cell death.[1078] Optimal heating time is probably less than one hour and may be as little as five minutes.[1076] Pulsed heating that lasts only a few minutes at a time may be even more effective than longer bouts of hyperthermia. The efficacy of hyperthermia on c-FLIP appears not to be mitigated by the adaptation to hyperthermia that occurs with heat shock proteins.[1074]

After hyperthermia, cFLIP levels are restored through new protein production in about 3 hours.[1079] Thus, another pulse of heat treatment can be repeated after this much time. It is noteworthy that hyperthermia at 42° C had no effect on cancer cell death in *in vitro* experiments when a Fas-ligand to stimulate TRAIL was not present.

Recall that Coley's vaccine was effective when fever temperatures from 38° – 40° C were achieved. Those levels seem too low to have a strong and optimal effect on most heat shock proteins or on c-FLIP. Perhaps it was not the sustained temperature, but only the spikes in temperatures to 42° C, even if only for minutes, and easily missed without a continuously recording thermometer that provided effective treatment. Heat also increases the activity of aSMAse and ceramide production. (Appendix B)

39: Non-Genotoxic Medications

Can we repurpose non-genotoxic medications for cancer treatment? Could we use the erectile dysfunction medication, Viagra, the anti-inflammatory drug, Celebrex, or the gout medication, allopurinol, for the treatment of cancer?

Viagra and Cialis, phosphodiesterase-5 inhibitors, enhance the effect of the arthritis medicine celecoxib (Celebrex) in the killing of multiple types of cancer cells. Celecoxib acts through several pathways, including the degradation of HSP 5 causing protein misfolding in the ER,[1080] but also by impairing c-FLIP and activating FADD induced activation of caspase 8.[1081] (Figure 38-1) It also promotes ceramide production.

Antabuse (disulfiram), used to treat alcohol abuse, is a proteasome inhibitor, and thus inhibits the breakdown of ubiquitinated proteins. The accumulation of these proteins both limits the recycling of amino acids for building new proteins and slows the breakdown of p53, Nrf2, the pro-apoptotic factors Bim, BAX, and the caspases. Proteasome inhibitors inhibit the ubiquitination and destruction of IκB kinase, the enzyme that inhibits NF-κB activation. Thus, disulfiram and other proteasome inhibitors promote apoptosis. Melatonin has similar activity, and may also be a proteasome inhibitor.[1082] [1083]

Epigallocatechin-3-gallate and other phenolic compounds in green teas are also proteasome inhibitors that promote cancer cell apoptosis.[1084] [1085]

Proteasome inhibitors prevent the destruction of c-FLIP, and thus may not be ideal during hyperthermia therapy.[1079] However, c-FLIP degradation is not required for pro-apoptotic activity through hyperthermia. It appears that when c-FLIP disassociate sufficiently from FADD, they tend to bind to other c-FLIP molecules and form inactive complexes.[1076]

As mentioned in a previous chapter, the corticosteroid medication dexamethasone, used for severe allergic reactions and inflammatory disorders, was originally used in some chemotherapeutic regimens to decrease toxicity. However, it additionally has multiple anti-growth effects, including inhibiting GADD45 and cyclin promotion via induction of cyclin kinase inhibitor proteins, and promotion of ceramide.[1086] Dexamethasone also induces AMPK, and decreases the formation of prostaglandin E.[1087] Thus, dexamethasone impedes survival influences.

GSK-3 is part of the Beta-catenin/Wnt pathway cascade that signals cell division and proliferation. (Sorry, this was one of the many pathways left out of this book.) GSK3B - tau-protein kinase inhibitors include lithium chloride, a medication long used in the treatment of bipolar disorder. This enzyme is also inhibited by caffeic acid, a phenolic compound found in sunflower seeds, many spices, olives, and other plant-based foods.[1088]

Akt promotes cell survival via mTOR and by promoting the induction of survival proteins and NF-κB activation. Atk1 inhibitors include luteolin, ellagic acid, baicalin, and apigenin.[1089] Ellagic acid is a hydroxybenzoic acid that may also inhibit AMPK, and thus, inhibit mTOR at another site.

The old anti-malarial drug chloroquine inhibits autophagy by inhibiting lysosomal degradation of proteins and thus may promote apoptosis.[1090] Its use in cancer treatment is under investigation.

Vitamin D3, betaine, and certain "FIASMA" medications, including amitriptyline, loratadine, and tomatidine from green tomatoes inhibit TLR4 and thus may downregulate NF-κB induced cell proliferation and survival in inflammatory conditions and in cancer. Opiates, often used for pain in patients with inflammation or cancer, activate TLR4, and thus, increase NF-κB activation. FIASMA medications may, however, interfere with ceramide production during cell stress such as during chemo. Ceramide is desirable in this circumstance as it promotes programmed cell death.

Allopurinol is a medication used in the treatment of gout that lowers uric acid levels. Allopurinol prevents uric acid synthesis and several hormonal changes that occur with fructose consumption and in the development of metabolic syndrome. (See Chapter 12) Allopurinol helps prevent insulin resistance and the reduction in adiponectin associated with high uric acid levels.[1091] Allopurinol has been shown to lower the risk of colorectal cancer in patients with gout and improve survival among patients with advanced colon cancer.[1092] Allopurinol can also be used to prevent injury from tumor lysis syndrome during chemo.[1093] Allopurinol can thus be a reasonable medication to use in patients with metabolic syndrome or isolated hyperuricemia in preparation for chemotherapy to increase treatment efficacy. The phenolic compounds quercetin and rutin have been found to be as effective in preventing insulin resistance from fructose as is allopurinol, in mitigating fructose-induced hyperlipidemia and inflammation. They also lowering uric acid levels, but to a lesser degree than allopurinol does.[1094]

40: After the Diagnosis

By this point, I hope that those interested in stopping a cancer after it has been diagnosed understand that the early chapters on cancer prevention were not a waste of shelf space. The same factors that cause cancer in the first place keep it going and make it worse.

Prevention is Half the Cure

Pretty much everything that causes cancer causes new mutations or helps the cancer avoid apoptosis and stimulates its growth. After the diagnosis comes treatment; the most effective cancer treatments rely on programmed cell death, and preferably pyroptosis of cancer cells. If a person is exposed to cancer risk factors that impair apoptosis, it is more likely the cancer cells will survive chemo or radiation. Those that survive are more likely to resist further treatment, and risk factors that support cell proliferation will assist these more resistant cancer cells with growth.

Individuals who have developed cancer have proven themselves to be highly susceptible to cancer. They are at high risk of developing independent, new cancers. Cancer may even arise from a different tissue. Women who carry a mutated BRCA1 gene and develop breast cancer are not suddenly excluded from getting ovarian or other BRCA1-associated cancers. The development of a tobacco-smoke related cancer only limits the development of other tobacco-related cancers by limiting the lifespan the patient has to develop them. The diagnosis of cancer should put a person on notice that they need to lower their cancer risk profile.

I am not suggesting that diet and lifestyle changes will cure cancer or make it disappear. Equally, however, don't expect a cancer cure to stick if the risk factors for the development of cancer continue.

If forces that caused or added to the risk for a cancer remain present, the cancer is more likely to come back, and new cancers are more likely to arise. Perhaps most dangerously, primary cancer risk factors raise the risk of cancer becoming more aggressive and spreading. If a person (other than children with embryonic cancers) develops cancer, it is strong evidence that their genetic makeup places them at increased susceptibility to it; that will not change. If a person remains exposed to carcinogens that induced the development of the first cancer are still present, expect more cancer induction. If the factors that induced rapid growth of the primary cancer cell are still present, expect other hidden cancer cells to grow rapidly. If the factors that inhibited effective immune response are still around, expect new cancer cells to escape immune destruction. On the other hand, since inflammatory cytokines induce cancer cell invasion and metastasis, it is reasonable to expect that lowering inflammatory cytokine levels through sufficient, quality sleep, exercise, and a healthy diet can slow cancer growth and deter metastasis.

By their very nature, cancers are genetically unstable. They are much more susceptible to carcinogens, and much more likely to undergo mutations when exposed to mutagens. Persons with cancer are those with the highest risk of mutations from carcinogens.

Earlier in my career, I had a medical practice in a small town, and I made house calls for my patients. I saw lung cancer patients, even those on oxygen where there was a high risk of fire, who still had an ashtray with cigarette butts next to the Lazy-boy, to which their days were confined. Smokers would tell me that it was too late to quit; they already had cancer and their death warrant. Even though I did not agree, I had little chance of convincing them otherwise. Smoking was not only an addiction, but it was also their self-identity, and in their eyes, they had little else left.

Even in advanced disease, quitting smoking improves the quality of life for the patient and decreases risk for his or her family members. It allows them better oxygenation, sleep, and appetite, and less fatigue after the nicotine withdrawal abates.

By the time hospice takes over, the chances of changing the long-term outcome of cancer through treatment and risk reduction are slim. But this certainly is not the case in early disease. Changing habits and exposures affect cancer outcome, especially when the change takes place before the cancer has had a chance to metastasize to other organs.

I pointed out smoking and lung cancer as a clear example of the relationship between smoking and cancer risk. Over 90 percent of lung cancer can be attributed to smoking, so it is easy to see the association of this risk and outcomes. A meta-analysis of available studies showed that a 65-year-old with non-small cell lung cancer (NSCLC) diagnosed during early stages of the disease, who continued to smoke had a 33 percent five-year survival rate. Only one in three such patients lives 5 years. These patients have a 70 percent five-year survival rate if they quit smoking. Those diagnosed with small-cell lung cancer, who continue to smoke, have a 29 percent 5-year survival rate as compared to a 63 percent rate for those who quit. Since most patients who survive 5 years are cured, this means that most lung cancer patients who are diagnosed and treated early and quit smoking beat the cancer. Even when the disease is discovered and treated early enough to be cured, those who continue to smoke are 4.3 times more likely to develop a completely *new primary* lung cancer![1095]

Smoking not only decreases survival but actually decreases the efficacy of treatment. It increases the resistance of cancer cells to certain chemotherapy agents, making chemo less effective.[1096] It makes healing after surgery slower and more difficult.

People often forget that less than half of the cancer deaths caused by tobacco are from lung cancers. Tobacco exposure after the diagnosis of other cancers also increases the risk of recurrence and invasive disease for those cancers. Men who continue to smoke *after the diagnosis* of prostate cancer are 2.5 times more likely to develop metastatic disease, 2.67 times more likely to develop disease that is resistant to hormonal control, and twice as likely to die of prostate cancer.[1097]

Even after the diagnosis of cancer, risk factor avoidance can reduce cancer recurrence, spread, and death. The genetic, lifestyle, and environmental risks factors along with immune susceptibilities that favored the cancer development, if still present, continue to favor cancer proliferation. Another example is gastro-esophageal acid reflux (GERD), which promotes inflammation and turnover of cells of the esophagus and throat. GERD is a risk factor for squamous cell carcinoma in these areas. Use of histamine-2 (H2) blocker medications that block acid production, such as Zantac and Pepcid, decrease the risk of death in patients with head and neck squamous cell carcinoma by a third; PPI medications, such as Prilosec and Nexium, that decrease acid production more effectively than H2 blockers do, decrease mortality in these patients by 45 percent during the follow-up period,[1098] nearly cutting the risk of death in half for these patients.

> Here is an natural treatment for gastro-esophageal reflux disease that is often helps:[135]
>
> elatonin 3 mg at bedtime, with
>
> 7 mg of an organic zinc supplement, such as zinc citrate.
>
> If this combination eliminates reflux symptoms, the additional use of an H2 blocker or PPI likely adds little benefit. Follow your doctor's advice here; as new data becomes available, so do more effective treatments.

Recall the study of overweight women supplementing their diet with extra virgin olive oil (EVOL) or tree nuts? Two tablespoons of

EVOL a day cut breast cancer risk by two-thirds during the follow-up period of about 5 years. In another group, an ounce of tree nuts cut risk by nearly one-half.[1] We can assume that at least of third of women the age of this cohort have tiny, clinically undetectable breast cancers.[40] Many of the women, who were asymptomatic and apparently free of cancer at the beginning of the study but developed it in the course of the following years, already had tiny, dormant breast cancers when the study began. It is most likely that the consumption of olive oil and nuts impeded the growth or helped eliminate cancers that were already present, rather than acting to prevent new lesions over the short duration of the study. Similarly, olive oil and nuts may prevent the growth of tiny metastatic lesions that have not yet developed their own blood supply.

In America, studies on the consumption of broccoli or other cruciferous vegetables (CV) reveal that those consuming CV twice have a decrease in cancer risk by around 20%. But I have never come across an epidemiologic study of CV and cancer where they asked if the CV were prepared in a manner that did not destroy the active compounds. Perhaps more than half of those people consuming CV were overcooking them, and destroying the active compounds. Preparing CV and allium vegetables such as garlic and onions properly, as described in Chapter 24, might cut cancer risk by over 40 percent.

Lifestyle, diet, and other risk factors that increase the risk of cancer continue to favor the development of cancer, even after a diagnosis, and even after a cure. The factors that lower the risk favor a cure. Nearly one-in-five new cancers diagnosed in the United States occurs in a previous cancer patient.[2] For most cancers, early diagnosis and treatment give a better chance of survival. The earlier that risk reduction begins, the more likely that cancer can be prevented, its progression slowed, and remission extended into a long-term cure. If the immune system is compromised, normalizing it can help the immune system recover so that it can eliminate cancer cells that may be lurking about. Avoiding inflammation can limit the stimulus for angiogenesis that cancers need for growth. Cancer can be prevented, even after diagnosis.

"Action is the Antidote to Despair."

Joan Baez

Appendix A: Foods Allowed in the *Sanafast*™ Diet

The *Sanafast*™ is a restricted diet for use in the days leading up to and during chemotherapy. It is intended to create famine-like conditions that starve rapidly growing cells of nutrients required for growth and promote autophagy in normal cells and apoptosis of cancer cells that are subjected to stress by chemotherapy.

- Tier One foods are those ingredients that contain no protein, betaine, or choline. They include fats, refined starches, and sugars. They can be used to add calories to the *Sanafast*™ diet.

- Tier Two foods are whole foods that have very low levels of methionine, choline, betaine, and leucine (MCBL) and can be consumed to satisfy appetite without the risk of exceeding the dietary limits.

- Tier Three foods are low in MCBL, and unlikely to exceed the *Sanafast*™ diet limits as long as the diet is kept to the normal caloric needs of the individual.

- Tier Four foods can be consumed in moderation as a part of a meal, as long as Tier One to Three components make up at least a third of the calories in the meal. For example, potatoes have too high a protein-to-calorie ratio for the *Sanafast*™, but if consumed with butter or olive oil the protein-to-calorie ratio becomes acceptable for the diet.

- Tier Five foods do not comply with the low MCBL to calorie criteria but are consumed in such small amounts that they can be included and are added because they bring anticarcinogenic effects.

- The Prepared Foods list meets the diet's criteria and includes some foods that might be used as emergency foods when a patient is unable to have a meal prepared for their needs.

Criteria

- Leucine: Less than 51 mg per 100 Cal
- Methionine: Less than 22 mg per 100 Cal
- Choline + (Betaine/3.375) no more than 15 mg per 100 Cal, preferably less than half this amount

Tier One Foods (Ingredients)*

Oils and fats: Extra virgin olive oil, coconut oil, cocoa butter
Vinegars
Sugar: Dextrose highly preferred. Maltose and table sugar
Baking soda, baking powder
Vanilla extract

Tier Two Foods

Cassava (Yuca, manioc, tapioca) root, flour
Tapioca: Pearls, flour (starch)
Arrowroot: flour, noodles
Cornstarch
Poi
Chinese mung bean (cellophane) noodles
Sweet potato noodles
Butter, ghee
Burdock root

Tier Three Foods

Apples, pears, cherries, quinces
Nectarines, plums, prunes
Blueberries, figs,
Seedless grapes, seedless raisins, dates
Honeydew melons, papayas,
Orange juice (no additives) tangerines, grapefruit**
Loquats, persimmons sapodilla, prickly pears, feijoa (pineapple guava),
Plantains
Small to large green or ripe olives (not jumbo olives)

Tier Four

Mangos, pineapple, cherimoya, oranges, cranberries, sapote
Fresh European Chestnuts (Only European and fresh),
Strawberries, black currants, blackberries
Water chestnuts
Onions (dry bulbs, not green onions or scallions)
Jicama
Coconut meat and milk and cream (not coconut flour†)
Butter, ghee (Butter has 19 mg and ghee, 22 mg choline/100 Cal)
Heavy Whipping cream (58 mg leucine, 17 betaine per 100 Cal.)
Acorn Squash

Tier Five Foods:

Tea: chamomile, green, black, oolong, cinnamon
Coffee
Garlic, Ginger, Capers
Cocoa, Dark and baking chocolate, semisweet chocolate chips
(Caution: Chocolate made with lecithin is high in choline)
Coriander, Mustard and Broccoli seeds and sprouts

Emergency Prepared Foods:
"Jello®" type gelatin dessert
Gingersnaps, Fig bars
Canned Pie Filling: apple, berry, cherry
Sweet cucumber pickles and pickle relish (not dill pickles)
Potato puffs and French Fried Potatoes (overwhelmed by fat)
Pumpkin Pie Mix
Fruit Pies (wheat protein is overwhelmed by sugar)

* Olive, coconut, palm kernel, cocoa butter oils and butter are the preferred fats for the is the preferred fat for use in the *Sanafast*™ diet for their low contents of linoleic and linolenic acids, as these fatty acids promote phospholipase D activity.[1099] Ghee or clarified butter is preferable to butter, as it has a lower protein and choline content. Dextrose if preferred as an added sugar over sucrose as it does not contain fructose. Dextrose should provide quicker satiety.

** Grapefruit should be avoided before chemotherapy as it can cause toxicity and medication interactions. See box in Chapter 26.

† Coconut flour has the fat removed, concentrating its protein content to several times the criteria for the *Sanafast*™ diet.

APPENDIX B: CERAMIDE AND S1P

Ceramide, sphingosine, sphingosine-1-phosphate (S1P), and ceramide-1-phosphate (C1P) are bioactive lipids that mediate cell proliferation, differentiation, apoptosis, adhesion, angiogenesis, and migration, principally through their activity as signaling molecules. They are integral to the regulation of immune cell activity and for protection and growth of the nervous system. Dysfunction in the regulation of these sphingolipid metabolites is seen in and may be the cause of various cancers, autoimmune diseases, and mood disorders.

Sphingolipids mediate various opposing actions; for example, ceramide promotes arrest of growth and apoptosis, as shown in Figure 37-1. In contrast, S1P and C1P promote cell proliferation and survival. Ceramide promotes atherosclerosis and the damage caused by ischemic events. Ceramide-1-phosphate (C1P) prevents apoptosis and promotes survival of inflammatory cells. High levels of S1P are seen in ovarian cancer, where it promotes not only cell proliferation but also adhesion, angiogenesis, and metastasis.[1100] S1P promotes NF-κB activity and promotes cell survival and proliferation. The sphingosine pathway is shown in Figure AB-1.

During cellular and oxidative stress, enzymatic lysis of sphingomyelin occurs via one of several sphingomyelinase isoenzymes, forming ceramide which can be further metabolized to other signaling or non-signaling molecules. Intracellular ROS, hydrogen peroxide production, elevated temperature, alcohol-related toxicity,[1101] or osmotic stress can increase the formation of ceramide and its products. Betaine prevents osmotic stress that provokes ceramide formation. Extracellular TNF-α activates SMase through membrane TNF receptors and thus, acts as a secondary messenger for inflammation.

The major source of ceramide during cellular stress is from sphingomyelin from cell membranes. Sphingomyelin (SPM) is a phospholipid found in high concentrations in the interior "leaf" of lipid rafts within the cell membrane and in the outer leaf of the nuclear, bilipid membrane. Thus, SPM tends to be found in high concentrations in membranes facing the cytosol, where intracellular enzymes can interact with it. Lipid rafts are also found in some organelle membranes, such as in lysosomal membranes. SPM is also a major component of the myelin sheath. Ceramide is formed from the lysis of SPM via the enzyme sphingomyelinase (SMase). Most of the time, we are not fans of ceramide. But when we want to eliminate cancer cells or cells breeding viruses, it is our buddy. It is there to do a dirty job. Ceramide starves cells by down-regulating nutrient transporters. Elevated 16:0 ceramide prevents neuronal growth, proliferation, maturation, and survival by intracellular nutrient deprivation.[1102]

Although there is one SMase gene, there are five different forms of SMase. Alterations in the protein created by alternative splicing allows for different mRNA to be created from one gene. The alternative splicing mechanism allows a smaller genome to produce a wider array of proteins and to tune metabolism more finely. Two of the SMases, lysosomal acid SMase (aSMase herein) and magnesium-dependent neutral SMase (nSMase) are those that appear most involved in the production of ceramide in response to cellular stress, and thus, most important in driving apoptosis. Another form of SMase secreted from cells promotes insulin resistance and cardiovascular disease.

Elevations in acid-SMase (aSMase) levels have been found in patients suffering from major depression, and many antidepressant medications have been found to be effective inhibitors of aSMase activity. Animals genetically or pharmaceutically treated to increase brain ceramide show depression-like behavior even in the absence of stress.[1103] Mast cell calcium channel activation is inhibited through aSMase inhibition by amitriptyline,[1104] and several antihistamine medications, including desloratadine, clemastine, and hydroxyzine, inhibit aSMase.[1105] Thus, these medications can inhibit ceramide production during cellular stress. Most of these medications act indirectly by decreasing the affinity of SMase to the lipid raft. The enzyme thus becomes ineffective and degrades. They are thus called Functional Inhibitors of SMAase, or FIASMA's. FIASMA medications should be avoided in the days leading up to and during chemotherapy.

When the cell has more energy and is more viable, ceramide released by SMase is further metabolized into C1P or S1P, and both of these inhibit apoptosis and promote survival and proliferation. S1P is essential for stimulating the immune system and for the proliferation and survival of white blood cells in inflammation. Extracellular S1P acts as an immune-stimulant for white blood cells, via various S1P receptors. Like an S-O-S distress signal, during infection or injury, stressed tissue produces S1P that acts as a signal, calling for immune cell activity.

TNF-α induces S1P production in endothelial cells, hepatocytes, neutrophils, monocytes, fibroblasts, and other cells by the induction of sphingosine kinase.[1106] S1P activates NF-κB and the transcription of inflammatory cytokines and induces the production of PGE2, NO, free radicals, chemoattractants, and adhesion molecules that promote neutrophil migration to the tissue. S1P further enhances the survival of neutrophils by preventing their apoptosis.

S1P aldolase (S1P lyase) stops S1P activity by hydrolyzing it into phosphoethanolamine and palmitaldehyde, thus irreversibly decommissioning it.

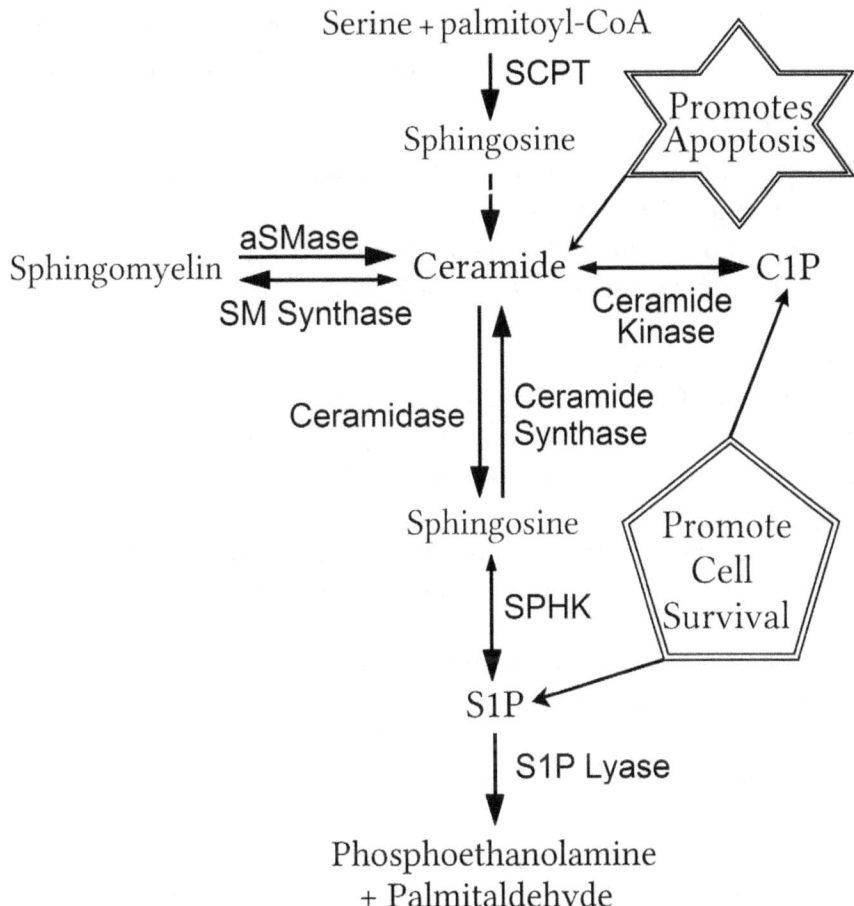

Enzymes Involved in the Ceramide-S1P pathway[1107]

Cancer chemotherapeutic agents are italicized.

Serine C-palmitoyltransferase (SPT, 2.3.1.50):
The rate-limiting enzyme in de novo ceramide biosynthesis.
- Cofactors: Pyridoxal 5'–phosphate, Mg^{++}
- Activators: *retinoic acid*, pioglitazone, certain cannabinoids, cell stress

Sphingomyelin Synthase (2.7.8.27): (a two-way reaction)
Ceramide + phosphatidylcholine ‹–› sphingomyelin + diacyl-glycerol
- Cofactors: Mg^{++}
- Inhibitors: Zn^{++}, TNF-α,

Sphingomyelinase (SMase, 3.1.4.12):
A sphingomyelin + H2O → a ceramide + phosphocholine

- Cofactors: Mg^{++}, requires Zn^{++} for full activity.
- Activators: Cu^{++}, arachidonic acid, cardiolipin, H_2O_2, bile acids, TNF-α, ethanol, *adriamycin* up-regulates endogenous nSMase expression. *Daunorubicin* and *doxorubicin*, via generation of reactive oxygen species.
- Inhibitors: reduced glutathione, lipoic acid, and FIASMA drugs such as: emetine, tamoxifen, trifluoperazine, amitriptyline, sertraline, amlodipine, and clemastine may impede apoptosis.

Ceramide Kinase (2.7.1.138):
ATP + ceramide → ADP + ceramide 1-phosphate
- Cofactors: Ca^{++}, Mg^{++}
- Activators: calmodulin, IL-1β, PPARβ
- Inhibitors: *all-trans retinoic acid*, calcitriol[1108]

Ceramidase (3.5.1.23):
A ceramide + H2O → a fatty acid + sphingosine
There are 5 human ceramidases. Blocking acid ceramidase activity in alveolar macrophages impedes Akt and ERK activity and induces apoptotic cell death.
- Activators: *all-trans retinoic acid*, CREB, IL-1β
- Inhibitors: Cu^{++}, Fe^{++}, Zn^{++}, desipramine, primary bile acids

Ceramide Synthase (2.3.1.24, Sphingosine N-acyltransferase):
acyl-CoA + sphingosine → Ceramide + CoA
- Activators: Celecoxib,[1109] *daunorubicin*
- Inhibitors: Fumonisin B1 (Chapter 21)

Sphingosine Kinase (SPHK, 2.7.1.91):
Sphingosine + ATP → ADP + sphinganine 1-phosphate (S1P)
- Cofactors: ATP, Mg^{++}
- Activator: cardiolipin, phosphatidic acid (PA)*, LPS, TNF-α,
- Inhibitors: *Docetaxel*, melatonin, phytosphingosine, Zn^{++}

S1P Aldolase (4.1.2.27):
Irreversibly breaks down S1P → phosphoethanolamine + palmitaldehyde.
- Cofactor: Pyridoxal 5'-phosphate (vitamin B6)
- Inhibitors: *cisplatin*, cyanide, *doxorubicin*, fingolimod, Zn^{++}

Phosphatidate Phosphate (PAP, 3.1.3.4)
C1P + H2O → ceramide + phosphate
S1P + H2O → ceramide + phosphate
Phosphatidic acid (PA) + H2O → diacyl-sn-glycerol + phosphate
- Cofactors: Mg^{++}
- Activator: Insulin, epinephrine, polyamines, fasting

- Inhibitors: ATP, chlorpromazine, alcohol, propranolol, Zn^{++}

*PA is formed when phosphatidylcholine is hydrolyzed into PA and choline by the enzyme PLD. PLD activity is enhanced by ATP and GTP, linoleic and linolenic acids, sphingosine, and histamine. PLD is inhibited in humans by ceramide, curcumin, oleic acid, resveratrol, and alcohol.

In light of the role of ceramide in apoptosis during cellular stress, its considerable role in the elimination of cancer cells, and the opposing role of S1P, the action of sphingolipid enzyme activators and inhibitors can be used to enhance the cancer-killing effect of chemotherapy.

Recall that kinase enzymes require ATP, and thus are dependent on energy availability. In a simplified explanation, these kinases require energy; healthy cells have sufficient energy reserves to phosphorylate sphingosine into S1P that supports growth and repair. Meanwhile, in debilitated or severely injured cells, ceramide is more likely to remain unphosphorylated, and cell destruction is promoted.

Vitamin B_6, pyridoxal-5'-phosphate (PLP), is a cofactor in ceramide production and the destruction of S1P and thus favors apoptosis. PLP, however, gets sequestered during inflammation, and so inflammation should be avoided. The proinflammatory cytokine, IL-1β promotes the conversion of ceramide to S1P.

IL-1β promotes cell survival via ceramide kinase and ceramidase, pushing ceramide towards S1P. IL-1β production is increased by leptin; a high-fat diet, especially n-6 fats and cholesterol; sleep deprivation; and by even mild, chronic stress. It is also elevated by LPS, a component of gram-negative bacteria cell walls. LPS may be present from bacterial overgrowth in the colon. LPS also enhances the formation of S1P. IL-1β transcription is lowered by melatonin.

Homocysteine (HCY), a cause of heart disease and cancer, exerts its effect via its activation of acid sphingomyelinase, which promotes intracellular ceramide formation,[1110] and the production of S1P. Reduced glutathione is a strong inhibitor of sphingomyelinase.[1111] Lipoic acid prevents H_2O_2 induced aSMase activation and may help stabilize lipid rafts.

The active form of vitamin D_3, calcitriol, decreases acid SMase activity and inhibits ceramide kinase but activates sphingosine kinase, thereby giving a net increase in S1P, and protecting cells from apoptosis.[1112] The vitamin A compound retinol increases ceramide production but also its conversion to S1P. All-trans-retinoic acid is used as a second line chemotherapeutic agent. However, it is not an ideal ceramide enhancer. Resveratrol, found in red wine, increases ceramide but also increases its conversion to

S1P.[1113] Resveratrol, however, also inhibits NF-κB, and thus, likely has an overall anti-proliferative effect. It also inhibits phospholipase D (PLD) activity. Magnesium is a cofactor or activator for many of the enzymes in this pathway. Zinc acts both as an activator and inhibitor and appears to act on balance to increase ceramide.

Estrogen receptor agonists and genistein increase S1P in epithelial cells by increasing ceramidase expression and by inhibition of S1P Aldolase.[1114] Estrogen should be avoided during chemotherapy even for non-breast and non-reproductive organ cancers. Fertile women may benefit from having chemo timed to the menstrual cycle when estrogen levels are at their lowest, or by the use of anti-estrogens.

The *Sanafast*™ diet favors the formation of homocysteine through the restriction of choline, betaine, and methionine, and thus should favor the activation of aSMase and the formation of ceramide. The *Sanafast* also includes phenolic compounds that down-regulate NF-κB and thus decrease the induction of IL-1β. The *Sanafast* includes saturated and monounsaturated fats but limits essential polyunsaturated fats (PUFA) that are needed for growth. The PUFA also promote PLD activity. As a preconditioning phase, the *Sanafast*™ diet recommends a low-fat, low-n-6 fat, high n-3 fat, low-cholesterol diet, with restrictions on fructose, to lower leptin resistance. This limits leptin resistance and leptin levels that raise IL-1β. This diet also promotes adequate dietary fiber to lower the risk of pathogenic bacteria overgrowth in the colon and the production of LPS. Furthermore, adequate sleep and avoidance of night shift work are highly encouraged during the preconditioning and treatment of cancer.

Additionally, in the days leading up to and including the days of chemotherapy, the following steps may be taken to increase ceramide and limit S1P:

- ❖ Low doses of zinc (e.g. 15 mg zinc citrate daily with a meal, or spread across meals) may increase ceramide-induced apoptosis. Larger doses of zinc may cause nausea.
- ❖ Celecobix effectively increases ceramide. Celecobix (Celebrex) increases ceramide levels and has pro-apoptotic potential.
- ❖ Pyridoxal 5'-phosphate (PLP) or other forms of vitamin B6 may be helpful in the formation of ceramide.
- ❖ Medications, notably the FIASMA medications, should be avoided during chemo as they may limit ceramide formation.
- ❖ Melatonin may be used for sleep (a dose of about 3 mg)

APPENDIX C: STRESS MANAGEMENT

Along with the diagnosis of cancer comes other problems; one of these is psychological stress. Diagnosing stress makes it much easier to treat. Here are strategies for stress management.[135]

1. To reduce stress, first, one must acknowledge the stress.

2. Identify the things causing the stress. This may not be easy, as our brains lie to us, and look for proximal rather than real causes. What are your fears and worries, and are they rational? It is not only O.K. to have rational fears; it is healthy. Make a list of the things that you are angry about, afraid of, worried about, frustrated, and annoyed by. Many times, there is no real cause, and it is just anxiety. That is O.K. too. We can deal with that too.

3. Sort out which items from your list that you have control over and what you do not control. Figure out what you can fix, what you cannot fix, where you can gain control, and if it is worth the effort.

4. Take control of the things that you can control. If you can fix the problem, act on it. Put your energy here.

5. If you cannot remedy the situation, then acknowledge that it is out of your hands, and thus, *it is not your responsibility*. Give it to the person or entity where responsibility lies. Faith in a high power is helpful, as you can cede your lack of control and accept that the outcome falls under the jurisdiction of God. Oftentimes we need to just let go. If you are sick, you may have to let go and put your faith in your doctor and other caregivers. Creating unhappiness and stress over things you cannot change or control does not just waste energy; it turns that energy against you.

> "Give me the courage to do what needs be done,
> Serenity to accept what cannot be remedied,
> And the insight to know one from the other."

6. Make a plan of action with a schedule or calendar. This can help take control of stressful situations. Missing from the prayer of serenity is a request for serenity during the unfolding of time; having too little time to accomplish what needs to be done, as well as having to wait for things to happen, is stressful. Having a plan can help organize time, and give some relief from it. When everything is arranged on a schedule, the problems may become more manageable. In the plan, try to deal with each stressor as an independent issue. The plan may include accepting loss and contingency plans.

7. Choose battles wisely. Choose battles that are winnable, and avoid those that cannot be. Only take on those in between after considering the risk and benefits of the struggle. Decline opportunities for stress by saying, "No, thank you" to people who treat you as if you were a source of cheap or free therapy or labor, or as an emotional dumping ground.

8. Avoid unneeded stressors that come into your life through electrical wires. These include:

- Telephone calls from relatives or others who drain you like vampires do;
- Media filled demagoguery that spew fear and loathing;
- Media that show graphic ugliness and violence;
- Internet time killers like social media and video games that keep you indoors sitting;
- Being a couch potato;
- Avoid rumination and focusing on the negative.

9. Focus on the present. You only have control over the present. Talk to a friend or counselor about how you feel to acknowledge and describe the stressors and your feelings. Be in the moment. Watch your body and relax when you notice defensive posturing. Remember to breathe. Yoga may be helpful. When you feel anxious, try to sit back, and watch it; ask yourself what event in your past it reminds you of. Most anxiety comes from situations that remind you of something that happened in the past. Are you in danger now? If you are in danger, take care of it, if not; consider it to be like a bad dream that you have now awakened from.

10. Take care of yourself. When you fell down or blue you can change your mood with exercise or a shower or a hot bath: walk, swim, jog, play with a puppy, get some sun. Get a massage. Regular, vigorous exercise helps reduce stress; walking or running 3 miles, at least three times a week is helpful. Remember to have fun. Give yourself enough time for sleep, but trying to bury your sorrows in bed does not work any better than burying them in booze.

11. Forgive and ask for forgiveness. Forgive yourself while you are at it.

> "Resentment is like drinking poison and waiting for it to kill your enemy."
> ~Nelson Mandela
>
> "Malice drinks one-half of its own poison."
> ~Seneca

12. Don't sweat the little stuff. Remember, it is almost all little stuff.

13. Cancer will not make you a better person, but you can use it as an opportunity to review your priorities and values. Approach a crisis as an opportunity for change.

14. Remember, a masterpiece can be painted on any canvas.

What Not to Do

Short-term fixes do not resolve chronic problems. Medications, such as benzodiazepines may be helpful for getting through a short-term crisis; however, they are not appropriate as a chronic fix, rather they are like buying on credit; you pay more later. For chronic problems, the payment just builds up. Use of tobacco, alcohol, and medications, such as benzodiazepines for relief from stress is like spending more than you earn and relying on credit cards to make payments. Alcohol is a poor substitute for courage. Drugs will not resolve social or financial problems and will likely worsen it. Most medications or herbs that relieve anxiety should only be used as short-term bridges over storm-swollen rivers.

Haste and intense emotions are the enemies of accuracy and wisdom. Avoid making decisions while upset or during emotionally charged circumstances. Better decisions are made when we are calm and thinking clearly, not under the influence of norepinephrine. In a study of patients that had attempted suicide, 24% had deliberated their decision less than 5 minutes, and 71% had spent less than an hour contemplating it.[1115] If you feel your heart pounding against your chest wall, you might want to wait on any life-altering decisions.

A short-term break in activities, vacation, or taking the time to adjust to a new situation can be helpful to recover from stress or a traumatic event. Taking a break to recover from illness, injury or trauma makes sense. However, avoiding friends and family; withdrawing from the world and procrastination is unlikely to help in the long run. It makes sense to catch your breath and take the time to review important decisions, but just delaying unpleasant situations that will not go away can just add stress.

Acceptance-Based Therapy teaches that rather than trying to control negative thoughts and emotions, it helps to observe them dispassionately; let them come and go. The goal is to change one's relationship with their thoughts and feelings, rather than the impossible task of changing emotions created in response to a situation.

Try to view emotions only as information that is being presented to you. Anxiety and fear are temporary feelings that will pass. Try to remember that those emotions may be more related to events that occurred long in the past than to the present situation. Anxiety is an alarm, triggered by something that reminds the subconscious of a frightening event. Every time the smoke detector goes off, it does not mean your house is on fire. A smoke detector may alarm because of a fire, burnt toast, or just dust or humidity. Take a look and see what is causing the alarm to activate before you go screaming and running from the building. That is what these emotions are for – they are an alarm to let you know there may be danger.

Anxiety often results from resisting the experience of anxiety. It is an alarm, and the brain wants you to check out why it is going off. Look to see what danger may be present and what actions, if any, are appropriate, and make a decision to act or not. If you give the brain a reason for the alarm, and you do not get upset about the alarm going off, it will usually turn itself off within a couple of minutes. Freaking out that the alarm is sounding just makes it worse.

Be receptive and look for humor in every scene you play in life. Sometimes life presents dark humor, but if you cast it as a comedy, it is much more likely to have a happy ending.

As a young man, I got caught in a strong rip current swimming at an isolated beach on the Pacific coast of Mexico that I later learned was notorious for frequent drownings. As I tried to swim back to the beach, it was becoming surprisingly smaller in the distance. I was getting exhausted and realized I could not overcome the force of the current. I must have actually listened to my father at least once, as I remembered his advice on rip currents: to relax and to take a new and leisurely, diagonal tact towards shore. The goal was not to get back to where I started, but rather to get to a piece of safe, dry ground. I swam diagonally towards the shore, and I ended up a half mile down from where I had left my gear. If I had fought the current with all my might, I likely would have joined other victims of the tide. When I just went for a ride, all I had to do was relax and keep moving with my goal in sight.

If you are diagnosed with cancer, you will probably never get back to the same place you were in life before it. Life moves under our feet. Sometimes you can control your destiny, and sometimes all you can do is stay afloat, and let life take you for a ride. If you take a realistic approach and focus on what is truly important, you are more likely to land on safe, dry ground, in a place from which you can restart your journey.

REFERENCES

Type "Pubmed" or "PMID" and the PMID number into a search engine to bring up the abstract and links to many of the full articles.

---

[1] Mediterranean Diet and Invasive Breast Cancer Risk Among Women at High Cardiovascular Risk in the PREDIMED Trial: A Randomized Clinical Trial. Toledo E, Salas-Salvadó J, Donat-Vargas C, et al. JAMA Intern Med. 2015 Nov;175(11):1752-60. PMID:26365989

[2] Aetiology, genetics and prevention of secondary neoplasms in adult cancer survivors. Travis LB, Demark Wahnefried W, et al. Nat Rev Clin Oncol. 2013 May;10(5):289-301. PMID: 23529000

[3] Influence of smoking cessation after diagnosis of early stage lung cancer on prognosis: systematic review of observational studies with meta-analysis. Parsons A, Daley A, Begh R, Aveyard P. BMJ. 2010 Jan 21;340:b5569. PMID:20093278

[4] Vegetarian dietary patterns and mortality in Adventist Health Study 2. Orlich MJ, Singh PN, Sabaté J, et al. JAMA Intern Med. 2013 Jul 8;173(13):1230-8. PMID:23836264

[5] Complementary Medicine, Refusal of Conventional Cancer Therapy, and Survival Among Patients With Curable Cancers. Johnson SB, Park HS, Gross CP, Yu JB. JAMA Oncol. 2018 Oct 1;4(10):1375-1381. doi: 10.1001/jamaoncol.2018.2487. PMID: 30027204

[6] Use of Alternative Medicine for Cancer and Its Impact on Survival. Johnson SB, Park HS, Gross CP, Yu JB. J Natl Cancer Inst. 2018 Jan 1;110(1). PMID:28922780

[7] The frightful evolution from tubercle to mass. Lewis EJ, Lewis CA. Cutis. 1998 Feb;61(2):100A. PMID: 9515218

[8] TNM staging system – Wikipedia: https://en.wikipedia.org/wiki/TNM_staging (Feb. 2015)

[9] https://en.wikipedia.org/wiki/User:Evolution_and_evolvability Thomas Shafee

[10] Drawing by Maria Ruis Villarreal. Used with permission.

[11] An estimation of the number of cells in the human body. Bianconi E, Piovesan A, Facchin F, et al. Ann Hum Biol. 2013 Nov-Dec;40(6):463-71. PMID:23829164

[12] Retrospective birth dating of cells in humans. Spalding KL, Bhardwaj RD, Buchholz BA, Druid H, Frisén J. Cell. 2005 Jul 15;122(1):133-43. PMID:16009139

[13] Implication of cell kinetic changes during the progression of human prostatic cancer. Berges RR, Vukanovic J, Epstein JI, CarMichel M, Cisek L, Johnson DE, Veltri RW, Walsh PC, Isaacs JT. Clin Cancer Res. 1995 May;1(5):473-80. PMID:9816006

[14] Retrospective birth dating of cells in humans. Spalding KL, Bhardwaj RD, Buchholz BA, Druid H, Frisén J. Cell. 2005 Jul 15;122(1):133-43. PMID:16009139

[15] Evidence for cardiomyocyte renewal in humans. Bergmann O, Bhardwaj RD, Bernard S, et al. Science. 2009 Apr 3;324(5923):98-102. PMID:19342590

[16] Mammalian heart renewal by pre-existing cardiomyocytes. Senyo SE, Steinhauser ML, Pizzimenti CL, et al. Nature. 2013 Jan 17;493(7432):433-6. PMID:23222518

[17] Rates of spontaneous mutation. Drake JW, Charlesworth B, Charlesworth D, Crow JF. Genetics. 1998 Apr;148(4):1667-86. PMID: 9560386

[18] MicroRNAs in cancer: biomarkers, functions and therapy. Hayes J, Peruzzi PP, Lawler S. Trends Mol Med. 2014 Aug;20(8):460-9. PMID:25027972

[19] Cancer etiology. Variation in cancer risk among tissues can be explained by the number of stem cell divisions. Tomasetti C, Vogelstein B. Science. 2015 Jan 2;347(6217):78-81. PMID: 25554788

[20] Breast cancer risk factors and second primary malignancies among women with breast cancer. Trentham-Dietz A, Newcomb PA, Nichols HB, Hampton JM. Breast Cancer Res Treat. 2007 Oct;105(2):195-207. PMID: 17186360

[21] http://www.cdc.gov/nchs/data/vsushistorical/mortcancer_1914.pdf

[22] US Mortality Volumes 1930 to 1959, US Mortality Data 1960 to 2011, National Center for Health Statistics, Centers for Disease Control and Prevention.

[23] The epidemiological enigma of gastric cancer rates in the US: was grandmother's sausage the cause? Paik DC, Saborio DV, Oropeza R, Freeman HP. Int J Epidemiol. 2001 Feb;30(1):181-2. PMID: 11171883

[24] Colorectal Cancer on the Decline--Why Screening Can't Explain It All. Welch HG, Robertson DJ. N Engl J Med. 2016 Apr 28;374(17):1605-7. PMID:27119236

[25] Red and processed meat and colorectal cancer incidence: meta-analysis of prospective studies. Chan DS, Lau R, Aune D, et al. PLoS One. 2011;6(6):e20456. PMID:21674008

[26] http://www.ers.usda.gov/data-products/chart-gallery/detail.aspx?chartId=40060

[27] Where can colorectal cancer screening interventions have the most impact? Siegel RL, Sahar L, Robbins A, etal. Cancer Epidemiol Biomarkers Prev. 2015 Aug;24(8):1151-6. PMID:26156973

[28] http://seer.cancer.gov/archive/csr/1975_2011/results_merged/sect_24_stomach.pdf

[29] NIH image bank: https://www.nih.gov/news-events/images

[30] Cyclin D activates the Rb tumor suppressor by mono-phosphorylation. Narasimha AM, Kaulich M, Shapiro GS, et al. Elife. 2014 Jun 4;3. PMID:24876129

[31] Recent progress with microtubule stabilizers: new compounds, binding modes and cellular activities. Rohena CC, Mooberry SL. Nat Prod Rep. 2014 Mar;31(3):335-55. PMID:24481420

[32] Survivin counteracts the therapeutic effect of microtubule de-stabilizers by stabilizing tubulin polymers. Cheung CH, Chen HH, Kuo CC, et al. Mol Cancer. 2009 Jul 3;8:43. PMID: 19575780

[33] Key Characteristics of Carcinogens as a Basis for Organizing Data on Mechanisms of Carcinogenesis. Smith MT, Guyton KZ, Gibbons CF, et al. Environ Health Perspect. 2015 Nov 24. PMID: 26600562

[34] Erythrocyte Glut1 triggers dehydroascorbic acid uptake in mammals unable to synthesize vitamin C. Montel-Hagen A, Kinet S, Manel N, Mongellaz C, et al. Cell. 2008 Mar 21;132(6):1039-48. PMID:18358815

[35] Vitamin C. Biosynthesis, recycling and degradation in mammals. Linster CL, Van Schaftingen E. FEBS J. 2007 Jan;274(1):1-22. PMID:17222174

[36] Antioxidant supplements for prevention of mortality in healthy participants and patients with various diseases. Bjelakovic G, Nikolova D, Gluud LL, Simonetti RG, Gluud C. Sao Paulo Med J. 2015 Mar-Apr;133(2):164-5. PMID:26018887

[37] Comprehensive identification of mutational cancer driver genes across 12 tumor types. Tamborero D, Gonzalez-Perez A, Perez-Llamas C, et al. Sci Rep. 2013 Oct 2;3:2650. PMID: 24084849

[38] Cancer genome landscapes. Vogelstein B, Papadopoulos N, Velculescu VE, et al. Science. 2013 Mar 29;339(6127):1546-58. PMID:23539594

[39] Proteome folding kinetics is limited by protein halflife. Zou T, Williams N, Ozkan SB, Ghosh K. PLoS One. 2014 Nov 13;9(11):e112701. PMID:25393560

[40] Breast cancer and atypia among young and middle-aged women: a study of 110 medicolegal autopsies. Nielsen M, Thomsen JL, Primdahl S, Dyreborg U, Andersen JA. Br J Cancer. 1987 Dec;56(6):814-9. PMID:2829956

[41] Tumor dormancy due to failure of angiogenesis: role of the microenvironment. Naumov GN, Folkman J, Straume O. Clin Exp Metastasis. 2009;26(1):51-60. PMID:18563595

[42] Cancer is a preventable disease that requires major lifestyle changes. Anand P, Kunnumakkara AB, Sundaram C, et al. Pharm Res. 2008 Sep;25(9):2097-116. PMID:18626751

[43] http://ghr.nlm.nih.gov/conditionCategory/cancers

44 Study of a single BRCA2 mutation with high carrier frequency in a small population. Thorlacius S, Sigurdsson S, Bjarnadottir H, et al. Am J Hum Genet. 1997 May;60(5):1079-84. PMID: 9150155

45 Cancers associated with BRCA1 and BRCA2 mutations other than breast and ovarian. Mersch J, Jackson MA, Park M et al. Cancer. 2015 Jan 15;121(2):269-75. PMID: 25224030

46 Second neoplasms in survivors of childhood cancer: findings from the Childhood Cancer Survivor Study cohort. Meadows AT, Friedman DL, Neglia JP, et al. J Clin Oncol. 2009 May 10;27(14):2356-62. PMID:19255307

47 Integrated Oncogene Genomics Database: http://www.intogen.org/search (Oct. 2016)

48 Report on Carcinogens(RoC)Concept:Selected Viruses. National Toxicology Program, US Dept of Health and Human Services

49 "Virus Replication" by YK Times wikimedia.org Virus_Replication.svg

50 Infection and Cancer: Global Distribution and Burden of Diseases. Oh JK, Weiderpass E. Ann Glob Health. 2014 September - October;80(5):384-392. PMID: 25512154

51 Hepatitis B seropositivity and risk of developing multiple myeloma or Hodgkin lymphoma: A meta-analysis of observational studies. Dalia S, Dunker K, Sokol L, Mhaskar R. Leuk Res. 2015 Dec;39(12):1325-33. PMID:26394533

52 Human papillomavirus-related diseases of the female lower genital tract: oncogenic aspects and molecular interaction. Zekan J, Skerlev M, Milić L, Karelović D. Coll Antropol. 2014 Jun;38(2):779-86. PMID:25145023

53 http://www.albawaba.com/news/highest-rates-hepatitis-c-virus-transmission-found-egypt (accessed Jan. 2015)

54 Evidence of intense ongoing endemic transmission of hepatitis C virus in Egypt. Miller FD, Abu-Raddad LJ. Proc Natl Acad Sci U S A. 2010 Aug 17;107(33):14757-62. PMID: 20696911

55 Hepatitis B or C viral infection and risk of pancreatic cancer: a meta-analysis of observational studies. Xu JH, Fu JJ, Wang XL, Zhu JY, Ye XH, Chen SD. World J Gastroenterol. 2013 Jul 14;19(26):4234-41. PMID:23864789

56 http://healthaffairs.org/blog/2014/06/05/the-cost-of-a-cure-medicares-role-in-treating-hepatitis-c/

57 http://www.medscape.com/viewarticle/862085#vp_2 (accessed Oct 2016)

58 Hepatitis B virus status and the risk of pancreatic cancer: a meta-analysis. Wang Y, Yang S, Song F, et al. Eur J Cancer Prev. 2013 Jul;22(4):328-34. PMID: 23165286

59 http://www.who.int/mediacentre/factsheets/fs204/en/

60 On the dynamics of acute EBV infection and the pathogenesis of infectious mononucleosis. Hadinoto V, Shapiro M, Greenough TC, et al. Blood. 2008 Feb 1;111(3):1420-7. PMID: 17991806

61 Human natural killer cells prevent infectious mononucleosis features by targeting lytic Epstein-Barr virus infection. Chijioke O, Müller A, Feederle R, et al. Cell Rep. 2013 Dec 26;5(6):1489-98. PMID: 24360958

62 http://www.cdc.gov/epstein-barr/hcp.html

63 Survey of Epstein Barr virus (EBV) immunogenic proteins and their epitopes: implications for vaccine preparation. Rajcani J, Szenthe K, Banati F, Szathmary S. Recent Pat Antiinfect Drug Discov. 2014;9(1):62-76. PMID: 25164057

64 Age-specific seroprevalence of Merkel cell polyomavirus, BK virus, and JC virus. Viscidi RP, Rollison DE, Sondak VK, et al.Clin Vaccine Immunol. 2011 Oct;18(10):1737-43. PMID:21880855

65 Photo by By Klaus D. Peter, Gummersbach, Germany

66 Xenophagy in Helicobacter pylori- and Epstein-Barr virus-induced gastric cancer. Zhang L, Sung JJ, Yu J, et al. J Pathol. 2014 Jun;233(2):103-12. PMID: 24633785

67 Epstein Barr virus and Helicobacter pylori co-infection are positively associated with severe gastritis in pediatric patients. Cárdenas-Mondragón MG, Carreón-Talavera R, Camorlinga-Ponce M, et al. PLoS One. 2013 Apr 24;8(4):e62850. PMID: 23638154

68 Association of Helicobacter pylori and Epstein-Barr virus with gastric cancer and peptic ulcer disease. Saxena A, Nath Prasad K, et al. Scand J Gastroenterol. 2008;43(6):669-74. PMID: 18569983

69 Pathogenesis of Helicobacter pylori infection. Kusters JG, van Vliet AH, Kuipers EJ. Clin Microbiol Rev. 2006 Jul;19(3):449-90. PMID: 16847081

70 Missing Microbes Martin Blaser. 2014, New York, Henry Holt and Company

71 American College of Gastroenterology: http://patients.gi.org/topics/barretts-esophagus/

72 Chronic bacterial and parasitic infections and cancer: a review. Samaras V, Rafailidis PI, Mourtzoukou EG, et al. J Infect Dev Ctries. 2010 Jun 3;4(5):267-81. PMID: 20539059

73 Chlamydia pneumoniae infection and risk for lung cancer. Chaturvedi AK, Gaydos CA, Agreda P, et al. Cancer Epidemiol Biomarkers Prev. 2010 Jun;19(6):1498-505. PMID: 20501758

74 Centers for Disease control. http://www.cdc.gov/parasites/schistosomiasis/biology.html

75 Smoking-attributable mortality, years of potential life lost, and productivity losses--United States, 2000-2004. Centers for Disease Control and Prevention (CDC). MMWR Morb Mortal Wkly Rep. 2008 Nov 14;57(45):1226-8. PMID:19008791

76 Smokeless Tobacco (SLT) associated cancers: A systematic review and meta-analysis of Indian studies. Sinha DN, Suliankatchi AR, Gupta PC. Int J Cancer. 2015 Oct 7. PMID:26443187

77 Alcohol and Tobacco Increases Risk of High Risk HPV Infection in Head and Neck Cancer Patients: Study from North-East Region of India. Kumar R, Rai AK, Das D, et al. PLoS One. 2015 Oct 16;10(10):e0140700. PMID:26473489

78 National Vital Statistics Report: Centers for Disease control. Vol 65, No.4. June 30, 2016

79 Smoking as a risk factor for accident death: a meta-analysis of cohort studies. Leistikow BN, Martin DC, Jacobs J, et al. Accid Anal Prev. 2000 May;32(3):397-405. PMID:10776858

80 Waking a sleeping giant: the tobacco industry's response to the polonium-210 issue. Muggli ME, Ebbert JO, Robertson C, Hurt RD. Am J Public Health. 2008 Sep;98(9):1643-50. PMID:18633078

81 Cigarette smoke radioactivity and lung cancer risk. Karagueuzian HS, White C, Sayre J, Norman A. Nicotine Tob Res. 2012 Jan; 14(1):79-90. PMID:21956761

82 Probing the smoking-suicide association: do smoking policy interventions affect suicide risk? Grucza RA, Plunk AD, Krauss MJ, Cavazos-Rehg PA, Deak J, Gebhardt K, Chaloupka FJ, Bierut LJ. Nicotine Tob Res. 2014 Nov;16(11):1487-94. PMID: 25031313

83 http://www.cdc.gov/tobacco/data_statistics/sgr/2001/index.htm

84 Parental smoking during pregnancy and ADHD in children: the Danish national birth cohort. Zhu JL, Olsen J, Liew Z, Li J, Niclasen J, Obel C. Pediatrics. 2014 Aug;134(2):e382-8. PMID:25049343

85 Relationship of environmental tobacco smoke to otitis media (OM) in children. Csákányi Z, Czinner A, Spangler J, Rogers T, Katona G. Int J Pediatr Otorhinolaryngol. 2012 Jul;76(7):989-93. PMID:22510576

86 Maternal prenatal smoking and hearing loss among adolescents. Weitzman M, Govil N, Liu YH, et al. JAMA Otolaryngol Head Neck Surg. 2013 Jul;139(7):669-77. PMID:23788030

87 Secondhand smoke and sensorineural hearing loss in adolescents. Lalwani AK, Liu YH, Weitzman M. Arch Otolaryngol Head Neck Surg. 2011 Jul;137(7):655-62. PMID:21768409

88 Tobacco smoke exposure and the risk of childhood acute lymphoblastic and myeloid leukemias by cytogenetic subtype. Metayer C, Zhang L, Wiemels JL, et al. Cancer Epidemiol Biomarkers Prev. 2013 Sep;22(9):1600-11. PMID:23853208

[89] Childhood passive smoke exposure is associated with adult head and neck cancer. Troy JD, Grandis JR, Youk AO, et al. Cancer Epidemiol. 2013 Aug;37(4):417-23. PMID:23619143

[90] Active smoking and secondhand smoke increase breast cancer risk: the report of the Canadian Expert Panel on Tobacco Smoke and Breast Cancer Risk (2009). Johnson KC, Miller AB, Collishaw NE, et al. Tob Control. 2011 Jan;20(1):e2. PMID:21148114

[91] Alcohol-attributable cancer deaths and years of potential life lost in the United States. Nelson DE, Jarman DW, Rehm J, et al. Am J Public Health. 2013 Apr;103(4):641-8. PMID:23409916

[92] The burden of cancer attributable to alcohol consumption. Testino G. Maedica (Buchar). 2011 Oct;6(4):313-20. PMID:22879847

[93] European Code against Cancer 4th Edition: Alcohol drinking and cancer. Scoccianti C, Cecchini M, Anderson AS, et al. Cancer Epidemiol. 2015 Jun 24. pii: S1877-7821(15)00023-5. PMID:26115567

[94] Alcohol consumption and risk of cancer: a systematic literature review. de Menezes RF, Bergmann A, Thuler LC. Asian Pac J Cancer Prev. 2013;14(9):4965-72. PMID:24175760

[95] Sloan Kettering Cancer Center https://www.mskcc.org/cancer-care/types/head-neck/about-head-neck (Accessed Jan. 2016).

[96] Alcohol and cancer. Blot WJ. Cancer Res. 1992 Apr 1;52(7 Suppl):2119s-2123s. PMID:1544150

[97] Esophageal cancer among black men in Washington, D.C. II. Role of nutrition. Ziegler RG, Morris LE, Blot WJ, et al. J Natl Cancer Inst. 1981 Dec;67(6):1199-206. PMID:6947105

[98] Acetaldehyde as an underestimated risk factor for cancer development: role of genetics in ethanol metabolism. Seitz HK, Stickel F. Genes Nutr. 2010 Jun;5(2):121-8. PMID:19847467

[99] ADH1B Arg47His polymorphism is associated with esophageal cancer risk in high-incidence Asian population: evidence from a meta-analysis. Zhang G, Mai R, Huang B. PLoS One. 2010 Oct 27;5(10):e13679. PMID:21048924

[100] Alcohol-related cancers and aldehyde dehydrogenase-2 in Japanese alcoholics. Yokoyama A, Muramatsu T, Ohmori T, et al. Carcinogenesis. 1998 Aug;19(8):1383-7. PMID:9744533

[101] Transgenic mouse models for alcohol metabolism, toxicity, and cancer. Heit C, Dong H, Chen Y, et al. Adv Exp Med Biol. 2015;815:375-87. PMID:25427919

[102] CYP2E1 and risk of chemically mediated cancers. Trafalis DT, Panteli ES, Grivas A, et al. Expert Opin Drug Metab Toxicol. 2010 Mar;6(3):307-19. PMID:20073996

[103] New perspectives on folate transport in relation to alcoholism-induced folate malabsorption--association with epigenome stability and cancer development. Hamid A, Wani NA, Kaur J. FEBS J. 2009 Apr;276(8):2175-91. PMID:19292860

[104] One-carbon metabolism related gene polymorphisms interact with alcohol drinking to influence the risk of colorectal cancer in Japan. Matsuo K, Ito H, Wakai K, et al. Carcinogenesis. 2005 Dec;26(12):2164-71. PMID:16051637

[105] Molecular mechanisms of alcohol-mediated carcinogenesis. Seitz HK, Stickel F. Nat Rev Cancer. 2007 Aug;7(8):599-612. PMID:17646865

[106] Alcohol drinking and one-carbon metabolism-related gene polymorphisms on pancreatic cancer risk. Suzuki T, Matsuo K, Sawaki A, et al. Cancer Epidemiol Biomarkers Prev. 2008 Oct;17(10):2742-7. PMID:18843018

[107] One-carbon metabolism-related gene polymorphisms and risk of breast cancer. Suzuki T, Matsuo K, Hirose K, et al. Carcinogenesis. 2008 Feb;29(2):356-62. PMID:18174236

[108] Alcohol and cancer: an overview with special emphasis on the role of acetaldehyde and cytochrome P450 2E1. Seitz HK, Mueller S. Adv Exp Med Biol. 2015;815:59-70. PMID:25427901

[109] The total margin of exposure of ethanol and acetaldehyde for heavy drinkers consuming cider or vodka. Lachenmeier DW, Gill JS, Chick J, Rehm J. Food Chem Toxicol. 2015 Sep;83:210-4. PMID:26116882

110 An overview of formation and roles of acetaldehyde in winemaking with emphasis on microbiological implications. Shao-Quan Liu SQ, Pilone GJ. International Journal of Food Science & Technology Volume 35, Issue 1, p. 49–61, Feb 2000

111 Gender differences in the pharmacokinetics of ethanol in saliva and blood after oral ingestion. Gubała W, Zuba D. Pol J Pharmacol. 2003 Jul-Aug;55(4):639-44. PMID:14581724

112 Alcohol metabolism by oral streptococci and interaction with human papillomavirus leads to malignant transformation of oral keratinocytes. Tao L, Pavlova SI, Gasparovich SR, Jin L, Schwartz J. Adv Exp Med Biol. 2015;815:239-64. PMID:25427911

113 Analysis of methanol and its derivatives in illegally produced alcoholic beverages. Arslan MM, Zeren C, Aydin Z, et al. J Forensic Leg Med. 2015 Jul;33:56-60. PMID:6048498

114 Formaldehyde in alcoholic beverages: large chemical survey using purpald screening followed by chromotropic acid spectrophotometry with multivariate curve resolution. Jendral JA, Monakhova YB, Lachenmeier DW. Int J Anal Chem. 2011;2011:797604. PMID:21760790

115 http://www.winegrowers.info/wine_making/Enzymes.htm

116 Influence of dietary folic acid on the developmental toxicity of methanol and the frequency of chromosomal breakage in the CD-1 mouse. Fu SS, Sakanashi TM, Rogers JM, Hong KH, Keen CL. Reprod Toxicol. 1996 Nov-Dec;10(6):455-63. PMID:8946559

117 Dietary methanol regulates human gene activity. Shindyapina AV, Petrunia IV, Komarova TV, et al. PLoS One. 2014 Jul 17;9(7):e102837. PMID:25033451

118 Alcoholic diseases in hepato-gastroenterology: a point of view. Testino G. Hepatogastroenterology. 2008 Mar-Apr;55(82-83):371-7. PMID:18613369

119 Epidemiology and pathophysiology of alcohol and breast cancer: Update 2012. Seitz HK, Pelucchi C, Bagnardi V, La Vecchia C. Alcohol Alcohol. 2012 May-Jun;47(3):204-12. PMID:22459019

120 European Code against Cancer 4th Edition: Alcohol drinking and cancer. Scoccianti C, Cecchini M, Anderson et al. Cancer Epidemiol. 2015 Jun 24. pii: S1877-7821(15)00023-5. PMID:26115567

121 Alcohol intake between menarche and first pregnancy: a prospective study of breast cancer risk. Liu Y, Colditz GA, Rosner B, et al. J Natl Cancer Inst. 2013 Oct 16;105(20):1571-8. PMID:23985142

122 Moderate alcohol consumption during adult life, drinking patterns, and breast cancer risk. Chen WY, Rosner B, Hankinson SE, Colditz GA, Willett WC. JAMA. 2011 Nov 2;306(17):1884-90. PMID:22045766

123 Relationship between established breast cancer risk factors and risk of seven different histologic types of invasive breast cancer. Li CI, Daling JR, Malone KE, et al. Cancer Epidemiol Biomarkers Prev. 2006 May;15(5):946-54. PMID:16702375

124 Postdiagnosis alcohol consumption and breast cancer prognosis in the after breast cancer pooling project. Kwan ML, Chen WY, Flatt SW, et al. Cancer Epidemiol Biomarkers Prev. 2013 Jan;22(1):32-41. PMID:23150063

125 Light alcohol drinking and cancer: a meta-analysis. Bagnardi V, Rota M, Botteri E, et al. Ann Oncol. 2013 Feb;24(2):301-8. PMID:22910838

126 Ethanol versus Phytochemicals in Wine: Oral Cancer Risk in a Light Drinking Perspective. Varoni EM, Lodi G, Iriti M. Int J Mol Sci. 2015 Jul 27;16(8):17029-47. PMID:26225960

127 Second cancers following oral and pharyngeal cancers: role of tobacco and alcohol. Day GL, Blot WJ, Shore RE, et al. J Natl Cancer Inst. 1994 Jan 19;86(2):131-7. PMID:8271296

128 Alcoholism: independent predictor of survival in patients with head and neck cancer. Deleyiannis FW, Thomas DB, Vaughan TL, Davis S. J Natl Cancer Inst. 1996 Apr 17;88(8):542-9. PMID:8606383

129 Understanding why aspirin prevents cancer and why consuming very hot beverages and foods increases esophageal cancer risk. Controlling the division rates of stem cells is an

important strategy to prevent cancer. López-Lázaro M. Oncoscience. 2015 Nov 10;2(10):849-56. eCollection 2015. PMID:26682276

[130] Effects of anatomical position on esophageal transit time: a biomagnetic diagnostic technique. Cordova-Fraga T, Sosa M, Wiechers C, et al. World J Gastroenterol. 2008 Oct 7;14(37):5707-11. PMID:18837088

[131] http://www.iarc.fr/en/media-centre/pr/2016/pdfs/pr244_E.pdf

[132] http://burnprevention.org/scald-prevention/

[133] Light alcohol drinking and cancer: a meta-analysis. Bagnardi V, Rota M, Botteri E, et al. Ann Oncol. 2013 Feb;24(2):301-8. PMID:22910838

[134] Association between alcohol consumption and the risk of ovarian cancer: a meta-analysis of prospective observational studies. Yan-Hong H, Jing L, Hong L, Shan-Shan H, Yan L, Ju L. BMC Public Health. 2015 Mar 7;15:223. PMID:25885863

[135] Enteroimmunology: A Guide to the Prevention and Treatment of Chronic Inflammatory Disease. Charles A. Lewis. Psy Press. 2015

[136] Formation of biogenic amines throughout the industrial manufacture of red wine. Marcobal A, Martín-Alvarez PJ, Polo MC, et al. J Food Prot. 2006 Feb;69(2):397-404. PMID:16496582

[137] Analysis of neuroactive amines in fermented beverages using a portable microchip capillary electrophoresis system. Jayarajah CN, Skelley AM, Fortner AD, Mathies RA. Anal Chem. 2007 Nov 1;79(21):8162-9. PMID:17892274

[138] The epidemiology of fetal alcohol syndrome and partial FAS in a South African community. May PA, Gossage JP, Marais AS, et al. Drug Alcohol Depend. 2007 May 11;88(2-3):259-71. PMID:17127017

[139] Maternal risk factors for fetal alcohol syndrome and partial fetal alcohol syndrome in South Africa: a third study. May PA, Gossage JP, Marais AS, et al. Alcohol Clin Exp Res. 2008 May;32(5):738-53. PMID:18336634

[140] Prenatal alcohol exposure and childhood behavior at age 6 to 7 years: I. dose-response effect. Sood B, Delaney-Black V, Covington C, Nordstrom-Klee B, Ager J, Templin T, Janisse J, Martier S, Sokol RJ. Pediatrics. 2001 Aug;108(2):E34. PMID:11483844

[141] Fetal alcohol exposure increases mammary tumor susceptibility and alters tumor phenotype in rats. Polanco TA, Crismale-Gann C, Reuhl KR, Sarkar DK, Cohick WS. Alcohol Clin Exp Res. 2010 Nov;34(11):1879-87. PMID:20662802

[142] Ethanol induces TLR4/TLR2 association, triggering an inflammatory response in microglial cells. Fernandez-Lizarbe S, Montesinos J, Guerri C. J Neurochem. 2013 Jul;126(2):261-73. PMID:23600947

[143] Effect of alcohol consumption on CpG methylation in the differentially methylated regions of H19 and IG-DMR in male gametes: implications for fetal alcohol spectrum disorders. Ouko LA, Shantikumar K, Knezovich J, Haycock P, Schnugh DJ, Ramsay M. Alcohol Clin Exp Res. 2009 Sep;33(9):1615-27. PMID:19519716

[144] Prenatal exposure to ethanol: a specific effect on the H19 gene in sperm. Stouder C, Somm E, Paoloni-Giacobino A. Reprod Toxicol. 2011 May;31(4):507-12. PMID:21382472

[145] An epidemiologic review of marijuana and cancer: an update. Huang YH, Zhang ZF, Tashkin DP, et al. Cancer Epidemiol Biomarkers Prev. 2015 Jan;24(1):15-31. PMID:25587109

[146] Red wine antioxidants protect hippocampal neurons against ethanol-induced damage: a biochemical, morphological and behavioral study. Assunção M, Santos-Marques MJ, de Freitas V, Carvalho F, et al. Neuroscience. 2007 Jun 8;146(4):1581-92. PMID:17490820

[147] Antioxidant capacities and phenolics levels of French wines from different varieties and vintages. Landrault N, Poucheret P, Ravel P, Gasc F, Cros G, Teissedre PL. J Agric Food Chem. 2001 Jul;49(7):3341-8. PMID:11453773

148 Grape seed flavanols, but not Port wine, prevent ethanol-induced neuronal lipofuscin formation.. Assunção M, de Freitas V, Paula-Barbosa M. Brain Res. 2007 Jan 19;1129(1):72-80. PMID:17156755

149 Red Wine, but not port wine, protects rat hippocampal dentate gyrus against ethanol-induced neuronal damage--relevance of the sugar content. Carneiro A, Assunção M, De Freitas V, et al. Alcohol & Alcoholism. 2008 Jul-Aug;43(4):408-15. PMID:18445757

150 Betaine treatment attenuates chronic ethanol-induced hepatic steatosis and alterations to the mitochondrial respiratory chain proteome. Kharbanda KK, Todero SL, King AL, Osna NA, et al. Int J Hepatol. 2012;2012:962183. PMID:22187660

151 Centers for Disease Control, Injury Prvention and Control, Accessed Jan. 2016. http://www.cdc.gov/motorvehiclesafety/impaired_driving/impaired-drv_factsheet.html

152 Prevalence of obesity in the United States, 2009-2010. Ogden CL, Carroll MD, Kit BK, Flegal KM. NCHS Data Brief. 2012 Jan;(82):1-8. PMID: 22617494

153 Obesity and the risk of myocardial infarction in 27,000 participants from 52 countries: a case-control study. Yusuf S, Hawken S, Ounpuu S, et al; INTERHEART Study Investigators. Lancet. 2005 Nov 5;366(9497):1640-9. PMID:16271645

154 Large waist circumference and risk of hypertension. Guagnano MT, Ballone E, Colagrande V, Della Vecchia R, Manigrasso MR, Merlitti D, Riccioni G, Sensi S. Int J Obes Relat Metab Disord. 2001 Sep;25(9):1360-4. PMID:11571600

155 Overall and central adiposity and breast cancer risk in the sister study. White AJ, Nichols HB, Bradshaw PT, Sandler DP. Cancer. 2015 Oct 15;121(20):3700-8. PMID:26193782

156 Body fat distribution and risk of premenopausal breast cancer in the Nurses' Health Study II. Harris HR, Willett WC, Terry KL, Michels KB. J Natl Cancer Inst. 2011 Feb 2;103(3):273-8. PMID:21163903

157 Weight gain prior to diagnosis and survival from breast cancer. Cleveland RJ, Eng SM, Abrahamson PE, Britton JA, Teitelbaum SL, Neugut AI, Gammon MD. Cancer Epidemiol Biomarkers Prev. 2007 Sep;16(9):1803-11. PMID: 17855698

158 Body weight and risk of breast cancer in BRCA1/2 mutation carriers. Manders P, Pijpe A, Hooning MJ, et al. Breast Cancer Res Treat. 2011 Feb;126(1):193-202. PMID: 20730487

159 Post-diagnosis adiposity and survival among breast cancer patients: influence of breast cancer subtype. Sun X, Nichols HB, Robinson W, Sherman ME, Olshan AF, Troester MA. Cancer Causes Control. 2015 Dec;26(12):1803-11. PMID:26428518

160 Weight, weight gain, and survival after breast cancer diagnosis. Kroenke CH, Chen WY, Rosner B, Holmes MD. J Clin Oncol. 2005 Mar 1;23(7):1370-8. PMID: 15684320

161 Dietary patterns and survival after breast cancer diagnosis. Kroenke CH, Fung TT, Hu FB, Holmes MD. J Clin Oncol. 2005 Dec 20;23(36):9295-303. PMID: 16361628

162 Dietary factors and the survival of women with breast carcinoma. Holmes MD, Stampfer MJ, Colditz GA, et al. Cancer. 1999 Sep 1;86(5):826-35. PMID:10463982

163 Weight change and survival after breast cancer in the after breast cancer pooling project. Caan BJ, Kwan ML, Shu XO, et al. Cancer Epidemiol Biomarkers Prev. 2012 Aug;21(8):1260-71. PMID:22695738

164 Favorable changes in serum estrogens and other biologic factors after weight loss in breast cancer survivors who are overweight or obese. Rock CL, Pande C, Flatt SW, et al. Clin Breast Cancer. 2013 Jun;13(3):188-95. PMID: 23375717

165 A pooled analysis of 14 cohort studies of anthropometric factors and pancreatic cancer risk. Genkinger JM, Spiegelman D, Anderson KE, et al. Int J Cancer. 2011 Oct 1;129(7):1708-17PMID:21105029

166 Central adiposity, obesity during early adulthood, and pancreatic cancer mortality in a pooled analysis of cohort studies. Genkinger JM, Kitahara CM, Bernstein L, et al. Ann Oncol. 2015 Nov;26(11):2257-66. PMID:26347100

[167] Body mass index and mortality in men with prostate cancer. Cantarutti A, Bonn SE, Adami HO, Grönberg H, Bellocco R, Bälter K. Prostate. 2015 Aug 1;75(11):1129-36. PMID:25929695

[168] Weight gain is associated with an increased risk of prostate cancer recurrence after prostatectomy in the PSA era. Joshu CE, Mondul AM, Menke A, Meinhold C et al. Cancer Prev Res (Phila). 2011 Apr;4(4):544-51. PMID:21325564

[169] Fructose-induced leptin resistance exacerbates weight gain in response to subsequent high-fat feeding. Shapiro A, Mu W, Roncal C, et al. Am J Physiol Regul Integr Comp Physiol. 2008 Nov;295(5):R1370-5. PMID: 18703413

[170] Anti-inflammatory effect of atorvastatin on vascular reactivity and insulin resistance in fructose fed rats. Mahmoud MF, El-Nagar M, El-Bassossy HM. Arch Pharm Res. 2012 Jan;35(1):155-62. PMID:22297754

[171] Modulation of hypothalamic PTP1B in the TNF-alpha-induced insulin and leptin resistance. Picardi PK, Caricilli AM, de Abreu LL, et al. FEBS Lett. 2010 Jul 16;584(14):3179-84. PMID: 20576518

[172] Insulin resistance induced by tumor necrosis factor-alpha in myocytes and brown adipocytes. Lorenzo M, Fernández-Veledo S, Vila-Bedmar R, et al. J Anim Sci. 2008 Apr;86(14 Suppl):E94-104. PMID:17940160

[173] Leptin resistance: a predisposing factor for diet-induced obesity. Scarpace PJ, Zhang Y. Am J Physiol Regul Integr Comp Physiol. 2009 Mar;296(3):R493-500. PMID: 19091915

[174] Hedonic and incentive signals for body weight control. Egecioglu E, Skibicka KP, Hansson C, et al. Rev Endocr Metab Disord. 2011 Sep;12(3):141-51. PMID:21340584

[175] Role of ghrelin in drug abuse and reward-relevant behaviors: a burgeoning field and gaps in the literature. Revitsky AR, Klein LC. Curr Drug Abuse Rev. 2013 Sep;6(3):231-44. PMID:24502454

[176] Meta-analysis of short sleep duration and obesity in children and adults. Cappuccio FP, Taggart FM, Kandala NB, et al. Sleep. 2008 May 1;31(5):619-26. PMID: 18517032

[177] Adverse effects of modest sleep restriction on sleepiness, performance, and inflammatory cytokines. Vgontzas AN, Zoumakis E, Bixler EO, Lin HM, Follett H, Kales A, Chrousos GP. J Clin Endocrinol Metab. 2004 May;89(5):2119-26. PMID: 15126529

[178] Polycyclic aromatic hydrocarbons potentiate high-fat diet effects on intestinal inflammation. Khalil A, Villard PH, Dao MA, et al.. Toxicol Lett. 2010 Jul 15;196(3):161-7.. PMID: 20412841

[179] The effects of insulin-like growth factors on tumorigenesis and neoplastic growth. Khandwala HM, McCutcheon IE, Flyvbjerg A, Friend KE. Endocr Rev. 2000 Jun;21(3):215-44. PMID:10857553

[180] Obesity-induced metabolic stresses in breast and colon cancer. Sung MK, Yeon JY, Park SY, Park JH, Choi MS. Ann N Y Acad Sci. 2011 Jul;1229:61-8. PMID:21793840

[181] The metabolic syndrome and risk of prostate cancer in Italy. Pelucchi C, Serraino D, Negri E, et al. Ann Epidemiol. 2011 Nov;21(11):835-41. PMID:21982487

[182] Metabolic syndrome and pancreatic cancer risk: a case-control study in Italy and meta-analysis. Rosato V, Tavani A, Bosetti C, et al. Metabolism. 2011 Oct;60(10):1372-8. PMID:21550085

[183] Dietary and genetic obesity promote liver inflammation and tumorigenesis by enhancing IL-6 and TNF expression. Park EJ, Lee JH, Yu Gy et al. Cell. 2010 Jan 22;140(2):197-208. PMID:20141834

[184] Visceral fat adipokine secretion is associated with systemic inflammation in obese humans. Fontana L, Eagon JC, Trujillo ME, et al. Diabetes. 2007 Apr;56(4):1010-3. PMID:17287468

[185] Visceral fat resection in humans: effect on insulin sensitivity, beta-cell function, adipokines, and inflammatory markers. Lima MM, Pareja JC, Alegre SM, et al. Obesity (Silver Spring). 2013 Mar;21(3):E182-9. PMID:23404948

186 A prospective randomized study comparing patients with morbid obesity submitted to sleeve gastrectomy with or without omentectomy. Sdralis E, Argentou M, Mead N, et al. Obes Surg. 2013 Jul;23(7):965-71. PMID:23526069

187 Omentectomy in addition to gastric bypass surgery and influence on insulin sensitivity: a randomized double blind controlled trial. Andersson DP, Thorell A, Löfgren P, et al. Clin Nutr. 2014 Dec;33(6):991-6. PMID:24485000

188 Degree of weight loss required to improve adipokine concentrations and decrease fat cell size in severely obese women. Varady KA, Tussing L, Bhutani S, Braunschweig CL. Metabolism. 2009 Aug;58(8):1096-101. PMID:19477470

189 Fructose metabolism in humans - what isotopic tracer studies tell us. Sun SZ, Empie MW. Nutr Metab (Lond). 2012 Oct 2;9(1):89. PMID:23031075

190 http://themedicalbiochemistrypage.org/fructose.php. King, MW

191 Sugar, uric acid, and the etiology of diabetes and obesity. Johnson RJ, Nakagawa T, Sanchez-Lozada LG, et al. Diabetes. 2013 Oct;62(10):3307-15. PMID:24065788

192 Enteroimmunology: A Guide to the Prevention and Treatment of Chronic Inflammatory Disease. Chapter 9. Charles A. Lewis. Psy Press. 2015

193 A review of phytotherapy of gout: perspective of new pharmacological treatments. Ling X, Bochu W. Pharmazie. 2014 Apr;69(4):243-56. PMID:24791587

194 Sucrose induces fatty liver and pancreatic inflammation in male breeder rats independent of excess energy intake. Roncal-Jimenez CA, Lanaspa MA, Rivard CJ, et al. Metabolism. 2011 Sep;60(9):1259-70. PMID:21489572

195 Sucrose-sweetened beverages increase fat storage in the liver, muscle, and visceral fat depot: a 6-mo randomized intervention study. Maersk M, Belza A, Stødkilde-Jørgensen H, et al. Am J Clin Nutr. 2012 Feb;95(2):283-9. PMID:22205311

196 Sugar-sweetened soft drinks, diet soft drinks, and serum uric acid level: the Third National Health and Nutrition Examination Survey. Choi JW, Ford ES, Gao X, Choi HK. Arthritis Rheum. 2008 Jan 15;59(1):109-16. PMID:18163396

197 Consumption of fructose- but not glucose-sweetened beverages for 10 weeks increases circulating concentrations of uric acid, retinol binding protein-4, and gamma-glutamyl transferase activity in overweight/obese humans. Cox CL, Stanhope KL, Schwarz JM, et al. Nutr Metab (Lond). 2012 Jul 24;9(1):68. PMID:22828276

198 Excessive fructose intake induces the features of metabolic syndrome in healthy adult men: role of uric acid in the hypertensive response. Perez-Pozo SE, Schold J, Nakagawa T, et al. Int J Obes (Lond). 2010 Mar;34(3):454-61. PMID:20029377

199 Fructose, exercise, and health. Johnson RJ, Murray R. Curr Sports Med Rep. 2010 Jul-Aug;9(4):253-8 PMID:20622544

200 Associations of recreational physical activity and leisure time spent sitting with colorectal cancer survival. Campbell PT, Patel AV, Newton CC, Jacobs EJ, Gapstur SM. J Clin Oncol. 2013 Mar 1;31(7):876-85. PMID:23341510

201 Physical activity and survival after colorectal cancer diagnosis. Meyerhardt JA, Giovannucci EL, Holmes MD, Chan AT, Chan JA, Colditz GA, Fuchs CS. J Clin Oncol. 006 Aug 1;24(22):3527-34. PMID:16822844

202 https://sites.google.com/site/compendiumofphysicalactivities/ Accessed Nov. 2015

203 Association between physical activity and mortality among breast cancer and colorectal cancer survivors: a systematic review and meta-analysis. Schmid D, Leitzmann MF. Ann Oncol. 2014 Jul;25(7):1293-311. PMID:24644304

204 Metabolic equivalents (METS) in exercise testing, exercise prescription, and evaluation of functional capacity. Jetté M, Sidney K, Blümchen G. Clin Cardiol. 1990 Aug;13(8):555-65. PMID:2204507

205 Physical activity and survival after prostate cancer diagnosis in the health professionals follow-up study. Kenfield SA, Stampfer MJ, Giovannucci E, Chan JM. J Clin Oncol. 2011 Feb 20;29(6):726-32. PMID:21205749

206 Physical activity after diagnosis and risk of prostate cancer progression: data from the cancer of the prostate strategic urologic research endeavor. Richman EL, Kenfield SA, Stampfer MJ, et al. Cancer Res. 2011 Jun 1;71(11):3889-95. PMID:21610110

207 Heat stress, cytokines, and the immune response to exercise. Starkie RL, Hargreaves M, Rolland J, Febbraio MA. Brain Behav Immun. 2005 Sep;19(5):404-12. PMID:16061150

208 Muscle as an endocrine organ: focus on muscle-derived interleukin-6. Pedersen BK, Febbraio MA. Physiol Rev. 2008 Oct;88(4):1379-406. PMID:18923185

209 Exercise alters the IGF axis in vivo and increases p53 protein in prostate tumor cells in vitro. Leung PS, Aronson WJ, Ngo TH, Golding LA, Barnard RJ. J Appl Physiol (1985). 2004 Feb;96(2):450-4. PMID:14715676

210 p53 is necessary for the adaptive changes in cellular milieu subsequent to an acute bout of endurance exercise. Saleem A, Carter HN, Hood DA. Am J Physiol Cell Physiol. 2014 Feb 1;306(3):C241-9. PMID:24284795

211 Reduced carbohydrate availability enhances exercise-induced p53 signaling in human skeletal muscle: implications for mitochondrial biogenesis. Bartlett JD, Louhelainen J, Iqbal Z, et al. Am J Physiol Regul Integr Comp Physiol. 2013 Mar 15;304(6):R450-8. PMID:23364526

212 A metabolic switch in brain: glucose and lactate metabolism modulation by ascorbic acid. Castro MA, Beltrán FA, Brauchi S, Concha II. J Neurochem. 2009 Jul;110(2):423-40. PMID:19457103

213 Lactate administration reproduces specific brain and liver exercise-related changes. E L, Lu J, Selfridge JE, Burns JM, et al. J Neurochem. 2013 Oct;127(1):91-100. PMID:23927032

214 Lactate sensitive transcription factor network in L6 cells: activation of MCT1 and mitochondrial biogenesis. Hashimoto T, Hussien R, Oommen S, Gohil K, Brooks GA. FASEB J. 2007 Aug;21(10):2602-12. PMID:17395833

215 Pathway of programmed cell death and oxidative stress induced by β-hydroxybutyrate in dairy cow abomasum smooth muscle cells and in mouse gastric smooth muscle. Tian W, Wei T, Li B, Wang Z, Zhang N, Xie G. PLoS One. 2014 May 6;9(5):e96775. PMID:24801711

216 Exercise promotes the expression of brain derived neurotrophic factor (BDNF) through the action of the ketone body β-hydroxybutyrate. Sleiman SF, Henry J, Al-Haddad R, et al. Elife. 2016 Jun 2;5. pii: e15092. PMID:27253067

217 Impact of epigenetic dietary compounds on transgenerational prevention of human diseases. Li Y, Saldanha SN, Tollefsbol TO. AAPS J. 2014 Jan;16(1):27-36. PMID:24114450

218 Fatty acids and epigenetics. Burdge GC, Lillycrop KA. Curr Opin Clin Nutr Metab Care. 2013 Dec 7. PMID:24322369

219 Histone deacetylases as targets for dietary cancer preventive agents: lessons learned with butyrate, diallyl disulfide, and sulforaphane. Myzak MC, Dashwood RH. Curr Drug Targets. 2006 Apr;7(4):443-52. PMID:16611031

220 Identification of HDAC Inhibitors Using a Cell-Based HDAC I/II Assay. Hsu CW, Shou D, Huang R, Khuc T, Dai S, Zheng W, Klumpp-Thomas C, Xia M. J Biomol Screen. 2016 Jul;21(6):643-52. PMID:26858181

221 Roles of melatonin in fetal programming in compromised pregnancies. Chen YC, Sheen JM, Tiao MM, Tain YL, Huang LT. Int J Mol Sci. 2013 Mar 6;14(3):5380-401. PMID:23466884

222 The neuroprotective effects of β-hydroxybutyrate on Aβ-injected rat hippocampus in vivo and in Aβ-treated PC-12 cells in vitro. Xie G, Tian W, Wei T, Liu F. Free Radic Res. 2015 Feb;49(2):139-50. PMID:25410532

223 A practical model of low-volume high-intensity interval training induces mitochondrial biogenesis in human skeletal muscle: potential mechanisms. Little JP, Safdar A, Wilkin GP, Tarnopolsky MA, Gibala MJ. J Physiol. 2010 Mar 15;588(Pt 6):1011-22. PMID:20100740

224 Short-term sprint interval versus traditional endurance training: similar initial adaptations in human skeletal muscle and exercise performance. Gibala MJ, Little JP, van Essen M, et al. J Physiol. 2006 Sep 15;575(Pt 3):901-11. PMID:16825308

225 Improvements in exercise performance with high-intensity interval training coincide with an increase in skeletal muscle mitochondrial content and function. Jacobs RA, Flück D, Bonne TC, et al. J Appl Physiol (1985). 2013 Sep;115(6):785-93. PMID:23788574

226 Mitochondrial gene expression in elite cyclists: effects of high-intensity interval exercise. Psilander N, Wang L, Westergren J, et al. Eur J Appl Physiol. 2010 Oct;110(3):597-606. PMID:20571821

227 Impact of various exercise modalities on hepatic mitochondrial function. Fletcher JA, Meers GM, Linden MA, Kearney ML, Morris EM, Thyfault JP, Rector RS. Med Sci Sports Exerc. 2014 Jun;46(6):1089-97. PMID:24263979

228 Age-related maximal heart rate: examination and refinement of prediction equations. Shargal E, Kislev-Cohen R, Zigel L, Epstein S, Pilz-Burstein R, Tenenbaum G. J Sports Med Phys Fitness. 2014 Nov 12. PMID:25389634

229 Perceptions and the role of group exercise among New York City adults, 2010-2011: an examination of interpersonal factors and leisure-time physical activity. Firestone MJ, Yi SS, Bartley KF, Eisenhower DL. Prev Med. 2015 Mar;72:50-5. PMID:25584986

230 Human blood neutrophil responses to prolonged exercise with and without a thermal clamp. Laing SJ, Jackson AR, Walters R, Lloyd-Jones E, Whitham M, Maassen N, Walsh NP. J Appl Physiol. 2008 Jan;104(1):20-6. PMID:17901240

231 Elevation of body temperature is an essential factor for exercise-increased extracellular heat shock protein 72 level in rat plasma. Ogura Y, Naito H, Akin S, Ichinoseki-Sekine N, etal. Am J Physiol Regul Integr Comp Physiol. 2008 May;294(5):R1600-7. PMID:18367652

232 Metabolic and hormonal responses to exogenous hyperthermia in man. Møller N, Beckwith R, Butler PC, et al. Clin Endocrinol (Oxf). 1989 Jun;30(6):651-60. PMID:2686866

233 Additive protective effects of the addition of lactic acid and adrenaline on excitability and force in isolated rat skeletal muscle depressed by elevated extracellular K+. de Paoli FV, Overgaard K, Pedersen TH, et al. J Physiol. 2007 Jun 1;581(Pt 2):829-39. PMID: 17347268

234 HSP72 protects against obesity-induced insulin resistance. Chung J, Nguyen AK, Henstridge DC, Holmes AG, Chan MH, Mesa JL, etal. Proc Natl Acad Sci U S A. 2008 Feb 5;105(5):1739-44. PMID:18223156

235 Heat treatment improves glucose tolerance and prevents skeletal muscle insulin resistance in rats fed a high-fat diet. Gupte AA, Bomhoff GL, Swerdlow RH, Geiger PC. Diabetes. 2009 Mar;58(3):567-78. PMID:19073766

236 Hot-tub therapy for type 2 diabetes mellitus. Hooper PL. N Engl J Med. 1999 Sep 16;341(12):924-5. PMID:10498473

237 Complementary and alternative medicine in the treatment of pain in fibromyalgia: a systematic review of randomized controlled trials. Terhorst L, Schneider MJ, Kim KH, et al. J Manipulative Physiol Ther. 2011 Sep;34(7):483-96. PMID:21875523

238 Concurrent detection of autolysosome formation and lysosomal degradation by flow cytometry in a high-content screen for inducers of autophagy. Hundeshagen P, Hamacher-Brady A, Eils R, Brady NR. BMC Biol. 2011 Jun 2;9:38. PMID:21635740

239 Folate deficiency and cervical dysplasia. Butterworth CE Jr, Hatch KD, Macaluso M, Cole P, Sauberlich HE, Soong SJ, Borst M, Baker VV. JAMA. 1992 Jan 22-29;267(4):528-33. PMID:1729576

240 Lower red blood cell folate enhances the HPV-16-associated risk of cervical intraepithelial neoplasia. Piyathilake CJ, Macaluso M, Brill I, Heimburger DC, Partridge EE. Nutrition. 2007 Mar;23(3):203-10. PMID:17276035

241 Diet and cancer. Willett WC. Oncologist. 2000;5(5):393-404. PMID:11040276

242 Nutrition and bladder cancer. La Vecchia C, Negri E. Cancer Causes Control. 1996 Jan;7(1):95-100. PMID:8850438

243 Systematic review of studies investigating the association between dietary habits and cutaneous malignant melanoma. de Waure C, Quaranta G, Gualano MR,et al. Public Health. 2015 Aug;129(8):1099-113. PMID:26212104

244 Patterns of food consumption among vegetarians and non-vegetarians. Orlich MJ, Jaceldo-Siegl K, Sabaté J, Fan J, Singh PN, Fraser GE. Br J Nutr. 2014 Nov 28;112(10):1644-53. PMID:25247790

245 MTHFR gene polymorphism, homocysteine and cardiovascular disease. Cortese C, Motti C. Public Health Nutr. 2001 Apr;4(2B):493-7. PMID:11683544

246 Methylenetetrahydrofolate reductase (MTHFR) polymorphism increases the risk of cervical intraepithelial neoplasia. Piyathilake CJ, Macaluso M, Johanning GL, Whiteside M, Heimburger DC, Giuliano A. Anticancer Res. 2000 May-Jun;20(3A):1751-7. PMID:10928104

247 Vitamin C and vitamin E supplement use and bladder cancer mortality in a large cohort of US men and women. Jacobs EJ, Henion AK, Briggs PJ, et al. Am J Epidemiol. 2002 Dec 1;156(11):1002-10. PMID:12446256

248 Vitamin E and the risk of prostate cancer: the Selenium and Vitamin E Cancer Prevention Trial (SELECT). Klein EA, Thompson IM Jr, Tangen CM, et al. JAMA. 2011 Oct 12;306(14):1549-56. PMID:21990298

249 Staphylococcus aureus is More Prevalent in Retail Beef Livers than in Pork and other Beef Cuts. Abdalrahman LS, Wells H, Fakhr MK. Pathogens. 2015 Apr 28;4(2):182-98. PMID:25927961

250 Prevalence and characterization of methicillin-resistant Staphylococcus aureus isolates from retail meat and humans in Georgia. Jackson CR, Davis JA, Barrett JB. J Clin Microbiol. 2013 Apr;51(4):1199-207. PMID:23363837

251 A higher prevalence rate of Campylobacter in retail beef livers compared to other beef and pork meat cuts. Noormohamed A, Fakhr MK. Int J Environ Res Public Health. 2013 May 21;10(5):2058-68. PMID:23698698

252 Incidence and antimicrobial resistance profiling of Campylobacter in retail chicken livers and gizzards. Noormohamed A, Fakhr MK. Foodborne Pathog Dis. 2012 Jul;9(7):617-24. PMID:22545960

253 Dietary patterns as identified by factor analysis and colorectal cancer among middle-aged Americans. Flood A, Rastogi T, Wirfält et al. Am J Clin Nutr. 2008 Jul;88(1):176-84. PMID:18614739

254 A review and meta-analysis of red and processed meat consumption and breast cancer. Alexander DD, Morimoto LM, Mink PJ, Cushing CA. Nutr Res Rev. 2010 Dec;23(2):349-65. PMID:21110906

255 A high ratio of dietary n-6/n-3 polyunsaturated fatty acids is associated with increased risk of prostate cancer. Williams CD, Whitley BM, Hoyo C, Grant DJ, etal. Nutr Res. 2011 Jan;31(1):1-8. PMID:21310299

256 Intake of polyunsaturated fatty acids and distal large bowel cancer risk in whites and African Americans. Kim S, Sandler DP, Galanko J, et al. Am J Epidemiol. 2010 May 1;171(9):969-79. PMID:20392864

257 Occupation and cancer - follow-up of 15 million people in five Nordic countries. Pukkala E, Martinsen JI, Lynge E, Gunnarsdottir HK, Sparén P, Tryggvadottir L, Weiderpass E, Kjaerheim K. Acta Oncol. 2009;48(5):646-790. PMID:19925375

258 Preferential formation of benzo[a]pyrene adducts at lung cancer mutational hotspots in P53. Denissenko MF, Pao A, Tang M, Pfeifer GP. Science. 1996 Oct 18;274(5286):430-2. PMID:8832894

259 Oral benzo[a]pyrene: understanding pharmacokinetics, detoxication, and consequences-- Cyp1 knockout mouse lines as a paradigm. Nebert DW, Shi Z, Gálvez-Peralta M, Uno S, Dragin N. Mol Pharmacol. 2013 Sep;84(3):304-13. PMID:23761301

260 Prenatal airborne polycyclic aromatic hydrocarbon exposure and child IQ at age 5 years. Perera FP, Li Z, Whyatt R, Hoepner L, Wang S, Camann D, Rauh V. Pediatrics. 2009 Aug;124(2):e195-202. PMID:19620194

261 Prenatal exposure to airborne polycyclic aromatic hydrocarbons and risk of intrauterine growth restriction. Choi H, Rauh V, Garfinkel R, Tu Y, Perera FP. Environ Health Perspect. 2008 May;116(5):658-65. PMID:18470316

262 Polycyclic aromatic hydrocarbons potentiate high-fat diet effects on intestinal inflammation. Khalil A, Villard PH, Dao MA, et al. Toxicol Lett. 2010 Jul 15;196(3):161-7. PMID:20412841

263 Carcinogenic food contaminants. Abnet CC. Cancer Invest. 2007 Apr-May;25(3):189-96. PMID:17530489

264 Cooking smoke: a silent killer. Schwela D. People Planet. 1997;6(3):24-5. PMID:12321046

265 Lung cancer and indoor air pollution in rural china. Kleinerman R, Wang Z, Lubin J, Zhang S, Metayer C, Brenner A. Ann Epidemiol. 2000 Oct 1;10(7):469. PMID:11018397

266 Well-done meat intake and meat-derived mutagen exposures in relation to breast cancer risk: the Nashville Breast Health Study. Fu Z, Deming SL, Fair AM, et al. Breast Cancer Res Treat. 2011 Oct;129(3):919-28. PMID:21537933

267 Association of meat intake and meat-derived mutagen exposure with the risk of colorectal polyps by histologic type. Fu Z, Shrubsole MJ, Smalley WE, et al. Cancer Prev Res (Phila). 2011 Oct;4(10):1686-97. PMID:21803984

268 Well-done red meat, metabolic phenotypes and colorectal cancer in Hawaii. Le Marchand L, Hankin JH, Pierce LM, et al. Mutat Res. 2002 Sep 30;506-507:205-14. PMID:12351160

269 Modification by N-acetyltransferase 1 genotype on the association between dietary heterocyclic amines and colon cancer in a multiethnic study. Butler LM, Millikan RC, Sinha R, et al. Mutat Res. 2008 Feb 1;638(1-2):162-74. PMID:18022202

270 Effect of NAT1 and NAT2 genetic polymorphisms on colorectal cancer risk associated with exposure to tobacco smoke and meat consumption. Lilla C, Verla-Tebit E, Risch A, et al. Cancer Epidemiol Biomarkers Prev. 2006 Jan;15(1):99-107. PMID:16434594

271 Smoke carcinogens cause bone loss through the aryl hydrocarbon receptor and induction of Cyp1 enzymes. Iqbal J, Sun L, Cao J, rt al. Proc Natl Acad Sci U S A. 2013 Jul 2;110(27):11115-20. PMID:23776235

272 DNA adducts of heterocyclic amine food mutagens: implications for mutagenesis and carcinogenesis. Schut HA, Snyderwine EG. Carcinogenesis. 1999 Mar;20(3):353-68. PMID:10190547

273 Well-done meat intake, heterocyclic amine exposure, and cancer risk. Zheng W, Lee SA. Nutr Cancer. 2009;61(4):437-46. PMID:19838915

274 Heterocyclic amines: Mutagens/carcinogens produced during cooking of meat and fish. Sugimura T, Wakabayashi K, Nakagama H, Nagao M. Cancer Sci. 2004 Apr;95(4):290-9. PMID:15072585

275 Human exposure to heterocyclic amine food mutagens/carcinogens: relevance to breast cancer. Felton JS, Knize MG, Salmon CP, Malfatti MA, Kulp KS. Environ Mol Mutagen. 2002;39(2-3):112-8. PMID:11921178

276 Dietary patterns as identified by factor analysis and colorectal cancer among middle-aged Americans. Flood A, Rastogi T, Wirfält E, et al. Am J Clin Nutr. 2008 Jul;88(1):176-84. PMID:18614739

277 Meat consumption, cooking practices, meat mutagens, and risk of prostate cancer. John EM, Stern MC, Sinha R, Koo J. Nutr Cancer. 2011 May;63(4):525-37. PMID:21526454

278 Intakes of red meat, processed meat, and meat mutagens increase lung cancer risk. Lam TK, Cross AJ, Consonni D, Randi G, Bagnardi V, Bertazzi PA, Caporaso NE, Sinha R, Subar AF, Landi MT. Cancer Res. 2009 Feb 1;69(3):932-9. PMID:19141639

279 Adolescent meat intake and breast cancer risk. Farvid MS, Cho E, Chen WY, Eliassen AH, Willett WC. Int J Cancer. 2015 Apr 15;136(8):1909-20. PMID:25220168

280 Metabolism of the food-derived carcinogen 2-amino-1-methyl-6-phenylimidazo[4,5-b]pyridine by lactating Fischer 344 rats and their nursing pups. Davis CD, Ghoshal A, Schut HA, Snyderwine EG. J Natl Cancer Inst. 1994 Jul 20;86(14):1065-70. PMID:8021955

281 Evidence for the presence of mutagenic arylamines in human breast milk and DNA adducts in exfoliated breast ductal epithelial cells. Thompson PA, DeMarini DM, Kadlubar FF, et al. Environ Mol Mutagen. 2002;39(2-3):134-42. PMID:11921181

282 DNA adducts of 2-amino-3-methylimidazo[4,5-f]quinoline (IQ) in fetal tissues of patas monkeys after transplacental exposure. Josyula S, Lu LJ, Salazar JJ, et al. Toxicol Appl Pharmacol. 2000 Aug 1;166(3):151-60. PMID:10906279

283 Comparative carcinogenicity of 4-aminobiphenyl and the food pyrolysates, Glu-P-1, IQ, PhIP, and MeIQx in the neonatal B6C3F1 male mouse. Dooley KL, Von Tungeln LS, Bucci T, Fu PP, Kadlubar FF. Cancer Lett. 1992 Mar 15;62(3):205-9. PMID:1596864

284 Polycyclic aromatic hydrocarbon-DNA adducts in human sperm as a marker of DNA damage and infertility. Gaspari L, Chang SS, Santella RM, Garte S, Pedotti P, Taioli E. Mutat Res. 2003 Mar 3;535(2):155-60. PMID:12581533

285 Relationship between seminal ascorbic acid and sperm DNA integrity in infertile men. Song GJ, Norkus EP, Lewis V. Int J Androl. 2006 Dec;29(6):569-75. PMID:17121654

286 Chronic high-fat diet in fathers programs β-cell dysfunction in female rat offspring. Ng SF, Lin RC, Laybutt DR, Barres R, Owens JA, Morris MJ. Nature. 2010 Oct 21;467(7318):963-6. PMID:20962845

287 Creatine and creatinine metabolism. Wyss M, Kaddurah-Daouk R. Physiol Rev. 2000 Jul;80(3):1107-213. PMID:10893433

288 Factors Affecting U.S. Beef Consumption. Davis GC, Lin BH. USDA LDP-M-135-02 October 2005

289 [Heterocyclic amines in cooked meat]. Vikse R, Reistad R, Steffensen IL, Paulsen JE, Nyholm SH, Alexander J. Tidsskr Nor Laegeforen. 1999 Jan 10;119(1):45-9. PMID:10025205

290 Effect of cooking methods on the formation of heterocyclic aromatic amines in chicken and duck breast. Liao GZ, Wang GY, Xu XL, Zhou GH. Meat Sci. 2010 May;85(1):149-54. PMID:20374878

291 Heterocyclic amines: occurrence and prevention in cooked food. Robbana-Barnat S, Rabache M, Rialland E, Fradin J. Environ Health Perspect. 1996 Mar;104(3):280-8. PMID:8919766

292 Effects of traditional Chinese cooking methods on formation of heterocyclic aromatic amines in lamb patties. Haitao Guo, Zhenyu Wang, Han Pan, et al. Food Science and Biotechnology June 2014, Volume 23, Issue 3, pp 747-753

293 On Food and Cooking, the Science and Lore of the Kitchen. Harold McGee. Scribner, New York, 2004

294 Minimization of heterocyclic amines and thermal inactivation of Escherichia coli in fried ground beef. Salmon CP, Knize MG, Panteleakos FN, Wu RW, Nelson DO, Felton JS. J Natl Cancer Inst. 2000 Nov 1;92(21):1773-8. PMID: 11058620

295 A Taste of Paradise Susana and Charles Lewis, Psy Press 2012 Carrabelle, FL

296 Mutagenicity of wood smoke condensates in the Salmonella/microsome assay. Asita AO, Matsui M, Nohmi T, et al. Mutat Res. 1991 Sep;264(1):7-14. PMID:1881415

[297] Direct mutagenicity of the polycylcic aromatic hydrocarbon-containing fraction of smoked and charcoal-broiled foods treated with nitrite in acid solution. Kangsadalampai K, Butryee C, Manoonphol K. Food Chem Toxicol. 1997 Feb;35(2):213-8. PMID:9146734

[298] Airborne mutagens produced by frying beef, pork and a soy-based food. Thiébaud HP, Knize MG, Kuzmicky PA, Hsieh DP, Felton JS. Food Chem Toxicol. 1995 Oct;33(10):821-8. PMID:7590526

[299] Mutagenicity of cooked hamburger is controlled delicately by reducing sugar content in ground beef. Kato T, Michikoshi K, Minowa Y, Kikugawa K. Mutat Res. 2000 Nov 20;471(1-2):1-6. PMID:11080655

[300] Effects of marinating with Asian marinades or western barbecue sauce on PhIP and MeIQx formation in barbecued beef. Nerurkar PV, Le Marchand L, Cooney RV. Nutr Cancer. 1999;34(2):147-52. PMID:10578481

[301] Effect of microwave pretreatment on heterocyclic aromatic amine mutagens/carcinogens in fried beef patties. Felton JS, Fultz E, Dolbeare FA, Knize MG. Food Chem Toxicol. 1994 Oct;32(10):897-903. PMID:7959444

[302] Occurrence of mutagenic/carcinogenic heterocyclic amines in meat and fish products, including pan residues, prepared under domestic conditions. Johansson MA, Jägerstad M. Carcinogenesis. 1994 Aug;15(8):1511-8. PMID:8055627

[303] Effect of marinades on the formation of heterocyclic amines in grilled beef steaks. Smith JS, Ameri F, Gadgil P. J Food Sci. 2008 Aug;73(6):T100-5. PMID:19241593

[304] Effect of red wine marinades on the formation of heterocyclic amines in fried chicken breast. Busquets R, Puignou L, Galceran MT, Skog K. J Agric Food Chem. 2006 Oct 18;54(21):8376-84. PMID:17032054

[305] Effect of beer/red wine marinades on the formation of heterocyclic aromatic amines in pan-fried beef. Melo A, Viegas O, Petisca C, Pinho O, Ferreira IM. J Agric Food Chem. 2008 Nov 26;56(22):10625-32. PMID:18950185

[306] Effect of marinades on the formation of heterocyclic amines in grilled beef steaks. Smith JS, Ameri F, Gadgil P. J Food Sci. 2008 Aug;73(6):T100-5. PMID:19241593

[307] Effect of oil marinades with garlic, onion, and lemon juice on the formation of heterocyclic aromatic amines in fried beef patties. Gibis M. J Agric Food Chem. 2007 Dec 12;55(25):10240-7. PMID:17988088

[308] Prevention of the formation of mutagenic and/or carcinogenic heterocyclic amines by food factors.. Kikugawa K, Hiramoto K, Kato T. Biofactors. 2000;12(1-4):123-7. PMID:11216472

[309] Heterocyclic Amines: 2. Inhibitory Effects of Natural Extracts on the Formation of Polar andNonpolar Heterocyclic Amines in Cooked Beef. Ahn J, Grun IU, J Food Science 70:(4)C263-68, 2005

[310] Influence of frying fat on the formation of heterocyclic amines in fried beefburgers and pan residues. Johansson MA, Fredholm L, Bjerne I, Jägerstad M. Food Chem Toxicol. 1995 Dec;33(12):993-1004. PMID:8847005

[311] Induction of human arylamine N-acetyltransferase type I by androgens in human prostate cancer cells. Butcher NJ, Tetlow NL, Cheung C, Broadhurst GM, Minchin RF. Cancer Res. 2007 Jan 1;67(1):85-92. PMID:17210686

[312] Direct reduction of N-acetoxy-PhIP by tea polyphenols: a possible mechanism for chemoprevention against PhIP-DNA adduct formation. Lin DX, Thompson PA, Teitel C, Chen JS, Kadlubar FF. Mutat Res. 2003 Feb-Mar;523-524:193-200. PMID:12628517

[313] Inhibition of the genotoxic effects of heterocyclic amines in human derived hepatoma cells by dietary bioantimutagens. Sanyal R, Darroudi F, Parzefall W, Nagao M, Knasmüller S. Mutagenesis. 1997 Jul;12(4):297-303. PMID:9237777

[314] Minimization of heterocyclic amines and thermal inactivation of Escherichia coli in fried ground beef. Salmon CP, Knize MG, Panteleakos FN, Wu RW, Nelson DO, Felton JS. J Natl Cancer Inst. 2000 Nov 1;92(21):1773-8. PMID:11058620

315 Diet-induced endogenous formation of nitroso compounds in the GI tract. Kuhnle GG, Story GW, Reda T, Mani AR, Moore KP, Lunn JC, Bingham SA. Free Radic Biol Med. 2007 Oct 1;43(7):1040-7. PMID:17761300

316 Application of toxicological risk assessment principles to the chemical constituents of cigarette smoke. Fowles J, Dybing E. Tob Control. 2003 Dec;12(4):424-30. PMID:14660781

317 Development of a food database of nitrosamines, heterocyclic amines, and polycyclic aromatic hydrocarbons. (Database) Jakszyn P, Agudo A, Ibáñez R, García-Closas R, Pera G, Amiano P, González CA. J Nutr. 2004 Aug;134(8):2011-4. PMID:15284391

318 Risk factors for esophageal cancer: a case-control study in South-western China. Yang CX, Wang HY, et al. Asian Pac J Cancer Prev. 2005 Jan-Mar;6(1):48-53. PMID: 15780032

319 Pickled vegetables and the risk of oesophageal cancer: a meta-analysis. Islami F, Ren JS, Taylor PR, Kamangar F. Br J Cancer. 2009 Nov 3;101(9):1641-7. PMID:19862003

320 Pickled food and risk of gastric cancer--a systematic review and meta-analysis of English and Chinese literature. Ren JS, Kamangar F, Forman D, Islami F. Cancer Epidemiol Biomarkers Prev. 2012 Jun;21(6):905-15. PMID:22499775

321 Kimchi and soybean pastes are risk factors of gastric cancer. Nan HM, Park JW, Song YJ, Yun HY, Park JS, Hyun T, Youn SJ, Kim YD, Kang JW, Kim H. World J Gastroenterol. 2005 Jun 7;11(21):3175-81. PMID:15929164

322 Occurrence of nitroso compounds in fungi-contaminated foods: a review. Li MH, Ji C, Cheng SJ. Nutr Cancer. 1986;8(1):63-9. PMID:3520493

323 Biogenic amines in meat and fermented meat products. Stadnik J, Dolatowski ZJ. Acta Sci. Pol., Technol. Aliment. 9(3) 2010, 251-263

324 The Formation of N-Nitrosamine in Kimchi and Salt-fermented Fish Under Simulated Gastric Digestion. Nan HG, Park JW, Song YJ et al. Journal of food hygiene and safety; ISSN:1229-1153; v.17; NO.2; p.94-100; (2002)

325 The effect of haem in red and processed meat on the endogenous formation of N-nitroso compounds in the upper gastrointestinal tract. Lunn JC, Kuhnle G, Mai V, et al. Carcinogenesis. 2007 Mar;28(3):685-90. PMID:17052997

326 Red meat consumption during adolescence among premenopausal women and risk of breast cancer. Linos E, Willett WC, Cho E, Colditz G, Frazier LA. Cancer Epidemiol Biomarkers Prev. 2008 Aug;17(8):2146-51PMID:18669582

327 Formation of N-nitrosamines in microwaved versus skillet-fried bacon containing nitrite. Miller BJ, Billedeau SM, Miller DW. Food Chem Toxicol. 1989 May;27(5):295-9. PMID:2744660

328 Effect of Frying and Other Cooking Conditions on Nitrosopyrrolidine Formation in Bacon. Pensabaine JW, Fidler W, Gates RA, etal. J of Food Sci., v 39, p 314-316.

329 Current trends in levels of volatile N-nitrosamines in fried bacon and fried-out bacon fat. Canas BJ, Havery DC, Joe FL Jr, Fazio T. J Assoc Off Anal Chem. 1986 Nov-Dec;69(6):1020-1. PMID:3804941

330 Distribution of Seven N-Nitrosamines in Food. Park JE, Seo JE, Lee JY, Kwon H. Toxicol Res. 2015 Sep;31(3):279-88. PMID:26483887

331 Biogenic amines in fish: roles in intoxication, spoilage, and nitrosamine formation--a review. Al Bulushi I, Poole S, Deeth HC, Dykes GA. Crit Rev Food Sci Nutr. 2009 Apr;49(4):369-77. PMID:19234946

332 N-nitrosamines and residual nitrite in cured meats from the Dutch market. Ellen G, Egmond E, Sahertian ET. Z Lebensm Unters Forsch. 1986 Jan;182(1):14-8. PMID:3953157

333 N-Nitroso compounds in the diet. Lijinsky W. Mutat Res. 1999 Jul 15;443(1-2):129-38. PMID:10415436

334 Effect of processed and red meat on endogenous nitrosation and DNA damage. Joosen AM, Kuhnle GG, Aspinall SM, Barrow TM, Lecommandeur E, Azqueta A, Collins AR, Bingham SA. Carcinogenesis. 2009 Aug;30(8):1402-7. PMID:19498009

335 Quantitative assessment of red meat or processed meat consumption and kidney cancer. Alexander DD, Cushing CA. Cancer Detect Prev. 2009;32(5-6):340-51. PMID:19303221

336 A review and meta-analysis of red and processed meat consumption and breast cancer. Alexander DD, Morimoto LM, Mink PJ, Cushing CA. Nutr Res Rev. 2010 Dec;23(2):349-65. PMID:21110906

337 Red and processed meat consumption and risk of ovarian cancer: a dose-response meta-analysis of prospective studies. Wallin A, Orsini N, Wolk A. Br J Cancer. 2011 Mar 29;104(7):1196-201. PMID:21343939

338 A review and meta-analysis of prospective studies of red and processed meat intake and prostate cancer. Alexander DD, Mink PJ, Cushing CA, Sceurman B. Nutr J. 2010 Nov 2;9:50. PMID:21044319

339 Red meat, dietary nitrosamines, and heme iron and risk of bladder cancer in the European Prospective Investigation into Cancer and Nutrition (EPIC). Jakszyn P, González CA, Luján-Barroso L, et al. Cancer Epidemiol Biomarkers Prev. 2011 Mar;20(3):555-9. PMID:21239687

340 Processed meat consumption and stomach cancer risk: a meta-analysis. Larsson SC, Orsini N, Wolk A. J Natl Cancer Inst. 2006 Aug 2;98(15):1078-87. PMID:16882945

341 Red and processed meat and colorectal cancer incidence: meta-analysis of prospective studies. Chan DS, Lau R, Aune D, Vieira R, Greenwood DC, Kampman E, Norat T. PLoS One. 2011;6(6):e20456. PMID:21674008

342 Lack of the DNA repair protein O6-methylguanine-DNA methyltransferase in histologically normal brain adjacent to primary human brain tumors. Silber JR, Blank A, Bobola MS, et al. Proc Natl Acad Sci U S A. 1996 Jul 9;93(14):6941-6. PMID:8692923

343 O6-methylguanine-DNA methyltransferase deficiency in developing brain: implications for brain tumorigenesis. Bobola MS, Blank A, Berger MS, Silber JR. DNA Repair (Amst). 2007 Aug 1;6(8):1127-33. PMID:17500046

344 An international case-control study of maternal diet during pregnancy and childhood brain tumor risk: a histology-specific analysis by food group. Pogoda JM, Preston-Martin S, Howe G, et al. Ann Epidemiol. 2009 Mar;19(3):148-60. PMID:19216997

345 Diet and risk of adult glioma in eastern Nebraska, United States. Chen H, Ward MH, Tucker KL, et al. Cancer Causes Control. 2002 Sep;13(7):647-55. PMID:12296512

346 Diet and brain cancer in adults: a case-control study in northeast China. Hu J, La Vecchia C, Negri E, et al. Int J Cancer. 1999 Mar 31;81(1):20-3. PMID:10077146

347 N-Nitroso compounds in the diet. Lijinsky W. Mutat Res. 1999 Jul 15;443(1-2):129-38. PMID:10415436

348 Childhood cancer in relation to cured meat intake: review of the epidemiological evidence. Blot WJ, Henderson BE, Boice JD Jr. Nutr Cancer. 1999;34(1):111-8. PMID:10453449

349 The chemistry of nitrosamine formation, inhibition and destruction. M. L. Douglass, B. L. Kabacoff, G. A. Anderson, M. C. Cheng Journal of the Society of Cosmetic Chemists, Vol. 29, No. 9, 581-606

350 A central role for heme iron in colon carcinogenesis associated with red meat intake. Bastide NM, Chenni F, Audebert M, et al. Cancer Res. 2015 Mar 1;75(5):870-9. PMID:25592152

351 Effect of vegetables, tea, and soy on endogenous N-nitrosation, fecal ammonia, and fecal water genotoxicity during a high red meat diet in humans. Hughes R, Pollock JR, Bingham S. Nutr Cancer. 2002;42(1):70-7. PMID:12235653

352 Evaluation of the genotoxic potential of 3-monochloropropane-1,2-diol (3-MCPD) and its metabolites, glycidol and beta-chlorolactic acid, using the single cell gel/comet assay. El Ramy

R, Ould Elhkim M, Lezmi S, Poul JM. Food Chem Toxicol. 2007 Jan;45(1):41-8. PMID:16971032

353 Occurrence of 3-MCPD and glycidyl esters in edible oils in the United States. MacMahon S, Begley TH, Diachenko GW. Food Addit Contam Part A Chem Anal Control Expo Risk Assess. 2013;30(12):2081-92. PMID:24138540

354 Occurrence of fatty acid esters of 3-MCPD, 2-MCPD and glycidol in infant formula. Wöhrlin F, Fry H, Lahrssen-Wiederholt M, Preiß-Weigert A. Food Addit Contam Part A Chem Anal Control Expo Risk Assess. 2015 Nov;32(11):1810-22. PMID:26179516

355 Fatty acid esters of monochloropropanediol (MCPD) and glycidol in refined edible oils. Craft BD, Chiodini A, Garst J, Granvogl M. Food Addit Contam Part A Chem Anal Control Expo Risk Assess. 2013;30(1):46-51. PMID:23020600

356 Acrylamide exposure and incidence of breast cancer among postmenopausal women in the Danish Diet, Cancer and Health Study. Olesen PT, Olsen A, Frandsen H, Frederiksen K, Overvad K, Tjønneland A. Int J Cancer. 2008 May 1;122(9):2094-100. PMID:18183576

357 Association among acrylamide, blood insulin, and insulin resistance in adults. Lin CY, Lin YC, Kuo HK, Hwang JJ, Lin JL, Chen PC, Lin LY. Diabetes Care. 2009 Dec;32(12):2206-11. PMID:19729525

358 The contribution of DNA single-strand breaks to the formation of chromosome aberrations and SCEs. Speit G, Hochsattel R, Vogel W. Basic Life Sci. 1984;29 Pt A:229-44. PMID:6085260

359 Genotoxicity of acrylamide and glycidamide. Besaratinia A, Pfeifer GP. J Natl Cancer Inst. 2004 Jul 7;96(13):1023-9. PMID:15240786

360 Lung cancer risk in relation to dietary acrylamide intake. Hogervorst JG, Schouten LJ, Konings EJ, Goldbohm RA, van den Brandt PA. J Natl Cancer Inst. 2009 May 6;101(9):651-62. PMID:19401552

361 Acrylamide and glycidamide hemoglobin adduct levels and endometrial cancer risk: A nested case-control study in nonsmoking postmenopausal women from the EPIC cohort. Obón-Santacana M, Freisling H, Peeters PH, et al. Int J Cancer. 2015 Sep 16. PMID:26376083

362 Acrylamide hemoglobin adduct levels and ovarian cancer risk: a nested case-control study. Xie J, Terry KL, Poole EM, Wilson KM, Rosner BA, Willett WC, Vesper HW, Tworoger SS. Cancer Epidemiol Biomarkers Prev. 2013 Apr;22(4):653-60. PMID:23417989

363 The genetic consequences of paternal acrylamide exposure and potential for amelioration. Katen AL, Roman SD. Mutat Res. 2015 Jul;777:91-100. PMID:25989052

364 Effect of cooking method (baking compared with frying) on acrylamide level of potato chips. Palazoğlu TK, Savran D, Gökmen V. J Food Sci. 2010 Jan-Feb;75(1):E25-9. PMID:20492162

365 The effect of domestic preparation of some potato products on acrylamide content. Michalak J, Gujska E, Klepacka J. Plant Foods Hum Nutr. 2011 Nov;66(4):307-12. PMID:2185329

366 Effects of storage temperature on the contents of sugars and free amino acids in tubers from different potato cultivars and acrylamide in chips. Matsuura-Endo C, Ohara-Takada A, Chuda Y, et al. Biosci Biotechnol Biochem. 2006 May;70(5):1173-80. PMID:16717419

367 Change in content of sugars and free amino acids in potato tubers under short-term storage at low temperature and the effect on acrylamide level after frying. Ohara-Takada A, Matsuura-Endo C, Chuda Y, et al. Biosci Biotechnol Biochem. 2005 Jul;69(7):1232-8. PMID:16041124

368 Acrylamide reduction in processed foods. Hanley AB, Offen C, Clarke M, Ing B, Roberts M, Burch R. Adv Exp Med Biol. 2005;561:387-92. PMID:16438313

369 Effective ways of decreasing acrylamide content in potato crisps during processing. Kita A, Bråthen E, Knutsen SH, Wicklund T. J Agric Food Chem. 2004 Nov 17;52(23):7011-6. PMID:15537311

370 Non-enzymatic browning and estimated acrylamide in roots, tubers and plantain products. Quason ET, Ayerson GS. Food Chen. Volume 105, Issue 4, 2007, Pages 1525–1529

371 Processing treatments for mitigating acrylamide formation in sweetpotato French fries. Truong VD, Pascua YT, Reynolds R, Thompson RL, Palazoğlu TK, Mogol BA, Gökmen V. J Agric Food Chem. 2014 Jan 8;62(1):310-6. PMID:24328312

372 Comparison of volatile aldehydes present in the cooking fumes of extra virgin olive, olive, and canola oils. Fullana A, Carbonell-Barrachina AA, Sidhu S. J Agric Food Chem. 2004 Aug 11;52(16):5207-14. PMID:15291498

373 Effect of carcinogenic acrolein on DNA repair and mutagenic susceptibility. Wang HT, Hu Y, Tong D, Huang J, Gu L, Wu XR, Chung FL, Li GM, Tang MS. J Biol Chem. 2012 Apr 6;287(15):12379-86. PMID:22275365

374 Acrolein cytotoxicity in hepatocytes involves endoplasmic reticulum stress, mitochondrial dysfunction and oxidative stress. Mohammad MK, Avila D, Zhang J, Barve S, Arteel G, McClain C, Joshi-Barve S. Toxicol Appl Pharmacol. 2012 Nov 15;265(1):73-82. PMID:23026831

375 Molecular mechanisms of acrolein toxicity: relevance to human disease. Moghe A, Ghare S, Lamoreau B, Mohammad M, Barve S, McClain C, Joshi-Barve S. Toxicol Sci. 2015 Feb;143(2):242-55. PMID:25628402

376 Biogenic amine formation in turkey meat under modified atmosphere packaging with extended shelf life: Index of freshness. Fraqueza MJ, Alfaia CM, Barreto AS. Poult Sci. 2012 Jun;91(6):1465-72. PMID:22582308

377 Effect of dietary meat and fish on endogenous nitrosation, inflammation and genotoxicity of faecal water. Joosen AM, Lecommandeur E, Kuhnle GG, Aspinall SM, Kap L, Rodwell SA. Mutagenesis. 2010 May;25(3):243-7. PMID:20106932

378 Heme-induced biomarkers associated with red meat promotion of colon cancer are not modulated by the intake of nitrite. Chenni FZ, Taché S, Naud N, Guéraud F, Hobbs DA, Kunhle GG, Pierre FH, Corpet DE. Nutr Cancer. 2013;65(2):227-33. PMID:23441609

379 A central role for heme iron in colon carcinogenesis associated with red meat intake. Bastide NM, Chenni F, Audebert M, et al. Cancer Res. 2015 Mar 1;75(5):870-9. PMID:25592152

380 Iron overload syndrome in the black rhinoceros (Diceros bicornis): microscopical lesions and comparison with other rhinoceros species. Olias P, Mundhenk L, Bothe M, Ochs A, Gruber AD, Klopfleisch R. J Comp Pathol. 2012 Nov;147(4):542-9. PMID:22935088

381 The risk of new-onset cancer associated with HFE C282Y and H63D mutations: evidence from 87,028 participants. Lv YF, Chang X, Hua RX, Yan GN, Meng G, Liao XY, Zhang X, Guo QN. J Cell Mol Med. 2016 Feb 19. PMID:26893171

382 Meta-Analysis of the Association between H63D and C282Y Polymorphisms in HFE and Cancer Risk. Zhang M, Xiong H, Fang L, Lu W, Wu X, Wang YQ, Cai ZM, Wu S. Asian Pac J Cancer Prev. 2015;16(11):4633-9. PMID:26107216

383 Hepatocellular carcinoma: epidemiology and risk factors. Kew MC. J Hepatocell Carcinoma. 2014 Aug 13;1:115-25. PMID:27508181

384 Mycotoxins in botanicals and dried fruits: a review. Trucksess MW, Scott PM. Food Addit Contam Part A Chem Anal Control Expo Risk Assess. 2008 Feb;25(2):181-92. PMID:18286408

385 Guidance for Industry: Action Levels for Poisonous or Deleterious Substances in Human Food and Animal Feed. August 2000.

386 Aflatoxin and PAH exposure biomarkers in a U.S. population with a high incidence of hepatocellular carcinoma. Johnson NM, Qian G, Xu L, et al. Sci Total Environ. 2010 Nov 1;408(23):6027-31. PMID:20870273

387 Costs and efficacy of public health interventions to reduce aflatoxin-induced human disease. Khlangwiset P, Wu F. Food Addit Contam Part A Chem Anal Control Expo Risk Assess. 2010 Jul;27(7):998-1014. PMID:20419532

388 Mycotoxins and human disease: a largely ignored global health issue. Wild CP, Gong YY. Carcinogenesis. 2010 Jan;31(1):71-82. PMID:19875698

389 Fortified by Global Warming, Deadly Fungus Poisons Corn Crops, Causes Cancer. Mollie Bloudoff-Indelicato Scientific American Jan. 15, 2013

390 Aflatoxin genotoxicity is associated with a defective DNA damage response bypassing p53 activation. Gursoy-Yuzugullu O, Yuzugullu H, Yilmaz M, Ozturk M. Liver Int. 2011 Apr;31(4):561-71. PMID:21382167

391 A follow-up study of urinary markers of aflatoxin exposure and liver cancer risk in Shanghai, People's Republic of China. Qian GS, Ross RK, Yu MC, Yuan JM, Gao YT, Henderson BE, Wogan GN, Groopman JD. Cancer Epidemiol Biomarkers Prev. 1994 Jan-Feb;3(1):3-10. PMID:8118382

392 Hepatitis B, aflatoxin B(1), and p53 codon 249 mutation in hepatocellular carcinomas from Guangxi, People's Republic of China, and a meta-analysis of existing studies. Stern MC, Umbach DM, Yu MC, et al. Cancer Epidemiol Biomarkers Prev. 2001 Jun;10(6):617-25. PMID:11401911

393 p53 mutations, chronic hepatitis B virus infection, and aflatoxin exposure in hepatocellular carcinoma in Taiwan. Lunn RM, Zhang YJ, Wang LY, et al. Cancer Res. 1997 Aug 15;57(16):3471-7. PMID:9270015

394 http://globocan.iarc.fr/Pages/fact_sheets_cancer.aspx Accessed Oct. 2015

395 Population attributable risk of aflatoxin-related liver cancer: systematic review and meta-analysis. Liu Y, Chang CC, Marsh GM, Wu F. Eur J Cancer. 2012 Sep;48(14):2125-36. PMID:22405700

396 Hepatic aflatoxin B1-DNA adducts and TP53 mutations in patients with hepatocellular carcinoma despite low exposure to aflatoxin B1 in southern Japan. Shirabe K, Toshima T, Taketomi A, et al. Liver Int. 2011 Oct;31(9):1366-72. PMID:21745313

397 Does aflatoxin B1 play a role in the etiology of hepatocellular carcinoma in the United States? Hoque A, Patt YZ, Yoffe B, Groopman JD, Greenblatt MS, Zhang YJ, Santella RM. Nutr Cancer. 1999;35(1):27-33. PMID:10624703

398 Photo by S.K. Mohan, Bugwood.org

399 Mycotoxins. Bennett JW, Klich M. Clin Microbiol Rev. 2003 Jul;16(3):497-516. PMID:12857779

400 Modulation of aflatoxin biomarkers in human blood and urine by green tea polyphenols intervention. Tang L, Tang M, Xu L, Luo H, Huang T, Yu J, Zhang L, Gao W, Cox SB, Wang JS. Carcinogenesis. 2008 Feb;29(2):411-7. PMID:18192689

401 Inhibitory effect(s) of polymeric black tea polyphenols on the formation of B(a)P-derived DNA adducts in mouse skin. Krishnan R, Maru GB. J Environ Pathol Toxicol Oncol. 2005;24(2):79-90. PMID:15831081

402 Modulation of aflatoxin toxicity and biomarkers by lycopene in F344 rats. Tang L, Guan H, Ding X, Wang JS. Toxicol Appl Pharmacol. 2007 Feb 15;219(1):10-7. PMID:17229449

403 Antimutagenic effects of lycopene and tomato purée. Polívková Z, Šmerák P, Demová H, Houška M. J Med Food. 2010 Dec;13(6):1443-50. PMID:20874227

404 Dietary carotenoids inhibit aflatoxin B1-induced liver preneoplastic foci and DNA damage in the rat: role of the modulation of aflatoxin B1 metabolism. Gradelet S, Le Bon AM, Bergès R, Suschetet M, Astorg P. Carcinogenesis. 1998 Mar;19(3):403-11. PMID:9525273

405 Natural chlorophyll inhibits aflatoxin B1-induced multi-organ carcinogenesis in the rat. Simonich MT, Egner PA, Roebuck BD, et al. Carcinogenesis. 2007 Jun;28(6):1294-302. PMID:17290047

406 Recent developments in mushrooms as anti-cancer therapeutics: a review. Patel S, Goyal A. 3 Biotech. 2012 Mar;2(1):1-15. PMID:22582152

407 Positive associations between ionizing radiation and lymphoma mortality among men. Richardson DB, Sugiyama H, Wing S, et al. Am J Epidemiol. 2009 Apr 15;169(8):969-76. PMID:19270049

[408] Solid cancer incidence in atomic bomb survivors exposed in utero or as young children. Preston DL, Cullings H, Suyama A, Funamoto S, Nishi N, Soda M, Mabuchi K, Kodama K, Kasagi F, Shore RE. J Natl Cancer Inst. 2008 Mar 19;100(6):428-36. PMID:18334707

[409] Reanalysis of cancer mortality in Japanese A-bomb survivors exposed to low doses of radiation: bootstrap and simulation methods. Dropkin G. Environ Health. 2009 Dec 9;8:56. PMID:20003238

[410] Low dose radiation and cancer in A-bomb survivors: latency and non-linear dose-response in the 1950-90 mortality cohort. Dropkin G. Environ Health. 2007 Jan 18;6:1. PMID:17233918

[411] Long-term radiation-related health effects in a unique human population: lessons learned from the atomic bomb survivors of Hiroshima and Nagasaki. Douple EB, Mabuchi K, Cullings HM, Preston DL, Kodama K, Shimizu Y, Fujiwara S, Shore RE. Disaster Med Public Health Prep. 2011 Mar;5 Suppl 1:S122-33. PMID:21402804

[412] Hepatocellular carcinoma among atomic bomb survivors: significant interaction of radiation with hepatitis C virus infections. Sharp GB, Mizuno T, Cologne JB, Fukuhara T, Fujiwara S, Tokuoka S, Mabuchi K. Int J Cancer. 2003 Feb 10;103(4):531-7. PMID:12478671

[413] Second malignancies in breast cancer patients following radiotherapy: a study in Florence, Italy. Zhang W, Becciolini A, Biggeri A, Pacini P, Muirhead CR. Breast Cancer Res. 2011 Apr 4;13(2):R38. PMID:21463502

[414] Proportion of second cancers attributable to radiotherapy treatment in adults: a cohort study in the US SEER cancer registries. Berrington de Gonzalez A, Curtis RE, Kry SF, Gilbert E, Lamart S, Berg CD, Stovall M, Ron E. Lancet Oncol. 2011 Apr;12(4):353-60. PMID:21454129

[415] Second cancers among 40,576 testicular cancer patients: focus on long-term survivors. Travis LB, Fosså SD, Schonfeld SJ, et al. J Natl Cancer Inst. 2005 Sep 21;97(18):1354-65. PMID:16174857

[416] Medical radiation exposure and breast cancer risk: findings from the Breast Cancer Family Registry. John EM, Phipps AI, Knight JA, Milne RL, Dite GS, Hopper JL, Andrulis IL, Southey M, Giles GG, West DW, Whittemore AS. Int J Cancer. 2007 Jul 15;121(2):386-94. PMID:17372900

[417] Exposure to diagnostic radiation and risk of breast cancer among carriers of BRCA1/2 mutations: retrospective cohort study (GENE-RAD-RISK). Pijpe A, Andrieu N, Easton DF, et al. BMJ. 2012 Sep 6;345:e5660. PMID:22956590

[418] Vitamin E and the Risk of Prostate Cancer: Updated Results of The Selenium and Vitamin E Cancer Prevention Trial (SELECT). Klein EA, Thompson IM, Tangen CM, et al. JAMA. Author manuscript; available in PMC 2014 September 19. PMC4169010

[419] Antioxidant supplements for prevention of mortality in healthy participants and patients with various diseases. Bjelakovic G, Nikolova D, Gluud LL, Simonetti RG, Gluud C. Cochrane Database Syst Rev. 2008 Apr 16;(2):CD007176. PMID:18425980

[420] Unleashing the untold and misunderstood observations on vitamin E. Gee PT. Genes Nutr. 2011 Feb;6(1):5-16. PMID:21437026

[421] Folic acid and risk of prostate cancer: results from a randomized clinical trial. Figueiredo JC, Grau MV, Haile RW, et al. J Natl Cancer Inst. 2009 Mar 18;101(6):432-5. PMID:19276452

[422] Dietary supplements and mortality in older women: the Iowa Women's Health Study. Mursu J, Robien K, Harnack LJ, Park K, Jacobs DR Jr. Arch Intern Med. 2011 Oct 10;171(18):1625-33. PMID:21987192

[423] Dietary regulation of Keap1/Nrf2/ARE pathway: focus on plant-derived compounds and trace minerals. Stefanson AL, Bakovic M. Nutrients. 2014 Sep 19;6(9):3777-801. PMID:25244368

[424] Fundamental flaws of hormesis for public health decisions. Thayer KA, Melnick R, Burns K, Davis D, Huff J. Environ Health Perspect. 2005 Oct;113(10):1271-6. PMID:16203233

[425] Antioxidant responses and cellular adjustments to oxidative stress. Espinosa-Diez C, Miguel V, Mennerich D, et al. Redox Biol. 2015 Dec;6:183-97. PMID:26233704

[426] Arsenic-mediated activation of the Nrf2-Keap1 antioxidant pathway. Lau A, Whitman SA, Jaramillo MC, Zhang DD. J Biochem Mol Toxicol. 2013 Feb;27(2):99-105. PMID:23188707

[427] Reactive oxygen species, redox signaling and neuroinflammation in Alzheimer's disease: the NF-κB connection. Kaur U, Banerjee P, Bir A, Sinha M, Biswas A, Chakrabarti S. Curr Top Med Chem. 2015;15(5):446-57. PMID:25620241

[428] Antiproliferative effects of celecoxib in Hep-2 cells through telomerase inhibition and induction of apoptosis. Zhao YQ, Feng HW, Jia T, et al. Asian Pac J Cancer Prev. 2014;15(12):4919-23. PMID:24998564

[429] COX-2-independent effects of celecoxib sensitize lymphoma B cells to TRAIL-mediated apoptosis. Gallouet AS, Travert M, Bresson-Bepoldin L, et al T.Clin Cancer Res. 2014 May 15;20(10):2663-73. PMID:24637636

[430] Antiproliferative effects of celecoxib in Hep-2 cells through telomerase inhibition and induction of apoptosis. Zhao YQ, Feng HW, Jia T, et al. Asian Pac J Cancer Prev. 2014;15(12):4919-23. PMID:24998564

[431] Melatonin signaling and cell protection function. Luchetti F, Canonico B, Betti M, et al. FASEB J. 2010 Oct;24(10):3603-24. PMID:20534884

[432] Sulforaphane induces antioxidative and antiproliferative responses by generating reactive oxygen species in human bronchial epithelial BEAS-2B cells. Lee YJ, Lee SH. J Korean Med Sci. 2011 Nov;26(11):1474-82. PMID: 22065904

[433] Sulforaphane induces autophagy through ERK activation in neuronal cells. Jo C, Kim S, Cho SJ, Choi KJ, Yun SM, Koh YH, Johnson GV, Park SI. FEBS Lett. 2014 Aug 25;588(17):3081-8. PMID: 24952354

[434] The involvement of Nrf2 in the protective effects of diallyl disulfide on carbon tetrachloride-induced hepatic oxidative damage and inflammatory response in rats. Lee IC, Kim SH, Baek HS, et al. Food Chem Toxicol. 2014 Jan;63:174-85. PMID:24246655

[435] Coffee modulates transcription factor Nrf2 and highly increases the activity of antioxidant enzymes in rats. Vicente SJ, Ishimoto EY, Torres EA. J Agric Food Chem. 2014 Jan 8;62(1):116-22. PMID:24328189

[436] Increase of the activity of phase II antioxidant enzymes in rats after a single dose of coffee. Vicente SJ, Ishimoto EY, Cruz RJ, Pereira CD, Torres EA. J Agric Food Chem. 2011 Oct 26;59(20):10887-92. PMID:21942680

[437] Degree of roasting is the main determinant of the effects of coffee on NF-kappaB and EpRE. Paur I, Balstad TR, Blomhoff R. Free Radic Biol Med. 2010 May 1;48(9):1218-27. PMID:20176103

[438] Consumption of a dark roast coffee decreases the level of spontaneous DNA strand breaks: a randomized controlled trial. Bakuradze T, Lang R, Hofmann T, Eisenbrand G, Schipp D, Galan J, Richling E. Eur J Nutr. 2015 Feb;54(1):149-56. PMID:24740588

[439] Dark roast coffee is more effective than light roast coffee in reducing body weight, and in restoring red blood cell vitamin E and glutathione concentrations in healthy volunteers. Kotyczka C, Boettler U, Lang R, Stiebitz H, Bytof G, Lantz I, Hofmann T, Marko D, Somoza V. Mol Nutr Food Res. 2011 Oct;55(10):1582-6. PMID:21809439

[440] A dark brown roast coffee blend is less effective at stimulating gastric acid secretion in healthy volunteers compared to a medium roast market blend. Rubach M, Lang R, Bytof G, Stiebitz H, Lantz I, Hofmann T, Somoza V. Mol Nutr Food Res. 2014 Jun;58(6):1370-3. PMID:24510512

[441] Potential antioxidant response to coffee - A matter of genotype? Hassmann U, Haupt LM, Smith RA, Winkler S, Bytof G, Lantz I, Griffiths LR, Marko D. Meta Gene. 2014 Aug 7;2:525-39. PMID:25606436

[442] Influence of feeding malt, bread crust, and a pronylated protein on the activity of chemopreventive enzymes and antioxidative defense parameters in vivo. Somoza V, Wenzel E,

Lindenmeier M, Grothe D, Erbersdobler HF, Hofmann T. J Agric Food Chem. 2005 Oct 19;53(21):8176-82. PMID:16218661

443 Inhibitory effect of bread crust antioxidant pronyl-lysine on two different categories of colonic premalignant lesions induced by 1,2-dimethylhydrazine. Panneerselvam J, Aranganathan S, Nalini N. Eur J Cancer Prev. 2009 Aug;18(4):291-302. PMID:19417676

444 Blackberry extract attenuates oxidative stress through up-regulation of Nrf2-dependent antioxidant enzymes in carbon tetrachloride-treated rats. Cho BO, Ryu HW, et al. J Agric Food Chem. 2011 Nov 9;59(21):11442-8. PMID:21888405

445 Oleuropein and oleacein may restore biological functions of endothelial progenitor cells impaired by angiotensin II via activation of Nrf2/heme oxygenase-1 pathway. Parzonko A, Czerwińska ME, Kiss AK, et al. Phytomedicine. 2013 Sep 15;20(12):1088-94. PMID:23809250

446 http://phenol-explorer.eu/contents/food/749 vs. http://phenol-explorer.eu/contents/food/822

447 The involvement of Nrf2 in the protective effects of diallyl disulfide on carbon tetrachloride-induced hepatic oxidative damage and inflammatory response in rats. Lee IC, Kim SH, Baek HS, et al. Food Chem Toxicol. 2014 Jan;63:174-85PMID:24246655

448 Anthocyanins from purple sweet potato attenuate dimethylnitrosamine-induced liver injury in rats by inducing Nrf2-mediated antioxidant enzymes and reducing COX-2 and iNOS expression. Hwang YP, Choi JH, et al. Food Chem Toxicol. 2011 Jan;49(1):93-9. PMID:20934476

449 Black currant anthocyanins abrogate oxidative stress through Nrf2- mediated antioxidant mechanisms in a rat model of hepatocellular carcinoma. Thoppil RJ, Bhatia D, Barnes KF, et al. Curr Cancer Drug Targets. 2012 Nov 1;12(9):1244-57. PMID:22873220

450 Berry anthocyanins suppress the expression and secretion of proinflammatory mediators in macrophages by inhibiting nuclear translocation of NF-κB independent of Nrf2-mediated mechanism. Lee SG, Kim B, Yang Y, et al. J Nutr Biochem. 2014 Apr;25(4):404-11. PMID:24565673

451 Protective effects of ursolic acid in an experimental model of liver fibrosis through Nrf2/ARE pathway. Ma JQ, Ding J, Zhang L, Liu CM. Clin Res Hepatol Gastroenterol. 2015 Apr;39(2):188-97. PMID:25459994

452 Naringenin attenuates CCl4 -induced hepatic inflammation by the activation of an Nrf2-mediated pathway in rats. Esmaeili MA, Alilou M.Clin Exp Pharmacol Physiol. 2014 Jun;41(6):416-22. PMID:24684352

453 BRCA1 interacts with Nrf2 to regulate antioxidant signaling and cell survival. Gorrini C, Baniasadi PS, Harris IS, et al. J Exp Med. 2013 Jul 29;210(8):1529-44. 23857982

454 Bioactive food components prevent carcinogenic stress via Nrf2 activation in BRCA1 deficient breast epithelial cells. Kang HJ, Hong YB, Kim HJ, Wang A, Bae I. Toxicol Lett. 2012 Mar 7;209(2):154-60. PMID:22192953

455 Indole-3-carbinol as a chemoprotective agent in breast and prostate cancer. Bradlow HL. In Vivo. 2008 Jul-Aug;22(4):441-5. PMID:18712169

456 Molecular targets and anticancer potential of indole-3-carbinol and its derivatives. Aggarwal BB, Ichikawa H. Cell Cycle. 2005 Sep;4(9):1201-15. PMID:16082211

457 Indole-3-carbinol suppresses NF-kappaB and IkappaBalpha kinase activation, causing inhibition of expression of NF-kappaB-regulated antiapoptotic and metastatic gene products and enhancement of apoptosis in myeloid and leukemia cells. Takada Y, Andreeff M, Aggarwal BB. Blood. 2005 Jul 15;106(2):641-9. PMID:15811958

458 Plant-derived 3,3'-Diindolylmethane is a strong androgen antagonist in human prostate cancer cells. Le HT, Schaldach CM, Firestone GL, Bjeldanes LF. J Biol Chem. 2003 Jun 6;278(23):21136-45. PMID:12665522

459 CXCR4 is a novel target of cancer chemopreventative isothiocyanates in prostate cancer cells. Sakao K, Vyas AR, Chinni SR, Amjad AI, Parikh R, Singh SV. Cancer Prev Res (Phila). 2015 May;8(5):365-74. PMID:25712054

460 D,L-sulforaphane-induced apoptosis in human breast cancer cells is regulated by the adapter protein p66Shc. Sakao K, Singh SV. J Cell Biochem. 2012 Feb;113(2):599-610. PMID:21956685

461 Sulforaphane inhibits mitochondrial permeability transition and oxidative stress.. Greco T, Shafer J, Fiskum G. Free Radic Biol Med. 2011 Sep 21. PMID:21986339

462 Comparison of the protective effects of steamed and cooked broccolis on ischaemia-reperfusion-induced cardiac injury. Mukherjee S, Lekli I, Ray D, Gangopadhyay H, Raychaudhuri U, Das DK. Br J Nutr. 2010 Mar;103(6):815-23. PMID:19857366

463 Sulforophane glucosinolate. Monograph. Altern Med Rev. 2010 Dec;15(4):352-60. PMID:2119425

464 Cruciferous vegetable consumption and lung cancer risk: a systematic review. Lam TK, Gallicchio L, Lindsley K, et al. Cancer Epidemiol Biomarkers Prev. 2009 Jan;18(1):184-95. PMID:19124497

465 Cruciferous vegetables and risk of colorectal neoplasms: a systematic review and meta-analysis. Tse G, Eslick GD. Nutr Cancer. 2014;66(1):128-39. PMID:24341734

466 Cruciferous vegetables, the GSTP1 Ile105Val genetic polymorphism, and breast cancer risk. Lee SA, Fowke JH, Lu W, et al. Am J Clin Nutr. 2008 Mar;87(3):753-60. PMID:18326615

467 GST polymorphism and excretion of heterocyclic aromatic amine and isothiocyanate metabolites after Brassica consumption. Steck SE, Hebert JR. Environ Mol Mutagen. 2009 Apr;50(3):238-46. PMID:19197987

468 A diet rich in high-glucoraphanin broccoli interacts with genotype to reduce discordance in plasma metabolite profiles by modulating mitochondrial function. Armah CN, Traka MH, Dainty JR, et al. Am J Clin Nutr. 2013 Sep;98(3):712-22. PMID: 23964055

469 A single mutation in human mitochondrial DNA polymerase Pol gammaA affects both polymerization and proofreading activities of only the holoenzyme. Lee YS, Johnson KA, Molineux IJ, Yin YW. J Biol Chem. 2010 Sep 3;285(36):28105-16. PMID: 20513922

470 Amelioration of Alzheimer's disease by neuroprotective effect of sulforaphane in animal model. Kim HV, Kim HY, Ehrlich HY, Choi SY, Kim DJ, Kim Y. Amyloid. 2013 Mar;20(1):7-12. PMID: 23253046

471 Glutathione Transferase (GST)-Activated Prodrugs. Ruzza P, Calderan A. Pharmaceutics. 2013 Apr 2;5(2):220-31. PMID:24300447

472 Allyl isothiocyanate triggers G2/M phase arrest and apoptosis in human brain malignant glioma GBM 8401 cells through a mitochondria-dependent pathway. Chen NG, Chen KT, Lu CC, Lan YH, Lai CH, Chung YT, Yang JS, Lin YC. Oncol Rep. 2010 Aug;24(2):449-55. PMID:20596632

473 Allyl isothiocyanate, a constituent of cruciferous vegetables, inhibits proliferation of human prostate cancer cells by causing G2/M arrest and inducing apoptosis. Xiao D, Srivastava SK, Lew KL, et al. Carcinogenesis. 2003 May;24(5):891-7. PMID:12771033

474 Sulforaphane suppresses in vitro and in vivo lung tumorigenesis through downregulation of HDAC activity. Jiang LL, Zhou SJ, Zhang XM, Chen HQ, Liu W. Biomed Pharmacother. 2016 Mar;78:74-80. PMID:26898427

475 Sulforaphane-induced apoptosis in human leukemia HL-60 cells through extrinsic and intrinsic signal pathways and altering associated genes expression assayed by cDNA microarray. Shang HS, Shih YL, Lee CH, et al. Environ Toxicol. 2016 Feb 2. PMID:26833863

476 Dietary Sulforaphane in Cancer Chemoprevention: The Role of Epigenetic Regulation and HDAC Inhibition. Tortorella SM, Royce SG, Licciardi PV, Karagiannis TC. Antioxid Redox Signal. 2015 Jun 1;22(16):1382-424. PMID:25364882

477 Phenethyl isothiocyanate sensitizes glioma cells to TRAIL-induced apoptosis. Lee DH, Kim DW, Lee HC, etal. Biochem Biophys Res Commun. 2014 Apr 18;446(4):815-21. PMID:24491546

478 Phenethyl isothiocyanate enhances TRAIL-induced apoptosis in oral cancer cells and xenografts. Yeh CC, Ko HH, Hsieh YP, et al. Clin Oral Investig. 2016 Jan 29. PMID:26822174

479 3,3'-diindolylmethane potentiates tumor necrosis factor-related apoptosis-inducing ligand-induced apoptosis of gastric cancer cells. Ye Y, Miao S, Wang Y, Zhou J, Lu R. Oncol Lett. 2015 May;9(5):2393-2397. PMID:26137077

480 In vitro studies of phenethyl isothiocyanate against the growth of LN229 human glioma cells. Su JC, Lin K, Wang Y, Sui SH, Gao ZY, Wang ZG. Int J Clin Exp Pathol. 2015 Apr 1;8(4):4269-76. PMID:26097624

481 ROS Accumulation by PEITC Selectively Kills Ovarian Cancer Cells via UPR-Mediated Apoptosis. Hong YH, Uddin MH, Jo U, Kim B, Song J, Suh DH, Kim HS, Song YS. Front Oncol. 2015 Jul 28;5:167. PMID:26284193

482 Synergy between sulforaphane and selenium in protection against oxidative damage in colonic CCD841 cells. Wang Y, Dacosta C, Wang W, Zhou Z, Liu M, Bao Y. Nutr Res. 2015 Jul;35(7):610-7. PMID:26094214

483 Sulforaphane prevents doxorubicin-induced oxidative stress and cell death in rat H9c2 cells. Li B, Kim do S, Yadav RK, et al. Int J Mol Med. 2015 Jul;36(1):53-64. PMID:25936432

484 Sulforaphane preconditioning of the Nrf2/HO-1 defense pathway protects the cerebral vasculature against blood-brain barrier disruption and neurological deficits in stroke. Alfieri A, Srivastava S, Siow RC, et al. Free Radic Biol Med. 2013 Dec;65:1012-22. PMID:24017972

485 Curcumin upregulates transcription factor Nrf2, HO-1 expression and protects rat brains against focal ischemia. Yang C, Zhang X, Fan H, Liu Y. Brain Res. 2009 Jul 28;1282:133-41. PMID:19445907

486 Sensitization of estrogen receptor-positive breast cancer cell lines to 4-hydroxytamoxifen by isothiocyanates present in cruciferous plants. Pawlik A, Słomińska-Wojewódzka M, Herman-Antosiewicz A. Eur J Nutr. 2016 Apr;55(3):1165-80. PMID:26014809

487 Phenylethyl isothiocyanate reverses cisplatin resistance in biliary tract cancer cells via glutathionylation-dependent degradation of Mcl-1. Li Q, Zhan M, Chen W, Zhao B, et al. Oncotarget. 2016 Mar 1;7(9):10271-82. PMID:26848531

488 Phenethyl isothiocyanate potentiates anti-tumour effect of doxorubicin through Akt-dependent pathway. Eisa NH, ElSherbiny NM, Shebl AM, Eissa LA, El-Shishtawy MM. Cell Biochem Funct. 2015 Dec;33(8):541-51. PMID:26548747

489 Phenethyl isothiocyanate enhances adriamycin-induced apoptosis in osteosarcoma cells. Fan Q, Zhan X, Xiao Z, Liu C. Mol Med Rep. 2015 Oct;12(4):5945-50. PMID:26252906

490 Frugal chemoprevention: targeting Nrf2 with foods rich in sulforaphane. Yang L, Palliyaguru DL, Kensler TW. Semin Oncol. 2016 Feb;43(1):146-53. PMID:26970133

491 Cruciferous vegetables and colo-rectal cancer. Lynn A, Collins A, Fuller Z, Hillman K, Ratcliffe B. Proc Nutr Soc. 2006 Feb;65(1):135-44. PMID:16441953

492 Cruciferous vegetables intake is associated with lower risk of renal cell carcinoma: evidence from a meta-analysis of observational studies. Zhao J, Zhao L. PLoS One. 2013 Oct 28;8(10):e75732. PMID:24204579

493 The activity of myrosinase from broccoli (Brassica oleracea L. cv. Italica): influence of intrinsic and extrinsic factors. Ludikhuyze L, Rodrigo L, Hendrickx M. J Food Prot. 2000 Mar;63(3):400-3. PMID:10716572

494 Effect of meal composition and cooking duration on the fate of sulforaphane following consumption of broccoli by healthy human subjects. Rungapamestry V, Duncan AJ, Fuller Z, Ratcliffe B. Br J Nutr. 2007 Apr;97(4):644-52. PMID:17349076

495 Changes in glucosinolate concentrations, myrosinase activity, and production of metabolites of glucosinolates in cabbage (Brassica oleracea Var. capitata) cooked for different durations. Rungapamestry V, Duncan AJ, Fuller Z, Ratcliffe B. J Agric Food Chem. 2006 Oct 4;54(20):7628-34. PMID:17002432

496 Kinetics of the stability of broccoli (Brassica oleracea Cv. Italica) myrosinase and isothiocyanates in broccoli juice during pressure/temperature treatments. Van Eylen D, Oey I, Hendrickx M, Van Loey A. J Agric Food Chem. 2007 Mar 21;55(6):2163-70. PMID:17305356

497 Heating decreases epithiospecifier protein activity and increases sulforaphane formation in broccoli. Matusheski NV, Juvik JA, Jeffery EH. Phytochemistry. 2004 May;65(9):1273-81. PMID:15184012

498 Chemoprotective glucosinolates and isothiocyanates of broccoli sprouts: metabolism and excretion in humans. Shapiro TA, Fahey JW, Wade KL, et al. Cancer Epidemiol Biomarkers Prev. 2001 May;10(5):501-8. PMID:11352861

499 [Sulforaphane (1-isothiocyanato-4-(methylsulfinyl)-butane) content in cruciferous vegetables]. Campas-Baypoli ON, Bueno-Solano C, Martínez-Ibarra DM, et al. Arch Latinoam Nutr. 2009 Mar;59(1):95-100. PMID:19480351

500 Bioavailability of Sulforaphane from two broccoli sprout beverages: results of a short-term, cross-over clinical trial in Qidong, China.. Egner PA, Chen JG, Wang JB, Wu Y et al. Cancer Prev Res (Phila). 2011 Mar;4(3):384-95. PMID:21372038

501 Prospective study of fruit and vegetable intake and risk of prostate cancer. Kirsh VA, Peters U, Mayne ST, et al; Prostate, Lung, Colorectal and Ovarian Cancer Screening Trial. J Natl Cancer Inst. 2007 Aug 1;99(15):1200-9. PMID:17652276

502 Vegetable and fruit intake after diagnosis and risk of prostate cancer progression.. Richman EL, Carroll PR, Chan JM. Int J Cancer. 2011 Aug 5. PMID:21823116

503 Safety, tolerance, and metabolism of broccoli sprout glucosinolates and isothiocyanates: a clinical phase I study. Shapiro TA, Fahey JW, Dinkova-Kostova AT, et al. Nutr Cancer. 2006;55(1):53-62. PMID:16965241

504 Garlic in health and disease. Rana SV, Pal R, Vaiphei K, Sharma SK, Ola RP. Nutr Res Rev. 2011 Jun;24(1):60-71. PMID:24725925

505 Comparison of the chemopreventive efficacies of garlic powders with different alliin contents against aflatoxin B1 carcinogenicity in rats. Bergès R, Siess MH, Arnault I, Auger J, Kahane R, Pinnert MF, Vernevaut MF, le Bon AM. Carcinogenesis. 2004 Oct;25(10):1953-9. PMID:15180943

506 Alleviation by garlic of antitumor drug-induced damage to the intestine. Horie T, Awazu S, Itakura Y, Fuwa T. J Nutr. 2001 Mar;131(3s):1071S-4S. PMID:11238819

507 Evidence of a novel docetaxel sensitizer, garlic-derived S-allylmercaptocysteine, as a treatment option for hormone refractory prostate cancer. Howard EW, Lee DT, Chiu YT, Chua CW, Wang X, Wong YC. Int J Cancer. 2008 May 1;122(9):1941-8. PMID:18183597

508 Clarifying the real bioactive constituents of garlic. Amagase H. J Nutr. 2006 Mar;136(3 Suppl):716S-725S. PMID:16484550

509 Garlic Phytocompounds Possess Anticancer Activity by Specifically Targeting Breast Cancer Biomarkers - an in Silico Study. Roy N, Davis S, Narayanankutty A, Nazeem P, Babu T, Abida P, Valsala P, Raghavamenon AC. Asian Pac J Cancer Prev. 2016;17(6):2883-8. PMID:27356707

510 Garlic: a review of potential therapeutic effects. Bayan L, Koulivand PH, Gorji A. Avicenna J Phytomed. 2014 Jan;4(1):1-14. PMID:25050296

511 Raw Garlic Consumption and Lung Cancer in a Chinese Population. Myneni AA, Chang SC, Niu R, Liu L, Swanson MK, Li J, Su J, Giovino GA, Yu S, Zhang ZF, Mu L. Cancer Epidemiol Biomarkers Prev. 2016 Apr;25(4):624-33. PMID:26809277

512 Correlation between antioxidant activity of garlic extracts and WEHI-164 fibrosarcoma tumor growth in BALB/c mice. Shirzad H, Taji F, Rafieian-Kopaei M. J Med Food. 2011 Sep;14(9):969-74. PMID:21812650

513 Steam-cooking rapidly destroys and reverses onion-induced antiplatelet activity. Hansen EA, Folts JD, Goldman IL. Nutr J. 2012 Sep 20;11:76. PMID:22992282

514 Effect of raw versus boiled aqueous extract of garlic and onion on platelet aggregation. Ali M, Bordia T, Mustafa T. Prostaglandins Leukot Essent Fatty Acids. 1999 Jan;60(1):43-7. PMID:10319916

515 Effect of cooking on garlic (Allium sativum L.) antiplatelet activity and thiosulfinates content. Cavagnaro PF, Camargo A, Galmarini CR, Simon PW. J Agric Food Chem. 2007 Feb 21;55(4):1280-8. PMID:17256959

516 Thermostability of allicin determined by chemical and biological assays. Fujisawa H, Suma K, Origuchi K, Seki T, Ariga T. Biosci Biotechnol Biochem. 2008 Nov;72(11):2877-83. PMID:18997429

517 Intake of garlic and its bioactive components. Amagase H, Petesch BL, Matsuura H, Kasuga S, Itakura Y. J Nutr. 2001 Mar;131(3s):955S-62S. PMID:11238796

518 Guidance for Industry Estimating the Maximum Safe Starting Dose in Initial Clinical Trials for Therapeutics in Adult Healthy Volunteers. FDA July 2005

519 USDA Nutrient database: http://www.ars.usda.gov/Services/docs.htm?docid=8964

520 Long-term effect of aspirin on cancer risk in carriers of hereditary colorectal cancer: an analysis from the CAPP2 randomised controlled trial. Burn J, Gerdes AM, Macrae F, et al. Lancet. 2011 Dec 17;378(9809):2081-7. PMID:22036019

521 Celecoxib for the prevention of sporadic colorectal adenomas. Bertagnolli MM, Eagle CJ, Zauber AG, et al; APC Study Investigators. N Engl J Med. 2006 Aug 31;355(9):873-84. PMID:16943400

522 Effects of flavonoids on prostaglandin E2 production and on COX-2 and mPGES-1 expressions in activated macrophages. Hämäläinen M, Nieminen R, Asmawi MZ, Vuorela P, Vapaatalo H, Moilanen E. Planta Med. 2011 Sep;77(13):1504-11. PMID:21341175

523 Vitamin E increases production of vasodilator prostanoids in human aortic endothelial cells through opposing effects on cyclooxygenase-2 and phospholipase A2. Wu D, Liu L, Meydani M, Meydani SN. J Nutr. 2005 Aug;135(8):1847-53. PMID:16046707

524 Cyclooxygenase-2 in tumorigenesis of gastrointestinal cancers: an update on the molecular mechanisms. Wu WK, Sung JJ, Lee CW, Yu J, Cho CH. Cancer Lett. 2010 Sep 1;295(1):7-16. PMID:20381235

525 Primary prevention of colorectal cancer. Chan AT, Giovannucci EL. Gastroenterology. 2010 Jun;138(6):2029-2043.e10. PMID:20420944

526 CTNNB1 catenin (cadherin-associated protein), beta 1, 88kDa [Homo sapiens] Gene ID: 1499, 23-Oct-2011 NCBI http://www.ncbi.nlm.nih.gov

527 Mechanical induction of PGE2 in osteocytes blocks glucocorticoid-induced apoptosis through both the β-catenin and PKA pathways. Kitase Y, Barragan L, Qing H, et al. J Bone Miner Res. 2010 Dec;25(12):2657-68. PMID:20578217

528 PGE2 Stimulates VEGF Production through the EP2 Receptor in Cultured Human Lung Fibroblasts. Nakanishi M, Sato T, Li Y, et al. Am J Respir Cell Mol Biol. 2011 Sep 15 PMID:21921240

529 Aspirin use after diagnosis but not prediagnosis improves established colorectal cancer survival: a meta-analysis. Li P, Wu H, Zhang H, Shi Y, Xu J, Ye Y, Xia D, Yang J, Cai J, Wu Y. Gut. 2015 Sep;64(9):1419-25. PMID:25239119

530 Effect of daily aspirin on risk of cancer metastasis: a study of incident cancers during randomised controlled trials. Rothwell PM, Wilson M, Price JF, Belch JF, Meade TW, Mehta Z. Lancet. 2012 Apr 28;379(9826):1591-601. PMID:22440947

531 Selective inhibition of cyclooxygenase-2 (COX-2) by 1alpha,25-dihydroxy-16-ene-23-yne-vitamin D3, a less calcemic vitamin D analog.Aparna R, Subhashini J, Roy KR, et al. J Cell Biochem. 2008 Aug 1;104(5):1832-42. PMID:18348265

532 Tocotrienols suppress proinflammatory markers and cyclooxygenase-2 expression in RAW264.7 macrophages.. Yam ML, Abdul Hafid SR, Cheng HM, Nesaretnam K. Lipids. 2009 Sep;44(9):787-97. PMID:19655189

533 gamma-tocopherol and its major metabolite, in contrast to alpha-tocopherol, inhibit cyclooxygenase activity in macrophages and epithelial cells. Jiang Q, Elson-Schwab I, Courtemanche C, Ames BN. Proc Natl Acad Sci U S A. 2000 Oct 10;97(21):11494-9. PMID:11005841

534 Tissue-specific, nutritional, and developmental regulation of rat fatty acid elongases. Wang Y, Botolin D, Christian B, et al. J Lipid Res. 2005 Apr;46(4):706-15.. PMID:15654130

535 Omega-3 polyunsaturated fatty acids inhibit hepatocellular carcinoma cell growth through blocking beta-catenin and cyclooxygenase-2. Lim K, Han C, Dai Y, Shen M, Wu T. Mol Cancer Ther. 2009 Nov;8(11):3046-55. PMID:19887546

536 Inhibition of prostaglandin synthesis and actions contributes to the beneficial effects of calcitriol in prostate cancer. Krishnan AV, Srinivas S, Feldman D. Dermatoendocrinol. 2009 Jan;1(1):7-11. PMID:20046582

537 γ-Tocotrienol inhibits cell viability through suppression of β-catenin/Tcf signaling in human colon carcinoma HT-29 cells. Xu W, Du M, Zhao Y, Wang Q, Sun W, Chen B. J Nutr Biochem. 2011 Aug 16. PMID:21852086

538 A paraptosis-like cell death induced by δ-tocotrienol in human colon carcinoma SW620 cells is associated with the suppression of the Wnt signaling pathway. Zhang JS, Li DM, He N, et al. Toxicology. 2011 Jul 11;285(1-2):8-17. PMID:21453743

539 Tocotrienols inhibit AKT and ERK activation and suppress pancreatic cancer cell proliferation by suppressing the ErbB2 pathway. Shin-Kang S, Ramsauer VP, Lightner J, et al. Free Radic Biol Med. 2011 Sep 15;51(6):1164-74.. PMID:21723941

540 d-δ-Tocotrienol-mediated cell cycle arrest and apoptosis in human melanoma cells. Fernandes NV, Guntipalli PK, Mo H. Anticancer Res. 2010 Dec;30(12):4937-44. PMID: 21187473

541 delta-Tocotrienol suppresses VEGF induced angiogenesis whereas alpha-tocopherol does not.. Shibata A, Nakagawa K, Sookwong P, Tsuduki T, Oikawa S, Miyazawa T. J Agric Food Chem. 2009 Sep 23;57(18):8696-704. PMID:19702331

542 alpha-Tocopherol attenuates the cytotoxic effect of delta-tocotrienol in human colorectal adenocarcinoma cells. Shibata A, Nakagawa K, Sookwong P, et al. Biochem Biophys Res Commun. 2010 Jun 25;397(2):214-9. PMID:20493172

543 Arachidonic acid impairs hypothalamic leptin signaling and hepatic energy homeostasis in mice. Cheng L, Yu Y, Zhang Q, Szabo A, Wang H, Huang XF. Mol Cell Endocrinol. 2015 Sep 5;412:12-8. PMID:25986657

544 http://www.kegg.jp/kegg-bin/show_pathway?k004923+K04265

545 An Increase in the Omega-6/Omega-3 Fatty Acid Ratio Increases the Risk for Obesity. Simopoulos AP. Nutrients. 2016 Mar 2;8(3). pii: E128. PMID:26950145

546 A high ratio of dietary n-3/n-6 polyunsaturated fatty acids improves obesity-linked inflammation and insulin resistance through suppressing activation of TLR4 in SD rats. Liu HQ, Qiu Y, Mu Y,et al. Nutr Res. 2013 Oct;33(10):849-58. PMID:24074743

547 n-6:n-3 PUFA ratio is involved in regulating lipid metabolism and inflammation in pigs. Duan Y, Li F, Li L, Fan J, Sun X, Yin Y. Br J Nutr. 2014 Feb;111(3):445-51. PMID:23947577

548 Conjugated Linoleic Acid and Postmenopausal Women's Health. Kim JH, Kim YJ, Park Y. J Food Sci. 2015 Jun;80(6):R1137-43. PMID:25962640

549 The influence of linoleic and linolenic acid on the activity and intracellular localisation of phospholipase D in COS-1 cells. Gemeinhardt A, Alfalah M, Gück T, Naim HY, Fuhrmann H. Biol Chem. 2009 Mar;390(3):253-8. PMID:19090716

550 Fruits, vegetables, and bladder cancer risk: a systematic review and meta-analysis. Vieira AR, Vingeliene S, Chan DS, et al. Cancer Med. 2015 Jan;4(1):136-46. PMID:25461441

551 Impact of folic acid fortification of flour on neural tube defects: a systematic review. Castillo-Lancellotti C, Tur JA, Uauy R. Public Health Nutr. 2013 May;16(5):901-11. PMID:22850218

552 Effect of Folic Acid Food Fortification in Canada on Congenital Heart Disease Subtypes. Liu S, Joseph KS, Luo W, León JA, Lisonkova S, Van den Hof M, Evans J, Lim K, Little J, Sauve R, Kramer MS; Canadian Perinatal Surveillance System (Public Health Agency of Canada). Circulation. 2016 Aug 30;134(9):647-55 PMID:27572879

553 Will mandatory folic acid fortification prevent or promote cancer? Kim YI. Am J Clin Nutr. 2004 Nov;80(5):1123-8. PMID:15531657

554 Naturally occurring folates in selected traditionally prepared foods in Southern India. Vishnumohan S, Pickford R, Arcot J. J Food Sci Technol. 2017 Dec;54(13):4173-4180. PMID:29184222

555 Influence of high-pressure processing on the profile of polyglutamyl 5-methyltetrahydrofolate in selected vegetables. Wang C, Riedl KM, Somerville J, Balasubramaniam VM, Schwartz SJ. J Agric Food Chem. 2011 Aug 24;59(16):8709-17. doi: 10.1021/jf201120n. Epub 2011 Aug 2. PMID:21770413

556 Folate content and retention in commonly consumed vegetables in the South Pacific. Maharaj PP, Prasad S, Devi R, Gopalan R. Food Chem. 2015 Sep 1;182:327-32. PMID:25842344

557 Folate content and retention in selected raw and processed foods. Bassett MN, Sammán NC. Arch Latinoam Nutr. 2010 Sep;60(3):298-305. PMID:21612148

558 Capillary electrophoresis and high-performance liquid chromatography determination of polyglutamyl 5-methyltetrahydrofolate forms in citrus products. Matella NJ, Braddock RJ, Gregory JF 3rd, Goodrich RM. J Agric Food Chem. 2005 Mar 23;53(6):2268-74. PMID:15769167

559 Nutrients, foods, and colorectal cancer prevention. Song M, Garrett WS, Chan AT. Gastroenterology. 2015 May;148(6):1244-60.e16. PMID:25575572

560 Folic acid handling by the human gut: implications for food fortification and supplementation. Patanwala I, King MJ, Barrett DA, et al. Am J Clin Nutr. 2014 Aug;100(2):593-9. PMID:24944062

561 High concentrations of folate and unmetabolized folic acid in a cohort of pregnant Canadian women and umbilical cord blood. Plumptre L, Masih SP, Ly A, Aufreiter S, Sohn KJ, Croxford R, Lausman AY, Berger H, O'Connor DL, Kim YI. Am J Clin Nutr. 2015 Oct;102(4):848-57. PMID:26269367

562 Total folate and unmetabolized folic acid in the breast milk of a cross-section of Canadian women. Page R, Robichaud A, Arbuckle TE, Fraser WD, MacFarlane AJ. Am J Clin Nutr. 2017 May;105(5):1101-1109. PMID:28298392

563 A Daily Dose of 5 mg Folic Acid for 90 Days Is Associated with Increased Serum Unmetabolized Folic Acid and Reduced Natural Killer Cell Cytotoxicity in Healthy Brazilian Adults. Paniz C, Bertinato JF, Lucena MR et al. J Nutr. 2017 Sep;147(9):1677-1685. PMID:28724658

564 Heterogenous Distribution of MTHFR Gene Variants among Mestizos and Diverse Amerindian Groups from Mexico. Contreras-Cubas C, Sánchez-Hernández BE, et al. PLoS One. 2016 Sep 20;11(9):e0163248. PMID:27649570

565 One-carbon metabolism-related gene polymorphisms and risk of breast cancer. Suzuki T, Matsuo K, Hirose K, et al. Carcinogenesis. 2008 Feb;29(2):356-62. PMID:18174236

566 Gene polymorphisms involved in folate and methionine metabolism and increased risk of sporadic colorectal adenocarcinoma. Guimarães JL, Ayrizono Mde L, Coy CS, Lima CS. Tumour Biol. 2011 Oct;32(5):853-61. PMID:21603981

567 Meta-analyses of the methylenetetrahydrofolate reductase C677T and A1298C polymorphisms and risk of head and neck and lung cancer. Boccia S, Boffetta P, Brennan P, et al. Cancer Lett. 2009 Jan 8;273(1):55-61. PMID:18789576

568 Alcohol drinking and one-carbon metabolism-related gene polymorphisms on pancreatic cancer risk. Suzuki T, Matsuo K, Sawaki A, et al. Cancer Epidemiol Biomarkers Prev. 2008 Oct;17(10):2742-7. PMID:18843018

569 Meta- and pooled analyses of the methylenetetrahydrofolate reductase C677T and A1298C polymorphisms and gastric cancer risk: a huge-GSEC review. Boccia S, Hung R, Ricciardi G et al. Am J Epidemiol. 2008 Mar 1;167(5):505-16. PMID:18162478

570 Association between serum folate level and cervical cancer: a meta-analysis. Zhou X, Meng Y. Arch Gynecol Obstet. 2016 Apr;293(4):871-7. PMID:26319154

571 Gene-gene interactions in the folate metabolic pathway influence the risk for acute lymphoblastic leukemia in children. Petra BG, Janez J, Vita D. Leuk Lymphoma. 2007 Apr;48(4):786-92. PMID:17454638

572 Polymorphisms in genes involved in folate metabolism as maternal risk factors for Down syndrome. Hobbs CA, Sherman SL, Yi P, et al. Am J Hum Genet. 2000 Sep;67(3):623-30. PMID:10930360

573 Prenatal vitamins, one-carbon metabolism gene variants, and risk for autism. Schmidt RJ, Hansen RL, Hartiala J, Allayee H, Schmidt LC, Tancredi DJ, Tassone F, Hertz-Picciotto I. Epidemiology. 2011 Jul;22(4):476-85. PMID:21610500

574 The MTHFR C677T polymorphism contributes to increased risk of Alzheimer's disease: evidence based on 40 case-control studies. Peng Q, Lao X, Huang X, Qin X, Li S, Zeng Z. Neurosci Lett. 2015 Jan 23;586:36-42. PMID:25486592

575 Meta-analysis of MTHFR gene variants in schizophrenia, bipolar disorder and unipolar depressive disorder: evidence for a common genetic vulnerability? Peerbooms OL, van Os J, Drukker M, et al. Brain Behav Immun. 2011 Nov;25(8):1530-43. PMID:21185933

576 Homocysteine and depression in later life. Almeida OP, McCaul K, Hankey GJ, Norman P, Jamrozik K, Flicker L. Arch Gen Psychiatry. 2008 Nov;65(11):1286-94. PMID:18981340

577 Relationship of homocysteine levels with lumbar spine and femur neck BMD in postmenopausal women. Bahtiri E, Islami H, Rexhepi S, Qorraj-Bytyqi H, Thaçi K, Thaçi S, Karakulak C, Hoxha R. Acta Reumatol Port. 2015 Oct-Dec;40(4):355-362. PMID:26922199

578 Genetic polymorphism of MTHFR C677T and premature coronary artery disease susceptibility: A meta-analysis. Hou X, Chen X, Shi J. Gene. 2015 Jul 1;565(1):39-44. PMID:25839940

579 Genotypes of the MTHFR C677T and MTRR A66G genes act independently to reduce migraine disability in response to vitamin supplementation. Menon S, Lea RA, Roy B, et al. Pharmacogenet Genomics. 2012 Oct;22(10):741-9. PMID:22926161

580 MTHFR 677T is a strong determinant of the degree of hearing loss among Polish males with postlingual sensorineural hearing impairment. Pollak A, Mueller-Malesinska M, Lechowicz U, et al. DNA Cell Biol. 2012 Jul;31(7):1267-73. PMID:22424391

581 Effect of Folic Acid, Betaine, Vitamin B6, and Vitamin B12 on Homocysteine and Dimethylglycine Levels in Middle-Aged Men Drinking White Wine. Rajdl D, Racek J, Trefil L, Stehlik P, Dobra J, Babuska V. Nutrients. 2016 Jan 12;8(1). pii: E34. PMID:26771632

582 Folate and vitamin B6 intake and risk of colon cancer in relation to p53 expression. Schernhammer ES, Ogino S, Fuchs CS. Gastroenterology. 2008 Sep;135(3):770-80. PMID:18619459

583 Dietary intake of B vitamins and methionine and colorectal cancer risk. Bassett JK, Severi G, Hodge AM, et al. Nutr Cancer. 2013;65(5):659-67. PMID:23859033

584 Biochemical indicators of B vitamin status in the US population after folic acid fortification: results from the National Health and Nutrition Examination Survey 1999-2000. Pfeiffer CM,

Caudill SP, Gunter EW, Osterloh J, Sampson EJ. Am J Clin Nutr. 2005 Aug;82(2):442-50. PMID:16087991

585 Determinants of plasma methylmalonic acid in a large population: implications for assessment of vitamin B12 status. Vogiatzoglou A, Oulhaj A, Smith AD, et al. Clin Chem. 2009 Dec;55(12):2198-206. PMID:19833840

586 Pre-diagnostic high-sensitive C-reactive protein and breast cancer risk, recurrence, and survival. Frydenberg H, Thune I, Lofterød T, et al. Breast Cancer Res Treat. 2016 Jan;155(2):345-54. PMID:26740213

587 A quantitative assessment of plasma homocysteine as a risk factor for vascular disease. Probable benefits of increasing folic acid intakes. Boushey CJ, Beresford SA, Omenn GS, Motulsky AG. JAMA. 1995 Oct 4;274(13):1049-57. PMID:7563456

588 Homocysteine, B-vitamins and CVD. McNulty H, Pentieva K, Hoey L, Ward M. Proc Nutr Soc. 2008 May;67(2):232-7. PMID:18412997

589 5-methyltetrahydrofolate. Monograph. Altern Med Rev. 2006 Dec;11(4):330-7. PMID:17176169

590 Association of vitamin B6, vitamin B12 and methionine with risk of breast cancer: a dose-response meta-analysis. Wu W, Kang S, Zhang D. Br J Cancer. 2013 Oct 1;109(7):1926-44. PMID:23907430

591 Phosphatidylethanolamine N-methyltransferase (PEMT) gene expression is induced by estrogen in human and mouse primary hepatocytes. Resseguie M, Song J, Niculescu MD, da Costa KA, Randall TA, Zeisel SH. FASEB J. 2007 Aug;21(10):2622-32. PMID:17456783

592 Dietary choline requirements of women: effects of estrogen and genetic variation. Fischer LM, da Costa KA, Kwock L, Galanko J, Zeisel SH. Am J Clin Nutr. 2010 Nov;92(5):1113-9. PMID:20861172

593 Choline and hepatocarcinogenesis in the rat. Zeisel SH, da Costa KA, Albright CD, Shin OH. Adv Exp Med Biol. 1995;375:65-74. PMID:7645429

594 Choline deficiency increases lymphocyte apoptosis and DNA damage in humans. da Costa KA, Niculescu MD, Craciunescu CN, Fischer LM, Zeisel SH. Am J Clin Nutr. 2006 Jul;84(1):88-94. PMID:16825685

595 Choline and/or folic acid deficiency is associated with genomic damage and cell death in human lymphocytes in vitro. Lu L, Ni J, Zhou T, Xu W, Fenech M, Wang X. Nutr Cancer. 2012 Apr;64(3):481-7. PMID:22439759

596 Choline deficiency selects for resistance to p53-independent apoptosis and causes tumorigenic transformation of rat hepatocytes. Zeisel SH, Albright CD, Shin OH, Mar MH, Salganik RI, da Costa KA. Carcinogenesis. 1997 Apr;18(4):731-8. PMID:9111207

597 Nothing Boring About Boron. Pizzorno L. Integr Med (Encinitas). 2015 Aug;14(4):35-48. PMID:26770156

598 Sugar-borate esters--potential chemical agents in prostate cancer chemoprevention. Scorei RI, Popa R. Anticancer Agents Med Chem. 2013 Jul 1;13(6):901-9. PMID:23293883

599 Comparative effects of boric acid and calcium fructoborate on breast cancer cells. Scorei R, Ciubar R, Ciofrangeanu CM, et al. Biol Trace Elem Res. 2008 Jun;122(3):197-205. PMID:18176783

600 Boric acid as a protector against paclitaxel genotoxicity. Turkez H, Tatar A, Hacimuftuoglu A, Ozdemir E. Acta Biochim Pol. 2010;57(1):95-7. PMID:20300661

601 Effect of flavonoids in the prevention of lung cancer: systematic review. García-Tirado J, Rieger-Reyes C, Saz-Peiró P. Med Clin (Barc). 2012 Oct 6;139(8):358-63. PMID:22459574

602 Fruits and vegetables consumption and the risk of histological subtypes of lung cancer in the European Prospective Investigation into Cancer and Nutrition (EPIC). Büchner FL, Bueno-de-Mesquita HB, Linseisen J, et al. Cancer Causes Control. 2010 Mar;21(3):357-71. PMID:19924549

603 Fruits, vegetables and lung cancer risk: a systematic review and meta-analysis. Vieira AR, Abar L, Vingeliene S, et al. Ann Oncol. 2016 Jan;27(1):81-96. PMID:26371287

604 Fructose content in popular beverages made with and without high-fructose corn syrup. Walker RW, Dumke KA, Goran MI. Nutrition. 2014 Jul-Aug;30(7-8):928-35. PMID:24985013

605 Time course of recovery of cytochrome p450 3A function after single doses of grapefruit juice. Greenblatt DJ, von Moltke LL, Harmatz JS, et al. Clin Pharmacol Ther. 2003 Aug;74(2):121-9. PMID:12891222

606 Association between CYP2D6 polymorphisms and outcomes among women with early stage breast cancer treated with tamoxifen. Schroth W, Goetz MP, Hamann U, et al. JAMA. 2009 Oct 7;302(13):1429-36. PMID:19809024

607 The effect of grapefruit intake on endogenous serum estrogen levels in postmenopausal women. Monroe KR, Stanczyk FZ, Besinque KH, Pike MC. Nutr Cancer. 2013;65(5):644-52. PMID:23859031

608 Prospective study of grapefruit intake and risk of breast cancer in postmenopausal women: the Multiethnic Cohort Study. Monroe KR, Murphy SP, Kolonel LN, Pike MC. Br J Cancer. 2007 Aug 6;97(3):440-5. PMID:17622247

609 A prospective study of grapefruit and grapefruit juice intake and breast cancer risk. Kim EH, Hankinson SE, Eliassen AH, Willett WC. Br J Cancer. 2008 Jan 15;98(1):240-1. PMID:18026192

610 Prospective study of the association between grapefruit intake and risk of breast cancer in the European Prospective Investigation into Cancer and Nutrition (EPIC). Spencer EA, Key TJ, Appleby PN, et al. Cancer Causes Control. 2009 Aug;20(6):803-9. PMID:19224379

611 Estrone sulfate (E1S), a prognosis marker for tumor aggressiveness in prostate cancer (PCa). Giton F, de la Taille A, Allory Y, et al. J Steroid Biochem Mol Biol. 2008 Mar;109(1-2):158-67. PMID:18337090

612 Lycopene and lutein inhibit proliferation in rat prostate carcinoma cells. Gunasekera RS, Sewgobind K, Desai S, et al. Nutr Cancer. 2007;58(2):171-7. PMID:17640163

613 Inhibition of mammary cancer by citrus flavonoids. Guthrie N, Carroll KK. Adv Exp Med Biol. 1998;439:227-36. PMID:9781306

614 Lycopene and Risk of Prostate Cancer: A Systematic Review and Meta-Analysis. Chen P, Zhang W, Wang X, et al. Medicine (Baltimore). 2015 PMID:26287411

615 Tomato phytochemicals and prostate cancer risk. Campbell JK, Canene-Adams K, Lindshield BL, et al. J Nutr. 2004 Dec;134(12 Suppl):3486S-3492S. PMID:15570058

616 Immunosuppressive CD71+ erythroid cells compromise neonatal host defence against infection. Elahi S, Ertelt JM, Kinder JM, et al. Nature. 2013 Dec 5;504(7478):158-62. PMID:24196717

617 A human gut microbial gene catalogue established by metagenomic sequencing. Qin J, Li R, Raes J, et al. Nature. 2010 Mar 4;464(7285):59-65. PMID:20203603

618 Diet drives convergence in gut microbiome functions across mammalian phylogeny and within humans. Muegge BD, Kuczynski J, Knights D, et al. Science. 2011 May 20;332(6032):970-4. PMID:21596990

619 Dominant and diet-responsive groups of bacteria within the human colonic microbiota. Walker AW, Ince J, Duncan SH, et al. ISME J. 2011 Feb;5(2):220-30. PMID: 20686513

620 Intake of dietary fiber, especially from cereal foods, is associated with lower incidence of colon cancer in the HELGA cohort. Hansen L, Skeie G, Landberg R, et al. Int J Cancer. 2011 Aug 22. PMID:21866547

621 Dietary fiber and whole-grain consumption in relation to colorectal cancer in the NIH-AARP Diet and Health Study. Schatzkin A, Mouw T, Park Y, et al. Am J Clin Nutr. 2007 May;85(5):1353-60. PMID:17490973

622 Randomized, double-blinded, placebo-controlled study of effect of wheat bran fiber and calcium on fecal bile acids in patients with resected adenomatous colon polyps. Alberts DS, Ritenbaugh C, Story JA, et al. J Natl Cancer Inst. 1996 Jan 17;88(2):81-92. PMID:8537982

623 Dietary factors and the risks of oesophageal adenocarcinoma and Barrett's oesophagus. Kubo A, Corley DA, Jensen CD, Kaur R. Nutr Res Rev. 2010 Dec;23(2):230-46. PMID:20624335

624 Ileal recovery of starch from whole diets containing resistant starch measured in vitro and fermentation of ileal effluent. Silvester KR, Englyst HN, Cummings JH. Am J Clin Nutr. 1995 Aug;62(2):403-11. PMID: 7625349

625 A human gut microbial gene catalogue established by metagenomic sequencing. Qin J, Li R, Raes J, Arumugam M, et al. Nature. 2010 Mar 4;464(7285):59-65. PMID: 20203603

626 Dominant and diet-responsive groups of bacteria within the human colonic microbiota. Walker AW, Ince J, Duncan SH, et al. ISME J. 2011 Feb;5(2):220-30. PMID:20686513

627 Resistant starches types 2 and 4 have differential effects on the composition of the fecal microbiota in human subjects. Martínez I, Kim J, Duffy PR, Schlegel VL, Walter J. PLoS One. 2010 Nov 29;5(11):e15046. PMID:21151493

628 Effects of partial replacement of dietary starch from barley or corn with lactose on ruminal function, short-chain fatty acid absorption, nitrogen utilization, and production performance of dairy cows. Chibisa GE, Gorka P, Penner GB, Berthiaume R, Mutsvangwa T. J Dairy Sci. 2015 Apr;98(4):2627-40. PMID:25704977

629 Colonic health: fermentation and short chain fatty acids. Wong JM, de Souza R, Kendall CW, Emam A, Jenkins DJ. J Clin Gastroenterol. 2006 Mar;40(3):235-43. PMID: 16633129

630 http://www.guidetopharmacology.org/GRAC/LigandDisplayForward?tab=biology&ligandId=1059 (Accessed Oct. 2016)

631 https://www.ncbi.nlm.nih.gov/gene?Db=gene&Cmd=ShowDetailView&TermToSearch=55869 (Accessed Oct. 2016)

632 A review of the potential mechanisms for the lowering of colorectal oncogenesis by butyrate. Fung KY, Cosgrove L, Lockett T, et al. Br J Nutr. 2012 Sep;108(5):820-31. PMID:22676885

633 Study of human microecology by mass spectrometry of microbial markers. Osipov GA, Verkhovtseva NV. Benef Microbes. 2011 Mar;2(1):63-78. PMID:21831791

634 Bacterial metabolic 'toxins': a new mechanism for lactose and food intolerance, and irritable bowel syndrome. Campbell AK, Matthews SB, Vassel N, et al. Toxicology. 2010 Dec 30;278(3):268-76. PMID: 20851732

635 Glycation of LDL by methylglyoxal increases arterial atherogenicity: a possible contributor to increased risk of cardiovascular disease in diabetes. Rabbani N, Godfrey L, Xue M, et al. Diabetes. 2011 Jul;60(7):1973-80. PMID:21617182

636 Baseline microbiota activity and initial bifidobacteria counts influence responses to prebiotic dosing in healthy subjects. de Preter V, Vanhoutte T, Huys G, Swings J, Rutgeerts P, Verbeke K. Aliment Pharmacol Ther. 2008 Mar 15;27(6):504-13. PMID:18081736

637 Effects of lactulose on nitrogen metabolism. Weber FL Jr. Scand J Gastroenterol Suppl. 1997;222:83-7. PMID:9145455

638 Gut-brain axis: how the microbiome influences anxiety and depression. Foster JA, McVey Neufeld KA. Trends Neurosci. 2013 May;36(5):305-12. PMID:23384445

639 Effect of lactulose and Saccharomyces boulardii administration on the colonic urea-nitrogen metabolism and the bifidobacteria concentration in healthy human subjects. De Preter V, Vanhoutte T, Huys G, Swings J, Rutgeerts P, Verbeke K. Aliment Pharmacol Ther. 2006 Apr 1;23(7):963-74. PMID: 16573799

640 Ileal recovery of starch from whole diets containing resistant starch measured in vitro and fermentation of ileal effluent. Silvester KR, Englyst HN, Cummings JH. Am J Clin Nutr. 1995 Aug;62(2):403-11. Erratum in: Am J Clin Nutr 1996 Mar;63(3):407. PMID: 7625349

641 Linkage of gut microbiome with cognition in hepatic encephalopathy. Bajaj JS, Ridlon JM, Hylemon PB, et al. Am J Physiol Gastrointest Liver Physiol. 2011 Sep 22. PMID:21940902

642 Metabolism of estrogens in the gastrointestinal tract of swine. III. Estradiol-17 beta-D-glucuronide instilled into sections of intestine. Pohland RC, Coppoc GL, Bottoms GD, Moore AB. J Anim Sci. 1982 Jul;55(1):145-52. PMID:7118739

643 Fat/fiber intakes and sex hormones in healthy premenopausal women in USA. Aubertin-Leheudre M, Gorbach S, Woods M, et al. J Steroid Biochem Mol Biol. 2008 Nov;112(1-3):32-9. PMID:18761407

644 Metabolism of phytoestrogen conjugates. D'Alessandro TL, Boersma-Maland BJ, et al. Methods Enzymol. 2005;400:316-42. PMID:16399358

645 Effects of soy phytoestrogens genistein and daidzein on breast cancer growth. de Lemos ML. Ann Pharmacother. 2001 Sep;35(9):1118-21. PMID:11573864

646 Phytoestrogens and breast cancer: a complex story. Helferich WG, Andrade JE, Hoagland MS. Inflammopharmacology. 2008 Oct;16(5):219-26. PMID:18815740

647 Dietary fiber intake and endogenous serum hormone levels in naturally postmenopausal Mexican American women: the Multiethnic Cohort Study. Monroe KR, Murphy SP, Henderson BE, et al. Nutr Cancer. 2007;58(2):127-35. PMID:17640158

648 Effect of daily fiber intake on reproductive function: the BioCycle Study. Gaskins AJ, Mumford SL, Zhang et al. Am J Clin Nutr. 2009 Oct;90(4):1061-9. PMID:19692496

649 Lower serum oestrogen concentrations associated with faster intestinal transit. Lewis SJ, Heaton KW, Oakey RE, McGarrigle HH. Br J Cancer. 1997;76(3):395-400. PMID:9252210

650 Diet and the excretion and enterohepatic cycling of estrogens. Gorbach SL, Goldin BR. Prev Med. 1987 Jul;16(4):525-31. PMID:3628202

651 Dietary fiber intake and risk of breast cancer in postmenopausal women: the National Institutes of Health-AARP Diet and Health Study. Park Y, Brinton LA, Subar AF, Hollenbeck A, Schatzkin A. Am J Clin Nutr. 2009 Sep;90(3):664-71. PMID:19625685

652 Estimated enterolignans, lignan-rich foods, and fibre in relation to survival after postmenopausal breast cancer. Buck K, Zaineddin AK, Vrieling A, et al. Br J Cancer. 2011 Oct 11;105(8):1151-7. PMID:21915130

653 Estrogen excretion patterns and plasma levels in vegetarian and omnivorous women. Goldin BR, Adlercreutz H, Gorbach SL, Warram JH, Dwyer JT, Swenson L, Woods MN. N Engl J Med. 1982 Dec 16;307(25):1542-7. PMID:7144835

654 Dietary fibre consumption and insulin resistance - the role of body fat and physical activity. Breneman CB, Tucker L. Br J Nutr. 2013 Jul 28;110(2):375-83. PMID:23218116

655 Effects of a low-fat, high-fiber diet and exercise program on breast cancer risk factors in vivo and tumor cell growth and apoptosis in vitro. Barnard RJ, Gonzalez JH, Liva ME, Ngo TH. Nutr Cancer. 2006;55(1):28-34. PMID:16965238

656 Dietary fiber intake and risk of breast cancer in postmenopausal women: the National Institutes of Health-AARP Diet and Health Study. Park Y, Brinton LA, Subar AF, Hollenbeck A, Schatzkin A. Am J Clin Nutr. 2009 Sep;90(3):664-71. PMID:19625685

657 Dietary Fiber Intake in Young Adults and Breast Cancer Risk. Farvid MS, Eliassine AH, Cho E. Lio X, Chen WY, Willett WC. Pediatrics 137,3, Mar. 2016

658 Commensal Bifidobacterium promotes antitumor immunity and facilitates anti-PD-L1 efficacy. Sivan A, Corrales L, Hubert N, et al. Science. 2015 Nov 27;350(6264):1084-9. PMID:26541606

659 Anticancer immunotherapy by CTLA-4 blockade relies on the gut microbiota. Vétizou M, Pitt JM, Daillère R, et al. Science. 2015 Nov 27;350(6264):1079-84. PMID:26541610

660 Intake of dietary fiber, especially from cereal foods, is associated with lower incidence of colon cancer in the HELGA cohort. Hansen L, Skeie G, Landberg R, et al. Int J Cancer. 2011 Aug 22. PMID:21866547

[661] Dietary fiber and whole-grain consumption in relation to colorectal cancer in the NIH-AARP Diet and Health Study. Schatzkin A, Mouw T, Park Y, et al. Am J Clin Nutr. 2007 May;85(5):1353-60. PMID:17490973

[662] An apple a day may hold colorectal cancer at bay: recent evidence from a case-control study. Jedrychowski W, Maugeri U. Rev Environ Health. 2009 Jan-Mar;24(1):59-74. PMID:19476292

[663] Secondary bile acids: an underrecognized cause of colon cancer. Ajouz H, Mukherji D, Shamseddine A. World J Surg Oncol. 2014 May 24;12:164. PMID: 24884764

[664] The secondary bile acid, deoxycholate accelerates intestinal adenoma-adenocarcinoma sequence in Apc (min/+) mice through enhancing Wnt signaling. Cao H, Luo S, Xu M, Zhang Y, et al. Fam Cancer. 2014 Dec;13(4):563-71. PMID:25106466

[665] Fermentation of vegetable fiber in the intestinal tract of rats and effects on fecal bulking and bile acid excretion. Nyman M, Schweizer TF, Tyrén S, Reimann S, Asp NG. J Nutr. 1990 May;120(5):459-66. PMID:2160526

[666] Effect of the combinations between pea proteins and soluble fibres on cholesterolaemia and cholesterol metabolism in rats. Parolini C, Manzini S, Busnelli M, et al. Br J Nutr. 2013 Oct;110(8):1394-401. PMID:23458494

[667] Effect of fibre on bile acid metabolism by human faecal bacteria in batch and continuous culture. Fadden K, Hill MJ, Owen RW. Eur J Cancer Prev. 1997 Apr;6(2):175-94. PMID:9237069

[668] Cholesterol 7 alpha-hydroxylase activity is increased by dietary modification with psyllium hydrocolloid, pectin, cholesterol and cholestyramine in rats. Matheson HB, Colón IS, Story JA. J Nutr. 1995 Mar;125(3):454-8. PMID:7876920

[669] Short-chain fatty acids and human colonic function: roles of resistant starch and nonstarch polysaccharides. Topping DL, Clifton PM. Physiol Rev. 2001 Jul;81(3):1031-64. PMID: 11427691

[670] Dietary pea protein stimulates bile acid excretion and lowers hepatic cholesterol concentration in rats. Spielmann J, Stangl GI, Eder K. J Anim Physiol Anim Nutr (Berl). 2008 Dec;92(6):683-93. PMID:19012614

[671] Effect of pigeon pea (Cajanus cajan L.) on high-fat diet-induced hypercholesterolemia in hamsters. Dai FJ, Hsu WH, Huang JJ, Wu SC. Food Chem Toxicol. 2013 Mar;53:384-91. PMID:23287313

[672] Randomized, double-blinded, placebo-controlled study of effect of wheat bran fiber and calcium on fecal bile acids in patients with resected adenomatous colon polyps. Alberts DS, Ritenbaugh C, Story JA, Aickin et al. J Natl Cancer Inst. 1996 Jan 17;88(2):81-92. PMID:8537982

[673] Fecal bile acid concentrations in a subpopulation of the wheat bran fiber colon polyp trial. Alberts DS, Einspahr JG, Earnest DL, et al. Cancer Epidemiol Biomarkers Prev. 2003 Mar;12(3):197-200. PMID:12646507

[674] The adsorption of heterocyclic aromatic amines by model dietary fibres with contrasting compositions. Harris PJ, Triggs CM, Roberton AM, Watson ME, Ferguson LR. Chem Biol Interact. 1996 Mar 8;100(1):13-25. PMID:8599852

[675] Physicochemical characterisation of dietary fibre components and their ability to bind some process-induced mutagenic heterocyclic amines, Trp-P-1, Trp-P-2, AαC and MeAαC. Raman M, Nilsson U, Skog K, Lawther M, Nair B, Nyman M. Food Chem. 2013 Jun 15;138(4):2219-24. PMID:23497879

[676] The effects of soluble-fiber polysaccharides on the adsorption of a hydrophobic carcinogen to an insoluble dietary fiber. Harris PJ, Roberton AM, Watson ME, et al. Nutr Cancer. 1993;19(1):43-54. PMID:8446514

[677] Model studies of lignified fiber fermentation by human fecal microbiota and its impact on heterocyclic aromatic amine adsorption. Funk C, Braune A, Grabber JH, Steinhart H, Bunzel M. Mutat Res. 2007 Nov 1;624(1-2):41-8. PMID:17475287

678 Binding effect of polychlorinated compounds and environmental carcinogens on rice bran fiber. Sera N, Morita K, Nagasoe M, Tokieda H, Kitaura T, Tokiwa H. J Nutr Biochem. 2005 Jan;16(1):50-8. PMID:15629241

679 Effect of green vegetable on digestive tract absorption of polychlorinated dibenzo-p-dioxins and polychlorinated dibenzofurans in rats. Morita K, Matsueda T, Iida T. et al. 1999 May;90(5):171-83. PMID:10396873

680 Promotive excretion of causative agents of Yusho by fermented brown rice with Aspergillus oryze in Yusho patients. Nagayama J, Todaka T, Hirakawa H, et al. Fukuoka Igaku Zasshi. 2011 Apr;102(4):123-9. PMID:21706891

681 Dietary lignan intake and postmenopausal breast cancer risk by estrogen and progesterone receptor status. Touillaud MS, Thiébaut AC, Fournier A, et al. J Natl Cancer Inst. 2007 Mar 21;99(6):475-86. PMID: 17374837

682 Dietary lariciresinol attenuates mammary tumor growth and reduces blood vessel density in human MCF-7 breast cancer xenografts and carcinogen-induced mammary tumors in rats. Saarinen NM, Wärri A, Dings RP, Airio M, Smeds AI, Mäkelä S. Int J Cancer. 2008 Sep 1;123(5):1196-204. PMID:18528864

683 Flaxseed and its lignans inhibit estradiol-induced growth, angiogenesis, and secretion of vascular endothelial growth factor in human breast cancer xenografts in vivo. Bergman Jungeström M, Thompson LU, Dabrosin C. Clin Cancer Res. 2007 Feb 1;13(3):1061-7. PMID:17289903

684 Phytoestrogen consumption and endometrial cancer risk: a population-based case-control study in New Jersey. Bandera EV, Williams MG, Sima C, et al. Cancer Causes Control. 2009 Sep;20(7):1117-27. PMID:9353280

685 Phytoestrogen intake and endometrial cancer risk. Horn-Ross PL, John EM, Canchola AJ, Stewart SL, Lee MM. J Natl Cancer Inst. 2003 Aug 6;95(15):1158-64. PMID:12902445

686 Intake of dietary fiber, especially from cereal foods, is associated with lower incidence of colon cancer in the HELGA cohort. Hansen L, Skeie G, Landberg R, et al. Int J Cancer. 2012 Jul 15;131(2):469-78. PMID:21866547

687 Fruit and vegetable consumption and risk of distal gastric cancer in the Shanghai Women's and Men's Health studies. Epplein M, Shu XO, Xiang YB, et al Am J Epidemiol. 2010 Aug 15;172(4):397-406. PMID:20647333

688 Vegetables and fruits consumption and risk of esophageal and gastric cancer subtypes in the Netherlands Cohort Study. Steevens J, Schouten LJ, Goldbohm RA, van den Brandt PA. Int J Cancer. 2011 Dec 1;129(11):2681-93 PMID:21960262

689 Fermentation of vegetable fiber in the intestinal tract of rats and effects on fecal bulking and bile acid excretion. Nyman M, Schweizer TF, Tyrén S, Reimann S, Asp NG. J Nutr. 1990 May;120(5):459-66. PMID:2160526

690 Dietary patterns and risk of oesophageal cancers: a population-based case-control study. Ibiebele TI, Hughes MC, Whiteman DC, Webb PM. Br J Nutr. 2011 Sep 7:1-10. PMID:21899799

691 Nonlinear reduction in risk for colorectal cancer by fruit and vegetable intake based on meta-analysis of prospective studies. Aune D, Lau R, Chan DS, Vieira R, Greenwood DC, Kampman E, Norat T. Gastroenterology. 2011 Jul;141(1):106-18. PMID:21600207

692 The Global Nonalcoholic Fatty Liver Disease Epidemic: What a Radiologist Needs to Know. Pereira K, Salsamendi J, Casillas J. J Clin Imaging Sci. 2015 May 29;5:32. PMID:26167390

693 Prevalence of obesity in the United States, 2009-2010.. Ogden CL, Carroll MD. NCHS Data Brief No. 82 January 2012

694 Fructose as a key player in the development of fatty liver disease. Basaranoglu M, Basaranoglu G, Sabuncu T, Sentürk H. World J Gastroenterol. 2013 Feb 28;19(8):1166-72. PMID:23482247

695 Development of hepatocellular carcinoma in a murine model of nonalcoholic steatohepatitis induced by use of a high-fat/fructose diet and sedentary lifestyle. Dowman JK, Hopkins LJ, Reynolds et al. Am J Pathol. 2014 May;184(5):1550-61. PMID:24650559

696 *Enteroimmunology*. Chapter 9. Charles Lewis. Psy Press, Carrabelle, FL, 2015.

697 Obesity and hepatocellular carcinoma: targeting obesity-related inflammation for chemoprevention of liver carcinogenesis. Shimizu M, Tanaka T, Moriwaki H. Semin Immunopathol. 2013 Mar;35(2):191-202. PMID:22945457

698 Betaine prevented fructose-induced NAFLD by regulating LXRα/PPARα pathway and alleviating ER stress in rats. Ge CX, Yu R, Xu MX, Li PQ, Fan CY, Li JM, Kong LD. Eur J Pharmacol. 2016 Jan 5;770:154-64. PMID:26593707

699 Betaine treatment attenuates chronic ethanol-induced hepatic steatosis and alterations to the mitochondrial respiratory chain proteome. Kharbanda KK, Todero SL, King AL, et al. Int J Hepatol. 2012;2012:962183. PMID:22187660

700 Dietary reference intakes for folate, thiamin, riboflavin, niacin, vitamin B12, pantothenic acid, biotin, and choline. Vol. 1. Institute of Medicine and National Academy of Sciences. Washington D.C.: National Academy Press; 1998. pp. 390–422.

701 Dietary choline and betaine intakes in relation to concentrations of inflammatory markers in healthy adults: the ATTICA study. Detopoulou P, Panagiotakos DB, Antonopoulou S, Pitsavos C, Stefanadis C. Am J Clin Nutr. 2008 Feb;87(2):424-30. PMID:18258634

702 Estimation of usual intake and food sources of choline and betaine in New Zealand reproductive age women. Mygind VL, Evans SE, Peddie MC, Miller JC, Houghton LA. Asia Pac J Clin Nutr. 2013;22(2):319-24. PMID:23635379

703 The association between betaine and choline intakes and the plasma concentrations of homocysteine in women. Chiuve SE, Giovannucci EL, Hankinson SE, Zeisel SH, Dougherty LW, Willett WC, Rimm EB. Am J Clin Nutr. 2007 Oct;86(4):1073-81. PMID:17921386

704 Concentrations of choline-containing compounds and betaine in common foods. Zeisel SH, Mar MH, Howe JC, Holden JM. J Nutr. 2003 May;133(5):1302-7. Erratum in: J Nutr. 2003 Sep;133(9):2918. PMID:12730414

705 Citrulline and Nonessential Amino Acids Prevent Fructose-Induced Nonalcoholic Fatty Liver Disease in Rats. Jegatheesan P, Beutheu S, Ventura G, Nubret E, Sarfati G, Bergheim I, De Bandt JP. J Nutr. 2015 Oct;145(10):2273-9. PMID:26246323

706 Effects of oral branched-chain amino acids on hepatic encephalopathy and outcome in patients with liver cirrhosis. Kawaguchi T, Taniguchi E, Sata M. Nutr Clin Pract. 2013 Oct;28(5):580-8. PMID:23945292

707 Plasma citrulline level as a biomarker for cancer therapy-induced small bowel mucosal damage. Barzał JA, Szczylik C, Rzepecki P, Jaworska M, Anuszewska E. Acta Biochim Pol. 2014;61(4):615-31. PMID:25473654

708 Review article: hepatitis C virus-associated steatosis--pathogenic mechanisms and clinical implications. Adinolfi LE, Durante-Mangoni E, Zampino R, Ruggiero G. Aliment Pharmacol Ther. 2005 Nov;22 Suppl 2:52-5. PMID: 16225474

709 Study of the effect of antiviral therapy on homocysteinemia in hepatitis C virus- infected patients. Mustafa M, Hussain S, Qureshi S, Malik SA, Kazmi AR, Naeem M. BMC Gastroenterol. 2012 Aug 28;12:117. PMID: 22925702

710 Impact of coffee on liver diseases: a systematic review. Saab S, Mallam D, Cox GA 2nd, Tong MJ. Liver Int. 2014 Apr;34(4):495-504. PMID:24102757

711 Coffee consumption and risk of liver cancer: a meta-analysis. Larsson SC, Wolk A. Gastroenterology. 2007 May;132(5):1740-5. PMID:17484871

712 Trans fatty acids and cardiovascular disease. Mozaffarian D, Katan MB, Ascherio A, Stampfer MJ, Willett WC. N Engl J Med. 2006 Apr 13;354(15):1601-13. PMID:16611951

713 Trans fatty acids and coronary heart disease. Zaloga GP, Harvey KA, Stillwell W, Siddiqui R. Nutr Clin Pract. 2006 Oct;21(5):505-12. PMID:16998148

714 Consumption of trans-fatty acid and its association with colorectal adenomas. Vinikoor LC, Schroeder JC, Millikan RC, et al. Am J Epidemiol. 2008 Aug 1;168(3):289-97. PMID:1858713

715 Dietary fatty acid intakes and the risk of ovulatory infertility. Chavarro JE, Rich-Edwards JW, Rosner BA, Willett WC. Am J Clin Nutr. 2007 Jan;85(1):231-7. PMID:17209201

716 Severe NAFLD with hepatic necroinflammatory changes in mice fed trans fats and a high-fructose corn syrup equivalent. Tetri LH, Basaranoglu M, Brunt EM, et al. Am J Physiol Gastrointest Liver Physiol. 2008 Nov;295(5):G987-95. PMID:18772365

717 Dietary trans-fatty acid induced NASH is normalized following loss of trans-fatty acids from hepatic lipid pools. Neuschwander-Tetri BA, Ford DA, Acharya S, Gilkey G, Basaranoglu M, Tetri LH, Brunt EM. Lipids. 2012 Oct;47(10):941-50. PMID:22923371

718 trans Fatty acids in milk produced by women in the United States. Mosley EE, Wright AL, McGuire MK, McGuire MA. Am J Clin Nutr. 2005 Dec;82(6):1292-7. PMID:16332663

719 Trans Fat Now Listed With Saturated Fat and Cholesterol FDA Newsletter

720 n-3 fatty acid dietary recommendations and food sources to achieve essentiality and cardiovascular benefits. Gebauer SK, Psota TL, Harris WS, Kris-Etherton PM. Am J Clin Nutr. 2006 Jun;83(6 Suppl):1526S-1535S. PMID: 16841863

721 http://www.fda.gov/NewsEvents/Newsroom/PressAnnouncements/ucm451237.htm FDA website accessed Jan. 2016

722 Household air pollution and lung cancer in China: a review of studies in Xuanwei. Seow WJ, Hu W, Vermeulen R, et al. Chin J Cancer. 2014 Oct;33(10):471-5. PMID:25223911

723 In-home coal and wood use and lung cancer risk: a pooled analysis of the International Lung Cancer Consortium. Hosgood HD, Boffetta P, Greenland S, et al. Environ Health Perspect. 2010 Dec;118(12):1743-7. PMID:20846923

724 An evidence-based assessment for the association between long-term exposure to outdoor air pollution and the risk of lung cancer. Yang WS, Zhao H, Wang X, Deng Q, Fan WY, Wang L. Eur J Cancer Prev. 2015 Mar 9. PMID:25757194

725 Traffic-related air pollution and lung cancer: A meta-analysis. Chen G, Wan X, Yang G, Zou X. Thorac Cancer. 2015 May;6(3):307-18. PMID:26273377

726 Cancers of the lung, head and neck on the rise: perspectives on the genotoxicity of air pollution. Wong IC, Ng YK, Lui VW. Chin J Cancer. 2014 Oct;33(10):476-80. PMID:25011457

727 Residential traffic exposure and childhood leukemia: a systematic review and meta-analysis. Boothe VL, Boehmer TK, Wendel AM, Yip FY. Am J Prev Med. 2014 Apr;46(4):413-22. PMID:24650845

728 A review and meta-analysis of outdoor air pollution and risk of childhood leukemia. Filippini T, Heck JE, Malagoli C, Del Giovane C, Vinceti M. J Environ Sci Health C Environ Carcinog Ecotoxicol Rev. 2015;33(1):36-66. PMID:25803195

729 Air pollution in relation to U.S. cancer mortality rates: an ecological study; likely role of carbonaceous aerosols and polycyclic aromatic hydrocarbons. Grant WB. Anticancer Res. 2009 Sep;29(9):3537-45. PMID:19667146

730 Breast cancer risk in relation to occupations with exposure to carcinogens and endocrine disruptors: a Canadian case-control study. Brophy JT, Keith MM, Watterson A, et al. Environ Health. 2012 Nov 19;11:87. PMID:23164221

731 Updated epidemiology of workers exposed to metalworking fluids provides sufficient evidence for carcinogenicity. Mirer F. Appl Occup Environ Hyg. 2003 Nov;18(11):902-12. PMID:14555443

732 Risk of female breast cancer and serum concentrations of organochlorine pesticides and polychlorinated biphenyls: a case-control study in Tunisia. Arrebola JP, Belhassen H, Artacho-Cordón F, et al. Sci Total Environ. 2015 Jul 1;520:106-13. PMID:25804877

733 Exposure to polychlorinated biphenyls and hexachlorobenzene, semen quality and testicular cancer risk. Paoli D, Giannandrea F, Gallo M, Turci R, Cattaruzza MS, Lombardo F, Lenzi A, Gandini L. J Endocrinol Invest. 2015 Jul;38(7):745-52. PMID:25770454

734 Concentrations of organohalogen compounds and titres of antibodies to Epstein-Barr virus antigens and the risk for non-Hodgkin lymphoma. Hardell K, Carlberg M, Hardell L, et al. Oncol Rep. 2009 Jun;21(6):1567-76. PMID:19424638

735 Dietary exposure to polychlorinated biphenyls and risk of myocardial infarction - a population-based prospective cohort study. Bergkvist C, Berglund M, Glynn A, Wolk A, Åkesson A. Int J Cardiol. 2015 Mar 15;183:242-8. PMID:25679993

736 Dietary exposure to polychlorinated biphenyls is associated with increased risk of stroke in women. Bergkvist C, Kippler M, Larsson SC, Berglund M, Glynn A, Wolk A, Åkesson A. J Intern Med. 2014 Sep;276(3):248-59. PMID:24428778

737 A new chapter in the bisphenol A story: bisphenol S and bisphenol F are not safe alternatives to this compound. Eladak S, Grisin T, Moison D, et al. Fertil Steril. 2015 Jan;103(1):11-21. PMID:25475787

738 Are structural analogues to bisphenol a safe alternatives? Rosenmai AK, Dybdahl M, Pedersen M, et al. Toxicol Sci. 2014 May;139(1):35-47. PMID:24563381

739 Organochlorine pesticide levels and risk of Alzheimer's disease in north Indian population. Singh N, Chhillar N, Banerjee B, Bala K, Basu M, Mustafa M. Hum Exp Toxicol. 2013 Jan;32(1):24-30. PMID:22899726

740 Sleep deprivation: Impact on cognitive performance. Alhola P, Polo-Kantola P. Neuropsychiatr Dis Treat. 2007;3(5):553-67. PMID:19300585

741 Fatigue, alcohol and performance impairment. Dawson D, Reid K. Nature. 1997 Jul 17;388(6639):235. PMID:9230429

742 Does abnormal sleep impair memory consolidation in schizophrenia? Manoach DS, Stickgold R. Front Hum Neurosci. 2009 Sep 1;3:21. PMID:19750201

743 Micropillar arrays as a high-throughput screening platform for therapeutics in multiple sclerosis. Mei F, Fancy SP, Shen YA, et al. Nat Med. 2014 Aug;20(8):954-60. PMID:24997607

744 Systematic interindividual differences in neurobehavioral impairment from sleep loss: evidence of trait-like differential vulnerability. Van Dongen HP, Baynard MD, Maislin G, Dinges DF. Sleep. 2004 May 1;27(3):423-33. PMID: 15164894

745 The cumulative cost of additional wakefulness: dose-response effects on neurobehavioral functions and sleep physiology from chronic sleep restriction and total sleep deprivation. Van Dongen HP, Maislin G, et al. Sleep. 2003 Mar 15;26(2):117-26. PMID: 12683469

746 Sleep drives metabolite clearance from the adult brain. Xie L, Kang H, Xu Q, et al. Science. 2013 Oct 18;342(6156):373-7. PMID:24136970

747 CLOCK and BMAL1 regulate MyoD and are necessary for maintenance of skeletal muscle phenotype and function.Andrews JL, Zhang X, McCarthy JJ, et al. Proc Natl Acad Sci U S A. 2010 Nov 2;107(44):19090-5. PMID: 20956306

748 Paradoxical sleep deprivation impairs spatial learning and affects membrane excitability and mitochondrial protein in the hippocampus. Yang RH, Hu SJ, Wang Y, Zhang WB, Luo WJ, Chen JY. Brain Res. 2008 Sep 16;1230:224-32. 18674519

749 Why we sleep: the temporal organization of recovery. Mignot E. PLoS Biol. 2008 Apr 29;6(4):e106. PMID:18447584

750 Sleep depth and fatigue: role of cellular inflammatory activation. Thomas KS, Motivala S, Olmstead R, Irwin MR. Brain Behav Immun. 2011 Jan;25(1):53-8. PMID: 20656013

751 Retinoid-related orphan receptors (RORs): critical roles in development, immunity, circadian rhythm, and cellular metabolism. Jetten AM. Nucl Recept Signal. 2009;7:e003. PMID:19381306

752 Leptin levels are dependent on sleep duration: relationships with sympathovagal balance, carbohydrate regulation, cortisol, and thyrotropin. Spiegel K, Leproult R, L'hermite-Balériaux M, et al. J Clin Endocrinol Metab. 2004 Nov;89(11):5762-71. PMID: 15531540

753 Sleep restriction increases the risk of developing cardiovascular diseases by augmenting proinflammatory responses through IL-17 and CRP. van Leeuwen WM, Lehto M, Karisola P, Lindholm H, et al. PLoS One. 2009;4(2):e4589. PMID: 19240794

754 Short sleep duration is associated with reduced leptin, elevated ghrelin, and increased body mass index. Taheri S, Lin L, Austin D, Young T, Mignot E. PLoS Med. 2004 Dec;1(3):e62. PMID: 15602591

755 Polysomnographic sleep, growth hormone insulin-like growth factor-I axis, leptin, and weight loss. Rasmussen MH, Wildschiødtz G, Juul A, Hilsted J. Obesity (Silver Spring). 2008 Jul;16(7):1516-21. PMID: 18464752

756 Improved prediction of all-cause mortality by a combination of serum total testosterone and insulin-like growth factor I in adult men. Friedrich N, Schneider HJ, Haring R, et al. Steroids. 2012 Jan;77(1-2):52-8. PMID:22037276

757 Adverse effects of modest sleep restriction on sleepiness, performance, and inflammatory cytokines.. Vgontzas AN, Zoumakis E, Bixler EO, Lin HM, Follett H, Kales A, Chrousos GP. J Clin Endocrinol Metab. 2004 May;89(5):2119-26. PMID: 15126529

758 Effect of zinc and melatonin supplementation on cellular immunity in rats with toxoplasmosis. Baltaci AK, Bediz CS, Mogulkoc R, Kurtoglu E, Pekel A. Biol Trace Elem Res. 2003 Winter;96(1-3):237-45. PMID:14716103

759 Loss of glucocorticoid receptor activation is a hallmark of BRCA1-mutated breast tissue. Vilasco M, Communal L, Hugon-Rodin J, et al. Breast Cancer Res Treat. 2013 Nov;142(2):283-96. PMID:24166279

760 Increased risk of benign prostate hyperplasia in sleep apnea patients: a nationwide population-based study. Chou PS, Chang WC, Chou WP, et al. PLoS One. 2014 Mar 25;9(3):e93081. PMID:24667846

761 Risk of Cancer in Patients with Insomnia, Parasomnia, and Obstructive Sleep Apnea: A Nationwide Nested Case-Control Study. Fang HF, Miao NF, Chen CD, Sithole T, Chung MH. J Cancer. 2015 Sep 15;6(11):1140-7. PMID:26516362

762 Sleep apnea and the subsequent risk of breast cancer in women: a nationwide population-based cohort study. Chang WP, Liu ME, Chang WC, Yang AC, Ku YC, Pai JT, Lin YW, Tsai SJ. Sleep Med. 2014 Sep;15(9):1016-20. PMID:25085620

763 Sleep apnea increased incidence of primary central nervous system cancers: a nationwide cohort study. Chen JC, Hwang JH. Sleep Med. 2014 Jul;15(7):749-54. PMID:24891080

764 Night work, shift work: Breast cancer risk factor?. Benabu JC, Stoll F, Gonzalez M, Mathelin C. Gynecol Obstet Fertil. 2015 Dec;43(12):791-9. PMID:26597486

765 Rotating night shifts and risk of breast cancer in women participating in the nurses' health study. Schernhammer ES, Laden F, Speizer FE, Willett WC, Hunter DJ, Kawachi I, Colditz GA. J Natl Cancer Inst. 2001 Oct 17;93(20):1563-8. PMID:11604480

766 A meta-analysis on dose-response relationship between night shift work and the risk of breast cancer. Wang F, Yeung KL, Chan WC, Kwok CC, Leung SL, Wu C, Chan EY, Yu IT, Yang XR, Tse LA. Ann Oncol. 2013 Nov;24(11):2724-32. PMID:23975662

767 Work at night and breast cancer--report on evidence-based options for preventive actions. Bonde JP, Hansen J, Kolstad HA, et al. Scand J Work Environ Health. 2012 Jul;38(4):380-90. PMID:22349009

768 Does night-shift work increase the risk of prostate cancer? a systematic review and meta-analysis. Rao D, Yu H, Bai Y, Zheng X, Xie L. Onco Targets Ther. 2015 Oct 5;8:2817-26. PMID:26491356

769 A meta-analysis including dose-response relationship between night shift work and the risk of colorectal cancer. Wang X, Ji A, Zhu Y, Liang Z, Wu J, Li S, Meng S, Zheng X, Xie L. Oncotarget. 2015 Sep 22;6(28):25046-60. PMID:26208480

770 Role of clock genes in gastrointestinal motility. Hoogerwerf WA. Am J Physiol Gastrointest Liver Physiol. 2010 Sep;299(3):G549-55. PMID:20558764

771 Circadian variation in the propagation velocity of the migrating motor complex. Kumar D, Wingate D, Ruckebusch Y. Gastroenterology. 1986 Oct;91(4):926-30. PMID:3743969

772 Melatonin and serotonin effects on gastrointestinal motility. Thor PJ, Krolczyk G, Gil K, Zurowski D, Nowak L. J Physiol Pharmacol. 2007 Dec;58 Suppl 6:97-103. PMID:18212403

773 Functional bowel disorders in rotating shift nurses may be related to sleep disturbances.. Zhen Lu W, Ann Gwee K, Yu Ho K. Eur J Gastroenterol Hepatol. 2006 Jun;18(6):623-7. PMID:16702851

774 Feeding cues alter clock gene oscillations and photic responses in the suprachiasmatic nuclei of mice exposed to a light/dark cycle. Mendoza J, Graff C, Dardente H, Pevet P, Challet E. J Neurosci. 2005 Feb 9;25(6):1514-22. PMID:15703405

775 Restricted feeding uncouples circadian oscillators in peripheral tissues from the central pacemaker in the suprachiasmatic nucleus. Damiola F, Le Minh N, Preitner N, Kornmann B, Fleury-Olela F, Schibler U. Genes Dev. 2000 Dec 1;14(23):2950-61. PMID:11114885

776 Effect of a phase advance and phase delay of the 24-h cycle on energy metabolism, appetite, and related hormones. Gonnissen HK, Rutters F, Mazuy C, Martens EA, Adam TC, Westerterp-Plantenga MS. Am J Clin Nutr. 2012 Oct;96(4):689-97. PMID:22914550

777 Circadian aspects of postprandial metabolism. Morgan L, Hampton S, Gibbs M, Arendt J. Chronobiol Int. 2003 Sep;20(5):795-808. PMID:14535354

778 Dietary inflammatory index scores differ by shift work status: NHANES 2005 to 2010. Wirth MD, Burch J, Shivappa N, Steck SE, Hurley TG, Vena JE, Hébert JR. J Occup Environ Med. 2014 Feb;56(2):145-8. PMID:24451608

779 Appetite-regulating hormones from the upper gut: disrupted control of xenin and ghrelin in night workers. Schiavo-Cardozo D, Lima MM, Pareja JC, Geloneze B. Clin Endocrinol (Oxf). 2012 Dec 1. PMID:23199168

780 Total and cause-specific mortality of U.S. nurses working rotating night shifts. Gu F, Han J, Laden F, Pan A, et al. Am J Prev Med. 2015 Mar;48(3):241-52. PMID:25576495

781 Shifting eating to the circadian rest phase misaligns the peripheral clocks with the master SCN clock and leads to a metabolic syndrome. Mukherji A, Kobiita A, Damara M, et al. Proc Natl Acad Sci U S A. 2015 Dec 1;112(48):E6691-8. PMID:26627260

782 The impact of the circadian timing system on cardiovascular and metabolic function. Morris CJ, Yang JN, Scheer FA. Prog Brain Res. 2012;199:337-58. PMID:22877674

783 Alcohol use in shiftworkers. Dorrian J, Heath G, Sargent C, Banks S, Coates A. Accid Anal Prev. 2015 Nov 24. pii: S0001-4575(15)30127-5. PMID:26621201

784 Rotating night-shift work and lung cancer risk among female nurses in the United States. Schernhammer ES, Feskanich D, Liang G, Han J. Am J Epidemiol. 2013 Nov 1;178(9):1434-41. PMID:24049158

785 Light at night and breast cancer risk among California teachers. Hurley S, Goldberg D, Nelson D, et al. Epidemiology. 2014 Sep;25(5):697-706. PMID:25061924

786 Breast cancer cells: Modulation by melatonin and the ubiquitin-proteasome system - A review. Vriend J, Reiter RJ. Mol Cell Endocrinol. 2015 Dec 5;417:1-9. PMID:26363225

787 Light during darkness, melatonin suppression and cancer progression. Blask DE, Dauchy RT, Sauer LA, et al. Neuro Endocrinol Lett. 2002 Jul;23 Suppl 2:52-6. PMID:12163849

788 Melatonin: an inhibitor of breast cancer. Hill SM, Belancio VP, Dauchy RT, et al. Endocr Relat Cancer. 2015 Jun;22(3):R183-204 PMID:25876649

789 Circadian and melatonin disruption by exposure to light at night drives intrinsic resistance to tamoxifen therapy in breast cancer. Dauchy RT, Xiang S, Mao L, et al. Cancer Res. 2014 Aug 1;74(15):4099-110. PMID:25062775

790 Melatonin-depleted blood from premenopausal women exposed to light at night stimulates growth of human breast cancer xenografts in nude rats. Blask DE, Brainard GC, Dauchy RT, et al. Cancer Res. 2005 Dec 1;65(23):11174-84. PMID: 16322268

791 Predicting human nocturnal nonvisual responses to monochromatic and polychromatic light with a melanopsin photosensitivity function. Revell VL, Barrett DC, Schlangen LJ, Skene DJ. Chronobiol Int. 2010 Oct;27(9-10):1762-77. PMID:20969522

792 Work at night and breast cancer--report on evidence-based options for preventive actions. Bonde JP, Hansen J, Kolstad HA, et al. Scand J Work Environ Health. 2012 Jul;38(4):380-90. PMID:22349009

793 Daytime Blue Light Enhances the Nighttime Circadian Melatonin Inhibition of Human Prostate Cancer Growth. Dauchy RT, Hoffman AE, Wren-Dail MA, et al. Comp Med. 2015;65(6):473-85. PMID:26678364

794 The potential role of the transcription factor RZR/ROR as a mediator of nuclear melatonin signaling. Wiesenberg I, Missbach M, Carlberg C. Restor Neurol Neurosci. 1998 Jun;12(2-3):143-50. PMID:12671309

795 RORα and ROR γ are expressed in human skin and serve as receptors for endogenously produced noncalcemic 20-hydroxy- and 20,23-dihydroxyvitamin D. Slominski AT, Kim TK, Takeda Y, et al. FASEB J. 2014 Jul;28(7):2775-89. PMID:24668754

796 Vitamin B12 enhances the phase-response of circadian melatonin rhythm to a single bright light exposure in humans. Hashimoto S, Kohsaka M, Morita N, Fukuda N, Honma S, Honma K. Neurosci Lett. 1996 Dec 13;220(2):129-32. PMID: 8981490

797 A multicenter study of sleep-wake rhythm disorders: therapeutic effects of vitamin B12, bright light therapy, chronotherapy and hypnotics. Yamadera H, Takahashi K, Okawa M. Psychiatry Clin Neurosci. 1996 Aug;50(4):203-9. PMID:9201777

798 Sleep Sleep duration associated with mortality in elderly, but not middle-aged, adults in a large US sample. Gangwisch JE, Heymsfield SB, Boden-Albala B, et al. Sleep. 2008 Aug 1;31(8):1087-96. PMID: 18714780

799 Mortality associated with sleep duration and insomnia. Kripke DF, Garfinkel L, Wingard DL, Klauber MR, Marler MR. Arch Gen Psychiatry. 2002 Feb;59(2):131-6. PMID: 11825133

800 Habitual sleep duration and insomnia and the risk of cardiovascular events and all-cause death: report from a community-based cohort. Chien KL, Chen PC, Hsu HC, Su TC, Sung FC, Chen MF, Lee YT. Sleep. 2010 Feb 1;33(2):177-84. PMID: 20175401

801 Association of sleep duration with mortality from cardiovascular disease and other causes for Japanese men and women: the JACC study. Ikehara S, Iso H, Date C, et al; JACC Study Group. Sleep. 2009 Mar 1;32(3):295-301. PMID: 19294949

802 Sleep duration and all-cause mortality: a systematic review and meta-analysis of prospective studies.Cappuccio FP, D'Elia L, Strazzullo P, Miller MA. Sleep. 2010 May 1;33(5):585-92. PMID: 20469800

803 Melatonin decreases delirium in elderly patients: a randomized, placebo-controlled trial. Al-Aama T, Brymer C, Gutmanis I, e. Int J Geriatr Psychiatry. 2010 Sep 15. PMID: 20845391

804 Vitamin B6 and risk of colorectal cancer: a meta-analysis of prospective studies. Larsson SC, Orsini N, Wolk A. JAMA. 2010 Mar 17;303(11):1077-83. PMID:20233826

805 Clinical uses of melatonin: evaluation of human trials. Sánchez-Barceló EJ, Mediavilla MD, Tan DX, Reiter RJ. Curr Med Chem. 2010;17(19):2070-95. PMID:20423309

806 Melatonin improves metabolic syndrome induced by high fructose intake in rats.. Kitagawa A, Ohta Y, Ohashi K. J Pineal Res. 2011 Dec 7. PMID:22220562

807 The potential therapeutic effect of melatonin in Gastro-Esophageal Reflux Disease. Kandil TS, Mousa AA, El-Gendy AA, Abbas AM. BMC Gastroenterol. 2010 Jan 18;10:7. PMID:20082715

808 The therapeutic potential of melatonin in migraines and other headache types. Gagnier JJ. Altern Med Rev. 2001 Aug;6(4):383-9. PMID:11578254

809 Potential therapeutic use of melatonin in migraine and other headache disorders. Peres MF, Masruha MR, Zukerman E, Moreira-Filho CA, Cavalheiro EA. Expert Opin Investig Drugs. 2006 Apr;15(4):367-75. PMID:16548786

810 The association of nocturnal serum melatonin levels with major depression in patients with acute multiple sclerosis. Akpinar Z, Tokgöz S, Gökbel H, Okudan N, Uğuz F, Yilmaz G. Psychiatry Res. 2008 Nov 30;161(2):253-7. PMID:18848732

811 The effect of vitamin D supplements on the severity of restless legs syndrome. Wali S, Shukr A, Boudal A, et al. Sleep Breath. 2015 May;19(2):579-83. PMID:25148866

812 Optimal serum 25-hydroxyvitamin D levels for multiple health outcomes. Bischoff-Ferrari HA. Adv Exp Med Biol. 2008;624:55-71. PMID:18348447

813 Vitamin D and risk of cause specific death: systematic review and meta-analysis of observational cohort and randomised intervention studies. Chowdhury R, Kunutsor S, Vitezova A, et al. BMJ. 2014 Apr 1;348:g1903. PMID:24690623

814 Serum 25-hydroxyvitamin D, mortality, and incident cardiovascular disease, respiratory disease, cancers, and fractures: a 13-y prospective population study. Khaw KT, Luben R, Wareham N. Am J Clin Nutr. 2014 Nov;100(5):1361-70. PMID:25332334

815 Cognitive impairment associated with low ferritin responsive to iron supplementation. Qubty W, Renaud DL. Pediatr Neurol. 2014 Dec;51(6):831-3. PMID:25283751

816 Children with autism: effect of iron supplementation on sleep and ferritin. Dosman CF, Brian JA, Drmic IE, Senthilselvan A, Harford MM, Smith RW, Sharieff W, Zlotkin SH, Moldofsky H, Roberts SW. Pediatr Neurol. 2007 Mar;36(3):152-8. PMID: 17352947

817 Improvement of anemia with erythropoietin and intravenous iron reduces sleep-related breathing disorders and improves daytime sleepiness in anemic patients with congestive heart failure. Zilberman M, Silverberg DS, Bits I, et al. Am Heart J. 2007 Nov;154(5):870-6. PMID: 17967592

818 Diagnostic accuracy of behavioral, activity, ferritin, and clinical indicators of restless legs syndrome. Richards KC, Bost JE, Rogers VE, Hutchison LC, Beck CK, Bliwise DL, Kovach CR, Cuellar N, Allen RP. Sleep. 2015 Mar 1;38(3):371-80. PMID:25325464

819 Iron deficiency and infant motor development.. Shafir T, Angulo-Barroso R, Jing Y, et al. Early Hum Dev. 2008 Jul;84(7):479-85. PMID: 18272298

820 Dietary intake of B vitamins and methionine and colorectal cancer risk. Bassett JK, Severi G, Hodge AM, et al. Nutr Cancer. 2013;65(5):659-67. PMID:23859033

821 Acute ethanol modulates glutamatergic and serotonergic phase shifts of the mouse circadian clock in vitro. Prosser RA, Mangrum CA, Glass JD. Neuroscience. 2008 Mar 27;152(3):837-48. PMID: 18313277

822 Habitual moderate alcohol consumption desynchronizes circadian physiologic rhythms and affects reaction-time performance. Reinberg A, Touitou Y, Lewy H, Mechkouri M. Chronobiol Int. 2010 Oct.;27(9-10):1930-1942. PMID: 20969532

823 Circadian rhythm of hormones is extinguished during prolonged physical stress, sleep and energy deficiency in young men.. Opstad K. Eur J Endocrinol. 1994 Jul;131(1):56-66. PMID: 8038905

824 High intention to fall asleep causes sleep fragmentation. Rasskazova E, Zavalko I, Tkhostov A, Dorohov V. J Sleep Res. 2014 Jun;23(3):295-301. PMID:24387832

825 Evening use of light-emitting eReaders negatively affects sleep, circadian timing, and next-morning alertness. Chang AM, Aeschbach D, Duffy JF, Czeisler CA. Proc Natl Acad Sci U S A. 2015 Jan 27;112(4):1232-7. PMID:25535358

826 Blue blocker glasses as a countermeasure for alerting effects of evening light-emitting diode screen exposure in male teenagers. van der Lely S, Frey S, Garbazza C, Wirz-Justice A, et al. J Adolesc Health. 2015 Jan;56(1):113-9. PMID:25287985

827 Bigger, Brighter, Bluer-Better? Current Light-Emitting Devices - Adverse Sleep Properties and Preventative Strategies. Gringras P, Middleton B, Skene DJ, Revell VL. Front Public Health. 2015 Oct 13;3:233. PMID:26528465

828 Daytime napping after a night of sleep loss decreases sleepiness, improves performance, and causes beneficial changes in cortisol and interleukin-6 secretion. Vgontzas AN, Pejovic S, Zoumakis E, et al. Am J Physiol Endocrinol Metab. 2007 Jan;292(1):E253-61.PMID: 16940468

829 The impact of sleep duration and subject intelligence on declarative and motor memory performance: how much is enough? Tucker MA, Fishbein W. J Sleep Res. 2009 Sep;18(3):304-12. PMID:19702788

830 Enhancement of declarative memory performance following a daytime nap is contingent on strength of initial task acquisition. Tucker MA, Fishbein W. Sleep. 2008 Feb;31(2):197-203. PMID:18274266

831 Post-sleep inertia performance benefits of longer naps in simulated nightwork and extended operations. Mulrine HM, Signal TL, van den Berg MJ, Gander PH. Chronobiol Int. 2012 Nov;29(9):1249-57. PMID:23002951

832 Effects of physical positions on sleep architectures and post-nap functions among habitual nappers. Zhao D, Zhang Q, Fu M, Tang Y, Zhao Y. Biol Psychol. 2010 Mar;83(3):207-13. PMID:20064578

833 Korea's thyroid-cancer "epidemic"--screening and overdiagnosis. Ahn HS, Kim HJ, Welch HG. N Engl J Med. 2014 Nov 6;371(19):1765-7. PMID:25372084

834 South Korea's Thyroid-Cancer "Epidemic"--Turning the Tide. Ahn HS, Welch HG. N Engl J Med. 2015 Dec 10;373(24):2389-90. PMID:26650173

835 http://www.nytimes.com/2010/07/20/health/20cancer.html?pagewanted=all&_r=1

836 Short-term outcomes of screening mammography using computer-aided detection: a population-based study of medicare enrollees. Fenton JJ, Xing G, Elmore JG, Bang H, Chen SL, Lindfors KK, Baldwin LM. Ann Intern Med. 2013 Apr 16;158(8):580-7. PMID:23588746

837 Mammography for symptomless women--not so wise? Cutler WB, Burki RE, Kolter J, Chambliss C. Climacteric. 2013 Jun;16(3):313-5. PMID:23425505

838 Flawed assumptions used to defend screening mammography. Bleyer A, Thomas CR Jr, Baines C, Miller AB. Cancer. 2015 Jan 15;121(2):320-1. PMID:25272974

839 Reply to flawed assumptions used to defend screening mammography. Helvie MA, Chang JT, Hendrick RE, Banerjee M. Cancer. 2015 Jan 15;121(2):321-3. PMID:25274466

840 Effect of three decades of screening mammography on breast-cancer incidence. Bleyer A, Welch HG. N Engl J Med. 2012 Nov 22;367(21):1998-2005. PMID: 23171096

841 Breast tissue composition and susceptibility to breast cancer. Boyd NF, Martin LJ, Bronskill M, et al. J Natl Cancer Inst. 2010 Aug 18;102(16):1224-37. PMID:20616353

842 Personalizing mammography by breast density and other risk factors for breast cancer: analysis of health benefits and cost-effectiveness. Schousboe JT, Kerlikowske K, Loh A, Cummings SR. Ann Intern Med. 2011 Jul 5;155(1):10-20. PMID:21727289

843 Benefits and harms of mammography screening after age 74 years: model estimates of overdiagnosis. van Ravesteyn NT, Stout NK, Schechter CB, et al. J Natl Cancer Inst. 2015 May 6;107(7). PMID:25948872

844 Screening mammography in older women: a review. Walter LC, Schonberg MA. JAMA. 2014 Apr 2;311(13):1336-47. PMID:24691609

845 Photo courtesy of Brian Camazine, MD

846 Adenoma detection rate and risk of colorectal cancer and death. Corley DA, Levin TR, Doubeni CA. N Engl J Med. 2014 Jun 26;370(26):2541. PMID:24963577

847 Relationship between detection of adenomas by flexible sigmoidoscopy and interval distal colorectal cancer. Rogal SS, Pinsky PF, Schoen RE. Clin Gastroenterol Hepatol. 2013 Jan;11(1):73-8. PMID:22902761

848 Differences between morning and afternoon colonoscopies for adenoma detection in female and male patients. Singh S, Dhawan M, Chowdhry M, Babich M, Aoun E. Ann Gastroenterol. 2016 Oct-Dec;29(4):497-501. PMID:27708517

849 Screening for Colorectal Cancer: US Preventive Services Task Force Recommendation Statement. US Preventive Services Task Force. JAMA. 2016 Jun 21;315(23):2564-75. PMID:27304597

850 http://seer.cancer.gov/statfacts/html/colorect.html (Accessed 8/2016)

851 Determinants of age at menarche in the UK: analyses from the Breakthrough Generations Study. Morris DH, Jones ME, Schoemaker MJ, Ashworth A, Swerdlow AJ. Br J Cancer. 2010 Nov 23;103(11):1760-4. PMID:21045834

852 Recent data on pubertal milestones in United States children: the secular trend toward earlier development. Herman-Giddens ME. Int J Androl. 2006 Feb;29(1):241-6; discussion 286-90. PMID:16466545

853 Breast cancer risk accumulation starts early: prevention must also. Colditz GA, Bohlke K, Berkey CS. Breast Cancer Res Treat. 2014 Jun;145(3):567-79. PMID:24820413

854 Relationship between age maximum height is attained, age at menarche, and age at first full-term birth and breast cancer risk. Li CI, Littman AJ, White E. Cancer Epidemiol Biomarkers Prev. 2007 Oct;16(10):2144-9. PMID:17932363

855 Childhood soy intake and breast cancer risk in Asian American women. Korde LA, Wu AH, Fears T, Nomura AM, West DW, Kolonel LN, Pike MC, Hoover RN, Ziegler RG. Cancer Epidemiol Biomarkers Prev. 2009 Apr;18(4):1050-9. PMID: 19318430

856 Soy intake is associated with increased 2-hydroxylation and decreased 16alpha-hydroxylation of estrogens in Asian-American women. Fuhrman BJ, Pfeiffer R, Xu X, Wu AH, Korde L, Gail MH, Keefer LK, Veenstra TD, Hoover RN, Ziegler RG. Cancer Epidemiol Biomarkers Prev. 2009 Oct;18(10):2751-60. PMID:19789363

857 USDA-Iowa State University Database on the Isoflavone Content of Foods. www.ars.usda.gov/SP2UserFiles/Place/80400525/Data/isoflav/isoflav1-4.pdf

858 Adolescent diet and incidence of proliferative benign breast disease. Baer HJ, Schnitt SJ, Connolly JL, Byrne C, Cho E, Willett WC, Colditz GA. Cancer Epidemiol Biomarkers Prev. 2003 Nov;12(11 Pt 1):1159-67. PMID:14652275

859 Preadolescent and adolescent risk factors for benign breast disease. Frazier AL, Rosenberg SM. J Adolesc Health. 2013 May;52(5 Suppl):S36-40. PMID:23601609

860 Intakes of alcohol and folate during adolescence and risk of proliferative benign breast disease. Liu Y, Tamimi RM, Berkey CS, Willett WC, Collins LC, Schnitt SJ, Connolly JL, Colditz GA. Pediatrics. 2012 May;129(5):e1192-8. PMID:22492774

861 Adolescent intakes of vitamin D and calcium and incidence of proliferative benign breast disease. Su X, Colditz GA, Collins LC, Baer HJ, Sampson LA, Willett WC, Berkey CS, Schnitt SJ, Connolly JL, Rosner BA, Tamimi RM. Breast Cancer Res Treat. 2012 Jul;134(2):783-91. PMID:22622809

862 Vegetable protein and vegetable fat intakes in pre-adolescent and adolescent girls, and risk for benign breast disease in young women. Berkey CS, Willett WC, Tamimi RM, et al. Breast Cancer Res Treat. 2013 Sep;141(2):299-306. PMID:24043428

863 Dairy intakes in older girls and risk of benign breast disease in young women. Berkey CS, Willett WC, Tamimi RM, Rosner B, Frazier AL, Colditz GA. Cancer Epidemiol Biomarkers Prev. 2013 Apr;22(4):670-4. PMID:23542805

864 Intakes of fat and micronutrients between ages 13 and 18 years and the incidence of proliferative benign breast disease. Su X, Boeke CE, Collins LC, Baer HJ, Willett WC, Schnitt SJ, Connolly JL, Rosner B, Colditz GA, Tamimi RM. Cancer Causes Control. 2015 Jan;26(1):79-90. PMID:25376828

865 Il-6 signaling between ductal carcinoma in situ cells and carcinoma-associated fibroblasts mediates tumor cell growth and migration. Osuala KO, Sameni M, Shah S, et al. BMC Cancer. 2015 Aug 13;15:584. PMID:26268945

866 Vital Statistics of the United States: Ninth Census – Volume II.

867 Large-scale genomic analyses link reproductive aging to hypothalamic signaling, breast cancer susceptibility and BRCA1-mediated DNA repair. Day FR, Ruth KS, Thompson DJ, et al. Nat Genet. 2015 Nov;47(11):1294-303. PMID:26414677

868 The BOADICEA model of genetic susceptibility to breast and ovarian cancers: updates and extensions. Antoniou AC, Cunningham AP, Peto J, et al. Br J Cancer. 2008 Apr 22;98(8):1457-66. PMID:18349832

869 Contribution of Germline Mutations in the RAD51B, RAD51C, and RAD51D Genes to Ovarian Cancer in the Population. Song H, Dicks E, Ramus SJ, et al. J Clin Oncol. 2015 Sep 10;33(26):2901-7. PMID:26261251

870 Tubal ligation and risk of ovarian cancer in carriers of BRCA1 or BRCA2 mutations: a case-control study. Narod SA, Sun P, Ghadirian P, et al. Lancet. 2001 May 12;357(9267):1467-70. PMID:11377596

871 Modifiers of cancer risk in BRCA1 and BRCA2 mutation carriers: systematic review and meta analysis. Friebel TM, Domchek SM, Rebbeck TR. J Natl Cancer Inst. 2014 Jun;106(6):dju091. PMID:24824314

872 Reproductive and hormonal factors, and ovarian cancer risk for BRCA1 and BRCA2 mutation carriers: results from the International BRCA1/2 Carrier Cohort Study. Antoniou AC, Rookus M, Andrieu N, et al. Cancer Epidemiol Biomarkers Prev. 2009 Feb;18(2):601-10. PMID:19190154

873 Hormonal contraception and risk of endometrial cancer: a systematic review. Mueck AO, Seeger H, Rabe T. Endocr Relat Cancer. 2010 Sep 23;17(4):R263-71. PMID:20870686

874 Oral contraceptive use and risk of breast, cervical, colorectal, and endometrial cancers: a systematic review. Gierisch JM, Coeytaux RR, Urrutia RP, et al. Cancer Epidemiol Biomarkers Prev. 2013 Nov;22(11):1931-43. PMID:24014598

875 Oral contraceptive use and breast cancer: a prospective study of young women. Hunter DJ, Colditz GA, Hankinson SE, Malspeis S, Spiegelman D, Chen W, Stampfer MJ, Willett WC. Cancer Epidemiol Biomarkers Prev. 2010 Oct;19(10):2496-502. PMID:20802021

876 Recent oral contraceptive use by formulation and breast cancer risk among women 20 to 49 years of age. Beaber EF, Buist DS, Barlow WE, Malone KE, Reed SD, Li CI. Cancer Res. 2014 Aug 1;74(15):4078-89. PMID:25085875

877 Association of estrogen and progestin potency of oral contraceptives with ovarian carcinoma risk. Lurie G, Thompson P, McDuffie KE, Carney ME, Terada KY, Goodman MT. Obstet Gynecol. 2007 Mar;109(3):597-607. PMID: 17329510

878 Bladder Cancer: Etiology and Prevention. Gloka K, Goebell PJ, Rettenmeier. Dtsch Arztebl 2007; 104(11): A 719–23

879 Cancer risks in hairdressers: assessment of carcinogenicity of hair dyes and gels. Czene K, Tiikkaja S, Hemminki K. Int J Cancer. 2003 May 20;105(1):108-12. PMID:12672039

880 Basic Red 51, a permitted semi-permanent hair dye, is cytotoxic to human skin cells: Studies in monolayer and 3D skin model using human keratinocytes (HaCaT). Zanoni TB, Tiago M,

Faião-Flores F, de Moraes Barros SB, Bast A, Hageman G, de Oliveira DP, Maria-Engler SS. Toxicol Lett. 2014 Jun 5;227(2):139-49. PMID:24657526

[881] Cytotoxic and genotoxic effects of two hair dyes used in the formulation of black color. Tafurt-Cardona Y, Suares-Rocha P, Fernandes TC, Marin-Morales MA. Food Chem Toxicol. 2015 Dec;86:9-15. PMID:26404083

[882] Alterations of telomere length and DNA methylation in hairdressers: A cross-sectional study. Li H, Åkerman G, Lidén C, Alhamdow A, Wojdacz TK, Broberg K, Albin M. Environ Mol Mutagen. 2015 Dec 6. PMID:26637967

[883] Bladder cancer in crack testers applying azo dye-based sprays to metal bodies. Golka K, Kopps S, Prager HM, et al. J Toxicol Environ Health A. 2012;75(8-10):566-71. PMID:22686317

[884] Benzidine Dyes Action Plan: Dyes Derived from Benzidine and Its Congeners. U.S. Environmental Protection Agency. Aug.18, 2010

[885] Dyes metabolized to Bebzidine. IARC Mongraphs Vol. 99, 262-296, Nov. 1999.

[886] NIOSH POCKET GUIDE TO CHEMICAL HAZARDS: TOLUENEDIAMINE

[887] A meta-analysis on the association between bladder cancer and occupation. Reulen RC, Kellen E, Buntinx F, Brinkman M, Zeegers MP. Scand J Urol Nephrol Suppl. 2008 Sep;(218):64-78. PMID:18815919

[888] Meta-analysis of studies on individual consumption of chlorinated drinking water and bladder cancer. Villanueva CM, Fernández F, Malats N, Grimalt JO, Kogevinas M. J Epidemiol Community Health. 2003 Mar;57(3):166-73 PMID:12594192

[889] Effects of indoor drinking water handling on trihalomethanes and haloacetic acids. Levesque S, Rodriguez MJ, Serodes J, Beaulieu C, Proulx F. Water Res. 2006 Aug;40(15):2921-30. PMID:16889815

[890] mLST8 Promotes mTOR-Mediated Tumor Progression. Kakumoto K, Ikeda J, Okada M, Morii E, Oneyama C. PLoS One. 2015 Apr 23;10(4):e0119015. PMID:25906254

[891] Role of PRAS40 in Akt and mTOR signaling in health and disease. Wiza C, Nascimento EB, Ouwens DM. Am J Physiol Endocrinol Metab. 2012 Jun 15;302(12):E1453-60. PMID:22354785

[892] KEGG mTOR Pathway: http://www.kegg.jp/kegg-bin/show_pathway?map04150 7/2016

[893] Amino acid signaling to mTOR mediated by inositol polyphosphate multikinase. Kim S, Kim SF, Maag D, et al. Cell Metab. 2011 Feb 2;13(2):215-21. PMID:21284988

[894] Dietary branched chain amino acids ameliorate injury-induced cognitive impairment. Cole JT, Mitala CM, Kundu S, et al. Proc Natl Acad Sci U S A. 2010 Jan 5;107(1):366-71. PMID:19995960

[895] Molecular targets of dietary phenethyl isothiocyanate and sulforaphane for cancer chemoprevention. Cheung KL, Kong AN. AAPS J. 2010 Mar;12(1):87-97. PMID: 20013083

[896] Metformin and salicylate synergistically activate liver AMPK, inhibit lipogenesis and improve insulin sensitivity. Ford RJ, Fullerton MD, Pinkosky SL, et al. Biochem J. 2015 May 15;468(1):125-32. PMID:25742316

[897] Salicylate activates AMPK and synergizes with metformin to reduce the survival of prostate and lung cancer cells ex vivo through inhibition of de novo lipogenesis. O'Brien AJ, Villani LA, Broadfield LA, et al. Biochem J. 2015 May 5. PMID:25940306

[898] Leptin regulates energy metabolism in MCF-7 breast cancer cells. Blanquer-Rosselló Mdel M, Oliver J, Sastre-Serra J, et al. Int J Biochem Cell Biol. 2016 Mar;72:18-26. PMID:26772821

[899] New insight into adiponectin role in obesity and obesity-related diseases. Nigro E, Scudiero O, Monaco ML, Palmieri A, Mazzarella G, Costagliola C, Bianco A, Daniele A. Biomed Res Int. 2014;2014:658913. PMID:25110685

[900] The role of adiponectin in cancer: a review of current evidence. Dalamaga M, Diakopoulos KN, Mantzoros CS. Endocr Rev. 2012 Aug;33(4):547-94. PMID:22547160

901 CaMKKβ is involved in AMP-activated protein kinase activation by baicalin in LKB1 deficient cell lines. Ma Y, Yang F, Wang Y, Du Z, Liu D, Guo H, Shen J, Peng H. PLoS One. 2012;7(10):e47900. PMID: 23110126

902 Ca2+/calmodulin-dependent protein kinase kinase is involved in AMP-activated protein kinase activation by alpha-lipoic acid in C2C12 myotubes. Shen QW, Zhu MJ, Tong J, Ren J, Du M. Am J Physiol Cell Physiol. 2007 Oct;293(4):C1395-403. PMID: 17687000

903 S-allyl cysteine attenuates free fatty acid-induced lipogenesis in human HepG2 cells through activation of the AMP-activated protein kinase-dependent pathway. Hwang YP, Kim HG, Choi JH, et al. J Nutr Biochem. 2013 Aug;24(8):1469-78. PMID: 23465592

904 Thyroid hormone activates adenosine 5'-monophosphate-activated protein kinase via intracellular calcium mobilization and activation of calcium/calmodulin-dependent protein kinase kinase-beta. Yamauchi M, Kambe F, Cao X, Lu X, Kozaki Y, Oiso Y, Seo H. Mol Endocrinol. 2008 Apr;22(4):893-903. PMID: 18187603

905 AMPK: a target for drugs and natural products with effects on both diabetes and cancer. Hardie DG. Diabetes. 2013 Jul;62(7):2164-72. PMID: 23801715

906 Withdrawal of essential amino acids increases autophagy by a pathway involving Ca2+/calmodulin-dependent kinase kinase-β (CaMKK-β). Ghislat G, Patron M, Rizzuto R, Knecht E. J Biol Chem. 2012 Nov 9;287(46):38625-36. PMID: 23027865

907 Phosphorylation of tau proteins to a state like that in Alzheimer's brain is catalyzed by a calcium/calmodulin-dependent kinase and modulated by phospholipids. Baudier J, Cole RD. J Biol Chem. 1987 Dec 25;262(36):17577-83. PMID: 3121601

908 Regulation of the p21-activated kinase-related Dictyostelium myosin I heavy chain kinase by autophosphorylation, acidic phospholipids, and Ca2+-calmodulin. Lee SF, Mahasneh A, de la Roche M, Côté GP. J Biol Chem. 1998 Oct 23;273(43):27911-7. PMID: 9774403

909 Phospholipids are necessary for calmodulin-stimulated activation of the Ca(2+)-ATPase of erythrocytes. Gazzotti P, Gloor-Amrein M, Adebayo R. Eur J Biochem. 1994 Sep 15;224(3):873-6. PMID: 7925410

910 Fas-triggered phosphatidylserine exposure is modulated by intracellular ATP. Gleiss B, Gogvadze V, Orrenius S, Fadeel B. FEBS Lett. 2002 May 22;519(1-3):153-8. PMID:12023035

911 2-Deoxyglucose Reverses the Promoting Effect of Insulin on Colorectal Cancer Cells In Vitro. Zhang D, Fei Q, Li J, et al. PLoS One. 2016 Mar 3;11(3):e0151115. PMID:26939025

912 Clinical studies for improving radiotherapy with 2-deoxy-D-glucose: present status and future prospects. Dwarakanath BS, Singh D, Banerji AK, et al. J Cancer Res Ther. 2009 Sep;5 Suppl 1:S21-6. PMID:20009289

913 Phospholipase D meets Wnt signaling: a new target for cancer therapy. Kang DW, Choi KY, Min do S. Cancer Res. 2011 Jan 15;71(2):293-7.. PMID: 21224347

914 Vitamin D and Wnt/beta-catenin pathway in colon cancer: role and regulation of DICKKOPF genes. Pendás-Franco N, Aguilera O, Pereira F, González-Sancho JM, Muñoz A. Anticancer Res. 2008 Sep-Oct;28(5A):2613-23. PMID: 19035286

915 Quercetin inhibit human SW480 colon cancer growth in association with inhibition of cyclin D1 and survivin expression through Wnt/beta-catenin signaling pathway. Shan BE, Wang MX, Li RQ. Cancer Invest. 2009 Jul;27(6):604-12. PMID: 19440933

916 Caffeic acid phenethyl ester induces growth arrest and apoptosis of colon cancer cells via the beta-catenin/T-cell factor signaling. Xiang D, Wang D, He Y, Xie J, Zhong Z, Li Z, Xie J. Anticancer Drugs. 2006 Aug;17(7):753-62. PMID: 16926625

917 Resveratrol attenuates C5a-induced inflammatory responses in vitro and in vivo by inhibiting phospholipase D and sphingosine kinase activities. Issuree PD, Pushparaj PN, Pervaiz S, Melendez AJ. FASEB J. 2009 Aug;23(8):2412-24. PMID:19346296

918 alpha-Lipoic acid increases energy expenditure by enhancing adenosine monophosphate-activated protein kinase-peroxisome proliferator-activated receptor-gamma coactivator-1alpha

signaling in the skeletal muscle of aged mice. Wang Y, Li X, Guo Y, Chan L, Guan X. Metabolism. 2010 Jul;59(7):967-76. PMID:20015518

[919] Phospholipase D signaling pathways and phosphatidic acid as therapeutic targets in cancer. Bruntz RC, Lindsley CW, Brown HA. Pharmacol Rev. 2014 Oct;66(4):1033-79. PMID:25244928

[920] http://www.brenda-enzymes.org/enzyme.php?ecno=3.1.4.4

[921] Phospholipase D1 is required for lipopolysaccharide-induced tumor necrosis factor-α expression and production through S6K1/JNK/c-Jun pathway in Raw 264.7 cells. Oh CH, Park SY, Han JS. Cytokine. 2014 Mar;66(1):69-77. PMID: 24548427

[922] mu-opioid receptor-stimulated synthesis of reactive oxygen species is mediated via phospholipase D2. Koch T, Seifert A, Wu DF, Rankovic M, Kraus J, Börner C, Brandenburg LO, Schröder H, Höllt V. J Neurochem. 2009 Aug;110(4):1288-96. PMID: 19519662

[923] Suppression of the TRIF-dependent signaling pathway of Toll-like receptors by luteolin. Lee JK, Kim SY, Kim YS, Lee WH, Hwang DH, Lee JY. Biochem Pharmacol. 2009 Apr 15;77(8):1391-400. PMID: 19426678

[924] Inhibition of homodimerization of Toll-like receptor 4 by curcumin. Youn HS, Saitoh SI, Miyake K, Hwang DH. Biochem Pharmacol. 2006 Jun 28;72(1):62-9. PMID:16678799

[925] Cinnamaldehyde suppresses toll-like receptor 4 activation mediated through the inhibition of receptor oligomerization. Youn HS, Lee JK, Choi YJ, Saitoh SI, Miyake K, Hwang DH, Lee JY. Biochem Pharmacol. 2008 Jan 15;75(2):494-502. PMID: 17920563

[926] Glycyrrhizin inhibits lipopolysaccharide-induced inflammatory response by reducing TLR4 recruitment into lipid rafts in RAW264.7 cells. Fu Y, Zhou E, Wei Z, et al. Biochim Biophys Acta. 2014 Jun;1840(6):1755-64. PMID: 24462946

[927] Melatonin modulates TLR4-mediated inflammatory genes through MyD88- and TRIF-dependent signaling pathways in lipopolysaccharide-stimulated RAW264.7 cells. Xia MZ, Liang YL, Wang H, et al. J Pineal Res. 2012 Nov;53(4):325-34. PMID: 22537289

[928] Sensing of energy and nutrients by AMP-activated protein kinase. Hardie DG. Am J Clin Nutr. 2011 Apr;93(4):891S-6. PMID:21325438

[929] Gallic acid regulates body weight and glucose homeostasis through AMPK activation. Doan KV, Ko CM, Kinyua AW, et al. Endocrinology. 2015 Jan;156(1):157-68. PMID:25356824

[930] The ancient drug salicylate directly activates AMP-activated protein kinase. Hawley SA, Fullerton MD, Ross FA, et al. Science. 2012 May 18;336(6083): PMID:22517326

[931] Metformin may protect nondiabetic breast cancer women from metastasis. El-Haggar SM, El-Shitany NA, Mostafa MF, El-Bassiouny NA. Clin Exp Metastasis. 2016 Apr;33(4):339-57. PMID:26902691

[932] Repurposing of metformin and aspirin by targeting AMPK-mTOR and inflammation for pancreatic cancer prevention and treatment. Yue W, Yang CS, DiPaola RS, Tan XL. Cancer Prev Res (Phila). 2014 Apr;7(4):388-97. PMID: 24520038

[933] Ghrelin-AMPK Signaling Mediates the Neuroprotective Effects of Calorie Restriction in Parkinson's Disease. Bayliss JA, Lemus MB, Stark R, et al. J Neurosci. 2016 Mar 9;36(10):3049-63. PMID:26961958

[934] Effects of resistance training on cytokines. de Salles BF, Simão R, Fleck SJ, Dias I, Kraemer-Aguiar LG, Bouskela E. Int J Sports Med. 2010 Jul;31(7):441-50. PMID:20432196

[935] Perceived psychological stress and serum leptin concentrations in Japanese men. Otsuka R, Yatsuya H, Tamakoshi K, Matsushita K, Wada K, Toyoshima H. Obesity (Silver Spring). 2006 Oct;14(10):1832-8. PMID:17062814

[936] Comparison of serum adiponectin and tumor necrosis factor-alpha levels between patients with and without obstructive sleep apnea syndrome. Kanbay A, Kokturk O, Ciftci TU, Tavil Y, Bukan N. Respiration. 2008;76(3):324-30. PMID:18487876

937 The important role of sleep in metabolism. Copinschi G, Leproult R, Spiegel K. Front Horm Res. 2014;42:59-72. PMID:24732925

938 Leptin, obestatin and apelin levels in patients with obstructive sleep apnoea syndrome. Zirlik S, Hauck T, Fuchs FS, Neurath MF, Konturek PC, Harsch IA. Med Sci Monit. 2011 Feb 25;17(3):CR159-64. PMID:21358603

939 Improved insulin sensitivity and adiponectin level after exercise training in obese Korean youth. Kim ES, Im JA, Kim KC, et al. Obesity (Silver Spring). 2007 Dec;15(12):3023-30. PMID:18198311

940 Pinealectomy increases and exogenous melatonin decreases leptin production in rat anterior pituitary cells: an immunohistochemical study. Kus I, Sarsilmaz M, Colakoglu N, Kukne A, Ozen OA, Yilmaz B, Kelestimur H. Physiol Res. 2004;53(4):403-8. PMID:15311999

941 Intermittent and rhythmic exposure to melatonin in primary cultured adipocytes enhances the insulin and dexamethasone effects on leptin expression. Alonso-Vale MI, Andreotti S, Borges-Silva Cd, et al. J Pineal Res. 2006 Aug;41(1):28-34. PMID:16842538

942 Changes in glucose tolerance and leptin responsiveness of rats offered a choice of lard, sucrose, and chow. Harris RB, Apolzan JW. Am J Physiol Regul Integr Comp Physiol. 2012 Jun;302(11):R1327-39. PMID:22496363

943 Leptin Level and Skipping Breakfast: The National Health and Nutrition Examination Survey III (NHANES III). Asao K, Marekani AS, VanCleave J, Rothberg AE. Nutrients. 2016 Feb 25;8(3). pii: E115. PMID:26927164

944 Enteroimmunology, Chapter 17. Charles Lewis, Psy Press 2015

945 http://www.brenda-enzymes.info/enzyme.php?ecno=2.7.11.17

946 Genistein, EGCG, and capsaicin inhibit adipocyte differentiation process via activating AMP-activated protein kinase. Hwang JT, Park IJ, Shin JI, et al. Biochem Biophys Res Commun. 2005 Dec 16;338(2):694-9. PMID: 16236247

947 Catechin-induced activation of the LKB1/AMP-activated protein kinase pathway. Murase T, Misawa K, Haramizu S, Hase T. Biochem Pharmacol. 2009 Jul 1;78(1):78-84. PMID:19447226

948 Punicalagin induces apoptotic and autophagic cell death in human U87MG glioma cells. Wang SG, Huang MH, Li JH, Lai FI, Lee HM, Hsu YN. Acta Pharmacol Sin. 2013 Nov;34(11):1411-9. PMID: 24077634

949 Nootkatone, a characteristic constituent of grapefruit, stimulates energy metabolism and prevents diet-induced obesity by activating AMPK. Murase T, Misawa K, Haramizu S, et al. Am J Physiol Endocrinol Metab. 2010 Aug;299(2):E266-75. PMID: 20501876

950 Xylitol toxicosis in dogs. Murphy LA, Coleman AE. Vet Clin North Am Small Anim Pract. 2012 Mar;42(2):307-12, vii. PMID:22381181

951 http://www.petpoisonhelpline.com/poisons/

952 Cancer: beyond speciation. Vincent MD. Adv Cancer Res. 2011;112:283-350. PMID:21925308

953 Protecting the normal in order to better kill the cancer. Liu B, Ezeogu L, Zellmer L, Yu B, Xu N, Liao DJ. Cancer Med. 2015 Sep;4(9):1394-403. PMID:26177855

954 Targeting tumour-supportive cellular machineries in anticancer drug development. Dobbelstein M, Moll U. Nat Rev Drug Discov. 2014 Mar;13(3):179-96. PMID:24577400

955 Sphingosine contributes to glucocorticoid-induced apoptosis of thymocytes independently of the mitochondrial pathway. Lépine S, Lakatos B, Courageot MP, Le Stunff H, Sulpice JC, Giraud F. J Immunol. 2004 Sep 15;173(6):3783-90. PMID:15356125

956 Protecting the normal in order to better kill the cancer. Liu B, Ezeogu L, Zellmer L, Yu B, Xu N, Liao DJ. Cancer Med. 2015 Sep;4(9):1394-403. PMID:26177855

957 The double-edged sword: Neurotoxicity of chemotherapy. Magge RS, DeAngelis LM. Blood Rev. 2015 Mar;29(2):93-100. PMID:25445718

958 Evidence for acute neurotoxicity after chemotherapy. Petzold A, Mondria T, Kuhle J, et al. Ann Neurol. 2010 Dec;68(6):806-15. PMID:21194151

959 Juvenile exposure to anthracyclines impairs cardiac progenitor cell function and vascularization resulting in greater susceptibility to stress-induced myocardial injury in adult mice. Huang C, Zhang X, Ramil JM, et al. Circulation. 2010 Feb 9;121(5):675-83. PMID:20100968

960 Clinical management of oxaliplatin-associated neurotoxicity. Grothey A. Clin Colorectal Cancer. 2005 Apr;5 Suppl 1:S38-46. PMID:15871765

961 Ethical and value issues in insurance coverage for cancer treatment. Brock DW. Oncologist. 2010;15 Suppl 1:36-42. PMID:20237216

962 Chemotherapy-induced hair loss. Trüeb RM. Skin Therapy Lett. 2010 Jul-Aug;15(7):5-7. PMID:20700552

963 Mild cognitive impairment after adjuvant chemotherapy in breast cancer patients--evaluation of appropriate research design and methodology to measure symptoms. Matsuda T, Takayama T, Tashiro M, et al. Breast Cancer. 2005;12(4):279-87. PMID:16286908

964 Chemotherapy-induced peripheral neurotoxicity and complementary and alternative medicines: progress and perspective. Cheng XL, Liu HQ, Wang Q, Huo JG, Wang XN, Cao P. Front Pharmacol. 2015 Oct 23;6:234. PMID:26557088

965 The AIM2 inflammasome is essential for host defense against cytosolic bacteria and DNA viruses. Rathinam VA, Jiang Z, Waggoner SN, et al. Nat Immunol. 2010 May;11(5):395-402. PMID:20351692

966 Cutting edge: Cytosolic bacterial DNA activates the inflammasome via Aim2. Warren SE, Armstrong A, Hamilton MK, et al. Immunol. 2010 Jul 15;185(2):818-21. PMID:20562263

967 The caspase-1 digestome identifies the glycolysis pathway as a target during infection and septic shock. Shao W, Yeretssian G, Doiron K, Hussain SN, Saleh M. J Biol Chem. 2007 Dec 14;282(50):36321-9. PMID:17959595

968 Inflammasomes: mechanism of action, role in disease, and therapeutics. Guo H, Callaway JB, Ting JP. Nat Med. 2015 Jul;21(7):677-87. PMID:26121197

969 Toxic effect of chemotherapy dosing using actual body weight in obese versus normal-weight patients: a systematic review and meta-analysis. Hourdequin KC, Schpero WL, McKenna DR, Piazik BL, Larson RJ. Ann Oncol. 2013 Dec;24(12):2952-62. PMID:23965736

970 Individual fluorouracil dose adjustment in FOLFOX based on pharmacokinetic follow-up compared with conventional body-area-surface dosing: a phase II, proof-of-concept study. Capitain O, Asevoaia A, Boisdron-Celle M, et al. Clin Colorectal Cancer. 2012 Dec;11(4):263-7. PMID:22683364

971 Personalized dosing via pharmacokinetic monitoring of 5-fluorouracil might reduce toxicity in early- or late-stage colorectal cancer patients treated with infusional 5-fluorouracil-based chemotherapy regimens. Kline CL, Schiccitano A, Zhu J, et al. Clin Colorectal Cancer. 2014 Jun;13(2):119-26. PMID:24461492

972 Cost effectiveness analysis of pharmacokinetically-guided 5-fluorouracil in FOLFOX chemotherapy for metastatic colorectal cancer. Goldstein DA, Chen Q, Ayer T, et al. Clin Colorectal Cancer. 2014 Dec;13(4):219-25. PMID:25306485

973 Short-term exercise training attenuates acute doxorubicin cardiotoxicity. Lien CY, Jensen BT, Hydock DS, Hayward R. J Physiol Biochem. 2015 Dec;71(4):669-78. PMID:26403766

974 Exercise training does not affect anthracycline antitumor efficacy while attenuating cardiac dysfunction. Parry TL, Hayward R. Am J Physiol Regul Integr Comp Physiol. 2015 Sep 15;309(6):R675-83. PMID:26246505

975 Physical exercise mitigates doxorubicin-induced brain cortex and cerebellum mitochondrial alterations and cellular quality control signaling. Marques-Aleixo I, Santos-Alves E, Balça MM, et al. Mitochondrion. 2016 Jan;26:43-57. PMID:26678157

976 Effects of Chronic Endurance Exercise on Doxorubicin-Induced Thymic Damage. Quinn CJ, Burns PD, Gibson NM, Bashore A, Hayward R, Hydock DS. Integr Cancer Ther. 2015 Nov 20. pii: 1534735415617014. PMID:26590123

977 Physical exercise prior and during treatment reduces sub-chronic doxorubicin-induced mitochondrial toxicity and oxidative stress. Marques-Aleixo I, Santos-Alves E, et al. Mitochondrion. 2015 Jan;20:22-33. PMID:25446396

978 Divergent targets of glycolysis and oxidative phosphorylation result in additive effects of metformin and starvation in colon and breast cancer. Marini C, Bianchi G, Buschiazzo et al. Sci Rep. 2016 Jan 22;6:19569. PMID:26794854

979 Diet-derived phytochemicals: from cancer chemoprevention to cardio-oncological prevention. Ferrari N, Tosetti F, De Flora S, Donatelli F, Sogno I, Noonan DM, Albini A. Curr Drug Targets. 2011 Dec;12(13):1909-24. PMID:21158708

980 Selecting bioactive phenolic compounds as potential agents to inhibit proliferation and VEGF expression in human ovarian cancer cells. He Z, Li B, Rankin GO, Rojanasakul Y, Chen YC. Oncol Lett. 2015 Mar;9(3):1444-1450. PMID:25663929

981 Gallic acid induces apoptosis and enhances the anticancer effects of cisplatin in human small cell lung cancer H446 cell line via the ROS-dependent mitochondrial apoptotic pathway. Wang R, Ma L, Weng D, et al. Oncol Rep. 2016 May;35(5):3075-83. PMID:26987028

982 Synergistic Effect of Curcumin in Combination with Anticancer Agents in Human Retinoblastoma Cancer Cell Lines. Sreenivasan S, Krishnakumar S. Curr Eye Res. 2015;40(11):1153-65. PMID:25495096

983 Protection of retinal function by sulforaphane following retinal ischemic injury. Ambrecht LA, Perlman JI, et al P. Exp Eye Res. 2015 Sep;138:66-9. PMID:26142954

984 Nutrition and Traumatic Brain Injury: Improving Acute and Subacute Health Outcomes in Military Personnel (2011) Chapter 9. National Academies Press

985 Dietary Reference Intakes for Thiamin, Riboflavin, Niacin, Vitamin B6, Folate, Vitamin B12, Pantothenic Acid, Biotin, and Choline Chapter 12. National Academies Press.

986 Evaluation of vitamin B12 effects on DNA damage induced by paclitaxel. Alzoubi K, Khabour O, Khader M, et al. Drug Chem Toxicol. 2014 Jul;37(3):276-80. PMID:24215581

987 3,3'-Diindolylmethane potentiates paclitaxel-induced antitumor effects on gastric cancer cells through the Akt/FOXM1 signaling cascade. Jin H, Park MH, Kim SM. Oncol Rep. 2015 Apr;33(4):2031-6. PMID:25633416

988 Dietary phytochemicals, HDAC inhibition, and DNA damage/repair defects in cancer cells. Rajendran P, Ho E, Williams DE, et al. Clin Epigenetics. 2011;3(1):4. PMID:22247744

989 Sulforaphane Preconditioning Sensitizes Human Colon Cancer Cells towards the Bioreductive Anticancer Prodrug PR-104A. Erzinger MM, Bovet C, Hecht KM, et al. PLoS One. 2016 Mar 7;11(3):e0150219. PMID:26950072

990 Concurrent detection of autolysosome formation and lysosomal degradation by flow cytometry in a high-content screen for inducers of autophagy. Hundeshagen P, Hamacher-Brady A, Eils R, Brady NR. BMC Biol. 2011 Jun 2;9:38. PMID:21635740

991 Preconditioning chemotherapy with paclitaxel and cisplatin enhances the antitumor activity of cytokine induced-killer cells in a murine lung carcinoma model. Huang X, Huang G, Song H, Chen L. Int J Cancer. 2011 Aug 1;129(3):648-58. PMID:20878978

992 Elevated C-reactive protein in the diagnosis, prognosis, and cause of cancer. Allin KH, Nordestgaard BG. Crit Rev Clin Lab Sci. 2011 Jul-Aug;48(4):155-70. PMID:22035340

993 CRP identifies homeostatic immune oscillations in cancer patients: a potential treatment targeting tool? Coventry BJ, Ashdown ML, Quinn MA, Markovic SN, Yatomi-Clarke SL, Robinson AP. J Transl Med. 2009 Nov 30;7:102. PMID:19948067

994 Dexamethasone as a chemosensitizer for breast cancer chemotherapy: potentiation of the antitumor activity of adriamycin, modulation of cytokine expression, and pharmacokinetics. Int J Oncol. 2007 Apr;30(4):947-53. PMID:17332934

995 Pretreatment with dexamethasone increases antitumor activity of carboplatin and gemcitabine in mice bearing human cancer xenografts: in vivo activity, pharmacokinetics, and clinical implications for cancer chemotherapy. Wang H, Li M, Rinehart JJ, Zhang R. Clin Cancer Res. 2004 Mar 1;10(5):1633-44. PMID:15014014

996 The growth-inhibitory effects of dexamethasone on renal cell carcinoma in vivo and in vitro. Arai Y, Nonomura N, Nakai Y, et al. Cancer Invest. 2008 Feb;26(1):35-40. PMID:18181043

997 Glucocorticoid receptor repression mediated by BRCA1 inactivation in ovarian cancer. Fang YY, Li D, Cao C, Li CY, Li TT. BMC Cancer. 2014 Mar 14;14:188. PMID:24629067

998 Cardiotoxicity of anticancer drugs: the need for cardio-oncology and cardio-oncological prevention. Albini A, Pennesi G, Donatelli F, et al. J Natl Cancer Inst. 2010 Jan 6;102(1):14-25. PMID:20007921

999 Effect of type 1 insulin-like growth factor receptor targeted therapy on chemotherapy in human cancer and the mechanisms involved. Hopkins A, Crowe PJ, Yang JL. J Cancer Res Clin Oncol. 2010 May;136(5):639-50. PMID:20140624

1000 Dietary restriction reduces insulin-like growth factor I levels, which modulates apoptosis, cell proliferation, and tumor progression in p53-deficient mice. Dunn SE, Kari FW, French J, rt al. Cancer Res. 1997 Nov 1;57(21):4667-72. PMID:9354418

1001 Interrelationships between dietary restriction, the IGF-I axis, and expression of vascular endothelial growth factor by prostate adenocarcinoma in rats. Powolny AA, Wang S, Carlton PS, Hoot DR, Clinton SK. Mol Carcinog. 2008 Jun;47(6):458-65. PMID:18058807

1002 Fasting vs dietary restriction in cellular protection and cancer treatment: from model organisms to patients. Lee C, Longo VD. Oncogene. 2011 Jul 28;30(30):3305-16. PMID:21516129

1003 Improvements in body fat distribution and circulating adiponectin by alternate-day fasting versus calorie restriction. Varady KA, Allister CA, Roohk DJ, Hellerstein MK. J Nutr Biochem. 2010 Mar;21(3):188-95. PMID:19195863

1004 Effects of modified alternate-day fasting regimens on adipocyte size, triglyceride metabolism, and plasma adiponectin levels in mice. Varady KA, Roohk DJ, Loe YC, et al. J Lipid Res. 2007 Oct;48(10):2212-9. PMID:17607017

1005 Alternate day calorie restriction improves clinical findings and reduces markers of oxidative stress and inflammation in overweight adults with moderate asthma. Johnson JB, Summer W, Cutler RG, et al. Free Radic Biol Med. 2007 Mar 1;42(5):665-74. PMID:17291990

1006 Modified alternate-day fasting regimens reduce cell proliferation rates to a similar extent as daily calorie restriction in mice. Varady KA, Roohk DJ, McEvoy-Hein BK, et al. FASEB J. 2008 Jun;22(6):2090-6. PMID:18184721

1007 Pretreatment with alternate day modified fast will permit higher dose and frequency of cancer chemotherapy and better cure rates. Johnson JB, John S, Laub DR. Med Hypotheses. 2009 Apr;72(4):381-2. PMID:19135806

1008 Reduced levels of IGF-I mediate differential protection of normal and cancer cells in response to fasting and improve chemotherapeutic index. Lee C, Safdie FM, Raffaghello L, et al. Cancer Res. 2010 Feb 15;70(4):1564-72. PMID:20145127

1009 Fasting cycles retard growth of tumors and sensitize a range of cancer cell types to chemotherapy. Lee C, Raffaghello L, Brandhorst S, et al. Sci Transl Med. 2012 Mar 7;4(124):124ra27. PMID:22323820

1010 Fasting vs dietary restriction in cellular protection and cancer treatment: from model organisms to patients. Lee C, Longo VD. Oncogene. 2011 Jul 28;30(30):3305-16. PMID:21516129

1011 Fasting plus tyrosine kinase inhibitors in cancer. Caffa I, Longo VD, Nencioni A. Aging (Albany NY). 2015 Dec;7(12):1026-7. PMID:26645151

1012 Fasting protects mice from lethal DNA damage by promoting small intestinal epithelial stem cell survival. Tinkum KL, Stemler KM, White LS, et al. Proc Natl Acad Sci U S A. 2015 Dec 22;112(51):E7148-54. PMID:26644583

1013 Fasting and differential chemotherapy protection in patients. Raffaghello L, Safdie F, Bianchi G, et al. Cell Cycle. 2010 Nov 15;9(22):4474-6. PMID:21088487

1014 Short-term calorie and protein restriction provide partial protection from chemotoxicity but do not delay glioma progression. Brandhorst S, Wei M, Hwang S, Morgan TE, Longo VD. Exp Gerontol. 2013 Oct;48(10):1120-8. PMID:23454633

1015 In vivo half-life of a protein is a function of its amino-terminal residue. Bachmair A, Finley D, Varshavsky A. Science. 1986 Oct 10;234(4773):179-86. PMID:3018930

1016 Quantification of protein half-lives in the budding yeast proteome. Belle A, Tanay A, Bitincka L, et al. Proc Natl Acad Sci U S A. 2006 Aug 29;103(35):13004-9. PMID:16916930

1017 Proteome half-life dynamics in living human cells. Eden E, Geva-Zatorsky N, Issaeva I, et al. Science. 2011 Feb 11;331(6018):764-8. PMID:21233346

1018 Long-term effects of calorie or protein restriction on serum IGF-1 and IGFBP-3 concentration in humans. Fontana L, Weiss EP, Villareal DT, Klein S, Holloszy JO. Aging Cell. 2008 Oct;7(5):681-7. PMID:18843793

1019 Effects of caloric or protein restriction on insulin-like growth factor-I (IGF-I) and IGF-binding proteins in children and adults. Smith WJ, Underwood LE, Clemmons DR. J Clin Endocrinol Metab. 1995 Feb;80(2):443-9. PMID:7531712

1020 Methionine restriction extends lifespan of Drosophila melanogaster under conditions of low amino-acid status. Lee BC, Kaya A, Ma S, et al. Nat Commun. 2014 Apr 7;5:3592. PMID:24710037

1021 Reactive oxygen species in choline deficiency-induced apoptosis in rat hepatocytes. Guo WX, Pye QN, et al. Free Radic Biol Med. 2004 Oct 1;37(7):1081-9. PMID:15336324

1022 Regulation of choline deficiency apoptosis by epidermal growth factor in CWSV-1 rat hepatocytes. Albright CD, da Costa KA, Craciunescu CN, Klem E, Mar MH, Zeisel SH. Cell Physiol Biochem. 005;15(1-4):59-68. PMID:15665516

1023 Novel Small Molecule Inhibitors of Choline Kinase Identified by Fragment-Based Drug Discovery. Zech SG, Kohlmann A, Zhou T, et al. J Med Chem. 2016 Jan 28;59(2):671-86. PMID:26700752

1024 Sphingosine contributes to glucocorticoid-induced apoptosis of thymocytes independently of the mitochondrial pathway. Lépine S, Lakatos B, Courageot MP, Le Stunff H, Sulpice JC, Giraud F. J Immunol. 2004 Sep 15;173(6):3783-90. PMID:15356125

1025 http://www.brenda-enzymes.org/enzyme.php?ecno=3.1.3.4

1026 http://www.kegg.jp/kegg-bin/show_pathway?map04071

1027 Modulation of ceramide synthase activity via dimerization. Laviad EL, Kelly S, Merrill AH Jr, Futerman AH. J Biol Chem. 2012 Jun 15;287(25):21025-33. PMID:22539345

1028 http://www.kegg.jp/kegg-bin/show_pathway?map04071

1029 Dietary Reference Intakes for Thiamin, Riboflavin, Niacin, Vitamin B6, Folate, Vitamin B12, Pantothenic Acid, Biotin, and Choline Chapter 12. National Academies Press.

1030 Amino acid sufficiency and mTOR regulate p70 S6 kinase and eIF-4E BP1 through a common effector mechanism. Hara K, Yonezawa K, Weng QP, et al. J Biol Chem. 1998 Jun 5;273(23):14484-94. PMID:9603962

1031 Amino acid sensing in dietary-restriction-mediated longevity: roles of signal-transducing kinases GCN2 and TOR. Gallinetti J, Harputlugil E, Mitchell JR. Biochem J. 2013 Jan 1;449(1):1-10. PMID:23216249

[1032] Bidirectional transport of amino acids regulates mTOR and autophagy. Nicklin P, Bergman P, Zhang B, et al. Cell. 2009 Feb 6;136(3):521-34. PMID:19203585

[1033] SLC1A5 mediates glutamine transport required for lung cancer cell growth and survival. Hassanein M, Hoeksema MD, Shiota M, et al. Clin Cancer Res. 2013 Feb 1;19(3):560-70. PMID:23213057

[1034] Deficiency in glutamine but not glucose induces MYC-dependent apoptosis in human cells. Yuneva M, Zamboni N, Oefner P, Sachidanandam R, Lazebnik Y. J Cell Biol. 2007 Jul 2;178(1):93-105. PMID:17606868

[1035] Inhibiting glutamine uptake represents an attractive new strategy for treating acute myeloid leukemia. Willems L, Jacque N, Jacquel A, et al. Blood. 2013 Nov 14;122(20):3521-32. PMID:24014241

[1036] Targeting ASCT2-mediated glutamine uptake blocks prostate cancer growth and tumour development. Wang Q, Hardie RA, Hoy AJ, et al. J Pathol. 2015 Jul;236(3):278-89. PMID:25693838

[1037] Inhibitors of glutamine synthetase and their potential application in medicine. Berlicki Ł. Mini Rev Med Chem. 2008 Aug;8(9):869-78. PMID:18691144

[1038] Glutamine synthetase protects the spinal cord against hypoxia-induced and GABA(A) receptor-activated axonal depressions. Matsumoto M, Ichikawa T, Young W, Kodama N. Surg Neurol. 2008 Aug;70(2):122-8; discussion 128. PMID:18262603

[1039] Crystal structures of mammalian glutamine synthetases illustrate substrate-induced conformational changes and provide opportunities for drug and herbicide design. Krajewski WW, Collins R, Holmberg-Schiavone L, et al. J Mol Biol. 2008 Jan 4;375(1):217-28. PMID:18005987

[1040] http://www.brenda-enzymes.org/enzyme.php?ecno=6.3.1.2

[1041] Forty percent methionine restriction decreases mitochondrial oxygen radical production and leak at complex I during forward electron flow and lowers oxidative damage to proteins and mitochondrial DNA in rat kidney and brain mitochondria. Caro P, Gomez J, Sanchez I, Barja G, et al. Rejuvenation Res. 2009 Dec;12(6):421-34 PMID:20041736

[1042] Forty percent and eighty percent methionine restriction decrease mitochondrial ROS generation and oxidative stress in rat liver. Caro P, Gómez J, López-Torres M, Sánchez I, , Barja G. Biogerontology. 2008 Jun;9(3):183-96. PMID:18283555

[1043] Protein and Amino Acid Requirements in Human Nutrition: Report of a Joint WHO/FAO/UNU Expert Consultation. World Health Organization ISBN-13: 9789241209359 December 2007

[1044] Adequate Intake levels of choline are sufficient for preventing elevations in serum markers of liver dysfunction in Mexican American men but are not optimal for minimizing plasma total homocysteine increases after a methionine load. Veenema K, Solis C, Li R, et al. Am J Clin Nutr. 2008 Sep;88(3):685-92. PMID:18779284

[1045] Dietary emulsifiers impact the mouse gut microbiota promoting colitis and metabolic syndrome. Chassaing B, Koren O, Goodrich JK, et al. Nature. 2015 Mar 5;519(7541):92-6. PMID:25731162

[1046] Translocation of Crohn's disease Escherichia coli across M-cells: contrasting effects of soluble plant fibres and emulsifiers. Roberts CL, Keita AV, Duncan SH, et al. Gut. 2010 Oct;59(10):1331-9. PMID:20813719

[1047] Fever and the thermal regulation of immunity: the immune system feels the heat. Evans SS, Repasky EA, Fisher DT. Nat Rev Immunol. 2015 Jun;15(6):335-49. PMID:25976513

[1048] Association of body temperature and antipyretic treatments with mortality of critically ill patients with and without sepsis: multi-centered prospective observational study. Lee BH, Inui D, Suh GY, et al. Crit Care. 2012 Feb 28;16(1):R33. PMID:22373120

[1049] Clinical review: fever in septic ICU patients--friend or foe? Launey Y, Nesseler N, Mallédant Y, Seguin P. Crit Care. 2011;15(3):222. PMID:21672276

1050 Syphilology: Parenteral Milk Injection in Syphilis. Hollingsworth MW. Cal West Med. 1927 May;26(5):671. PMID:18740351

1051 II. Contribution to the Knowledge of Sarcoma. Coley WB. Ann Surg. 1891 Sep;14(3):199-220. PMID:17859590

1052 Local tumour hyperthermia as immunotherapy for metastatic cancer. Toraya-Brown S, Fiering S. Int J Hyperthermia. 2014 Dec;30(8):531-9. PMID:25430985

1053 Dr William Coley and tumour regression: a place in history or in the future. Hoption Cann SA, van Netten JP, van Netten C. Postgrad Med J. 2003 Dec;79(938):672-80. PMID:14707241

1054 Targeted near infrared hyperthermia combined with immune stimulation for optimized therapeutic efficacy in thyroid cancer treatment. Zhou L, Zhang M, Fu Q, Li J, Sun H. Oncotarget. 2016 Feb 9;7(6):6878-90. 26769848

1055 A genomics approach to identify susceptibilities of breast cancer cells to "fever-range" hyperthermia. Amaya C, Kurisetty V, Stiles J, et al. BMC Cancer. 2014 Feb 11;14:81. PMID:24511912

1056 Thermotolerance induced at a fever temperature of 40 degrees C protects cells against hyperthermia-induced apoptosis mediated by death receptor signalling. Bettaieb A, Averill-Bates DA. Biochem Cell Biol. 2008 Dec;86(6):521-38. PMID:19088800

1057 Thermotolerance induced at a mild temperature of 40°C alleviates heat shock-induced ER stress and apoptosis in HeLa cells. Bettaieb A, Averill-Bates DA. Biochim Biophys Acta. 2015 Jan;1853(1):52-62. PMID:25260982

1058 Fever and the thermal regulation of immunity: the immune system feels the heat. Evans SS, Repasky EA, Fisher DT. Nat Rev Immunol. 2015 Jun;15(6):335-49. PMID:25976513

1059 Heat shock proteins 27, 60 and 70 as prognostic markers of prostate cancer. Glaessgen A, Jonmarker S, Lindberg A, et al. APMIS. 2008 Oct;116(10):888-95. PMID:19132982

1060 Heat shock proteins HSP27, HSP60, HSP70, and HSP90: expression in bladder carcinoma. Lebret T, Watson RW, Molinié V, et al. Cancer. 2003 Sep 1;98(5):970-7. PMID:12942564

1061 Quercetin liposome sensitizes colon carcinoma to thermotherapy and thermochemotherapy in mice models. He B, Wang X, Shi HS, et al. Integr Cancer Ther. 2013 May;12(3):264-70. PMID:22740083

1062 Mathematical modeling of the heat-shock response in HeLa cells. Scheff JD, Stallings JD, Reifman J, Rakesh V. Biophys J. 2015 Jul 21;109(2):182-93. PMID:26200855

1063 Modelling the efficacy of hyperthermia treatment. Rybinski M, Szymanska Z, Lasota S, Gambin A. J R Soc Interface. 2013 Aug 28;10(88):20130527. PMID:23985732

1064 Fever-range hyperthermia vs. hypothermia effect on cancer cell viability, proliferation and HSP90 expression. Kalamida D, Karagounis IV, Mitrakas A, et al. PLoS One. 2015 Jan 30;10(1):e0116021. PMID:25635828

1065 Cross talk between cytokine and hyperthermia-induced pathways: identification of different subsets of NF-κB-dependent genes regulated by TNFα and heat shock. Janus P, Stokowy T, Jaksik R, et al. Mol Genet Genomics. 2015 Oct;290(5):1979-90. PMID:25944781

1066 Phosphorylation of CBP by IKKalpha promotes cell growth by switching the binding preference of CBP from p53 to NF-kappaB. Huang WC, Ju TK, Hung MC, Chen CC. Mol Cell. 2007 Apr 13;26(1):75-87. PMID:17434128

1067 Degree of roasting is the main determinant of the effects of coffee on NF-kappaB and EpRE. Paur I, Balstad TR, Blomhoff R. Free Radic Biol Med. 2010 May 1;48(9):1218-27. PMID:20176103

1068 Plant extracts of spices and coffee synergistically dampen nuclear factor-κB in U937 cells. Kolberg M, Paur I, Balstad TR, et al. Nutr Res. 2013 Oct;33(10):817-30. PMID:24074740

1069 Extract of oregano, coffee, thyme, clove, and walnuts inhibits NF-kappaB in monocytes and in transgenic reporter mice. Paur I, Balstad TR, Kolberg M, et al. Cancer Prev Res (Phila). 2010 May;3(5):653-63. PMID:20424131

1070 Anthocyanins from black soybean seed coat enhance wound healing.. Xu L, Choi TH, Kim S, et al. Ann Plast Surg. 2013 Feb 12. PMID:23407247

1071 Curcumin inhibits prostate cancer metastasis in vivo by targeting the inflammatory cytokines CXCL1 and -2.. Killian PH, Kronski E, Michalik KM, et al. Carcinogenesis. 2012 Dec;33(12):2507-19. PMID:23042094

1072 Resveratrol mitigates lipopolysaccharide- and Aβ-mediated microglial inflammation by inhibiting the TLR4/NF-κB/STAT signaling cascade. Capiralla H, Vingtdeux V, Zhao H, et al. J Neurochem. 2012 Feb;120(3):461-72. PMID:22118570

1073 Quercetin 3-O-beta-glucoside is better absorbed than other quercetin forms and is not present in rat plasma. Morand C, Manach C, Crespy V, Remesy C. Free Radic Res. 2000 Nov;33(5):667-76. PMID:11200097

1074 Hyperthermia enhances mapatumumab-induced apoptotic death through ubiquitin-mediated degradation of cellular FLIP(long) in human colon cancer cells. Song X, Kim SY, Zhou Z, Lagasse E, Kwon YT, Lee YJ. Cell Death Dis. 2013 Apr 4;4:e577. PMID:23559011

1075 Lipid rafts and nonrafts mediate tumor necrosis factor related apoptosis-inducing ligand induced apoptotic and nonapoptotic signals in non small cell lung carcinoma cells. Song JH, Tse MC, Bellail A, et al. Cancer Res. 2007 Jul 15;67(14):6946-55. PMID:17638906

1076 Hyperthermia restores apoptosis induced by death receptors through aggregation-induced c-FLIP cytosolic depletion. Morlé A, Garrido C, Micheau O. Cell Death Dis. 2015 Feb 12;6:e1633. PMID:25675293

1077 Hyperthermia Sensitizes Glioma Stem-like Cells to Radiation by Inhibiting AKT Signaling. Man J, Shoemake JD, Ma T, et al. Cancer Res. 2015 Apr 15;75(8):1760-9. PMID:25712125

1078 Fever-like hyperthermia controls T Lymphocyte persistence by inducing degradation of cellular FLIPshort. Meinander A, Söderström TS, Kaunisto A, et al. J Immunol. 2007 Mar 15;178(6):3944-53. PMID:17339495

1079 Hyperthermia enhances mapatumumab-induced apoptotic death through ubiquitin-mediated degradation of cellular FLIP(long) in human colon cancer cells. Song X, Kim SY, Zhou Z, Lagasse E, Kwon YT, Lee YJ. Cell Death Dis. 2013 Apr 4;4:e577. PMID:23559011

1080 Regulation of OSU-03012 toxicity by ER stress proteins and ER stress-inducing drugs. Booth L, Roberts JL, Cruickshanks N, Grant S, Poklepovic A, Dent P. Mol Cancer Ther. 2014 Oct;13(10):2384-98. PMID:25103559

1081 PDE5 inhibitors enhance celecoxib killing in multiple tumor types. Booth L, Roberts JL, Cruickshanks N, et al. J Cell Physiol. 2015 May;230(5):1115-27. PMID:25303541

1082 The Keap1-Nrf2-antioxidant response element pathway: a review of its regulation by melatonin and the proteasome. Vriend J, Reiter RJ. Mol Cell Endocrinol. 2015 Feb 5;401:213-20. PMID:25528518

1083 Melatonin as a proteasome inhibitor. Is there any clinical evidence? Vriend J, Reiter RJ. Life Sci. 2014 Oct 12;115(1-2):8-14. PMID:25219883

1084 Green tea polyphenols as a natural tumour cell proteasome inhibitor. Dou QP, Landis-Piwowar KR, Chen D, et al. Inflammopharmacology. 2008 Oct;16(5):208-12. PMID:18815743

1085 Epigallocatechin Gallate (EGCG) is the most effective cancer chemopreventive polyphenol in green tea. Du GJ, Zhang Z, Wen XD, Yu C, Calway T, Yuan CS, Wang CZ. Nutrients. 2012 Nov 8;4(11):1679-91. PMID:23201840

1086 Nuclear lipid microdomain as resting place of dexamethasone to impair cell proliferation. Cataldi S, Codini M, Cascianelli G, et al. Int J Mol Sci. 2014 Oct 31;15(11):19832-46. PMID:25365174

1087 http://www.brenda-enzymes.org/ligand.php?brenda_ligand_id=1159

1088 http://www.brenda-enzymes.org/enzyme.php?ecno=2.7.11.26

1089 http://www.brenda-enzymes.org/enzyme.php?ecno=2.7.11.1

1090 Misfolded proteins: from little villains to little helpers in the fight against cancer. Brüning A, Jückstock J. Front Oncol. 2015 Feb 24;5:47. PMID:25759792

1091 Hyperuricemia as a mediator of the proinflammatory endocrine imbalance in the adipose tissue in a murine model of the metabolic syndrome. Baldwin W, McRae S, Marek G, et al. Diabetes. 2011 Apr;60(4):1258-69. PMID:21346177

1092 Allopurinol in subjects with colorectal adenoma--response. Puntoni M, Decensi A. Cancer Prev Res (Phila). 2013 Apr;6(4):369. PMID:23447561

1093 Efficacy and safety of febuxostat for prevention of tumor lysis syndrome in patients with malignant tumors receiving chemotherapy: a phase III, randomized, multi-center trial comparing febuxostat and allopurinol. Tamura K, Kawai Y, Kiguchi T, et al. Int J Clin Oncol. 2016 Mar 26. PMID:27017611

1094 Allopurinol, rutin, and quercetin attenuate hyperuricemia and renal dysfunction in rats induced by fructose intake: renal organic ion transporter involvement. Hu QH, Wang C, Li JM, et al. Am J Physiol Renal Physiol. 2009 Oct;297(4):F1080-91. PMID:19605544

1095 Influence of smoking cessation after diagnosis of early stage lung cancer on prognosis: systematic review of observational studies with meta-analysis. Parsons A, Daley A, Begh R, Aveyard P. BMJ. 2010 Jan 21;340:b5569. PMID: 20093278

1096 Cigarette smoke promotes drug resistance and expansion of cancer stem cell-like side population. An Y, Kiang A, Lopez JP, et al. PLoS One. 2012;7(11):e47919. PMID: 23144836

1097 Cigarette smoking is associated with an increased risk of biochemical disease recurrence, metastasis, castration-resistant prostate cancer, and mortality after radical prostatectomy: results from the SEARCH database. Moreira DM, Aronson WJ, Terris MK, et al. Cancer. 2014 Jan 15;120(2):197-204. PMID: 4127391

1098 Proton pump inhibitors and histamine 2 blockers are associated with improved overall survival in patients with head and neck squamous carcinoma. Papagerakis S, Bellile E, Peterson LA, et al. Cancer Prev Res (Phila). 2014 Dec;7(12):1258-69. PMID: 25468899

1099 The influence of linoleic and linolenic acid on the activity and intracellular localisation of phospholipase D in COS-1 cells. Gemeinhardt A, Alfalah M, Gück T, Naim HY, Fuhrmann H. Biol Chem. 2009 Mar;390(3):253-8. PMID:19090716

1100 Sphingosine 1-phosphate signalling in cancer. Pyne NJ, Tonelli F, Lim KG, Long JS, Edwards J, Pyne S. Biochem Soc Trans. 2012 Feb;40(1):94-100. PMID:22260672

1101 ASMase is required for chronic alcohol induced hepatic endoplasmic reticulum stress and mitochondrial cholesterol loading. Fernandez A, Matias N, Fucho R, et al. J Hepatol. 2013 Oct;59(4):805-13. PMID:23707365

1102 A new take on ceramide: starving cells by cutting off the nutrient supply. Guenther GG, Edinger AL. Cell Cycle. 2009 Apr 15;8(8):1122-6. PMID:19282666

1103 Acid sphingomyelinase-ceramide system mediates effects of antidepressant drugs. Gulbins E, Palmada M, Reichel M, et al. Nat Med. 2013 Jul;19(7):934-8. PMID:23770692

1104 Role of acid sphingomyelinase in the regulation of mast cell function. Yang W, Schmid E, Nurbaeva MK, Set al. Clin Exp Allergy. 2014 Jan;44(1):79-90. PMID:24164338

1105 Identification of novel functional inhibitors of acid sphingomyelinase. Kornhuber J, Muehlbacher M, Trapp S, et al. PLoS One. 2011;6(8):e23852. PMID:21909365

1106 Activation of sphingosine kinase by tumor necrosis factor-alpha inhibits apoptosis in human endothelial cells. Xia P, Wang L, Gamble JR, Vadas MA. J Biol Chem. 1999 Nov 26;274(48):34499-505. PMID:10567432

1107 http://www.brenda-enzymes.org/index.php

1108 New signalling pathway involved in the anti-proliferative action of vitamin D3 and its analogues in human neuroblastoma cells. A role for ceramide kinase. Bini F, Frati A, Garcia-Gil M, et al. Neuropharmacology. 2012 Sep;63(4):524-37. PMID:22579669

[1109] Activation of ceramide synthase 6 by celecoxib leads to a selective induction of C16:0-ceramide. Schiffmann S, Ziebell S, Sandner J, et al. Biochem Pharmacol. 2010 Dec 1;80(11):1632-40. PMID:20735991

[1110] Homocysteine induces cerebral endothelial cell death by activating the acid sphingomyelinase ceramide pathway. Lee JT, Peng GS, Chen SY, et al. Prog Neuropsychopharmacol Biol Psychiatry. 2013 Aug 1;45:21-7. PMID:23665108

[1111] http://www.brenda-enzymes.org/php/result_flat.php4?ecno=3.1.4.12 Brenda, accessed June 2016.

[1112] 1Alpha,25-dihydroxyvitamin D3 protects human keratinocytes from apoptosis by the formation of sphingosine-1-phosphate. Manggau M, Kim DS, Ruwisch L, et al. J Invest Dermatol. 2001 Nov;117(5):1241-9. PMID:11710939

[1113] Resveratrol stimulates sphingosine-1-phosphate signaling of cathelicidin production. Park K, Elias PM, Hupe M, et al. J Invest Dermatol. 2013 Aug;133(8):1942-9. PMID:23856934

[1114] The dietary ingredient, genistein, stimulates cathelicidin antimicrobial peptide expression through a novel S1P-dependent mechanism. Park K, Kim YI, Shin KO, et al. J Nutr Biochem. 2014 Jul;25(7):734-40. PMID:24768661

[1115] Characteristics of impulsive suicide attempts and attempters. Simon OR, Swann AC, Powell KE, et al. Suicide Life Threat Behav. 2001;32(1 Suppl):49-59. PMID:11924695

Index

Acetaldehyde, 99- 117, 440
Acrolein, 185-188, 454
Aflatoxin, 159, 192-197, 230, 277
Akt, 68, 69, 128, 213, 214, 239, 240, 356-361, 379, 389, 395, 396, 403, 413, 416, 427
Alcohol, 2, 86, 91, **96-118**, 125, 162, 191, 211, 214, 248, 250, 276-280, 284, 292, 299, 307, 328, 331, 333, 357, 402, 415, 424, 428, 434
Ammonia, 262, 263, 271, 274-277, 2810
AMPK, 68, 129, 130, 137, 138, 142, 240, **348-366**, 382, 383, 380, 392-395, 398, 415- 416
Apoptosis, 11, 24, 32-34, 45-48, 50, 53, 55-57, 68, 69, 75, 76, 86, 90, 112, 126, 128, 136, 137, 139, 142, 156, 186, 193, 212, 213, 215, 216, 220, 223, 225, 226, 229, 230, 232, 236, 238, 239, 252, 269, 272, 296, 340, 344, 347, 351, 353, 354, 356, 357, 358, 359, 360, 369-430
Aspergillus, 103, 111, 192, 193, 194, 195
Asprin, 236-238, 350
ATP, 129, 130, 137, 138, 139, 189, 279, 346, 348, 349, 350-353, 357, 360, 383, 396, 402, 427, 428,
Autophagy, 32, 360, 393
Azo dyes, 337, 338
Barrett's esophagus, 8, 86
Benign Breast Disease (BBD), 106-107, 324- 329
Betaine, 246, 249, **279-281**, 395, 401, 421, 424
Bile, 86, 87, 207, 211, 249, 253, 259, **262- 274**, 277, 325, 427
Bladder Cancer, 89, 90, 176, 244, **337-339**,
Boron, 151, 252, 377, 384
BPA, 286-289
BRCA1, 39, 55, **65-71**, 122, 203, 219, 220, 248, 297, 325, **331-333**, 387, 417
BRCA2, 39, 55, 66-71, 122, 203, 325, 331-333
Breast Cancer, 1, 2, 14, 15, 36, 39, 47, 55, 65, 66, 68, 71, 96, 105-108, 110, 112, 117, 121, 122, 123, 133, 137, 161, 175, 190, 200-203, 214, 224, 226, 240-242, 248, 249, 252-255, 265-266, 272, 282, 286-289, 298-301, 307, 311, **313-336**, 361, 376, 385, 406, 417, 420
Burkitt lymphoma, 75, 82, 88
Centromere, 43
Ceramide, 195, 357, 373, 387, 396, 397, 403, 414- 416, 424-430
Checkpoint, **45- 48**, 66, 69, 229, 346, 359, 389
Chemo – see Chemotherapy
Chemotherapy, 3, 4, 6, 12-16, 55, 61-62, 95, 186, 203, 226, 229, 232, 252, 255, 281, 314, 321, 339, 342, 361, **368-388**, 389-406, 416-419, 421, 423, 428-430
Chocolate, 306, 366, 423
Choline, 250, 251, 256, 279-284, 331, 352- 359, 377, 384, 385, 395-403, 421-423, 428-429
Cigarette, 37, 60, 93-95, 97, 103, 157, 173, 181, 188, 299, 324, 418
Citrus fruit, 219, 245, 275
Colon Cancer - see Colorectal Cancer
Coffee, 2, 94, 109, 117, 144, 149, 180, 188, 195, 212, **217-220**, 283, 284, 291, 305, 305, 312, 331, 411, 423

Colorectal Cancer, 33, 36,38, 53, 68, 89, 90, 101, 133, 150, 154, 160, 189, 190, 231, 237, 240, 245, 249, 260, 262, 264, 268, 271-275, 279, 283, 290, 301, 304, **321-323**,333, 350, 353, 354, 381, 416
Commensal bacteria, 260-262, 267, 274
Contraceptive, **333-336**
Cruciferous Vegetables, 1, **216-220**, **221-233**, 244, 256, 272, 273, 331, 347, 383, 384, 385, 420
CYP1A1, 156-160, 176, 196, 229
CYP1A2, 159-160, 196, 229
CYP2E1, 99-105, 107, 176, 181
DCIS, 314, 315
Diabetes, 10, 60, **92-93**, 119-132, 148, 157, 161, 180, 184, 186, 190, 217, 277, 278, 282, 296, 299, 340, 351, 361, 362, 365, 404
Endocrine Disruptors, **287-290**
Epigenetic Reset, 143
Epstein Barr Virus (EBV), 73, 80-84, 88,
Estrogen Receptor, 108, 265, 300, 325,
Exercise, 2, 132, **133-148**, 305, 362, 382
Fasting, 3, 147, 365, 386, 387, **389-402**, 428
Fiber, 87, 132, 151, **253-275**, 279, 328-331, 364, 376, 429
Fish (oil), 5, 154, 163, 166, 167, 175, 177-179, 186, 189, 195, 235, 236, 240-242, 252, 288, 401
Flavonoids, 147, 252, 253, 255, 362, 387
Folate, 101-105, 108, 149, 150, 206, 244-249, 272, 277, 281, 304, 329, 370, 403
Fructose, 2, **124-132**, 138, 167, 182, 254, 256, 278-284, 331, 362, 363, 364, 384, 416, 423, 429
Fungal toxins, 192-197
G1 phase, 42, 138, 341, 346, 372
Garlic, 169, 174, 188, 195, 216, 219, 220, **229-233**, 256, 331, 352, 361, 367, 370, 383-385, 401, 420
Gastric cancer - **36-39**, 68, **84-85** 149, 174-178, 199, 273, 385
Glossary, **7-17**
Glycolysis, 137, **139-143**, 251, 346, 355, 360, 378, 402
Grapefruit, 208, 255, 423
H. pylori -see Helicobacter pylori
Hamburger, 163, **166-172**, 241-242
HBV – see Hepatitis B
Heterocyclic Amines (HCA), **159-172**, 173, 176, 178, 179, 180, 183, 186, 187, 207, 216, 218, 224, 229, 242, 271, 328, 331
HCC –see Hepatocellular Carcinoma
Helicobacter pylori, 38, 73, **83-85**, 149, 178, 358
Hemochromatosis, **189-191**
Hepatitis B, 3, 38, 73, 75, 78-80, 193-194, 358
Hepatitis C, 38, 78, 105, 276, 285
Hepatocellular Carcinoma, 78-80, 105, 190, 193, 200, 238, **274-284**
HDAC (Histone Deacetylase) Inhibitors, 142, 261
HIV, **75-79**, 82, 83, 89
Homocysteine, 249, 281, 331, 354, 396, 428
Human Papilloma Virus (HPV), 73-80, 90, 91, 103, 109, 117, 149, 333

Inflammasome, **378-379**, 394, 407
Iron, 50, 154, **189-191**, 206, 241, 304
Isothiocyanate (ITC), 170, 221-233, 347
KEAP1, **209-218**, 224
Liver cancer - see Hepatocellular Carcinoma
LKB1, 68, **349-352**, 361
Lung Cancer, 13, 36, 37, 38, 47, 60, 87, 92, 149, 157, 161, 166, 181, 199, 200, 223, 225, 230, 231, 252, 253, 285, 337, 368, 383, 418
Mammography, 203, **313-319**, 480
Mastectomy, 71, 313
Meat, 2, 4, 5, 38, 123, **149-154**, **157-191**, 224, 235, 240-242, 256, 262, 268, 273, 289, 303, 327, 392, 422
Melatonin, 19, 294, 298-303, 308, 310, 311, 358, 363, 364, 415, 419, 427-430
Menarche, 106, 108, **323-327**, 330, 332, 335
Menstrual cycle, 107, 110, 204, 323, **327-328**, 334
Merkel Cell Carcinoma, 75, 83
Methionine, 21, 101, 102, 246-254, 359, 395-401, 421, 429
microRNA, (miRNA), 30
Mitosis, **41-48**, 139, 215, 238, 341, 344, 371, 378, 389
MTHFR, 101-102, 150, **245-250**
mTOR, 230, 328, **340-360**, 365, 373, 379, 384, 389, 393, 395, 397, 403, 416
NASH, 277, 278, 282, 473
NF-κB, 113, 124, 130, **212-220**, 223-226, 236, 239, 329, 346, 347, 351, 353, 356, 358, 361, 379, 380, 383, 385, 387, 410, 411, 413-416, 424, 425, 429
Non-Alcoholic Steatohepatitis - see NASH
Nrf2, **209-220**, 223-224, 228-229, 232, 294, 330, 377, 415
Obesity, 2, 5, 72, 112, 116, **119-132**, 136, 161, 239, 240, 265, 276, 278, 282, 287, 296, 297, 299, 305, 318, 323-235, 329, 340, 3454, 361, 362, 363, 382
Oral Contraceptives, **333-336**
Olive oil, 1, 4, 185, 218, 238, 241, 242, 330, **419-422**
Ovarian Cancer, 2, 48, 68, 71, 88, **331-335**, 383, 424
p53 Protein, 32, 33, 45-47, 50, 54, 55, 68, 69, 76, 90, 137-144, 147, 156, 181, 193, 215, 220, 244, 248, 267, 355, 356, 389, 410, 411, 415
Polycyclic Aromatic Hydrocarbons (PAH), 155-158, 161, 165, 166, 289, 338
Pancreatic Cancer, 39, 68, 86, 87, 124, 129, 159, 199, 262, 269, 278, 287, 402
Pancreas, 26, 70, 91, 96, 332
Paraptosis, 32, 33
Polycyclic biphenyl (PCB), 272, 286, 288
Pharyngeal Cancer – see UART
Phenolic Compounds, 112, 116, 130, 147, 169, 170, 174, 178, 212, 218, 253, 255, 256, 274, 279, 331, 350, 354, 358, 361, 364, 366, 383, 385, 394, 401, 403, 411, 415, 416, 429
Phytochemicals, 383, 385
Preconditioning, 377, 382-384, 394, 402, 429
Programmed Cell Death, 11, 32, 55-58, 138, 213, 227, 340, 344, 373, 379, 380, 397, 402, 403, 416

Prostate Cancer, 8, 10, 13, 25, 27, 37, 40, 66, 68, 69, 71, 124, 128, 135-137, 149, 154, 159, 161, 176, 201, 206, 222, 223, 225, 228, 239, 252, 255, 257, 266, 274, 287, 292, 298, 301, 385, 3987, 419
Puberty, 71, 204, 265, 286, 289, **323-326**
Pyroptosis, 32, 40, 404, 417
Radiation, 3, 6, 8, 14, 15, 35, 49, 50, 63, 67, 69, 72, 92, 95, 164, **198-205**, 214, 215, 281, 314, 318, 320, 328, 353, 386, 389, 391, 402, 406, 413, 417
Reactive Oxygen Species, 50, 99, 105, 112, 138, 142, 216, 219, 226, 360, 361, 378, 379, 393, 395, 398, 408, 424, 427
RNS, 50, 216, 360
ROS – see Reactive Oxygen Species
S phase, 42-47, 67, 215, 225, 344-356, 371, 389
S6K1, 343-346, 397, 398
Schistosoma, 78, **88-89**, 214
Sleep, 2, 4, 5, 109, 119, 124-134, 144, 286, **292-312**, 331, 361-364, 384, 418, 428-430, 433
Smoking, 3, 4, 37, 54, 60, 91-95, 99, 113, 149, 151, 157, 160, 169, 173, 253, 337, 418
Sphingolipids, 424-430
Sphingomyelin, 251, 395, 396, 403, 424-430
Stem cells, 34-37, 53-54, 323
Stomach Cancer -see gastric Cancer
Stress (Psychological), 432-435
Sulforaphane, 216, 219, **221-227**, 383, 385
Thyroid, 13, 68, 69, 204, 293, 294, 296, 297, 298, 313, 314, 352, 382
Thyroid cancer, 313, 382
Tobacco, 3, 37, 64, 72, 86, **91-99**, 103, 105, 109, 110, 113, 117, 119, 154, 156, 157, 160, 169, 178, 185, 285, 307, 338, 417, 419, 434
Trans fats, 282-284, 331, 473
UADT (Upper Airway and Digestive Tract Cancers), 96-99, 102-105, 109, 113
Viruses, 27, 35, 58, **73-83**, 91, 103, 105, 149, 288, 358, 378, 404, 407, 424
Vitamin C, 30, 50-52, 161, 169, 174, 178, 189, 206, 222
Vitamin D3, 5, 101, 239, 243, 249, 302, 304, 328, 354, 358, 403, 416
Vitamins, 5, 50, 54, 159, 180, 194, 206, 210, 216, 239, 249, 256, 264, 268, 277, 279, 281, 304, 398, 403
X-rays, 35, 63, 92, 203, 204, 315

More extensive indexing is available by searching the use of the digital editions of this book, or searching within the "Look Inside" icon on the book's Amazon page.